# The New York Times

## BOOK OF

# WOMEN'S HEALTH

# 𝕿𝖍𝖊 𝕹𝖊𝖜 𝖄𝖔𝖗𝖐 𝕿𝖎𝖒𝖊𝖘

## BOOK OF

# WOMEN'S HEALTH

*The Latest on Feeling Fit, Eating Right, and Staying Well*

# JANE E. BRODY

AND REPORTERS OF *THE NEW YORK TIMES*

EDITED BY DENISE GRADY

INTRODUCTION BY JANE E. BRODY

Lebhar-Friedman Books

New York • Chicago • Los Angeles • London • Paris • Tokyo

Lebhar-Friedman Books
425 Park Avenue
New York, NY 10022

Published by Lebhar-Friedman Books
Lebhar-Friedman Books is a company of Lebhar-Friedman, Inc.

Printed in the United States of America

Library of Congress Cataloging-in-Publication Data

The New York Times book of women's health / Jane E. Brody and
reporters of the New York Times ; edited by Denise Grady ; introduced
by Jane E. Brody.
     p. cm.
  Includes bibliographical references and index.
  ISBN 0-86730-806-0 (alk. paper)
   1. Women--Health and hygiene. I. Brody, Jane E. II. Grady, Denise.

 RA778 .N713 2000
 613'.04244--dc21

                                                    00-020829

All figures and charts courtesy of *The New York Times*

Visit our Web site at lfbooks.com

**Volume Discounts**
This book makes a great gift and incentive. Call (212) 756-5240
for information on volume discounts

# ACKNOWLEDGMENTS

Much of the inspiration for the articles in this volume has come from our readers, from their unfailing curiosity, their high expectations and their spirited and incisive feedback.

Mitchel Levitas, editorial director of book development for *The New York Times*, provided the impetus for this project. Several editors deserve special credit for commissioning the work that appears here and helping to hone it: Cornelia Dean, editor of the science department, Dennis Overbye, deputy editor, their predecessors Nicholas Wade and James Gorman, science editors Laura Chang and John Wilson, former science editor William Dicke and former health editor Linda Villarosa.

Robert Saar provided invaluable help in editing the manuscript. Frank Scatoni, our editor at Lebhar-Friedman Books, contributed a fresh point of view and sharp editorial judgment.

The ideas, insights and abundant information in this book derive from the talents of the many writers whose work is gathered here.

—Denise Grady

# CONTRIBUTORS

The list below provides the initial key for the contributors who participated in this book. At the end of each article, a set of initials will correspond to one these entries:

| | |
|---|---|
| LKA | Lawrence K. Altman |
| NA | Natalie Angier |
| SB | Sandra Blakeslee |
| JEB | Jane E. Brody |
| DC | Dana Canedy |
| JAC | John A. Cutter |
| JD | Jennifer Dunning |
| KE | Kurt Eichenwald |
| JE | Janet Elder |
| LMF | Lawrence M. Fisher |
| JF | Jane Fritsch |
| WG | Winifred Gallagher |
| SG | Susan Gilbert |
| CG | Carey Goldberg |
| EG | Erica Goode |
| TG | Timothy Gower |
| DG | Denise Grady |
| JG | Jane Gross |
| TH | Tracey Harden |
| AH | Amanda Hesser |
| AHi | Andrea Higbie |
| ALK | Alice Lesch Kelly |
| GK | Gina Kolata |
| WM | Wendy Marston |
| KM | Kathleen McAuliffe |
| MM | Martha McCully |
| BRM | Bonnie Rothman Morris |
| HBN | Holcomb B. Noble |
| KRR | Katherine Russell Rich |
| MRo | Marion Roach |
| DR | David Rohde |
| MR | Marjorie Rosen |
| KS | Karen Stabiner |
| SGS | Sheryl Gay Stolberg |
| AZ | Abigail Zuger |

# CONTENTS

Introduction ................................................................. xiii

### SECTION 1
## Nutrition

#### LINKS BETWEEN FOOD, HEALTH AND DISEASE

People Who Skip Breakfast Pay a High Price ................................ 3

Calcium Takes Its Place as a Superstar of Nutrients ...................... 4

Finding Calcium Sources Outside the Dairy Case .......................... 7

Osteoporosis Linked to Vitamin D Deficiency ............................. 9

Diet-Diabetes Link Reported ............................................ 10

Fiber Does Not Help Prevent Colon Cancer, Study Finds ................. 12

Keep the Fiber Bandwagon Rolling, for Heart and Health ............... 13

Diet Is Not a Panacea, But It Cuts Risk of Cancer ...................... 15

Now, a Food Pyramid to Guide the Elderly ............................. 17

Women's Heart Risk Linked to Types of Fats, Not Total ................. 19

Fat Debates, Sustacal Shakes: It's Life in the Diet Blender ............. 22

### SECTION 2
## Life-style: Exercise for Health and Pleasure

#### EVEN A MODEST EXERCISE PROGRAM IS BENEFICIAL

A Leap from Childbirth to Ballet Stage ................................. 27

The Athlete's Secret to Warding Off Overuse Injuries: Good Technique ........ 28

After 100,000 Miles, Even Soles on Feet Wear Out ..................... 30

Female Bodybuilders Discover Curves .................................. 33

How to Build Abs of Undulating Steel ................................. 35

How Errol Flynn Made It Look So Easy ................................ 38

Persuading Potatoes to Get Off the Couches ........................... 39

Crunches, Not Devices, Help Tighten Abdomen ....................... 41

For Younger Muscles, Just Pump Away ................................ 42

Learning Pilates, One Stretch at a Time ................................ 44

Medicine Ball Pops Back Into Vogue .................................. 46

Some Shape Up by Surfing the Internet ................................ 48

## SECTION 3
# Gains and Losses: Women and Weight

### COMMON SENSE DIET AND EXERCISE WIN OUT OVER DRUGS AND SPECIAL FOODS

New Guide Puts Most Americans on the Fat Side ............................................. 53

The Fat Get Fatter; Overweight Was Bad Enough ........................................... 54

Scientists Unmask Diet Myth: Willpower .......................................................... 56

95% Regain Lost Weight. Or Do They? ............................................................. 58

Just How Perilous Can 25 Extra Pounds Be? .................................................... 60

Gaining Weight on Sugar-Free, Fat-Free Diets ................................................. 62

Doubts Fail to Deter "The Diet Revolution" ..................................................... 64

New Look at Dieting: Fat Can Be a Friend ....................................................... 67

F.D.A. Approves Fat-Blocking Anti-Obesity Drug ........................................... 70

Obesity Drug Can Lead to Modest Weight Loss, Study Finds ........................ 72

History Counsels Caution on Diet Pills ............................................................. 74

Weight Loss the Herbal Way: No All-Natural Silver Bullet ............................. 75

## SECTION 4
# Emotional Health

### STRESS AND DEPRESSION ARE WIDESPREAD

Human Nature: Some Fear Everything, Even Fear Itself ................................... 79

Study Challenges Idea of PMS as Emotional Disorder ................................... 81

Study Disputes Abortion Trauma ....................................................................... 82

Hypnosis May Cause False Memories ................................................................ 84

For Employed Moms, the Pinnacle of Stress Comes After Work Ends .......... 85

Rising Stress of Raising a Grandchild ............................................................... 87

When Symptoms Are Obvious, but Cause Is Not ............................................ 89

Trying to Cope When a Partner or a Loved One
Is Chronically Depressed ................................................................................... 91

Depressed Parent's Children at Risk ................................................................. 93

Some Still Despair in a Prozac Nation .............................................................. 94

New Tack Promising on Winter Depression ...................................................... 97

Coming to Terms With Grief After a Longtime Partner Dies .......................... 99

When a Loss Remains Unresolved ...................................................................102

SECTION 5
# Violence

### THREATS ARISE FROM INSIDE AND OUTSIDE THE HOME

Battered Women Face Pit Bulls and Cobras .......................................................107

Planning to Escape From an Abusive Relationship ...........................................110

Many Prostitutes Suffer Combat Disorder ........................................................112

A Fistful of Hostility Is Found in Women ........................................................113

Genetic Ties May Be Factor in Violence in Stepfamilies ..................................114

Researchers Unravel the Motives of Stalkers ...................................................117

Dos and Don'ts for Thwarting a Stalker ..........................................................120

Call for New Sex-Abuse Trial is Said to Harm Rape Shield Law .....................122

SECTION 6
# Sexuality

### DRUGS CAN HELP, BUT THE EMOTIONAL PART REMAINS KEY

Women and Sex: On This Topic, Science Blushes ..............................................125

The Pill at 40: Renewed, Improved and in Its Prime .......................................127

Morning-After Contraceptive To Be Marketed .................................................129

Better Loving Through Chemistry: Sure, We've Got a Pill for That ...................130

Male Hormone Molds Women, Too, in Mind and Body .....................................132

Facing Viagra's Emotional Ripples ...................................................................135

Sour Note in the Viagra Symphony .................................................................137

In the History of Gynecology, a Surprising Chapter ........................................139

Issues of Gender, From Pronouns to Murder ...................................................141

Group Sends Book on Gay Tolerance to Schools ............................................142

U.S. Awakes to Epidemic of Sexual Diseases ..................................................144

SECTION 7
# Pregnancy, Childbirth and Matters of the Womb

### MYSTERIES REMAIN AMID TECHNOLOGICAL ADVANCES

$50,000 Offered to Tall, Smart Egg Donor ........................................................149

Quandary on Donor Eggs: What to Tell the Children ........................................150

Researchers Report Success in Method to Pick Baby's Sex ..............................153

Dancer's Ovarian Tissue Transplant Gives Hope to
Other Young Women Facing Infertility ............................................................156

Big Study Finds No Link in Abortion and Cancer ............................................157

Drugs, Safe and Not Safe, in Pregnancy ..........................................................159

Herbal Remedies Tied to Pregnancy Risks .......................................................161

A Study Finds Link Between Birth Defects and Solvents ...................................162

No Benefit Found for Fetal Monitors ...................................163

Ultrasound and Fury: One Mother's Ordeal ...................................164

Why Babies Are Born Facing Backward, Helpless and Chubby ...................................167

What's Missing in Childbirth These Days? Often, the Pain ...................................171

Doctors Report Rise in Elective Caesareans ...................................173

Benefits of Assistant for Childbirth Go Far Beyond the Birthing Room ...................................175

Deaths Linked to Sex After Childbirth ...................................177

Breast Is Best for Babies, but Sometimes Mom Needs Help ...................................178

Estrogen Patch Appears to Lift Severe Depression in New Mothers ...................................180

Diagnosing Fibroids Is Simple; Deciding What to Do Is Hard ...................................182

A Less Invasive Alternative for Fibroids ...................................184

SECTION 8

# The Teenage Years: Raising Healthy Daughters

### PHYSICAL AND EMOTIONAL CHALLENGES DURING LIFE'S SECOND DECADE

A Sex Guide for Girls, Minus Homilies ...................................189

Eating Disorders Haunt Ballerinas ...................................191

Efforts to Fight Eating Disorders May Backfire ...................................193

Girls and Puberty: the Crisis Years ...................................195

Yesterday's Precocious Puberty Is Norm Today ...................................196

Parents Can Bolster Girls' Fragile Self-Esteem ...................................198

Emotional Ills Tied to Stunted Growth in Girls ...................................199

Study Finds TV Alters Fiji Girls' View of Body ...................................200

In Quest for the Perfect Look, More Girls Choose the Scalpel ...................................202

Birth Rate at New Low as Teenage Pregnancy Declines ...................................205

Teenagers and Sex: Younger and More at Risk ...................................206

Coping with Cold, Hard Facts on Teenage Drinking ...................................209

Steroid Use by Teenage Girls Is Rising ...................................210

SECTION 9

# Menopause and Aging

### BALANCING THE BODY'S CHEMISTRY LATER IN LIFE

Theorists See Evolutionary Advantages in Menopause ...................................215

Menopause Begins Silently, Before Its Symptoms ...................................218

Scientists Now Envision Life Without Menopause ...................................219

Weighing the Pros and Cons of Hormone Therapy ...................................221

A Study Plays Down Estrogen Link to Breast Cancers ...................................223

Hormone Use Helps Women, a Study Finds ...................................................225

A Tad of Testosterone Adds Zest to Menopause ........................................227

Keeping Clinical Depression Out of the Aging Formula ..........................228

Test at Onset of Menopause Can Avert Bone Loss ...................................231

Guidelines Offer an Earlier Blueprint for the Battle Against Bone Loss .........232

New Drug Helps Delay Bone Loss ...............................................................235

For Some Women, Losing Pounds Could Add Up to a Hip Fracture .............236

### SECTION 10
## Women's Greatest Fear: Breast Cancer

#### DETECTION AND TREATMENT CONTINUE TO IMPROVE

In Breast Cancer Data—Hope, Fear and Confusion .........................................241

Coping with Fear: Keeping Breast Cancer in Perspective .............................243

Software to Compute Women's Cancer Risk ...................................................245

Sorting Out Contradictory Findings About Fat and Health .........................246

Studies Confirm Relationship of Alcohol to Breast Cancer ........................248

Do Breast Self-Exams Save Lives? Science Still Doesn't Have Answer ...........250

Living Proof: Mammograms Are Not Always Enough ..................................252

Cancer Gene Tests Turn Out to Be Far From Simple ....................................254

Breast Cancer Drug Dilemma: Who Should Take It, and When? ...................257

Round 3 in Cancer Battle: A 5-Year Drug Regimen .....................................259

Drugs to Fight Breast Cancer Near Approval ................................................262

Hope for Sale: Business Thrives on Unproven Care,
Leaving Science Behind .....................................................................................265

Reactions of Women With Cancer ...................................................................270

Breast Surgeons Turn to a Gentler Biopsy .....................................................271

Removal of Healthy Breasts Is Found to Cut Cancer Risk ...........................272

Study Says Few Women Rue Preventive Breast Operation ...........................275

Breast Reconstruction: All at Once or Not at All? .........................................277

### SECTION 11
## Heart Disease

#### MORE NEEDS TO BE DONE TO CURB THE NUMBER ONE KILLER OF WOMEN

Paradox or Not, Cholesterol in France Is on the Rise ....................................281

What Women Can Do to Escape Heart Disease ............................................284

Protein May Be Heart Risk Factor ...................................................................285

Study Finds Secondhand Smoke Doubles Risk of Heart Disease ...............287

Study Cites Risks for Women Under 50 With Heart Attacks .........................288

Yet Another Reason to Fight the Fat ...................................................290

Savory Diet That's Good for the Heart? Let's Eat ...............................292

There's Plenty of Choice in a Diet for a Healthier Heart ...................295

Drink a Day Can Lower Death Rate By 20 Percent ............................297

High Intake of 2 Vitamins May Lower Coronary Risk .........................298

SECTION 12
# Image and Self-Image

### THE SURGICAL PATH TO APPEARANCE CHANGES

A Question of Beauty: Is It Good for You? ........................................303

Life's Wrinkles, Some of Them Ugly, Afflict the Beautiful, Too ..........306

Cosmetic Breast Enlargements Are Making a Comeback ...................308

Panel Confirms No Major Illness Tied to Implants . . . ....................310

. . . But Panel Calls for Study of Some Implant Risks ........................312

Via Microtechnology, an Alternative to Glasses and Contacts ...........313

Promise and Risks of Laser Eye Surgery ...........................................315

As Ethnic Pride Rises, Rhinoplasty Takes a Nose Dive .....................317

In the Golden Age of Teeth, a Smile Can Be Perfected ...................318

The Joy of a New Neck ...................................................................320

Doctors' Review of 5 Deaths Raises Concern
About the Safety of Liposuction ......................................................321

SECTION 13
# Herbs, Supplements and Alternative Medicine

### CAUTION IS NEEDED AS OFFERINGS MULTIPLY

Alternative Medicine Makes Inroads, but Watch Out for Curves .......325

Taking Stock of Mysteries of Medicine .............................................327

Articles Question Safety of Dietary Supplements ..............................328

Americans Gamble on Herbs as Medicine ........................................331

Seeking Help for the Body in the Well-Being of the Soul .................337

Puzzle in a Bottle: In Vitamin Mania, Millions Take a Gamble on Health ......339

U.S. Panel on Acupuncture Calls for Wider Acceptance ...................348

The Arthritis Is at Bay, Thank You ..................................................349

Kava May Soothe Jagged Nerves, but Is It Safe? .............................351

Study on Using Magnets to Treat Pain Surprises Skeptics ................353

Words of Caution About a Hot Potato .............................................355

Behind the Hoopla Over a Hormone ...............................................356

Index .............................................................................................359

**W**omen have long been the primary consumers of medical care, the ones who are most likely to read about health, go to doctors and see to it that family members get proper medical care. But until very recently in the history of medicine, research on women's health issues has lagged considerably behind that devoted to medical problems that beset men. The differences between men and women are significant, we now know, and findings in men cannot be assumed to apply equally to women. Besides, many of the health needs of women, who serve the species as its primary reproductive system, differ greatly from those of men. Henry Higgins' behest notwithstanding, women cannot be more like men, nor should they want to be.

Fortunately, women are no longer tolerating medical neglect. They are constantly asking questions about their health and demanding answers based on facts. As a result, research on women's health issues has skyrocketed in recent decades, and the way women's medical problems are handled has, in some cases, changed dramatically as a result of new findings. Witness the remarkable progress in the treatment of breast cancer. As recently as the late 1970s, radical mastectomy was the standard of care, regardless of how advanced a woman's tumor. Now, nearly no one is subjected to this mutilating surgery, thanks to a series of well-designed Government-financed clinical trials that proved that less extensive surgery, followed by chemotherapy or radiation therapy, or both, produced results just as good—in fact, better, in most cases.

Unfortunately, women's knowledge about their health too often lags behind the facts. In some cases, extensive publicity given to certain health issues—like breast cancer—has resulted in distorted views about the seriousness of various health risks. In other cases, publicity about conflicting findings has prompted many women to put their heads in the sand and wait for the researchers to make up their minds instead of acting now on the basis of the best available knowledge.

As the recipient of dozens of queries each month from readers of my Personal Health column and as a frequent lecturer on health to large audiences of women throughout the United States, I am regularly besieged by queries about women's health issues. While in general, women's concerns about their health are hardly trivial, I am struck by the fact that the concerns rarely focus on the most serious health threats or the most productive preventive steps women could take.

For example, most women are far more worried about breast cancer than they are about heart disease, even though the chances that heart disease will kill them is six times greater. Even lung cancer is a bigger killer than breast cancer, claiming 50 percent more women's lives each year than breast cancer does. Women are forever asking about which calcium supplements are best able to protect their bones, but almost no one asks about the foods that could keep their skeletons intact as they age. Women worry about food additives, pesticide residues, artificial sweeteners and vitamin-mineral supplements instead of focusing on how to consume a proper balance of foodstuffs: the kinds and amounts of proteins, fats and carbohydrates. Too often, weight loss diets seriously distort that balance and place women at risk of ending up a thin corpse. Only a minority of American women consume the minimal recommendation of five servings of fruits and vegetables daily, which can help to prevent everything from blinding eye diseases to cancer.

Even more serious is the still-large number of women who place their current and future health at risk by smoking. Currently, more teenaged girls and young women are smoking than are boys and men. To paraphrase the Virginia Slims slogan, "You've come a long way baby"—toward a shorter life. Not to mention wrinkles, a chronic cough and an obnoxious odor.

The good news is that there is a substantial body of facts now available on which women can act to preserve their health and, should that effort fail, to get the kind of medical care most likely to restore them to health with a minimum of trauma. We now know, for example, that there are two very good reasons why women should be more alert to heart disease: Heart attacks are twice as deadly in women as in men, and doctors often miss the signs of serious heart disease and even heart attack in women, whose symptoms are frequently vague and hard to interpret. Women having a heart attack are very likely to experience breathlessness, nausea and heartburn and to receive a diagnosis of anxiety attack, not heart attack. The delay in recognizing the true cause of symptoms can make a life-and-death difference.

Likewise, many women worry far more about their weight and outward appearance than about the tissues that support a healthy body. Concern about bones and calcium should begin in childhood, when the primary bone structure is being formed. While there are new treatments that can help build bone even in the sixth decade of life and beyond, it is far better to reach midlife with strong, healthy bones and keep them that way through proper nutrition and regular weight-bearing exercise.

Speaking of exercise, even many women who pay close attention to their diets often neglect the other end of the caloric equation: the calories used through physical activity. Optimal health cannot be achieved without regular exercise. Now that labor-saving devices have replaced strenuous physical activity in the daily lives of most women in this country, women must be purposeful about exercise and set aside time each day to work their bodies the way nature intended—the way that can keep them healthy and strong for the eight or nine or even 10 decades that women in this country now live. This book should help every health-conscious woman achieve that goal. So, read on...

— Jane E. Brody,
Personal Health Columnist,
*The New York Times*

# *Nutrition*

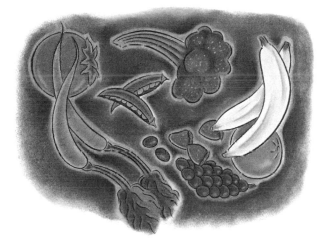

## LINKS BETWEEN FOOD, HEALTH AND DISEASE

We seem to be bombarded with so many conflicting theories about what to eat and what not to eat that at times it is tempting to give up, figure we've got to die of something anyway and abandon our fate to potato chips.

But nutrition research in recent years has been reassuringly consistent about the importance of certain components of the diet. Calcium, for instance, is vital, not only for the formation of bones and teeth; it may also play a significant role in preventing high blood pressure, colon cancer and premenstrual syndrome. Fiber can protect the heart and may also help to stabilize blood sugar and ward off diabetes. Vitamin D is essential for preventing osteoporosis—and yet many Americans are deficient in it.

But how to make sure we get the essentials? The best way is to adopt a diet rich in whole grains, fruits and vegetables, moderate in red meat and low in saturated fat, sugar, refined flour and alcohol. Eating "right" is not complicated, and it does not take the joy out of life. There is such a variety of tasty and nourishing foods that even the most finicky, armed with common sense, motivation and some basic information, can put together a diet that is healthful, delicious and satisfying.

# People Who Skip Breakfast Pay a High Price

The fall is that no-time-in-the-morning time of year. The kids are back in school, parents are back to work and breakfast in many households has become a catch-as-catch-can affair, if it is eaten at all. This decade has seen a steady decline in the proportion of Americans who regularly eat breakfast, long considered "the most important meal of the day."

Though you may not think so as you hit the snooze alarm to catch a few more winks of morning sleep, it would pay to get up 15 minutes earlier to make time for a nutritious breakfast. A sweet roll or bagel and coffee from a nearby deli is not an adequate breakfast. Nor is a so-called breakfast bar or Pop Tart or bag of chips munched on the way to school. These may temporarily suppress hunger pangs, but they will do little to enhance brain function and mood, not to mention nutritional status and overall health.

Given what most Americans call breakfast, a fast-food sandwich is actually an improvement even though it is likely to be much higher in fat, salt and calories than, say, cereal with fruit and low-fat or skim milk.

Performance questions aside, the goal of many breakfast skippers is to save on calories. However, calories consumed early in the day are least likely to put on pounds, and skipping any meal simply increases the temptation to eat a high-calorie snack or overeat at the next meal. In fact, the leanest people tend to be those who eat three or more meals a day.

Then there is the matter of nutrients. Breakfast may be the only time during the day when a child or adult consumes fruit juice and milk, making this meal an important source of vitamins C and D and calcium. Studies of teenagers have shown that those who skip breakfast have an intake of calcium and vitamin C that is 40 percent lower and an iron intake that is 10 percent lower than those who eat breakfast. These nutrients are most critical during the years of growth and development. Further, given the demands of modern lives, breakfast may be the only

meal teenagers regularly eat at home and the only one over which parents might have some say.

Ideally, breakfast should supply one-quarter to one-third of the day's protein plus fiber-rich complex carbohydrates and a small amount of fat. The breakfasts served in school generally strive to meet most, if not all, these nutrient needs. Simple homemade meals that fulfill these criteria include a whole-grain cereal (cold or hot) with fruit and low-fat or skim milk; low-fat or nonfat yogurt with fruit and whole-wheat bread with jam or margarine; a shake made with yogurt, fruit and skim milk plus whole-wheat toast, or a turkey, cheese or peanut butter sandwich on whole-grain bread with fruit juice and milk.

Parents should provide a good example by eating breakfast themselves. Children are most likely to eat breakfast if someone eats with them. If that is not possible, at least try to sit with children while they eat.

In families where mornings are already overly loaded with demands, it helps to set up breakfast the night before. When my sons were young and I had to get out early, I often made them sandwiches for breakfast or set up pita pizzas they could pop into the toaster oven in the morning. If the boys were running late, they could eat these foods on the way to school.

But on most days, breakfast was eaten at home. Sometimes I cooked French toast or pancakes in advance to be heated in the morning and topped with sliced bananas or berries and yogurt. Another make-ahead favorite was "Eggs Jane"—poached egg white and turkey on a whole-wheat pita topped with a slice of cheese, ready to heat in the toaster oven in the morning. Although hot cereal doesn't lend itself to advance preparation, it takes only two minutes (and no pots to wash) to cook quick oats with skim milk and raisins in the microwave oven.

Of course, school-age children can serve themselves ready-to-eat breakfast cereal. But it is up to parents to assure that the selection of cereals in the house is nutritious. The best cereals are well-stocked with nutrients and fiber and not overly rich in sugars or fats. Don't be misled by claims that a serving supplies 100 percent of lots of vitamins and minerals, since there is no need for anyone to consume the day's nutrient needs at breakfast. Look instead for whole grain cereals with no more than 6 grams of sugar per serving. Among good choices that young taste buds are likely to enjoy are Wheaties, Cheerios, Wheat Chex and Raisin Bran, perhaps with a sweeter cereal like Life or granola as a garnish.

And for those who can't bear to eat first thing in the morning, try a glass of juice and piece of bread before leaving home with a portable breakfast (like a container of yogurt or sandwich) to eat later when hunger strikes, often just before the school or work day starts.

[JEB, October 1998]

## Calcium Takes Its Place as a Superstar of Nutrients

Calcium emerged as the nutrient of the '90s, a substance with such diverse roles in the body that virtually no major organ system escapes its influence. As the most abundant mineral in the body, calcium has long been recognized as vital to the formation and maintenance of strong bones and teeth. But bones, rather than serving as the final destination of calcium, are in a sense, just a starting point. They continuously release the mineral into the system where new research suggests it may play a central role in controlling blood pressure and easing premenstrual syndrome, or PMS. In addition, new studies indicate that unused dietary calcium may help to prevent colon cancer.

The recent focus on calcium comes at a time when the nation is becoming increasingly deficient both in the mineral and in vitamin D, which enables the body to absorb and use it. While the most dire effects of too little calcium and vitamin D are seen in adults, it is the country's children who have drawn some of the most intense concern, because this calcium-diminished younger generation is putting itself at much greater risk for osteoporosis—the brittle-bone disease now plaguing many older Americans.

The new research has come in a flurry. Within two months of each other, one New York research group reported that eating more calcium-rich foods reduced the risk of colon cancer in men prone to the disease, and another New York-based team described a 50 percent reduction in life-disrupting premenstrual symptoms among hundreds of women who took daily calcium supplements.

Findings reported by Boston researchers supported earlier evidence that calcium was important in controlling high blood pressure. The researchers found that blood pressure fell in women with mild hypertension after brief exposures of their skin to ultraviolet-B radiation, which stimulates the production of vitamin D.

In another report, published in the *British Medical Journal* in August 1998, researchers in Argentina showed that women who were given calcium supplements during pregnancy had children whose blood pressure remained lower than average for at least the first seven years of life, which would lower their risk of later developing hypertension. And in the October 1998 issue of *The American Journal of Clinical Nutrition*, a research team at the University of Southern California in Los Angeles reported that adding calcium to the diet lowered blood pressure in 116 black teenagers who normally consumed little of the mineral.

The new work builds on a well-established body of research pointing to calcium's complex role in the body. Through the years, scientists have demonstrated that calcium is required for myriad body functions:

▶ Transmission of nerve impulses that control muscle contractions.
▶ Release of chemicals that carry messages between nerves.

- Binding together of cells to form organs.
- Production and activity of enzymes and hormones that regulate digestion, fat metabolism, energy release and saliva production.
- Clotting of the blood to initiate wound healing.
- Secretion of hormones and other substances from glands throughout the body.
- Chemical signaling within cells.
- Growth and maturation of lining cells throughout the body.

"It's not surprising that calcium plays so many roles," said Dr. Hector F. DeLuca, a biochemist at the University of Wisconsin who is an expert on vitamin D and calcium metabolism. "Since all life originated in the sea in a bath containing calcium, we all developed systems that depend on it."

Once animals emerged from the sea, leaving behind a steady supply of calcium, the body had to evolve a system for keeping calcium "at sea level" in the blood, Dr. DeLuca said. The result was the evolution of a calcium storage tank—the bones—for the body to draw on from minute to minute when blood levels of this essential mineral drop too low, as well as a mechanism to establish and replenish the body's calcium from outside sources—the diet. This mechanism involves vitamin D. In its activated form as a hormone, vitamin D enables calcium to enter the blood through the intestinal wall and be incorporated into bone.

But if the body does not receive enough dietary calcium to maintain the needed blood level, parathyroid hormone leaps to the rescue. Its job is to signal the release of calcium from the bones to restore a normal blood level of this life-sustaining mineral. If the diet is chronically deficient in calcium (or vitamin D), as it is for as many as three-fourths of Americans, the bones gradually get weaker and weaker.

A chronic deficiency or imbalance of calcium is what Dr. Susan Thys-Jacobs, an endocrinologist at St. Luke's-Roosevelt Hospital Center in New York, believes is largely responsible for the disruptive symptoms of PMS suffered by as many as 40 percent of women. In fact, Dr. Thys-Jacobs said, PMS may be a harbinger of osteoporosis, a warning that a woman is not getting enough calcium and, as a result, is constantly losing bone.

Buoyed by the promising results of a pilot study of calcium's ability to relieve premenstrual symptoms and menstrual pain, Dr. Thys-Jacobs and colleagues at 11 other medical centers enrolled nearly 500 women with debilitating PMS in a trial of calcium's ability to relieve their monthly discomfort. For two months, the women kept careful track of the occurrence and severity of 17 symptoms grouped under four categories: mood swings, bloating, food cravings and pain. Then they were randomly assigned to take either 1,200 milligrams of calcium daily (as calcium carbonate in Tums E-X) or a look-alike placebo. The women continued on their assigned regimens and evaluated their symptoms for the next three menstrual cycles.

By the third cycle, Dr. Thys-Jacobs and her collaborators reported in *The American Journal of Obstetrics and Gynecology* the overall severity of symptoms was reduced by 48 percent in the calcium group, compared with 30 percent in the placebo group. Improvement in the calcium group exceeded that of the placebo group in every category studied, both psychological and physical, and in 15 of the 17 symptoms evaluated. Most significantly, subjects in the calcium group noted a 54 percent reduction in aches and pains, while the placebo group had a 15 percent increase in pain symptoms. The study was financed by SmithKline Beecham, makers of Tums.

Dr. Thys-Jacobs concluded that women with PMS might have a form of "functional hypocalcemia"—calcium levels in their blood and urine are normal, but only because parathyroid hormone levels are abnormally high and the hormone is continually extracting calcium from their bones to replenish the blood's supply. She suggested that all women with PMS be assessed for deficiencies of calcium and vitamin D, as indicated by their blood levels of parathyroid hormone and 25-hydroxy vitamin D. She pointed out that "80 percent of a person's vitamin D is made in the skin when exposed to sunlight, but a lot of young women are now avoiding the sun and using sunscreens."

"Their vitamin D levels are very low," said Dr. Thys-Jacobs, "and therefore they're not absorbing enough calcium from their diet even if they consume enough, which most young women do not."

Tissues throughout the body are lined with epithelial cells like the ones that form the outer layer of skin. They grow, mature, slough off and are replaced by new ones. In the lining of the colon, where cancers arise, the turnover of epithelial cells normally takes a week. But in people prone to colon cancer, these cells fail to grow and mature normally and instead immature cells proliferate rapidly. Studies in people and animals have linked high-fat diets to colon cancer and shown that fatty acids and the bile acids released to process them are irritants that stimulate abnormal cell proliferation in the colon.

Dr. Martin Lipkin of the Strang Cancer Research Laboratory at Rockefeller University in New York described studies showing that calcium could bind tightly to these irritants and inhibit their ability to stimulate cell proliferation. With calcium present, as it would be on a calcium-rich diet, the cells differentiate and mature like normal epithelial cells.

Dr. Lipkin and his colleagues showed that calcium supplements could inhibit colonic cell proliferation in people susceptible to colon cancer. This finding gained support from population studies that found a link between consumption of dairy products and a reduced risk of colon cancer.

A study directed by Dr. Peter R. Holt of St. Luke's-Roosevelt and published in October 1998 in the *Journal of the American Medical Association* showed that calcium-rich foods worked as well or better than previously thought. When participants' consumption of low-fat, calcium-rich dairy products was doubled, reaching 1,200 milligrams of calcium a day, cell growth in the colon became normal. The 70 participants had undergone surgery earlier to remove benign polyps, common forerunners of colon cancer.

Dr. Lipkin, a co-author of the new study, said that animal research indicated that increasing calcium levels to protect epithelial cells might also help prevent cancer in such organs as the breast, prostate and pancreas. Raising the animals' intake of calcium and vitamin D reduced excessive cell proliferation and induced normal development of epithelial cells in these various organs, he said.

A person's blood pressure is influenced by many factors, including genetics, body weight, physical activity and, in some cases, salt intake. But dozens of studies since the early 1980s have also implicated calcium as a potentially important contributor to normal blood pressure, especially the calcium found in dairy

## How Much Calcium?

Experts remain divided over how much calcium is enough. Currently, the National Institutes of Health calls for higher intakes for women who are older than 50 and not using hormone replacement therapy (H.R.T.) and for pregnant and nursing women. The dietary reference intakes offered by the National Academy of Sciences do not account for these and other differences and are lower over all.

### National Academy of Sciences Recommendations

| AGE GROUP | MILLIGRAMS PER DAY |
|---|---|
| 0 to 6 months | 210 (solely from human milk) |
| 7 to 12 months | 270 (human milk and solid foods) |
| 1 to 3 years | 500 |
| 4 to 8 years | 800 |
| 9 to 18 years | 1,300 |
| 19 to 50 years | 1,000 |
| 51 and older | 1,200 |

*Source: Food and Nutrition Board, Institute of Medicine of the National Academy of Sciences*

### National Institutes of Health Recommendations

| AGE GROUP | MILLIGRAMS PER DAY |
|---|---|
| **INFANTS** | |
| Birth to 6 months | 400 |
| 6 months to 1 year | 600 |
| **CHILDREN** | |
| 1 to 5 years | 800 |
| 6 to 10 years | 800–1,200 |
| **ADOLESCENTS/YOUNG ADULTS** | |
| 11 to 24 years | 1,200–1,500 |
| **MEN** | |
| 25 to 65 years | 1,000 |
| Over 65 years | 1,500 |
| **WOMEN** | |
| 25 to 50 years | 1,000 |
| Pregnant or nursing | 1,200–1,500 |
| **Postmenopausal** | |
| Taking/not taking H.R.T. | 1,000/1,500 |
| Over 65 years | 1,500 |

*Source: National Institutes of Health Consensus Development Panel on Optimal Calcium Intake*

products. The findings suggest that a low intake of calcium-rich dairy products may partly account for the high rates of hypertension among African-Americans.

A shortage of calcium might also contribute to the rise in blood pressure that commonly accompanies aging. Even if calcium intake is adequate, which it usually is not, most older people are deficient in the active form of vitamin D needed to absorb calcium.

While the American Heart Association's latest assessment of the relationship between high blood pressure and dietary minerals strongly emphasized sodium chloride (i.e. salt) as the prime offender, it also noted that the harmful effects of a high-salt diet were most common among people whose diets are low in calcium. Though he was a co-author of the association's statement, which was published recently in the journal *Circulation*, Dr. David McCarron, a hypertension specialist at Oregon Health Sciences University in Portland, champions the view that calcium-rich milk products are more effective than a low-sodium diet in curbing hypertension.

In 1997, Dr. McCarron's view won major support from the surprising results of the large, Federally-financed DASH (Dietary Approaches to Stop Hypertension) trial. That study found that a diet rich in low-fat dairy products, fruits and vegetables significantly lowered blood pressure in adults with high-normal pressure or mild hypertension, although participants lost no weight and continued to consume ample amounts of salt. Also, the blood pressure benefits were noted within two weeks.

The DASH diet contains up to 1,200 milligrams of calcium; participants who continued on their regular diets got only about 450 milligrams of calcium. Nearly half of Americans consume less than 450 milligrams of calcium a day, "and it's getting worse," Dr. McCarron said.

His main concern now is the "seriously deficient" diet consumed by a very large proportion of American children. Children, he said, are drinking soda and juices, not milk, and they rarely come close to eating the recommended five servings a day of fruits and vegetables. He believes parents and schools are setting children up for a lifetime of ill health.

"Calcium is a lot more than simply bone health," Dr. McCarron concluded. "It may even influence behavior," he said, citing a space shuttle study in which rats bred to become hypertensive were "frantic" on a low-calcium diet, but when fed more calcium, "they relaxed and enjoyed the space flight."

[JEB, October 1998]

## Finding Calcium Sources Outside the Dairy Case

Photos of famous men and women sporting mustaches of milk have become familiar advertisements for a calcium-rich food that has fallen on hard times. Milk consumption has been dropping for the last three decades, and calcium nutrition among both young and old has collapsed with it. Some experts predict an epidemic of osteoporosis because today's children and teenagers, who guzzle sodas and juice drinks instead of milk, are consuming about half the amount of calcium from foods that youngsters did in 1950.

Peak bone mass, the single best predictor of osteoporosis, is largely achieved by age 20, so most of these young people will enter the years of gradual bone loss in their 30s with a glass that is already only half-full. Now, as new evidence points to the ever-widening role of calcium in preventing disease, it is even more important to be sure that everyone gets enough of this vital nutrient each day.

Achieving the recommended daily amounts of calcium is not difficult for people whose diets are rich in dairy products. Children who drink three or four glasses of milk a day, for example, would easily meet their needs. But there is much confusion about other food sources of calcium and the ability of calcium supplements to compensate for a dietary deficiency.

Food is nearly always a better source of calcium than supplements, if for no other reason than food provides more nutritional benefits than just calcium, including nutrients that help the body use calcium. A consensus conference convened by the National Institutes of Health concluded in 1994 that "to attain optimal calcium levels, a change in dietary habits, including increased consumption of dairy products and/or calcium-rich vegetable sources, is needed."

The experts might have also cautioned Americans about eating too much salt and protein, especially animal protein, which increases the loss of calcium in urine. Eating just one fast-food hamburger leads to a net loss of 23 milligrams of calcium, according to Dr. Robert P. Heaney, a calcium expert at Creighton University in Omaha. However, despite earlier concerns about caffeine, it only minimally increases calcium loss, by about 2 or 3 milligrams for a cup of coffee, Mr. Heaney said.

**Dairy Products.** Milk remains the best dietary source of calcium for two reasons: the lactose (milk sugar) naturally in milk and the vitamin D added to it enhance calcium absorption through the gut. (For those who have trouble digesting lactose, ample calcium is absorbed from lactose-reduced milk and from yogurt with active cultures, which is also low in lactose.) Ounce for ounce, nonfat plain yogurt has more calcium than milk, although it contains no vitamin D. Among frozen dairy desserts, nonfat frozen yogurt is a much better source of calcium than ice cream or ice milk.

Hard cheese, high or low in fat, is quite rich in calcium. Ricotta cheese is also an excellent source, but cottage cheese, creamed or otherwise, is not nearly as good a source as milk and yogurt unless calcium is added by the maker. Using less water when reconstituting dry milk and adding nonfat dry milk powder to other drinks and foods are excellent ways to increase calcium.

For children allergic to cow's milk or who become constipated when consuming it, soy milk fortified with calcium or a daily calcium supplement may be substituted.

**Vegetables.** Some of the best vegetable sources of calcium include kale, collard greens, turnip greens, mustard greens, Chinese cabbage, chicory and bok choy. Broccoli, chard and acorn squash, though not as rich in calcium, are more common sources. Although spinach has a lot of calcium, it also contains a substance—oxalic acid—that binds up its calcium and prevents absorption of all but about 5 percent of it. However, the oxalic acid in spinach and foods like rhubarb does not interfere with absorption of calcium from other foods eaten at the same time. Phytic acid, another substance in foods like dried beans and peas, also depresses calcium absorption somewhat, but less than oxalic acid.

Most forms of fiber have little or no effect on calcium absorption. Wheat bran, though, can partly block absorption of calcium from other foods, for example, the milk in a bowl of bran cereal.

**Other Food.** Canned sardines with their bones included are especially rich in calcium—3 ounces of sardines have more calcium than 8 ounces of milk. Canned salmon, also with bones, is about half as good. Other sources include dry-roasted soybeans, blackstrap molasses, figs, some beans and peas (black-eyed peas, white beans, great northern beans, navy beans and soybeans, although the calcium in beans is only about half as available to the body as that in milk), poppy and sesame seeds, tahini, almonds, oranges and calcium-fortified orange juice. The acid in the juice enhances calcium absorption, and is especially good for older people short on stomach acid.

For those who cannot or do not get enough calcium from foods, calcium supplements are the next best option. As long as the maximum does not exceed a total of 2,000 milligrams a day from foods and pills, supplementation appears to be safe, except perhaps for people who tend to form calcium-containing kidney stones. Amounts higher than 2,000 milligrams can cause drowsiness, impaired absorption of other minerals and calcium deposits in the tissues that may be mistaken for cancer on X-rays.

As for how well a calcium tablet is absorbed, there is no predictable relationship between a supplement's ability to dissolve in vinegar water and its usefulness to the body. Calcium carbonate (as in Tums and Rolaids as well as various supplements) is least expensive and as good a source when taken with meals as, say, calcium citrate, which can be taken between meals and is the preferred supplement for older people who are deficient in stomach acid. Avoid natural sources of calcium like bone meal, oyster shell or dolomite, since they may contain harmful contaminants.

Bedtime is another good time to take calcium, since it will remain in the stomach longer. If possible, avoid taking calcium with meals that contain a lot of wheat fiber. Also, if taking iron or a multivitamin with iron, take calcium at a different time since it interferes with iron absorption.

When buying a calcium supplement, check the label for the amount of elemental calcium in each tablet, not the total weight, to calculate the amount of calcium being consumed. Calcium supplements are best used by the body when taken in doses of 500 milligrams or less. Chewable and effervescent supplements are available for those who have trouble swallowing tablets.

And don't forget vitamin D. Many Americans do not get enough of this vitamin to assure optimal calcium absorption. And the latest studies suggest that adults need 800 International Units a day, not 400 as is now recommended. Although milk is supposed to be fortified with vitamin D (400 units per quart), the actual amount in milk varies widely. About 90 percent of the vitamin D people get is made in skin exposed to the sun's ultraviolet-B rays. Try to expose some part of your body (without sunscreen) to the sun for 10 or 15 minutes a day year-round. Alternatively, eat fatty fish or take cod-liver oil or a supplement with D.

[JEB, October 1998]

## Osteoporosis Linked to Vitamin D Deficiency

An important study strongly suggests that widespread deficiencies of vitamin D may play a big role in causing the bone-wasting disease osteoporosis among older Americans. The researchers attributed vitamin D deficiencies to two factors of growing importance: insufficient dietary intake and inadequate exposure to sunlight, which stimulates production of vitamin D in the skin.

The study findings, published in *The New England Journal of Medicine*, suggest not only that millions of American adults lack enough vitamin D in their blood to protect their bones but also that newly upgraded recommendations for vitamin D intake may be inadequate to prevent osteoporosis in many older people. Although calcium is the main nutrient of concern for preventing osteoporosis, vitamin D also plays an important role.

Deficient levels of vitamin D were found in the blood of 37 percent of those who reported consuming the newly recommended amounts of 400 International Units a day for people 51 to 70 years old and 600 International Units for those over 70. The previous recommendation for all adults had been 200 International Units.

The study was conducted by Dr. Melissa K. Thomas and colleagues at Massachusetts General Hospital among 290 hospitalized patients, who might be expected to have lower-than-average levels of vitamin D in their blood. And indeed more than half of them did. Using a conservative measure of deficiency, Dr. Thomas said 57 percent of the patients were deficient, including 22 percent who were severely deficient in this essential nutrient.

Asked whether the findings in hospital patients could be applied to the general population, Dr. Thomas said that although the percentage of people with vitamin D deficiency might be somewhat lower in healthy people, the problem was still likely to be widespread. Dr. Thomas based this judgment on a separate analysis of vitamin D levels among 44 patients who were younger and healthier and had none of the usual risk factors that might cause a vitamin D deficiency. Yet she found that 42 percent of them were deficient.

The results of this and other studies suggest that at least for adults living at northern latitudes where essentially no vitamin D is made in the skin all winter, a dietary supplement of 800 International Units a day may be needed to stave off a chronic deficiency. In an editorial accompanying the new report, Dr. Robert D. Utiger, a specialist in endocrinology, pointed out that low vitamin D levels had been found in 46 percent of those who reported taking multivitamins, most of which contain 400 International Units of vitamin D.

Vitamin D aids in the absorption of dietary calcium, but its most important role is in maintaining normal blood levels of calcium. In the patients labeled deficient, levels of vitamin D in the blood were low enough to cause calcium to be removed from their bones to supply the blood. Adults deficient in vitamin D cannot properly mineralize their bones, which gradually come to resemble a rubbery framework without cement.

A recent study of 3,270 healthy elderly French women showed that a dietary supplement of calcium plus 800 International Units of vitamin D a day decreased the risk of hip fractures by 43 percent in just two years.

Dr. Michael Horlick, chief of endocrinology at Boston University Medical Center, said there was now enough evidence to conclude that "vitamin D deficiency is an unrecognized epidemic in our middle-aged and older population—both in patients and in healthy people throughout the year." For example, in a recent study he did among 160 Bostonians 49 through 83 years old who visited the hospital clinics, 40 percent were deficient in vitamin D.

Dr. Horlick's studies have shown that the American diet is an unreliable and generally poor source of vitamin D. The only major dietary source is milk that has been fortified with vitamin D, supposedly at a minimum level of 400 International Units in each quart. But he said he found that "no more than 20 percent of milk samples throughout the nation contained at least 320 I.U. per quart and 15 percent of skim milk samples had no detectable vitamin D at all, even though the label said they were fortified with vitamin D."

"About 90 percent of the vitamin D in most people comes from casual exposure to sunlight," Dr. Horlick said. "But the concern about cancer risk has limited people's exposure to sunlight." Speaking of a sun protection factor, he added, "If you religiously apply sunscreen with an S.P.F. of 8 to your exposed skin, you will make no vitamin D."

[JEB, March 1998]

# Diet-Diabetes Link Reported

People who eat lots of potatoes, white bread and white rice in the mistaken belief that it is the best way to follow a low-fat diet may be doing themselves more harm than good. A steady diet of such foods may actually be a recipe for diabetes, according to a study by Harvard researchers published in the *Journal of the American Medical Association*.

The study, which tracked 65,173 women for six years, found that those who ate a starchy diet that was also low in fiber and drank a lot of soft drinks had two and a half times the rate of diabetes found in women who ate less of those foods and more fiber, or roughage, specifically, more fiber from whole-grain cereals. Information about diet came from surveys filled out by the women themselves as part of the 20-year-old Nurses' Health Study project.

The starchy, low-fiber diet increased the diabetes

risk in all the women, independent of other risk factors like age, obesity, exercise and family history. In separate research, the scientists have found a similar effect in men, said the study director, Dr. Walter C. Willett, a professor of epidemiology and nutrition at the Harvard School of Public Health.

The study participants who became diabetic developed the most common form of the disease, non-insulin-dependent diabetes, which has also been called adult-onset or Type II diabetes. Eight million Americans have been given a diagnosis of diabetes, and another eight million are thought to have the disease without knowing it. It is characterized by high levels of blood sugar, or glucose, that are caused by a shortage of the hormone insulin or an inability to use the hormone properly to metabolize glucose and control its levels in the blood.

The treatments for this type of diabetes include diet and exercise to control weight, because obesity is a major risk factor. Insulin injections and other medications are also used to control blood sugar, but severe complications often occur even in spite of treatment; they include heart disease, blindness, kidney failure and circulation problems that lead to amputation of feet and legs.

Dr. Willett, offering a possible explanation for the new dietary findings, suggested that too little fiber and too much of the wrong type of carbohydrate may be harmful. It has been known for at least 15 years that the carbohydrates in white bread, potatoes and white rice are quickly digested and absorbed, causing a big surge in blood sugar, or glucose, which in turns leads the pancreas to secrete high levels of insulin. Ounce for ounce, those foods increase blood glucose levels more than eating sugar itself.

Over time, high blood sugar and insulin levels may make the body less sensitive to insulin, a condition called insulin resistance, and greater and greater amounts of insulin are needed to metabolize glucose. Insulin resistance, thought to affect 25 percent of Americans, is often associated with obesity. In some people, the pancreas may eventually become unable to keep up with the demand, leading to diabetes.

The lack of fiber is detrimental because fiber can slow the absorption of carbohydrates and prevent surges in the levels of blood sugar and insulin. In addition, Dr. Willett said, micronutrients in fiber, particularly magnesium, may be important in preventing diabetes. Previous studies have suggested that magnesium can increase the body's sensitivity to insulin, easing the stress on the pancreas.

In this study, though, it was impossible to tell whether it was magnesium or some other fiber ingredient that protected people from diabetes, so Dr. Willett recommended eating foods rich in fiber rather than taking magnesium or other supplements.

Dr. Willett said he expected that people would be shocked to hear the bad news about white bread and rice, and especially potatoes. "Americans have been told to load up on those things as if they're magical foods because they're low in fat," he said. "It's what some very health-conscious people are doing. The base of the food pyramid is 11 servings a day of carbohydrates, and it includes potatoes."

But his findings do not challenge the basic idea of the food pyramid, he said, or support any of the popular diet books that urge people to abandon carbohydrates in favor of high-protein diets. Carbohydrates should still be the basis of the diet, Dr. Willett said, but he cautioned, "Be careful which ones you eat."

Cold breakfast cereals (the women in this study ate whole-grain cereals like bran flakes) were related to reduced risk. It is reasonable to think that other whole-grain breakfast cereals, cooked and uncooked, would have a similar effect, Dr. Willett said.

"Bread, rice and pasta should be in the whole-grain form: brown rice and whole-grain pastas and breads," he added. "And go easy on the potatoes. Potatoes have been a staple when people faced starvation and needed calories, but they're not a staple food for a relatively sedentary population like the United States'. I'd eat potatoes in small amounts, and not every day."

Although researchers have long known that eating too much is an important risk factor for diabetes because the disease can be brought on by obesity, there has never before been evidence linking it to specific types of foods, not even sweets.

The president-elect for health care and education at the American Diabetes Association, Christine

Beebe, a nutritionist in Chicago Heights, said: "At the American Diabetes Association, we're delighted that these authors attempted to get to the issue of the quality of the diet in diabetes. We haven't had a lot of information on exactly what in the diet could predispose you to diabetes."

But she also said, "This study only begins to suggest what we need to look at further." The findings need to be confirmed by other researchers, she said, noting that the study depended on the women's answers to questionnaires about their eating habits, which could have been inaccurate. The potential of their diets to raise blood sugar was calculated from their reports of what they ate, rather than being measured.

In the meantime, researchers say, there is no harm in advising people to eat enough fiber. The American Diabetes Association is already doing that. "Most people get about 5 grams a day," Ms. Beebe said, "and we're encouraging 10 or more."

[DG, February 1997]

## Fiber Does Not Help Prevent Colon Cancer, Study Finds

It has been nearly three decades since Dr. Denis P. Burkitt, a British missionary surgeon who studied the differences in diseases of poor Africans and affluent Westerners, postulated that the Africans' high-fiber diet protected them against colon cancer. He spread his thesis as dietary gospel, prompting millions to change their diets.

Now, the largest study ever to examine Dr. Burkitt's theory has found that, at least when it comes to preventing colon cancer, all those fruits, vegetables and cereals do not do any good.

The research, by a team from Harvard University and Brigham and Women's Hospital in Boston, tracked the eating habits of more than 88,000 female nurses over 16 years and found that women who ate a high-fiber diet were no less likely to develop colorectal cancer or polyps, which can be a precursor to cancer, than women who ate little fiber.

The findings, which appear in *The New England Journal of Medicine*, were, for the most part, the same no matter what type of fiber the subjects ate, or how fastidious their habits—whether they smoked or did not smoke, whether they dined on fatty steak or lean tofu, whether they exercised regularly or sat on the couch and watched television.

The researchers and others commenting on their findings noted that the study had its limitations. For example, many scientists believe that men and women respond differently to dietary fat and fiber, and the study group involved only women. Still, the new study adds to growing research that suggests when it comes to colorectal cancer, the benefits of fiber have yet to be proved.

"We really can't substantiate a protective effect of fiber on the rates and risk of colon cancer," said Dr. Charles S. Fuchs, a medical oncologist at Brigham and Women's and the lead author of the study. "That is not to say that fiber is not a good thing. It is still helpful, but not for colon cancer."

Indeed, experts were quick today to urge Americans to eat a diet rich in fruits, vegetables and whole grains, primarily because those fiber-rich foods protect against the nation's leading killer, heart disease. In addition, a high-fiber diet has been shown to prevent other types of cancer, including that of the mouth, pharynx, larynx, esophagus and stomach, said Dr. Michael Thun, vice president for epidemiology at the American Cancer Society.

But none of those are as common as colorectal cancer, which kills more Americans—an estimated 57,000 in 1998—than any other type of cancer except lung cancer. While experts say the best way to prevent colorectal cancer is to undergo regular screening, some interviewed today were unconvinced by the findings of Dr. Fuchs and his colleagues.

They argued that Dr. Burkitt's hypothesis might

indeed be true, just difficult to prove through a study that relied, as the Boston one did, on participants to recall their eating habits accurately. Or other factors, like consumption of sugar, which has been associated with an increased risk of colon cancer, could have confounded the study results.

"This is an experienced group," said Dr. Arthur Schatzkin, senior investigator in the nutritional epidemiology branch of the National Cancer Institute. "It's a study with a strong design, but it is by no means the last word on the subject. It is possible that there really is a true relationship between fiber intake and colorectal cancer, but it is just that the epidemiologic tools that we use are too crude to see it."

The final word, Dr. Schatzkin said, will come after scientists conduct controlled clinical trials comparing cancer rates in patients who eat fiber-rich diets against those who do not. He is conducting one such study: the Polyp Prevention Trial, financed by the cancer institute. It began in 1991 and involves 2,000 people; half have been eating a specially designed high-fiber diet, while the other half have eaten as they normally would. Dr. Schatzkin said he was currently analyzing the results.

The findings in *The New England Journal of Medicine* article were drawn from the Nurse's Health Study, which since 1976 has been chronicling the health and habits of 121,700 female registered nurses. The nurses, who were 30 to 55 when the study began, were sent detailed questionnaires about their eating habits; the questionnaires were updated every two to four years.

For their research, Dr. Fuchs and his colleagues broke the women into five groups according to their median intake of fiber in 1980. They then studied only those women who maintained a consistent fiber intake for the next six years, 88,757 nurses in all, and tracked them until 1996. While the average American eats 13.3 grams of fiber a day, the fiber intake among the nurses averaged 9.8 grams in the lowest quintile and 24.9 grams in the highest. (A bowl of oatmeal contains about 4 grams.)

During the 16 years of the study, 787, or roughly nine-tenths of 1 percent of the study population, developed colorectal cancer. An additional 1,012 women were found to have benign tumors among 27,530 participants who underwent procedures to detect them.

The percentage of patients who developed colorectal cancer was relatively consistent among the five groups. But there was one curious finding: When the researchers teased apart the cancer rates according to the type of fiber the women ate, it appeared that those who ate the most vegetables actually increased their risk of colon cancer by 35 percent. But Dr. Fuchs said that finding was probably the result of chance.

"The effect was small but statistically significant," Dr. Fuchs said. "I don't make much of it. I certainly would not tell anybody to be concerned about vegetables."

[SGS, January 1999]

## Keep the Fiber Bandwagon Rolling, for Heart and Health

You've heard it now for years: fiber is good for you. Eat more whole grains, dried peas and beans, fruits and vegetables if you want to stay healthy. Fiber protects the colon against cancer. It also helps the heart by lowering cholesterol, reduces the risk of developing diabetes and facilitates weight control.

Then along comes a widely publicized Harvard study of nearly 89,000 nurses that seems to derail the fiber bandwagon. The study, published in 1999 in *The New England Journal of Medicine*, found no greater protection from colon cancer among the women who consumed the highest amount of fiber, more than 25 grams a day, than among those who consumed the least fiber, less than 10 grams a day.

But before you decide that it is now okay to return

to pasty white bread, white rice and pasta and shun those greens, whole grains and other fiber-rich plant foods, it is important to put this disheartening study in perspective and appreciate the diverse benefits dietary fiber can bestow.

Fiber first gained celebrity in modern times in 1979 when Dr. Denis P. Burkitt reported that Africans who consumed lots of fiber had very low rates of cancer of the colon and rectum, a common and often fatal disease in this country. Dr. Burkitt and others realized that there were many differences besides fiber intake between Africans and Americans, but the logic behind fiber as a gut protector seemed overwhelming.

Fiber has long had a reputation as a natural laxative that helps to prevent disorders like diverticulosis and diverticulitis, caused by years of straining to eliminate hard, dry stools. Fiber softens and adds bulk to the stool and thus facilitates rapid elimination of solid wastes. This in turn should reduce the exposure of the gut to carcinogens in foods and to carcinogens that may form in the digestive tract. Fiber also favorably changes the balance of microorganisms that live in the gut and may even activate a gene that protects against cancer.

In the years since Dr. Burkitt's observation, dozens of studies have looked for corroborating evidence. In a review of 39 studies examining a possible link between fiber intake and colon cancer, 26 studies showed a protective effect of fiber, but the remaining 13 studies did not. A 1994 Harvard study of 47,000 men was among those showing no evidence that fiber prevented colon cancer.

The nurses' study, though the largest thus far to look into this relationship, is nonetheless just one more negative finding in a field that remains highly controversial as researchers struggle to decipher the links, if any, between diet and colorectal cancer.

Several experts say methodological flaws could account for the negative findings of the study, known as the Nurses' Health Study. But even if the study were perfect and its findings correct, that should not be an excuse to ignore the advice to eat more fiber. The average American ingests only 5 to 13 grams of fiber each day, whereas nutrition experts, including the American Dietetic Association and the National Cancer Institute, recommend a daily intake of 20 to 35 grams.

Dietary fiber comes in two forms: soluble and insoluble. Both are more or less indigestible. Insoluble fibers, like lignin, that form the structure of plants are well-established stimulants of the gut. Soluble fibers dissolve in water and include pectin, mucilages and gums. The soluble fiber in oats is what gives oatmeal its gummy texture. You may recall the mania for oat bran that swept the country just a few years ago after researchers reported that the soluble fiber in oats lowered blood cholesterol levels.

Just five months after publication of the colon cancer finding, researchers examining a different aspect of the nurses' study published a finding in *The Journal of the American Medical Association* that was unquestionably more important to American health. Data gathered over 10 years from nearly 69,000 nurses ages 37 to 64 showed that the risk of suffering a fatal or nonfatal heart attack was 23 percent lower among women who consumed an average of 23 grams of fiber a day than among those who averaged only 11.5 grams a day.

Only fiber from grains, like whole-grain cereals and breads, brown rice and corn, was linked to cardiac protection. For each five-gram increase in daily intake of grain-based fiber, there was a 37 percent decrease in coronary risk. An earlier study in men also showed a protective effect of fiber on the heart, though not as strong an effect as was observed in women.

The researchers, led by Dr. Alicja Wolk of the Karolinska Institute in Stockholm, pointed out that only a quarter of grain-based fiber was soluble fiber and thus its effects on cholesterol could not possibly account for the large benefit observed among those eating the most grain fiber. Clearly, other beneficial effects are involved, including a possible benefit from plant estrogens. But while researchers try to sort out the reasons, Dr. Wolk and colleagues concluded that their finding provided "further reason to replace refined forms of starch with whole-grain products."

Perhaps this is a good time to mention that unrefined grains are far richer in essential nutrients than those that have been stripped down to bare starch.

When a grain like wheat is refined, 22 nutrients and most of the fiber are removed. But when refined grains are enriched, only four nutrients and none of the fiber is returned. That leaves the wheat kernel deficient in 18 natural nutrients as well as fiber. Among the lost nutrients are magnesium and folate, both of which help prevent heart disease.

Two years earlier, the nurses' study weighed in with yet another benefit of fiber. Among 65,000 nurses followed for six years, those who ate a starchy diet that was low in fiber and drank a lot of soft drinks developed diabetes at a rate two and a half times greater than women who ate less of these foods. A similar effect was also found in men being followed in another Harvard study. And as with heart disease, whole-grain breakfast cereals were most strongly related to protection against diabetes.

Dr. Walter C. Willett, the director of the nurses' study, said fiber was protective because it could slow the absorption of carbohydrates and prevent surges in blood levels of sugar and insulin. And, he said, the micronutrients in unrefined foods, especially magnesium, which increases the body's sensitivity to insulin, may be important in preventing diabetes.

Finally, for those grappling with a weight problem, fiber helps to fill you up without filling you out. In other words, fiber gives you something—satiation—for nothing. Also, meals rich in fiber are digested more slowly and thus hunger is kept at bay longer.

Start the day with a whole-grain cereal (half a cup of bran flakes supplies 5.5 grams of fiber) and half a grapefruit; eat unpeeled fruits for desserts and snacks; add beans to soups, stews and salads; choose high-fiber vegetables like carrots, cabbage, broccoli and brussels sprouts; try barley, brown rice or whole-grain pasta or bulgur for the starch at dinner, and eat a mixed green salad most days.

[JEB, July 1999]

## Diet Is Not a Panacea, But It Cuts Risk of Cancer

When words like "cure" and "prevention" appear in the title of a book about a chronic, disabling or life-threatening disease, they often enrich authors and publishers at the public's expense. Such is likely the case with a best seller, *The Breast Cancer Prevention Diet* by Dr. Bob Arnot, the medical correspondent for NBC.

The book's premise—that adopting a diet rich in soy, flaxseed and fish oils can prevent breast cancer—has been soundly denounced by breast cancer researchers and patient advocates alike as promising something it cannot possibly deliver.

As Fran Visco, president of the National Breast Cancer Coalition put it, "There is no breast cancer prevention diet," and the basis for Dr. Arnot's assertion is too flimsy to warrant a radical dietary shift based on a "bet," as he put it, that it will deliver the goods.

Faced with an onslaught of criticism, Dr. Arnot now says he should have used the words "risk reduction" instead of "prevention" in his book title. Critics say the book overextends laboratory findings that have yet to be confirmed in women, suggests dietary changes that have not been tested for long-term safety and intimates that, counter to all rules of sound medical science, it is foolhardy to wait for definitive proof of the effectiveness and safety of the diet.

Dr. Arnot is not wrong in suggesting that diet plays an important role in reducing the risk of cancer, including breast cancer. The American Cancer Society estimates that diet is a primary factor in a third of cancer deaths. That estimate is derived from thousands of studies of people worldwide and is supported by findings in laboratory cell cultures and animal experiments.

These studies suggest that a reorientation of American eating habits—to emphasize fruits, vegetables and whole grains while minimizing red meats, total fat and especially saturated fats and alcohol—

can significantly reduce the likelihood of developing most of the common cancers like those of the colon and rectum, lung, bladder, stomach, esophagus, mouth, throat and breast.

What cannot be said is that adopting a particular diet can assure that you won't get cancer or that, if you do, the diet will prevent the cancer from recurring. In 1997 the American Institute for Cancer Research and the World Cancer Research Fund released an analysis of more than 4,500 studies that examined the relationship between cancer, diet and exercise. The conclusion, as summarized in a 1998 issue of *Nutrition Action Health Letter*: "While there are no guarantees, there is plenty you can do to cut your risk." Simply eating more fruits and vegetables, for example, can eliminate about 20 percent of cancers, the analysis suggests.

Perhaps most important is that the recommended anti-cancer diet is the very same diet that studies have shown can help to counter heart disease, high blood pressure, diabetes and obesity.

In other words, anyone who is interested in maximizing the chances of staying healthy would be wise to consider adopting a diet rich in whole grains, fruits and vegetables that are loaded with fiber, vitamins and minerals and other cancer-fighting chemicals that occur naturally in plant foods. A protective diet would also be moderate in animal protein—especially red meats—and low in fat, saturated fat, simple sugars and alcohol.

In contrast to the low-carbohydrate scheme advocated by Dr. Arnot, such a diet is rich in carbohydrates—not sugars, of course, but the complex carbohydrates, or starchy foods, particularly in their natural, unrefined, fiber-rich state. This is also a diet that can help fight obesity, which is strongly linked to an increased risk of breast, uterine and other cancers.

The cancers most directly linked to diet are those that arise in lining tissues throughout the body, especially cancers of the colon and rectum, lung, bladder, stomach and, to a lesser extent, the breast, uterus and prostate. The following dietary suggestions are based on the strongest associations established in studies:

**Fruits and Vegetables.** Evidence in people has accumulated rapidly in recent years to support the protective role of plant foods against most cancers. The average American eats only about three or four servings a day of vegetables and fruits, while five servings, and preferably nine, are recommended. Especially helpful are yellow, dark-green and orange vegetables rich in carotenoids; fruits like citrus, tomatoes and strawberries that are rich in vitamin C, and all the cabbage family vegetables like broccoli, brussels sprouts, cauliflower, collards, kale, bok choy and mustard and turnip greens. Such foods are linked to lower risks of lung, stomach, colon and rectum, oral cavity, esophagus and, to a lesser degree, breast, bladder, pancreas and larynx cancers.

Garlic, onions and leeks contain allium compounds that help ward off cancer, especially breast cancer. To reduce loss of the protective chemicals, these vegetables should be cut up and let stand for 10 minutes before they are cooked. Other recent findings suggest that the risk of prostate cancer can be reduced by eating lots of cooked tomato products, including ketchup, that are rich in a carotenoid called lycopene and foods rich in the mineral selenium, like meats, fish, grains and seeds.

**Soy and Other Dried Beans.** These contain plant estrogens that may be beneficial in reducing the risk of hormone-related cancers, including breast, uterine

## Eating to Reduce Cancer Risk

No food can prevent cancer, but a diet that emphasizes fruits, vegetables and whole grains lowers the risk. Experts recommend these foods:

- Dried beans
- Tomatoes
- Broccoli
- Cabbage
- Milk
- Salmon
- Carrots
- Green tea
- Garlic and onions

- All dark green leafy vegetables
- Whole grains
- All-bran cereal
- All fruits, especially apples, oranges, strawberries and grapes
- Red peppers
- Olive Oil

and possibly ovarian cancer. A soy-rich diet may in part explain why Asian women have a low risk of these cancers. Dried beans may also help against colon cancer. But experts say that beans are most likely to be protective when used in place of meats and when the rest of the diet is low in fat.

**Whole Grains.** Wheat bran in whole-grain cereals and breads is strongly linked to reducing the risk of developing colon and rectal cancers, probably because they speed the passage of wastes and limit exposure of the lower gut to cancer-causing substances.

**Other Helpful Foods.** The list of possible dietary cancer weapons keeps growing. Among recent additions are green tea, olive oil (linked to a lower risk of breast cancer when used in place of other fats) and milk and other foods rich in calcium and vitamin D (linked to a reduced risk of breast and colon cancer). Though the evidence that flaxseed and fish oils can reduce the risk of developing breast or any other cancer is still highly preliminary, there are many other health benefits associated with eating more fish.

[JEB, December 1998]

## Now, a Food Pyramid to Guide the Elderly

Many ailments that afflict older Americans are directly caused or indirectly worsened by poor nutrition—an inadequate intake of essential nutrients, dietary fiber and water. Health problems like heart disease, osteoporosis, diabetes, kidney disease and even cancer are influenced by the foods consumed, or not consumed, especially in older people.

Poor choice of foods, rather than a shortage of finances, is the usual reason. Studies indicate that nutritional shortcomings are common among the elderly who are well-to-do as well as those with limited resources.

Historically, the elderly have been sorely neglected by nutrition researchers. But in the last decade or so, experts have learned much about both nutritional needs of people over 70 and nutritional shortcomings they commonly experience. And studies have shown that just as a child's nutritional requirements differ in quantity and quality from an adult's, the nutritional needs of the elderly differ from those of younger adults.

The Food Guide Pyramid to good eating habits devised in 1992 by the United States Departments of Agriculture and Health and Human Services is now familiar to many households. It depicts the food groups and the number of recommended servings of each per day to be consumed by a healthy adult who wants to stay that way. The pyramid calls for a daily intake of 6 to 11 servings of grain-based foods, 3 to 5 servings of vegetables, 2 to 4 of fruits, 2 to 3 of a high-protein food (meat, poultry, fish, dried beans, eggs and nuts) and 2 to 3 of dairy foods. Fats, oils and sweets, at the tip of the pyramid, should be eaten sparingly.

But large numbers of elderly Americans fall seriously short of these recommendations, consuming the least nutritious choices in each food category, like white bread instead of whole grain and fruit juice instead of whole fruit. In addition, as energy needs decline with age, the elderly tend to eat fewer calories, and hence fewer servings, of the recommended food groups.

With these problems in mind, Dr. Robert M. Russell, a professor of medicine and nutrition at Tufts University in Boston and his colleagues at the Department of Agriculture's Human Nutrition Research Center on Aging at Tufts, Dr. Alice Lichtenstein and Helen Rasmussen, a registered dietitian, have developed a revised food guide pyramid for Americans over 70.

This guide has a new foundation: water, eight 8-ounce glasses of it (or its nonalcoholic, caffeine-free equivalent) each day. Dr. Russell said that "older people have a reduced thirst mechanism—they have to consciously think of drinking more and keeping well hydrated, especially if they live in warm climates." He explained that without enough water, blood pressure can fall dangerously low, clots may form and block blood vessels, kidney function may be compromised (and may result in toxic concentrations of drugs) and constipation can become chronic.

The next level—six or more servings a day of grain-based foods like bread, cereal, rice and pasta, which form the bulk of the elderly diet—must emphasize fiber-rich choices, the Tufts researchers insist. Fiber, Dr. Russell said, is important in preventing constipation and its complications, diverticulosis and diverticulitis. Certain fibers also help counter high cholesterol, protect against cancer and maintain a normal blood sugar level, which is especially important for people with diabetes. And the cereals in the grain group should be fortified with extra nutrients, especially B vitamins like folic acid and B-12. Folic acid can lower blood levels of homocysteine, a substance that increases the risk of heart disease.

Then come the fruits and vegetables, both of which are best consumed as fiber-rich whole foods,

not juice. They can be sliced, chopped or pureed and they can be fresh, canned or frozen, but fruits packed in syrup provide too many sweet calories, the researchers maintain. Furthermore, they say, the recommended three or more servings of vegetables and two or more servings of fruits should feature foods that are richly colored—dark green, orange, red or yellow. These are richest in essential nutrients. In addition, vegetables in the cabbage family like broccoli, cauliflower, kale and mustard greens, are rich in cancer-blocking chemicals.

In the dairy group, the three recommended servings a day should feature low-fat choices. Dr. Russell noted that people who were lactose intolerant could still consume lactose-reduced milk, low-fat hard cheeses and yogurt. Most adults in this country do not consume enough vital calcium or vitamin D nutrients.

Within the meat group, the two or more daily servings should emphasize variety and feature fish (which may reduce cardiac risk) and dried beans (rich in fiber) as well as lean cuts of meat and poultry, the new pyramid suggests.

Over all, the consumption of high-fat and highly sweetened foods should be limited since they provide

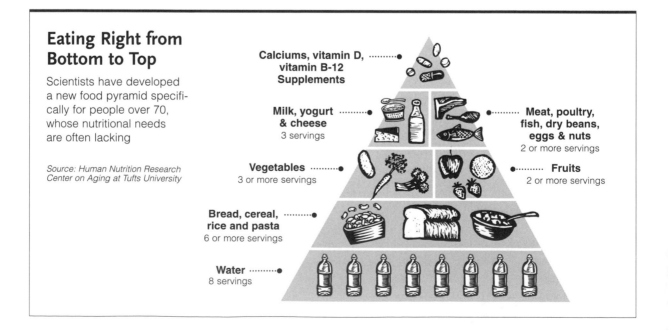

### Eating Right from Bottom to Top

Scientists have developed a new food pyramid specifically for people over 70, whose nutritional needs are often lacking

*Source: Human Nutrition Research Center on Aging at Tufts University*

Calciums, vitamin D, vitamin B-12 Supplements

Milk, yogurt & cheese
3 servings

Meat, poultry, fish, dry beans, eggs & nuts
2 or more servings

Vegetables
3 or more servings

Fruits
2 or more servings

Bread, cereal, rice and pasta
6 or more servings

Water
8 servings

nutritionally empty calories and leave less room in the daily energy quotient for nutrient-rich foods. As for the types of fats used in cooking, in dressings and as table spreads, the Tufts scientists recommend liquid oils and, if margarine is used it should be free of so-called trans fatty acids, which behave like artery-clogging saturated fat in the body.

The Tufts researchers, who are publishing their suggested food guide in the March 1999 issue of *The Journal of Nutrition*, have added something new to the pyramid: a supplement "flag" at the peak. Dr. Russell explained that few older people were able to get enough calcium, vitamin B-12 and vitamin D from their diets to achieve the recommended intake of these nutrients, and many would have to take supplements to fulfill these nutritional needs.

Based on studies of bone metabolism over the last two decades, older people are now being advised to consume 400 International Units of vitamin D daily (double the previous recommendation), the amount in a quart of milk. Though vitamin D is made in the skin when it is exposed to sunlight, many older people do not spend enough time outdoors with sunscreen-free skin exposed to meet their need for this nutrient.

It is also difficult for the elderly to achieve the recommended intake of calcium—1,200 to 1,400 milligrams a day (up from 800 milligrams), about the amount in a quart of milk. Other good sources are yogurt, hard cheese and calcium-fortified orange juice. Many older people would need to take a calcium supplement to get the recommended daily amount, Dr. Russell said. But he cautioned that multivitamin-mineral supplements did not contain enough calcium to meet nutritional needs.

As for vitamin B-12, a diet containing any animal foods supplies this nutrient. But among people over 60, 10 percent to 30 percent do not form enough acid in their stomachs to release the vitamin from the food protein that binds it. If the vitamin remains bound, it cannot be absorbed. B-12 that can be absorbed even by people with low stomach acid is found in supplements and in cereals fortified with the vitamin.

[JEB, March 1999]

## Women's Heart Risk Linked to Types of Fats, Not Total

The kinds of fats consumed, not the total amount of fat, determine a woman's risk of suffering a heart attack, according to the first major study of the effects of all dietary fats in women. The 14-year study, of more than 80,000 nurses, highlighted two types of fats as the bad actors in heart disease: saturated fats, found mainly in meat and dairy foods, and trans fats, found in most margarines, commercial baked goods and deep-fried foods prepared with hardened vegetable oils.

The research, which documented 939 heart attacks, fatal and nonfatal, among the participants, is one in a series of studies that have sought to define more carefully the effects of diet on heart disease. Earlier research focused mainly on saturated fat, cholesterol and total fat intake as the chief dietary factors.

The later findings, in contrast, confirm and extend those from a report, published in 1993 and also based on this study of nurses, about the risk of trans fats.

When the researchers took into account other influences on coronary risk like smoking, trans fats stood out as the most serious problem, and the authors said they believed that their finding would apply to men as well as to women. But a number of other experts reacted to the report skeptically, saying reduction of total fat ought to remain the focus of healthful eating.

Among the women in the study who consumed the largest amounts of trans fats, the chance of suffering a heart attack was found to be 53 percent higher than among those at the low end of trans fat consumption. But women in the group with the largest consumption of total fat (46 percent of calories) had no greater risk of heart attack than those in the group with the lowest consumption of total fat (29 percent of calories).

The researchers, from the Harvard School of Public Health and Brigham and Women's Hospital in Boston, said this suggested that limiting consumption of trans fats would be more effective in avoiding heart attacks than reducing overall fat intake. Some other experts pointed out that the study had not examined the effects of a diet any lower in fat than 29 percent of calories, and said they would continue to recommended that people reduce total fat.

Currently, about 5 to 10 percent of the fat in American diets is trans fat, which is produced when vegetable oils are artificially hydrogenated to increase their firmness and resistance to rancidity. Liquid vegetable oils, including olive, canola, soybean and corn oils, are free of trans fat.

Trans fats are not listed on food labels—the Food and Drug Administration is considering a petition that would require such listing—but a product is likely to contain them if hydrogenated fat is listed among the ingredients. The softer the fat, the fewer trans fats it contains.

Like earlier research, the new study found that polyunsaturates, which are highest in safflower, soybean, corn and sunflower oils, could lower coronary risk even below normal levels, and that monounsaturates, most prominent in olive and canola oil, had a small benefit.

By the time the study was published in *The New England Journal of Medicine*, it had already generated extensive comment, especially from advocates of a low-fat diet to prevent heart disease and those who say a high-fat diet promotes obesity and some cancers.

"How can they say what happens on a low-fat diet when no group in the study consumed less than 29 percent of calories from fat?" said Dr. Dean Ornish of Sausalito, California, who has demonstrated that a vegetarian diet in which only 10 percent of calories are derived from fat can reverse arterial clogging and

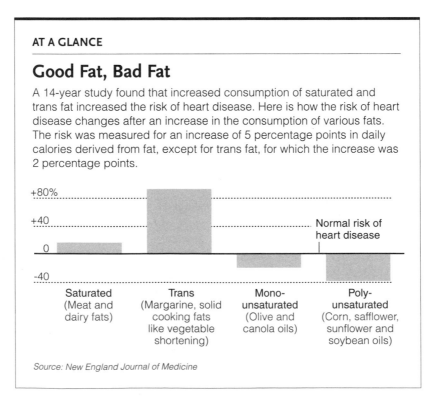

AT A GLANCE

## Good Fat, Bad Fat

A 14-year study found that increased consumption of saturated and trans fat increased the risk of heart disease. Here is how the risk of heart disease changes after an increase in the consumption of various fats. The risk was measured for an increase of 5 percentage points in daily calories derived from fat, except for trans fat, for which the increase was 2 percentage points.

+80%

+40　　　　　　　　　　　　　　　　　　　Normal risk of
　　　　　　　　　　　　　　　　　　　　heart disease
0

-40

| Saturated (Meat and dairy fats) | Trans (Margarine, solid cooking fats like vegetable shortening) | Mono-unsaturated (Olive and canola oils) | Poly-unsaturated (Corn, safflower, sunflower and soybean oils) |

*Source: New England Journal of Medicine*

reduce recurrent heart attacks by 50 percent in patients with advanced heart disease.

Two previous studies, in men, also linked the consumption of trans fats to an increase in coronary disease. And the earlier, less definitive report from the study on the nurses concluded that eating lots of trans fats raised a woman's risk of heart disease by as much as 50 percent. That report prompted some manufacturers to produce margarines free of trans fats and also led to a popular belief that butter is better than margarine, a conclusion that the researchers of the latest study say is wrong.

"Butter is bad for heart health," said Dr. Frank Hu, the lead author of the new report. "It dramatically raises LDLs"—low-density lipoproteins, the cholesterol-carrying proteins that result in fatty deposits in coronary arteries, the cause of most heart attacks and coronary deaths.

"You can't protect your heart by substituting butter for margarine or margarine for butter," Dr. Hu said in an interview "The best solution is to decrease saturated fats and avoid trans fats, and replace these unhealthy fats with healthy ones—monounsaturates and polyunsaturates from natural vegetable oils. The best solution is to use liquid vegetable oils for cooking, baking and frying wherever possible."

The researchers expressed concern about diets in which much less than 30 percent of calories come from fats, since lower-fat diets can reduce blood levels of heart-protecting HDLs (high-density lipoproteins) and raise heart-damaging triglycerides. But the coronary protection achieved by Dr. Ornish's very-low-fat diet occurred despite the accompanying drop in HDLs and rise in triglycerides, he said.

Dr. Ronald Krauss, chairman of the American Heart Association's nutrition committee, said: "The study supports previous evidence that trans fats, like saturated fats, should be reduced in the diet. But because Americans consume more saturated fat than trans fat, the opportunities to reduce saturated fat should still be emphasized."

Claire Regan, a registered dietitian who is director of scientific affairs for the Grocery Manufacturers of America, said: "I would continue to tell people to focus on total fat, because as total fat decreases, the intake of saturated and trans fats will decrease as well. The simpler the message to consumers, the more likely they will do the right thing."

Dr. Penny Kris-Etherton, nutrition professor at Pennsylvania State University, agreed that the main nutrition message should be to reduce total dietary fat. "I'm afraid the American people will again get confused and focus on trans fat and forget about everything else," Dr. Kris-Etherton said.

But Dr. Walter C. Willett, a co-author of the new study, said the problem with low-fat diets is that people replace fats with carbohydrates, primarily sugars and refined starches, which can have adverse effects on coronary risk, particularly among the sedentary.

"A high-carbohydrate diet doesn't have much of an adverse effect on someone who is lean and active," Dr. Willett said, "but it can be a problem for people who are overweight and inactive, which is true of a large percentage of Americans."

On the other hand, Dr. William Connor, an expert in diet and heart disease at the Oregon Health Sciences University in Portland, pointed out that a high-fat meal causes a temporary increase in fatty particles that can build up on artery walls. It can also cause blood clots, a finding that led Dr. William Castelli, former director of the Framingham Heart Study, to conclude that "the last fatty meal is the likely cause of most heart attacks."

The American Cancer Society, too, now advocates a diet that derives only 20 percent of its calories from fat. That is far less than is consumed by the average American, about 34 percent of whose diet is fat—a level that exceeds the 30 percent advised by the American Heart Association and most other major health organizations.

The cancer society, in a statement last year, pointed out that "high-fat diets have been associated with an increase in the risk of cancers of the colon and rectum, prostate and endometrium," and have also been linked to breast cancer, although much more weakly.

Dr. David Allison, an obesity researcher at St. Luke's-Roosevelt Hospital in New York, urged skepticism about the report, saying that an observational study, as opposed to a clinical trial, could not demonstrate cause and effect, and noting that another major study, in Europe, had found no association between trans fats and coronary disease.

"I don't think it's reasonable to eat as much fat as you want, even if it is heart-healthy fat," Dr. Allison said. "Obesity is a major killer, and there is ample data from well-controlled animal and human studies, and observational studies, showing that those consuming a diet with a higher percentage of calories from fat become fatter."

[JEB, November 1997]

## Fat Debates, Sustacal Shakes: It's Life in the Diet Blender

Reluctantly, I have agreed to go out to dinner with friends. This is going to be tricky. I plan to arrive at the restaurant early. When I get there, the antipasto table mocks me. I quickly head past it into the bathroom for refuge. In the privacy of the cramped room, I unpack my purse and create my liquid meal: eight ounces of skim milk, a packet of vitamin-rich Sustacal (the powder hospitals administer to patients whose jaws are wired shut) and two capfuls of fish oil, dispensed from a dark brown bottle. In my portable plastic container, I shake it up, then drink it down, praying no one comes in. Aaaah. I can now sit with my friends, pick on a dry salad and pretend I'm enjoying life.

Over the last two decades, I have tried every diet from Cambridge to Scarsdale and every weight-loss gimmick from inflatable leg massagers to acupuncture needles in my ears (which were supposed to enhance serotonin and suppress my appetite). My motivation was both personal (I am a former chemistry nerd who truly loves nutrition) and professional (for years, I was a beauty and health editor at a women's magazine, where it was my duty to experience the latest and greatest). I developed my nutritional acumen to the point where I stunned the folks promoting olestra when I was the only person in a series of meetings to detect the fake fat in a potato chip.

I was never trying to starve myself, or even to feel hungry. Unlike the Stairmaster-crazed, Snackwell's-obsessed thinnies in New York City, my travels from fat-free to fen-phen, from algae pills to acupuncture, protein to Rice Dream, were not mapped out simply to lose ten extra pounds. I wanted to be in control of my health. It's the modern version of mastering one's destiny.

Like all women, I was a little more than influenced by my parents in my food behavior. They were always focused on eating but truly in a healthy way. My father is a pioneer in the world of heart-disease research, and my mother has been preparing meals filled with antioxidants and B vitamins for 30 years. As a child, I was given frozen vegetables as snacks. I had never heard of candy before age six.

Like most teenagers, I needed to rebel, and I did so through food. Even though I was perfectly thin and athletic, I went to Diet Workshop, the Jenny Craig of the 1970s, for the sense of community. I begged my parents to send me to a hypnotist for weight loss (they sensibly refused). I lived on Tab. Granted, it's not at all unusual for a teenage girl to become fixated on food and eating, and one hopes that her food issues will never become life issues. But for me, my childhood fascination with food and nutrition developed into a 20-year pursuit.

At *Allure* magazine, I was a human guinea pig. I binged on books for foodies: *Outsmarting the Female Fat Cell*, *The Carbohydrate Addict's Diet*, *Fat Is a Family Affair*, *Super Nutrition for Women*. I turned diets into stories, gimmicks into trends. Acupuncture for Cellulite! Laci Le Beau Tea: Instant Diuretic! Colorad! Metabalance! Trident by the Value Pack!

Each new diet regime was accompanied by the thrill of hope. Maybe this blind date would be Mr. Right. When Chinese herbs were in vogue, I carried a Prada pouch filled with Herbaswee and Soy-Futura, dispensing dropperfuls of brown liquid into my Evian in four-star restaurants. (I still have an unidentifiable headache that I swear is an herbal hangover. Serves me right.)

I entered my 30s armed with more knowledge about nutrition than some nutritionists. My reading was more advanced: the *Berkeley Wellness Letter* replaced *When Food Is Love*. I gave up the gimmicks and flings and strove for committed relationships.

Fat-free was my first true love. I bought vintage balsamic vinegar in an attempt to glorify my oil-free salads, scoured cookbooks for lean cuisine recipes and substituted fat-free yogurt wherever I could. Like so many other women in the early 1990s, I believed in the mantra that fat makes you fat.

Going out in New York was no longer fun, it was a dare. If the vegetables were shiny (a telltale sign of oil), they were sent back. "Are you sure that's skim milk in my cappuccino?" Don't touch that dessert menu! Waiters feared me; friends were appalled. But if I remained virtuous, I won. Or so I thought.

Ultimately, fat-free wasn't for me. Cranky and constipated, I was living on Tasti D-Lite and scooped-out bagels. Steamed vegetables, steamed fish, steamed life. I remember the Easter when my mother, trying to accommodate my demands, abolished pasta and made a fat-free ricotta cheese pie. I would now like to apologize to the rest of my family for that.

After having lived fat-free, it was easy to give up other food groups. Over the years, I have abstained from more foods than most people indulge in. Coffee was the easiest, followed by soda, then fizzy water, pasta, alcohol, Nutrasweet, bread, flour and sugar. (What a blissful reunion I've had lately with Nutrasweet and San Pellegrino.)

Maintaining some sanity, I never attempted to give up chocolate. Visiting my parents, I would pack Wasa crackers, protein powder and herbs. "Just have some chicken," my mother would say—at every meal. Was I crazy? Not really. Extreme? Perhaps. But like so many other women in their teens, 20s, 30s, 40s (not our entire lives, I hope), my relationship with food is complex.

Traveling as a food fanatic was a challenge. What? No protein at breakfast in Venice? I'll pack powdered

egg whites. Snacks in Paris? I'll bring my own Laughing Cow Lite. The feeling of outsmarting the system was fulfilling. But who was I outsmarting? And for what? Still, with the strength of a stealth mission, I persevered. For months, my morning drink was a hot-water-lemon-cayenne-maple-syrup cocktail designed to cleanse the kidneys. Spending a night at a boyfriend's apartment, I packed clean underwear and a lemon. When in Europe for the fashion shows, I lived for days on protein powder frothed up by a battery-operated blender.

I should have found a better use of my energy years earlier, but I didn't. It was about not only calories and carbohydrates, but also enlightenment. The food gurus of New York—diet doctors and professional nutritionists—were my mentors. I could lecture on the pros and cons of orlistat, Optifast and olestra. I spent months seeing a hypnotist, who taught me to breathe deeply while in the back seat of a taxi, repeating to myself, "Sugar is not my friend." I wrote down every food that passed my lips for years at a time, each nutritionist scrutinizing my choices as if he was grading a test. My favorite of all was a sage of a doctor who made audio tapes to reprogram my mind: "If you eat it today, you'll wear it tomorrow"; "You didn't go to Princeton to take orders from a cookie."

Then one guru led me astray. Consuming upward of 40 vitamins, mineral supplements and thyroid pills a day, wondering about their calorie content, I overdosed. Literally. My legs hurt, my joints ached, I couldn't exercise, and I was having trouble walking. My internist took one look at me and knew what was going on. I had to stop the insanity.

I went cold turkey. No more supplements, no more pills. I sold my portable blender in a yard sale and threw out tubs of Designer Protein. I decided to listen to my body and to my mind. Combining the simplest, most intelligent information I had acquired over 20 years, I put together my own way of eating—mostly protein and vegetables, very few refined carbohydrates. Some would call it a protein diet, but since I no longer use the word diet, I just have to say this is the way I eat. And then something amazing happened. I actually started to feel different, better, not deprived, but satisfied. I lost weight; I felt more energetic.

I called my parents and excitedly described my insights: Limit refined carbs! Chicken at every meal! They listened patiently, just as they had for more than 30 years. They let me go on and on, just as parents do when their child decides, on her own, to go to their alma mater. They never once said, "We told you so." They promised to try my new regime, as my mother called it. Of course they really didn't have to change. After all, this was how they ate.

My food journey is over. For the last four years, I have eaten in a balanced, healthy way. I no longer crave peanut M & Ms; I don't plan tomorrow night's dinner at today's breakfast. I never found the pot of gold or the Holy Grail. But I did find the secret. Just like Dorothy's in *The Wizard of Oz*, it was there all the time. There is no place like home—especially when it comes to food.

[MM, August 1999]

# Life-style: Exercise for Health and Pleasure

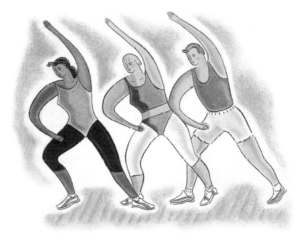

## EVEN A MODEST EXERCISE PROGRAM IS BENEFICIAL

We all know that exercise is good for us, and that the lack of it is unhealthy, even downright dangerous. And yet Americans do not exercise: fewer than a fifth engage in the kind of regular activity that has been proved to lower the risk of heart disease, diabetes, high blood pressure, osteoporosis and stroke. Anyone who has looked around at fellow customers in a shopping mall, restaurant or theater can see that the trend toward lethargy is taking its toll on waistlines as well: Americans are literally getting fatter every year.

People say they do not have time to exercise, or they admit that the thought of jogging, pacing on a treadmill or dashing about a tennis court, covered in sweat, is just not their idea of fun.

But there is good news: Exercise does not have to be torture to be beneficial. Just about anything that gets the body moving on a daily basis can help the heart and lungs, whether it is brisk walking, gardening, or even housework. And weight training to improve strength and muscle tone does not require the heroic exertions of a bodybuilder, either: Sets of 10 to 15 repetitions with small weights can accomplish a great deal. Fancy gadgets and glamorous gyms are also not a requirement, since research has shown that old-fashioned unaided "crunches," a type of sit-up with the knees bent, can strengthen the abdomen just as well as exercise devices specially marketed to do the same thing.

The luckiest people are the ones who find types of exercise that go beyond tolerable to genuinely enjoyable. The best way to discover an untapped passion or talent for a sport or other fitness activity is to try it out, at a gym or health club that will work with beginners. Even if it turns out not to be the dream activity of a lifetime, it will still be worthwhile to burn some calories and flex a few muscles.

# A Leap from Childbirth to Ballet Stage

As Margaret Tracey floated across the Lincoln Center stage on a Sunday afternoon, every line of a perfectly fit ballerina's body where every line ought to be, it was impossible to believe that little more than six months before she was, as grandmother used to say, great with child.

Ms. Tracey, 32, a principal with the New York City Ballet, gave birth to a son, Avery, in October 1998. Her friend Stacey Calvert, a 36-year-old soloist with the company, gave birth to a girl, Ayla, two weeks later. Six months later, both ballerinas had their post-baby debuts, and the experience makes it clear that it is far easier to get in great shape soon after pregnancy or other disruptive events if one was in great shape to begin with.

As for staying in shape during pregnancy, supervision, group interaction and organized fitness classes are invaluable aids, say fitness experts like Elizabeth Noble, author of *Essential Exercise for the Childbearing Year*.

Ms. Tracey had no problem with the group interaction part. She continued with the dance company during the first four months of her pregnancy. At the end of that period, with her waist expanding, she starred as the Pearly Queen in *Union Jack*. "But this is one of the easier roles I have," she said in an interview. She appeared, as a costermonger and streetwise entertainer, in a loose-fitting, camouflaging jacket. She then stopped performing but continued with ballet classes an hour and a half a day, five days a week until two months before the baby was due. After that, she continued rigorous stretching until the day she entered the hospital.

Her fitness regimen before the baby's birth was close to perfection, in the view of her trainer and physical therapist, Marika Molnar, director of Westside Dance Physical Therapy, which treats the company dancers. But Ms. Molnar also pointed out that both "Margaret and Stacey were in excellent shape before the pregnancy," and this enabled them to continue more rigorous activity than would otherwise be prudent.

The guidelines of the American College of Obstetricians and Gynecologists recommend exercise of moderate intensity and duration—stretching, stationary cycling, swimming and walking. Other types are either disapproved or require modification, but the college says: avoid "jerky, bouncy movements and exercises that involve straining, jumping or sudden changes in direction"—the very definition of ballet.

For these dancing mothers, "modification" and extraordinary conditioning were the keys. "Margaret and Stacey have been dancing all their lives," Ms. Molnar said. "They know what their bodies can and can't do. And they knew to take the easier roles that are doable and safe."

Experts agree that elevator, or Kegel, exercises, before and after delivery are essential to restore the muscles that are most weakened during pregnancy and delivery. "The first area to be worked, contracted and relaxed, can actually be started in the recovery room—within a half-hour of delivery," Ms. Molnar said, depending on difficulties in delivery or pregnancy.

Ms. Molnar described the Kegels as three sets of exercises: first as contractions of the lower pelvic muscles, holding the contraction for 10 seconds, relaxing, then repeating the exercise 50 times every hour. The second is a series of "quick flick" contractions of those muscles, with no holding, for one minute. The third is deep diaphragmatic breathing, inhaling and expanding the rib cage, filling the back part with air, which strengthens the lower-back muscles; then exhaling, contracting the abdominals between pubic bone and navel, which pushes the lower abdominal muscles toward the back. She recommends repeating this set for about five minutes every hour.

"These simple exercises are important for everyone, for the lungs, posture, for keeping the abdominals strong and the stomach flat," Ms. Molnar said. Sports-medicine experts and trainers stress the value of learning well-timed rhythmic breathing for peak performance, making difficult tasks—from weight lifting to golf swings to ballet steps—easier during exhalation when the body is more relaxed.

Ms. Calvert tried Kegels after delivery and did them sporadically in the days that followed. Ms. Tracey was quick to confess that she did not do them and waited eight weeks before starting any kind of workout regimen. The routine for the ballerinas intensified as the weeks of recovery passed and they added spring-resistance-weight training, especially well suited to dancers for strengthening muscles at the hip joint in particular, as well as legs, arms, chest and upper back. The spring weights are attached to a strong bedlike fabric on which the two ballerinas could safely perform all their routines, each spring

being tightened to increase resistance as they gained strength. Finally, Ms. Molnar readied her stars by insisting that they walk, walk and walk more. "Three times a week, 30 to 45 minutes, no errands, non-stop," Ms. Molnar said.

Ms. Calvert's post-baby debut came in a solo role in the new production of Peter Martin's *Swan Lake*. It was a good performance to start with: "It was not hard," said Ms. Calvert, who felt strong and happy to be back. Ms. Tracey said that when she stepped out to dance her solo as a muse in Stravinsky's *Apollo*, "I knew I was home, in a place where I belonged."

The applause was good to hear, they said. Which was better, they were asked, the applause of a full house at the New York State Theater, or the sound of two hands clapping at home? The smiles of the ballerinas left no doubt about the answer.

[HBN, May 1999]

## The Athlete's Secret to Warding Off Overuse Injuries: Good Technique

Overuse injuries happen to the very best of athletes. Just 16 days before the 1998 United States Open golf tournament Tiger Woods was forced to take a break from golf for a week to let a sore back heal. Soon after, during the United States Open semifinal tennis match, Pete Sampras was hobbled by a strained muscle in his thigh.

But for most of us amateurs on the playing fields, walking and running paths, and in swimming pools and weight rooms, overuse injuries are all too often the consequence of poor technique or misalignment of body parts. As the *Penn State Sports Medicine Newsletter* points out: "An injury caused by moving the body the wrong way over a period of time presents athletes with two problems. First, they have to recover from the injury. Then they have to retrain themselves so that it won't happen again."

But there is a better approach: To minimize the risk of injuries, learn how to perform your chosen activi-

ties correctly from the beginning and have your technique monitored periodically by an expert to be sure you haven't lapsed into body-damaging form. Although it is not possible in the space of this column to describe injury-provoking errors for all sports, several popular activities account for common problems.

**Tennis.** The elbow is the tennis player's Achilles' heel. Tennis elbow, a form of tendinitis, results from repeated vibrations through the playing arm whenever the ball hits the racquet. The usual cause: improper stroking of the backhand—leading with the elbow and using just the upper body to hit the ball. In a proper backhand, the elbow is in line with the racquet hand, and the muscles of the feet, legs, hips, shoulders, arms and hands participate in the stroke and contribute to its power and placement.

Pennsylvania State University experts cite two ways to fix a backhand. One is to use a grip that permits the inside of the thumb, not its bottom part, to stay in contact with the handle and allow the elbow to drop down and away from the body as you stroke. The second is to use a two-handed backhand, which forces the trunk and arms to move together and involves no movement at the elbows.

**Swimming.** Among swimmers, the shoulders are most likely to take a beating. Many swimmers use strokes that put their shoulders at risk of tendinitis. Pete Brown, the swim coach at Penn State, said the usual victims fail to keep their elbows high in relation to their hands and, instead of rotating the shoulder to get "over the stroke," they press downward too soon, which puts excess pressure on the shoulder. In a proper stroke when swimming the crawl, the elbow should be bent 90 degrees as the hand passes the face and, as if reaching over a barrel, the shoulder remains high while the hand is driven deep into the water.

**Running and Walking.** My knees took a beating both running and walking until I found a walking partner who teaches movement. She repeatedly reminds me to lift the weight off the knees by raising the torso like a dancer and keeping the knees and feet in alignment. But many runners and walkers are cursed with a built-in mechanical flaw: too much or too little pronation. In overpronation, the foot rolls inward too far after the heel strikes the ground. In underpronation, the foot doesn't roll over far enough. Thus, only one runner in four has a normal gait. Overpronation is the more serious problem because muscles from the toes to the hips are called upon to stabilize the feet. It can cause excessive torque of the knees and contributes to problems like tendinitis, plantar fasciitis and knee strain.

The usual solution is to use orthotics, shoe inserts that compensate for flat feet and other common causes of overpronation and enable the foot to absorb shock without becoming unstable. It is best to consult a podiatrist or orthopedic surgeon about the best kind of orthotic for your feet. Also, be sure your running and walking shoes have adequate support, reinforced heel counters and motion control features. For detailed advice, see *Runner's World* magazine's shoe issue.

**Weight Training.** With this activity, "any technique that does not allow the body to move in a biomechanically efficient way is potentially dangerous," says Dr. William J. Kraemer, associate editor of the Penn State newsletter. He cited as an example "cheat curls," explaining that some lifters doing bicep curls with free weights use their back muscles to lift the weight instead of only the muscles of their arms. This causes them to rock or swing the body back when they lift, which can result in lower back injuries. To do it properly, the head is up and facing forward, the torso erect, upper arms still and elbows close to the body.

In doing leg presses, a common error is to quickly extend the legs and lock the knees. With correct technique, the leg is extended slowly and the motion is stopped before the knee is straight.

**Golf.** In this sport, where strokes involve twisting at the hips, the lower back is most likely to suffer. When driving the ball, low-back pain is often caused by a side-to-side tilting of the body during the swing. A more upright stance and swing minimizes the twisting motion and resulting "crunch" on the spine. On the other hand, many golfers fail to rotate their hips at all during the backswing and instead generate power by sliding their hips back and then forward. This places the spine in a vulnerable position when the twisting motion occurs later in the swing. Keith Kennedy, a fitness professional for the Ladies Professional Golf Association, suggests that the risk of injury can be lessened if the hips are rotated instead of sliding them back and forth when transferring body weight during the swing.

**Cycling.** Most recreational cyclists worry about sore seats. But a more serious problem involves the hands, in particular the ulnar nerve that lies in the outer base of the hand below the pinky finger. This nerve can become irritated when the handlebars are gripped too tightly for too long, resulting in tingling, numbness and weakness that can travel up to the elbow. Wearing padded riding gloves helps but is not always enough. A better approach is frequently changing hand positions on the handlebars, loosening the grip and riding with elbows unlocked.

Of course, no matter what sport you do, it makes sense to do both warm-up and stretching exercises beforehand and to repeat the stretches afterward.

And if you haven't done an activity in a while, don't try to resume it immediately at full tilt. Build up gradually. Finally, if you start to feel discomfort associated with an activity, don't ignore it. When an injury is untreated or aggravated by continued misuse, you can end up with a long-lasting problem that may force you to abandon the activity altogether.

[JEB, October 1998]

# After 100,000 Miles, Even Soles on Feet Wear Out

There seems to be a week for just about every health problem that afflicts a significant number of Americans. But where is the week for those "poor, poor feet" celebrated in song a generation ago in *The Most Happy Fella*? Our feet take a beating, bearing our full weight for a lifetime of walking and running, often in shoes that squeeze, rub or deform them.

With age, the shape and condition of our feet change, setting the stage for a host of discomforting problems that can make it difficult to walk. People tell me I don't look my age (57), but there's no lying to my feet, which, according to estimates made by the American Podiatric Medical Association, have endured well over 100,000 miles, probably 200,000 or more. By the age of 50, the association figures, the average American has logged 75,000 miles, and my activity level is hardly average.

And do my feet know it! They have lengthened, growing a size and a half since adolescence, and widened at the forefoot. Three toenails have become weird-looking; I've developed tendinitis on the top of one foot and corns on the balls of both feet. And that's for starters. I have good reason to believe I am not alone. A survey conducted in April among 1,000 adults by Yankelovich Partners found that nearly half of Americans at any given time have some type of foot or ankle problem and that for one in five, foot or ankle problems have forced them to alter their activities.

As with shoes, the soles of the feet gradually lose their natural cushioning—and therefore, their shock-absorbing ability—because protective fat pads degenerate. Upon reaching the 75,000-mile mark, half the natural padding under the ball of the foot may have been lost, and beyond 75,000 miles the deterioration seems to accelerate, podiatrists say.

The scores of ligaments and tendons that hold together the 26 bones and 33 joints in each foot become stretched, resulting in feet that are wider and longer. Dr. Jonathan T. Deland, foot and ankle specialist at the Hospital for Special Surgery in New York, reports that age increases the risk for an often unrecognized condition called posterior tibial tendon insufficiency. If untreated in its early stages, it can make walking impossible.

You should expect your shoe size to change with age, probably to a size larger at 50 than it was at 20. You may also need a wider width at the forefoot (but probably not at the heel), which may necessitate buying more expensive shoes that are made with a combination—for example, a C width at the forefoot and a B at the heel. Alternatively, fit the forefoot properly and use pads on either side of the heel (but not a U-shaped insert) to keep the shoe from slipping off the heel.

Toe and joint deformities increase with age. For example, the podiatric association reports that after the age of 50, the incidence of problems like hammer toes, bunions, arthritis in the foot and ankle, and toenail abnormalities increases by 70 percent to 100 percent. The American Orthopedic Foot and Ankle Society describes these as often seen in older people.

**Hammer Toes and Claw Toes.** These deformities result from years of wearing shoes with overly short and narrow toe boxes, the shoes so many women force their feet to endure in the name of fashion. One or more toes eventually curl under the stress, resulting in bony protrusions that develop painful corns when they rub on shoes. While the toes remain flexible, the discomfort can be eased by using a toe pad (sold in pharmacies) and wearing shoes with roomier toe boxes.

**Bunions.** These are prominent bony bumps that develop on the side and base of the big toe, again usually the result of years of wearing narrow, pointed shoes and high heels. The toe itself turns inward, and the pressure of the shoe on the bump can cause painful swelling and inflammation. You can protect a bunion with a doughnut-shaped moleskin pad. Wear roomy shoes of soft leather or sandals that do not rub against the bunion. Sometimes custom-made orthotics (shoe inserts) can help. Severe cases may require surgery.

**Corns and Calluses.** These result from pressure of shoes when standing and walking. They most often occur on the ball of the foot and the toes. Doughnut-shaped pads can relieve the pressure, as well as wearing roomier shoes with padded innersoles. If a corn develops between the toes, a piece of lamb's wool can keep the toes from rubbing together. Soak your feet in warm water to soften corns and calluses and then file them down with a pumice stone (never use a razor). Experts are reluctant to recommend over-the-counter acids for corn removal since they sometimes cause complications, especially in diabetics.

**Ingrown Toenails.** These can happen at any age, usually because the nails were trimmed too short or in a curve instead of straight across. Shoes that compress the toes can compound the problem and result in the nail growing painfully into the soft tissue of the toe. Treat by soaking the foot in warm water twice a day and keeping a small piece of cotton between the nail and flesh. If an infection develops, a doctor may have to prescribe an antibiotic.

**Fallen Arches.** Those who were born with arches can lose them with age as the ligaments that support the arch become too loose or stretched to hold it up. If this results in fatigue or pain in the feet, legs or lower back, custom-made orthotics that support the arch may bring relief.

**Morton's Neuroma.** The nerve sheath between the base of two toes can become irritated and swell, causing burning, cramping, numbness or severe pain that may feel like you just stepped on a nail. The discomfort may force you to stop what you are doing, remove your shoes and massage the area for relief. Surgery, only sometimes necessary, is successful in at least 80 percent of cases, but the neuroma may recur. Usually all that is needed to relieve the irritation is to wear roomier shoes with low heels and place protective pads under the involved area.

You can foster flexibility in your feet and ankles with a brief series of daily exercises. While sitting on a chair, straighten your knees to raise your feet. Circle each foot to the right 10 times, then to the left. Next, extend and flex your feet by pointing the toes outward then toward your body. Repeat this exercise 10 times. Finally, stand on the balls of your feet and raise yourself up as high as you can, holding the position for a minute, then drop back on your heels. Repeat this exercise 10 times.

People with diabetes need to be especially careful about foot care because their disease can impair nerve sensations and circulation to their feet and greatly increase the risk of injuries and their ability to heal. Neglected foot problems can lead to amputation. The National Institute of Diabetes and Digestive and Kidney Diseases has produced a very helpful booklet, "Take Care of Your Feet for a Lifetime" that includes the following tips:

▶ Check your feet daily for cuts, blisters, red spots and swellings.

▸ Wash your feet daily in warm—not hot—water and dry them thoroughly.

▸ Apply a thin coating of skin lotion daily to the tops and bottoms of your feet, but not between the toes.

▸ Keep toenails trimmed straight across and use a pumice stone to smooth corns and calluses.

▸ Always protect your feet by wearing socks and comfortable shoes that "breathe" (avoid nylon socks and vinyl, plastic and rubber shoes). Keep slippers at bedside.

▸ Protect your feet from temperature extremes. For example, wear socks at night if your feet get cold and avoid walking barefoot on hot sand.

▸ Foster circulation through regular exercise, keeping your feet up while sitting, making circles with your feet and wiggling your toes twice a day and not sitting with legs crossed for prolonged periods.

▸ Call your doctor right away if any foot problem develops that does not begin to heal within a day.

To obtain a free copy of the booklet, write to "Take Care of Your Feet for a Lifetime," 1 Diabetes Way, Bethesda, MD 20892-3600 or call the message number, 800-438-5383 and leave your name and address and the name of the booklet.

[JEB, July 1998]

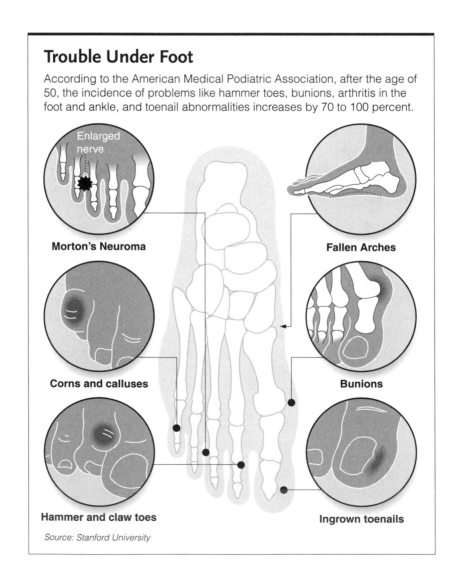

## Trouble Under Foot

According to the American Medical Podiatric Association, after the age of 50, the incidence of problems like hammer toes, bunions, arthritis in the foot and ankle, and toenail abnormalities increases by 70 to 100 percent.

**Enlarged nerve**

**Morton's Neuroma**

**Fallen Arches**

**Corns and calluses**

**Bunions**

**Hammer and claw toes**

**Ingrown toenails**

*Source: Stanford University*

# Female Bodybuilders Discover Curves

When the history of women's bodybuilding is written, 1998 will emerge as the year that the weights tipped in favor of the sport's old nemesis, femininity.

In the 20 years since women began publicly showing off their muscles in earnest, this issue—whether the muscles that make the man also make the woman manly—has hewn the sport more than any other. What has happened this year might have seemed, to some, inevitable: Fitness competition, a slenderized version of women's bodybuilding, has eclipsed some of the bulked-up muscle shows in participant and audience popularity.

What has surprised many in the field of strength and fitness, however, is the swiftness with which women's fitness competitions have swept the world. In the four years since the National Physique Committee's first National Bodybuilding and Fitness Championships in 1994, registration for the women's fitness competition has tripled. At the 1998 nationals in Atlanta, fitness competitors outnumbered their bodybuilding sisters for the first time. By the end of the year the committee had run 600 regional bodybuilding and fitness competitions.

This new version of women's bodybuilding is not news to everyone. Readers of fitness and muscle magazines knew things were changing by 1994, when women's fitness competitors had all but replaced traditional female bodybuilders as models on the magazines' pages.

And with that visibility came the controversy. Ridiculed by feminists, held in disdain by many women in power lifting, bodybuilding and strength training circles, the new women's fitness events have many detractors. As has always been the case with women's strength and the sports that display it, the criticism centers on how things look. With fitness, the criticism is directed at its portrayal in magazines that feature champions laid out in lingerie and publish special swimsuit issues.

Jim Manion, of the National Physique Committee, takes a Darwinian view of the evolution of the women's bodybuilding scene. "The difference between the two sports is right there in the name," he said. "Body builders build their bodies. In fitness we are looking for fit, toned bodies with good muscle shape, but not a lot of size."

Like traditional bodybuilding, fitness competitions require the athletes to pose in stances chosen to accent particular groups of muscles. While bodybuilders pose barefoot, fitness competitors do so in heels, in two of three required competitive rounds. In the first, they wear a two-piece bathing suit. In the third, it's a one-piece suit. In the Ms. Fitness contests, one of the rounds has an evening gown competition.

But, heels (and big hair) aside, what distinguishes fitness competitions is round two, in which the athletes are required to perform a three-minute choreographed routine. It is something of a breathtaking combination of aerobics, dancing and tumbling designed to show strength, flexibility and agility.

Preparing for fitness competitions involves many of the aspects of training for competitive bodybuilding, including lifting weights, reducing fat intake, increasing lean muscle mass and performing aerobic exercise. But the notion of a dance segment, to be sure, seems more Miss America than Ms. Olympia, far from the Arnold Schwarzenegger days of the sport of bodybuilding. It was the emergence of Mr. Schwarzenegger in the 1970s that catapulted men's bodybuilding to a mass market.

Women who were attracted to the sport late in that decade were competitive athletes who were able and willing to make their physiques look like dancers'. One was Lisa Lyon, a graduate of the University of California at Los Angeles who had studied kendo, a Japanese martial art, and who had been encouraged by Mr. Schwarzenegger to become a bodybuilder. In 1979, she won the first World Women's Bodybuilding Championship and became the sport's only media star, as well as its unofficial spokeswoman—a role

## Differing Approaches to the Body Beautiful

Fitness competitions have eclipsed traditional women's bodybuilding events in terms of audience and participants. A look at two of the competitions and their current champions highlights the differences.

### Comparing the Competitions

| MS. FITNESS: Susie Curry | | MS. OLYMPIA: Kim Chizevski | |
|---|---|---|---|
| **HEIGHT:** | 5'2" | **HEIGHT:** | 5'8" |
| **WEIGHT:** | 115 | **WEIGHT:** | Mid-150s |
| **COMPETITION:** | Three rounds—evening gown, swim suit, and 90 second fitness routine | **COMPETITION:** | A posing routine designed to best display the body's muscle groups. |
| **JUDGING CRITERION:** | Bodies should have lean muscularity and reasonable level of body fat. Strength and flexibility, endurance and beauty are also judged. | **JUDGING CRITERION:** | Muscular development and symmetry are stressed, and with low body fat (5% or 6%) for clear definition. Bulk is judged favorably. |

that led to a *Playboy* photo spread. But by 1980 she had stopped competing. She was too small.

That year, at the International Federation of Bodybuilders' first Miss Olympia competition (now Ms. Olympia), the easy winner was Rachel McLish, whose soap opera star looks were a perfect match for her long-waisted, rippled, hard body. For a time it seemed Ms. McLish was the epitome of the sport. In 1983, she again placed first in the Ms. Olympia competition, but was disqualified over a controversy involving padding in her swimsuit.

This was just one of the controversies the judges handled that year. The other involved Bev Francis, a former shot-putter and javelin and discus thrower from Australia who held six individual world power-lifting records. Her 24-inch thighs, planed chest and quilted abdomen rocked the world of women's bodybuilding and, some say, changed it forever. Ms. Francis was bigger and more muscular than any woman bodybuilding fans had ever seen.

That world was, of course, a small one. While the standard set by Ms. Francis made other competitors strive to reach that muscular mark, the evolution of the sport to emphasize a bigger female physique went unseen by the general sports fan.

But in the early 1990's, television brought the Ms. Olympia competition to a public outside the close-knit world of bodybuilding. "The calls and letters of fans reported an overall disgust at the women, their size and even their sport," said Maria Lowe, author of the book *Women of Steel: Female Bodybuilders and the Struggle for Self-Definition.* "In the early '80s, the women bodybuilders looked good and women wanted to look like them and men wanted to look at them. But when the women got big, that was not the case."

This just added to the already perplexing reality of a sport in which there are no sanctioned rules about size. For instance, a 24-inch thigh is not of more competitive value than a 20-inch thigh, but a woman who is considered too big is penalized.

Added to that are other troubling aspects of traditional competitive bodybuilding: drugs and nutritional supplements that hold out the promise of bigger bodies; the increasing appearance of breast implants to match the increased size of muscles (while muscle implants are banned for all bodybuilders, breast implants are not), and the radical pre-posing diet designed to make competitors look highly defined, or "cut," which many athletes consider antithetical to a healthy regimen. So it is not surprising that by the '90s, the posing stage was set for someone new to step in. And those who stepped in were wearing heels.

What is surprising is that this women's sport, so long in the shadows of the men, has given birth to a fast-growing male counterpart. After only a few years in existence, some male fitness competitions are expected to attract more participants than traditional bodybuilding competitions. This is not to say that traditional bodybuilding is disappearing.

Still, many in the sport are yielding to the new direction, including Carla Dunlap-Kann, one of the premiere bodybuilders of the '80s, who now helps train fitness competitors and judges Ms. Fitness contests. "The fitness competitions are the future," said Mr. Manion of the National Physique Committee. "It is something that almost everybody can relate to."

And lest anyone think that fitness competition is "bodybuilding lite," ask a champion. Susie Curry, 26, virtually lives at the gym. After graduating from the University of North Carolina, where she competed as a gymnast, she needed another outlet for her athletic drive. She found it in fitness competition. Ms. Curry works out five hours a day at a gym, where she is co-owner, in Bremen, Georgia. In March, 1998, she placed first in the International Federation of Bodybuilders Fitness International, known as the Arnold Classic.

"Fitness is healthier," said Ms. Curry, who competes about twice a year. "Bodybuilders cannot maintain their competitive sizes all year round. They have to strain before every competition to get into that shape for one day."

"The women who compete in the Ms. Olympia are incredibly fit by all standards," said Dr. Jan Todd, a professor of kinesiology at the University of Texas in Austin and a former national champion in weight lifting and power lifting. "But on the day of competition, they are probably not the healthiest people. They are dehydrated, have deprived themselves of food for considerable lengths of time. But the very nature of the aerobic competition insists that they not be all drawn down," she said. "So they might have a healthier edge."

But there remains that controversial edge, as well. "It's pornography," said Leslie Heywood, champion power lifter, professor of English and author of the books *Pretty Good for a Girl* and *Bodymakers: A Cultural Anatomy of Women's Body Building*. "In 1994, all the bodybuilding magazines started having all these spreads featuring fitness models in stock pornography poses, wearing lingerie. It's depressing."

"The hair, the heels, sure, it sells," Ms. Curry argued, "but if you want to see what the sport is all about, come and watch us work out. We are athletes."

[MRo, November 1998]

## How to Build Abs of Undulating Steel

**B**elly dancing has its place in dimly-lit clubs, thick with incense and the beat of drums. But it is certainly not what you expect to find in an urban gym. In fact, though, you can. Both Equinox and New York Health and Racquet Club in New York have started belly dancing programs, tailoring the dance into a legitimate workout. In fact, said Judy Taylor, the director of public relations for Equinox Fitness Clubs, "Any kind of ethnic dance is catching on nationally."

It's a strange confluence, and one that ever-insatiable gym goers are responding to enthusiastically. Curious, I signed up, too. I went to Equinox. When I arrived, the lights in the workout room were dimmed and there was pipe and drum music bouncing off the hardwood floor and mirrored walls. It was a weird scene.

Nathalie Levy-Koffer, a fit woman with large almond-shaped eyes and a great deal of wavy brown hair, came toward me waving a bright green piece of fabric. "Tie this around your waist," she instructed. I did as she said, making a sarong out of it over my gym shorts. There were about 10 people in the class. All women. Most of them were wearing tight shorts and half shirts. Their sarongs were all flag colors—red, blue, yellow, green—too. Ms. Levy-Koffer wore a printed one with a loose chain dangling across her waist.

We began slowly, rolling our heads, moving our shoulders in circles, and then our upper bodies, touching our ankles and sweeping our torsos up to standing position and around to our toes again. Ms. Levy-Koffer stopped for a minute to show us a few fundamental belly dancing moves. She stood before us with her left arm raised, her left leg bent slightly and her right leg forward, also bent but with just her toes touching the ground. "You must tuck in your belly," she said. It felt like posture class taken to the extreme.

In this position, though, the right hip is naturally positioned upward. From it, Ms. Levy-Koffer flung her hip upward further to the right and down, in a motion as crisp and quick as the snap of two fingers. "You must use your legs," she said. We followed, stiffly and slowly. She smiled, a look of pity.

"More quickly," she said, repeating the motion. We mimicked her for a minute or two, sweeping our hips from side to side. Then, she moved her waist in

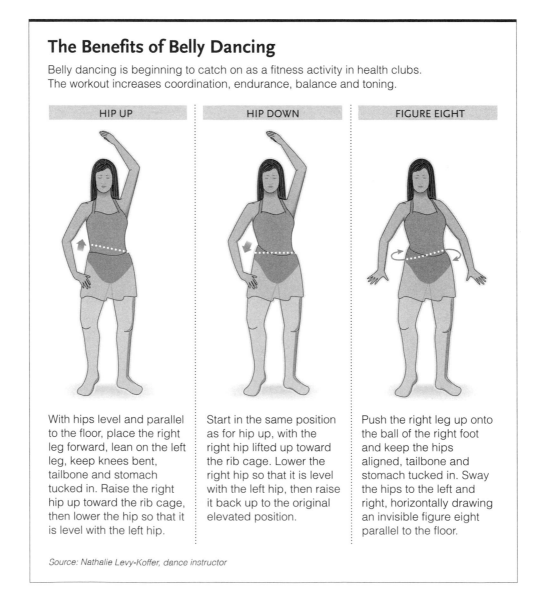

## The Benefits of Belly Dancing

Belly dancing is beginning to catch on as a fitness activity in health clubs. The workout increases coordination, endurance, balance and toning.

| HIP UP | HIP DOWN | FIGURE EIGHT |
|---|---|---|

With hips level and parallel to the floor, place the right leg forward, lean on the left leg, keep knees bent, tailbone and stomach tucked in. Raise the right hip up toward the rib cage, then lower the hip so that it is level with the left hip.

Start in the same position as for hip up, with the right hip lifted up toward the rib cage. Lower the right hip so that it is level with the left hip, then raise it back up to the original elevated position.

Push the right leg up onto the ball of the right foot and keep the hips aligned, tailbone and stomach tucked in. Sway the hips to the left and right, horizontally drawing an invisible figure eight parallel to the floor.

*Source: Nathalie Levy-Koffer, dance instructor*

a figure eight, a motion so smooth that it looked like ribbon undulating in the wind. Her arms flowed along. Again, we followed along, stiffly. "So we are ready now?" she asked. "Don't get scared. Feel the motion in your soul. This is your body."

My soul, I'm afraid, did not know my body was ever supposed to move this way. But I had company. The music sped up and Ms. Levy-Koffer did, too. The chain around her waist jingled to the music as her body shook and glided. I would have been just as happy to stop what I was doing and just watch her.

We did "the bird," moving our hips as we waved our arms fluidly like the wings of a bird. We did "the snake," joining our hands above our heads and moving our heads with our necks, from left to right. Just as she had warned, you must use your legs as much as you use your stomach muscles. It is the leg muscles that enable you to make more crisp, powerful movements. When watching a belly dancer, you often don't notice this because the legs are hidden by the sarong.

Belly dancing, said Stella Grey, a belly dancer who is an instructor at New York Health and Racquet Club, is believed to have originated in what is now northern India. It spread throughout eastern Europe and into northern Africa 700 years ago, she said, mixing with indigenous dance forms.

Ms. Levy-Koffer was born in Morocco and was raised in Israel, both cultures that revere the art of belly dancing. She learned many styles, and does not stick to any one during the one-hour workout classes.

In truth, the class wasn't at all what I expected. It felt a little gimmicky, a flashy way to keep fickle gym goers amused. A second class was more satisfying. I realized I was learning to move my body in ways I never knew it could. And it was refreshing to work my stomach muscles without doing sit-ups. The

workout is good for coordination, endurance, balance and toning. I think of belly dancing as a counterpoint to a higher energy workout like running. The second time around I went to a different Equinox gym. The class was more experienced, so Ms. Levy-Koffer taught less and paused less. We did longer, faster repetitions, flinging the hips not only left to right, but forward and back.

She was tougher, too. "Cut, cut!" she shouted to the beat as we moved left to right. "It's not disco; I want you to feel your belly a little," she said. We also learned to shimmy, which requires shaking your body, letting the muscles in your buttocks and upper legs flap loosely. "Think tush, tush, tush," she said. The class reluctantly shimmied. Ms. Levy-Koffer approached the only male, a thin man in black cycling shorts, in the class. "What's happening here?" she asked, watching him jiggle stiffly from side to side. "I have no tush," he said.

Most belly dancers do, though, and they are not stick thin. They have thick torsos, dense with muscle and flesh. Rounded bodies shake better and certainly appear to roll and swing more fluidly. More than that, in some belly dancing cultures, that body shape is desirable. "Belly dancing is not going to flatten your abs," Ms. Grey said. "The undulations that are so characteristic are not going to get your stomach concave. They build your lower abs so you can push out as much as you pull in." And yet, here I was, far from the culture of belly dancing, surrounded by people striving to be fit and thin. It was a lovely contradiction. One that may become more common.

Belly dancing is a new phenomenon at health clubs. Most classes are taught at dance studios. Expect more of an aerobic workout at health clubs and more technique at dance studios.

[AH, July 1999]

# How Errol Flynn Made It Look So Easy

"Just show up with a T-shirt, workout-type clothing," said Lee Roy Longenbach, a manager at Metropolis Fencing, when I called to sign up for a few classes. They were not the words I wanted to hear. Sure, I was interested in a good workout for my legs and improving my coordination, but I also wanted to get to wear one of those sleek-looking white body suits. That was just my first misconception.

I showed up at the studio in Manhattan and discovered that fencing was another world altogether from the romanticized one I had created in my head. And I soon learned not to call a sword a sword. "There are three weapons," Mr. Longenbach said. "There's the foil, the epee and the saber." All three are used in competition, but traditionally fencers are trained with the foil, which is flexible, making it easier to wield. The epee is much stiffer and has a larger hand guard for protection—they were once very sharp. The saber, is considered much more barbaric and a bit more obscure.

I changed into my rumpled gym clothes, then met Michael, the instructor, and Valerie, the only other student, for warm-up. Out of each one-hour session, the first 20 minutes are spent loosening up. It is not unlike high school gym class. You roll your neck, swing your arms, touch your toes and stretch your hamstrings. I began to wonder if I was ever going to get my hands on a foil.

Finally, Michael told us to get suited up. The fencing uniform, my motivation, was within grasp. Or, at least, half of it. Metropolis Fencing provides you with the jackets, which upon close inspection I discovered were something of a cross between a straitjacket and a catcher's chest guard. There is a strap between your legs and it zips up the back. You are also given soft leather gloves and a thimble-shaped helmet with a black face screen. I felt like I was wearing a bad Halloween costume. But there was no time to fret; it was time to get down to business.

"When you fence you must work all five fingers,"

Michael said, holding a foil to show us. "But it is these three that control the foil," he said referring to the thumb, index and middle fingers. It is a little like holding a large chopstick. Up until this point, the only knives I had ever wielded were in the kitchen. And even my largest fish knife suddenly seemed small and insignificant—but sharper: the weapons we used were dull, generally not sharp enough to cut the skin.

First, Michael taught us the *en garde* position. You stand with one foot forward, facing your opponent, one foot behind, perpendicular to the front foot, the foil out in front and your other arm held in the air for balance. The forward foot is for movement, the back foot for balance. At this angle, you give your opponent the narrowest target.

We began repetitions of various positions. Following Michael in the *en garde* position, we waddled forward, we waddled backward. We advanced, lunged and recovered. We jumped, lunged and recovered. This was fun until my thighs began to burn and my arm holding the foil turned to lead. Then Valerie and I stood opposite each other and learned how to defend ourselves. Rolling your wrist to the left and blocking the opponent's sword is one of fencing's most fundamental moves, the "four parry." To the right, it is the "six parry." Once we got that down, we learned, with a straight and fluid movement like a boxer's punch, to strike one another. This was difficult to get used to. Valerie was older; I felt like I was stabbing my mother.

At the very end, though, when Michael gave us the go ahead to bout, that feeling suddenly left me. I wanted to go in for the kill. Soon, my movements no longer resembled the jump-lunge-recover we had practiced. I was flailing my foil at Valerie. But Valerie was just as vicious. Her foil was a constant presence in my face. I forgot to four parry and six parry, and instead tried to swipe her weapon out of my way.

We charged and poked at each other for a few minutes, then Michael pulled us apart and told us our session was over. "Yeah," Mr. Longenbach shouted from across the studio, "It's not like it is on TV. It's more difficult than it looks." And I was not a natural. Fencing, I realized, requires a strong foundation of technique, a lot of strategy and incredible agility.

The grace and poise I had hoped for would come with time. But only after coordination and speed kicked in. And though it might not seem so when you're watching Errol Flynn, fencing requires aggressiveness. It is not just a matter of catching your opponent off guard. Like chess, it is about planning a few moves ahead to outwit her, then being extremely quick and agile on your feet so you can go in for the point.

What is perhaps unusual about fencing is its openness and equality. Fencing is a sport for all ages and, despite its image for attracting slim men, all body types. Professional foil fencers usually do not hit their prime until ages 25 to 35, and epee fencers continue for many years after that.

It is as much about strategy as it is about physical strength. The steel is the great equalizer, Mr. Longenbach said. At Metropolis Fencing, I once saw a skinny teenage girl take on a much older man, who looked like he belonged on a wrestling mat. It was a tight match, and each fencer, though aggressive, would score with just a gentle touch of the sword against the other's metallic vest to set off the scoring buzzer.

"It's not like punching with a knife," Mr. Longenbach said. "It's just the touch. It's like flicking the cigarette out of the person's mouth with a whip."

The second time I went was a Tuesday evening. The place was packed. Music thumped. Experienced fencers were bouting in every inch of the place. Some were charging at each other; some stood completely still, their foils just touching, tensely waiting for the other to make the first move. This time, the movements came easier for me, but only slightly. I don't think I'll be flicking cigarettes any time soon.

[AH, January 1999]

## Persuading Potatoes to Get Off the Couches

Exercise—you know you should be doing it, but something always seems to keep you from getting started. You don't have time, the weather's bad, there's no good place to work out, there's no one to watch the kids, it disrupts your day, you're too tired or, perhaps the most common and truthful excuse of them all, you hate to exercise.

You're not alone. More than 60 percent of Americans get little or no exercise, despite repeated reminders about the myriad rewards of regular physical activity to body and mind. But there's good news for you. According to two studies published in the *Journal of the American Medical Association*, you don't have to exercise in the traditional sense—as in jogging, aerobics and cycling—to glean many of the health benefits of activity, including weight control. All you have to do is incorporate more movement into your daily routines.

Despite a plethora of diets, in the last three decades Americans have become fatter and fatter even though national health surveys indicate that we actually consume fewer calories than in years past. Because body fat cannot appear out of thin air, the explanation for our increasing weight must be that we are using significantly fewer of the calories we consume.

And it doesn't take much to figure out why. Just look around you: television sets operated by remote control, motorized vehicles, elevators and escalators, clothes and dish washers, computers and fax machines, e-mail in the office, catalogue and Internet shopping, electric hedge clippers, chain saws, gas-powered lawn mowers, leaf and snow blowers, and so forth and so on. One hardly has to lift a finger to get through the day. And, to be sure, most people don't.

Dr. Steven Blair, director of research and epidemiology at the Cooper Institute of Aerobics Research in

Dallas, quotes a Scottish researcher's estimate that in Britain, average energy expenditures have dropped by 800 calories a day in the last 25 years. If anything, the decline has been more precipitous on this side of the Atlantic. Even if you used just 100 calories a day less and ate the same amount, you would gain about 10 pounds a year, nearly all of them as body fat unless you are physically active.

Dr. William Haskell, an exercise expert at Stanford University, has calculated that if you spend two minutes an hour of each workday sending e-mail to office mates instead of walking down the hall to talk to them, you would accumulate the caloric equivalent of 11 pounds of body fat in a decade.

And because body fat uses fewer calories than muscle to maintain itself, your metabolic rate—the number of calories you use up minute by minute—would drop and you would gain even more weight. And thus we have the vicious cycle of inactivity and weight gain that now plagues half the population.

Fewer than one-fifth of Americans engage in regular, sustained, vigorous physical activity, the kind that causes them to sweat a little, the kind that has been demonstrated to reduce the risk of chronic diseases and early death. The proportion of Americans who engage in this kind of exercise has not increased since the mid-1980s despite ever-mounting evidence that such activity can greatly reduce the risk of developing and dying of heart disease, stroke, diabetes, hypertension and osteoporosis and reduce the functional losses that accompany aging.

This lack of progress in getting more Americans on the move prompted leading health authorities a few years ago to modify their exercise advice. Rather than pushing everyone to exercise at their so-called target heart rate for at least 20 minutes at a time at least three times a week, the American Heart Association, the American College of Sports Medicine and the Centers for Disease Control and Prevention took a more practical tack. They now suggest that everyone do 30 minutes or more of moderately intense physical activity on most, and preferably all, days of the week. They further say that the 30 minutes of daily activity can be divided into as many as three 10-minute segments.

Possible choices include walking briskly all or part way to your destination, walking the dog (or a neighbor's dog), raking leaves, digging in the garden, swimming laps, riding an exercise bike, playing with the kids in the park, polishing furniture, washing the car, mopping the floor or sawing wood by hand. Additional calories can be burned and the benefits of activity gained by walking up—and down—stairs, parking at the far end of the lot, carrying groceries, even washing dishes and sweeping the floor.

Dr. Blair, among others, has pointed out that becoming more fit can take 20 years off a person's chronological age. In an interview in the current issue of *Nutrition Action Health Letter*, he noted that "unfit people start to develop limitations 20 to 25 years earlier than higher-fit people." He also cited evidence that exercise improves sleep, the ability to handle stress, the functioning of the immune system and mental outlook. People who exercise regularly feel better and have more energy, which would also contribute to a better sex life, he said.

Dr. Blair is a co-author of a study directed by Dr. Andrea L. Dunn at the Cooper Institute. The study involved 235 sedentary and slightly overweight men and women. Half were randomly assigned to a six-month structured exercise program in a gym and the other half were placed on a program involving routine activities like walking instead of riding and taking stairs instead of elevators. Two years later, both groups had about the same improvements in heart function and blood pressure and, while neither group lost weight, they both reduced their percentage of body fat. At least one-fourth of the participants maintained an improvement in cardiovascular fitness of 10 percent, which could translate into a 15 percent reduction in mortality, Dr. Dunn and his colleagues reported.

The second study also examined the effects of structured aerobic activity versus life-style activity, in this case among 40 obese women who also were placed on a moderate weight-reduction diet. The researchers, headed by Dr. Ross E. Anderson of the Johns Hopkins University School of Medicine, found that both groups lost about the same amount of weight, but that one year after completing the 16-

week program, the life-style activity group had regained less. In addition, the life-style program was as effective as aerobic activity in improving weight, blood pressure and cholesterol levels.

"This is good news for people who understand the role of physical activity in weight control but dislike vigorous physical activity or believe that they lack time to exercise," the researchers concluded. "Patients should strive to incorporate regular physical activity into their lives on a daily basis but should realize that even some physical activity, even if not performed regularly, is much better than being sedentary."

[JEB, February 1999]

## Crunches, Not Devices, Help Tighten Abdomen

**W**ant to flatten that tummy? Lose those love handles? Cultivate a washboard abdomen? If you have not already invested in an "ab" device, you might just save your money, get down on the floor and start doing some crunches to get as good an effect as that from any of the popular devices. A study sponsored by the American Council on Exercise has shown that old-fashioned bent-leg sit-ups are as effective as popular abdominal exercise gadgets in working those midriff muscles.

The study, directed by Dr. William C. Whiting, a specialist in biomechanics at California State University in Northridge, found no overall advantage to the devices, which cost from $75 to $120, unless their purchase motivates someone to adopt and stick with a fitness program. Dr. Whiting and his collaborators at Occidental College in Los Angeles took strong issue with "infomercial" assertions that ab devices could help someone shed "10 pounds in 10 days" or "four to six inches in a month." Dr. Whiting said that such advertising claims were based, not on the workout done using the devices, but on the nutrition and aerobic exercise program outlined in the brochures that accompany them.

Crunches, whether done on one's own or aided by a device, do not use enough calories to result in weight loss and cannot "spot reduce" accumulations of body fat, the researchers said in their report in the current issue of *ACE FitnessMatters*, the council's bimonthly publication. The council is a nonprofit agency based in San Diego that promotes physical activity, certifies fitness instructors and publishes training manuals.

What crunches can do is strengthen the muscles between the chest and the groin. In doing a basic crunch unaided, a person would lie on his back on the floor and, with knees raised, feet flat on the floor and fingers linked loosely behind the head, raise the torso toward the knees by contracting the abdominal muscles. The torso is then slowly lowered, though not quite to the floor, again using abdominal muscles. Crunches are also done obliquely, raising one shoulder at a time toward the opposite knee.

To assess the potential effectiveness of ab devices, the researchers measured the activity of five muscle groups during crunches done on each of four popular devices and compared the results with crunches done without any mechanical assistance. Nineteen young adults in good physical condition were hooked up to a machine that measured the activity of various muscles while doing a uniform series of sit-ups with and without the devices.

The muscle groups assessed were the central abdominal muscle, which can give the upper abdomen a washboard appearance; the lower abdominal muscle, which extends from the belt line to just above the pelvis; the muscles on the side of the stomach beneath the love handles; the main muscle along the top of the thigh, and the muscles in the back of the neck.

In theory, when doing crunches, the thigh muscles should not contract and the neck muscles should contract as little as possible. One claim made for ab devices is that they help to minimize strain on the neck. But when participants did an oblique crunch, one of the devices, Abworks by Nordic Track, actually resulted in much greater neck strain than the unaided crunch and those done with the other devices tested, the researchers reported. This device also resulted in greater involvement of the thigh muscles during an oblique crunch, according to the study. In doing a basic crunch with hands behind the head, the study showed there was slightly less neck strain associated with two devices—the Ab Roller Plus made by Quantum North America and the AB Trainer made by Precise—than occurred during an unaided crunch.

Michael Smith, a spokesperson for Nordic Track in Chaska, Minnesota, said that an independent study by Dr. James Dowling, an exercise physiologist at MacMaster University in Hamilton, Ontario,

showed that Abworks resulted in significantly greater abdominal muscle activity than an unaided crunch, at least among users who were able to do 20 unaided crunches.

But the California researchers concluded that there was "no apparent benefit or detriment" to the devices. They emphasized, however, that "performance of abdominal exercises, in the absence of proper aerobic exercise and nutrition, cannot be expected to result in weight loss." At best, they added, abdominal exercises will strengthen abdominal muscles "underneath the layers of fat."

Dr. Dowling agreed that no device by itself was going to give a person "the washboard abdomen seen on underwear models." To achieve that kind of development requires exercising against greater resistance than these devices can provide.

[JEB, January 1997]

## For Younger Muscles, Just Pump Away

I am not what anyone would call a typical sedentary middle-aged American. At 58, I still do at least one and usually two or three forms of physical activity every day. My regular year-round activities include fitness walking, singles tennis and lap swimming, as well as ice skating in winter and bike riding the rest of the year.

So I was a bit taken aback when an exercise physiologist asked if I did any form of strength training. Don't my regular activities keep me as strong as I'm likely to get? Don't swimming and tennis give my arms and shoulders enough of a workout to keep upper body muscles strong? And don't my other activities do the same for my legs and hips?

But when I tried to do a few bicep curls with a two-pound hand weight or lift myself up on a chinning bar, I learned otherwise. Could I save myself if I were hanging from a cliff? Might I have had an easier time biking the hills of southern Spain last fall if my leg muscles had been stronger at the start?

The exercise physiologist explained that to get strong and stay strong, muscles need to be worked regularly against resistance until they fatigue. Lest this sound forbidding, let me assure you that it is neither difficult nor particularly time-consuming to build and maintain muscle strength that can make an enormous difference in your lasting health and well-being.

You don't need to leave your house, join a gym or buy costly exercise equipment. Whether you are a man, woman or child, by devoting just 20 minutes two or three times a week to strength training, the rewards you can reap will more than make up for the time and effort. And it's never too late to start. Even people in their 80s and 90s can gain muscle strength that will help reduce their risk of injury and illness and improve their outlooks on life.

Many people have shunned the idea of muscle-building exercise because they harbor misconceptions about what it is, whom it is for and what it does to the body. Strength training is not the same as body-building, a "sport" that is more like a beauty contest of overdeveloped musculature.

Strength training can add tone and definition to the shape of your limbs and any other body part you work on, but it won't make you inflexibly muscle-bound or turn you into a Charles Atlas of bulging muscles. Nor will you be lifting heavy weights that make you grunt and groan. Rather, strength training involves using small weights or working against resistance such that you are able to repeat the movement 10 to 15 times before your muscles get too tired to continue.

Women are often inhibited by the fear that lifting weights will cause them to look too masculine. This can happen only if women take high doses of testosterone or, occasionally, if a woman with an inherited predisposition to develop big muscles does high-intensity workouts. For the vast majority of women, strength training offers an opportunity to reduce flab and improve appearance without detracting one iota from femininity.

Even children can do strength training without harm. Dr. Steven Fleck, an exercise physiologist in Colorado Springs and a consultant to the *Georgia Tech Sports Medicine & Performance Newsletter*, says any child old enough to participate in organized sports is old enough to do age-appropriate resistance training if the correct techniques are used. Such training not only can improve children's fitness levels but also their self-esteem and their athletic performance.

Aerobic exercise, like running, brisk walking, cycling or lap swimming, can improve your overall level of fitness and the functioning of your heart and lungs, but it won't necessarily make the muscles throughout your body significantly stronger or ward off the loss of muscle with age.

Strength training can prevent much of the muscle deterioration that otherwise inevitably occurs as people get older. As you age, the cells of the body's muscles, more than 600 of them, gradually decrease in size and number. Dr. Thomas D. Fahey, director of exercise physiology at California State University in Chico, noted in an article in *Healthline* that between the ages of 40 and 60, the average person loses up to

20 percent of muscle mass unless something is done to prevent or slow that loss.

In addition, he wrote, there is a gradual loss of connections between nerves and the muscle cells they control, making it more difficult for the nervous system to activate the muscles. "These changes rob you of the strength you need to climb stairs, run for a bus or prevent falls," Dr. Fahey said.

A study of nursing home residents aged 72 to 98 showed that 10 weeks of progressive strength training for the muscles in the thigh and lower leg increased their strength by an average of 113 percent and improved the participants' walking speed and ability to climb stairs.

The training also is likely to increase bone density, thereby reducing the risk of fracture. Any increase in bone density after menopause is a big plus, since most women lose bone throughout the second half of life.

Increased muscle strength is a guaranteed energy enhancer. But perhaps the biggest selling point for increasing your body's ratio of muscle to fat is that muscle tissue is metabolically far more active than fat tissue. This means you will burn more calories even at rest.

Furthermore, muscle tissue is more compact than the same weight of fat. So by replacing fat with muscle, you can lose inches and sizes without having to lose any weight at all. Just think of the difference in appearance of a 250-pound football player and a 250-pound sedentary desk executive.

Beginning strength trainers should definitely get professional guidance. There are a number of excellent, well-illustrated books that can help, but a few sessions with a trainer are better for teaching correct form and correcting mistakes. Check with your local exercise center. Many offer classes in strength training or have trainers available. To do the exercises, you can use hand and ankle weights in graduated sizes, elastic resistance bands, resistance machines found in most gyms, cans of soup or even your own body.

You should start out with a weight that you can lift or push against 10 to 15 times before your muscles fatigue. Then, as you get stronger, the weight is gradually increased to produce further strengthening.

Training more than three times a week may be counterproductive because the muscles need rest periods in which to recover and rebuild themselves. As with most good things in life, you have to continue working at strength training to maintain the gains.

[JEB, July 1999]

## Learning Pilates, One Stretch at a Time

It is called Pilates, and I had been hearing about it for some time but dismissed it as a faddish '90s workout. It fit the mold perfectly: It had the requisite exotic name (pronounced puh-LAH-tees), you had to go to a gym to do it, and celebrities hailed it as a miracle workout that managed, with perfect '90s perversity, to give shapely women the bodies of 12-year-old boys.

Pilates, I had heard, involved archaic equipment with names like "the reformer" and "the barrel," but that was about all I knew when I arrived at TriBeCa Bodyworks, a Pilates studio on Duane Street, determined to see if my bias was well-founded. A model-thin woman blew by me, a single line of sweat dripping down her radiant cheek. Great. I hated the place already.

Alycea Baylis-Ungaro, the owner of the studio, had instructed me to bring loose clothing and to wear socks. No sneakers were necessary. Showing me to the changing room, she whispered, "Even men do Pilates. We get a lot of them." It is true. During my workouts at least one-third were men. Besides, there is, as I soon learned, nothing feminine about Pilates.

The exercise method was invented by a man, Joseph Pilates, a boxer and physical therapist from Germany. Obsessed with body conditioning, he developed the framework for Pilates while serving as a nurse during World War I. So that patients could exercise in bed, he redesigned a hospital bed and developed simple exercises. Modern Pilates apparatus relies on the use of springs to provide resistance, much like weights, but easier on the body. He opened the first Pilates Studio in the United States in New York City in 1926.

A workout developed that long ago, when athletes smoked and tennis players wore long pants? Still, I signed up for three one-hour Pilates sessions. The first, Alycea said, would just be introductory. For $65, she would lead me through the fundamental exercises. Later sessions would get more intense, Alycea promised, at $55 a session. A bargain! I could not quite believe I was handing over this much money to exercise. I am a reasonable person. I live near a park. I own a pair of sneakers. Why not just put them on and run around the park?

The reason became clearer with each exercise. Alycea took me to the reformer, a long, low, bedlike apparatus with a flat, padded carriage that slid back and forth the length of the bed. It made a dentist's chair look friendly. Alycea had me lie face up on the carriage, with my knees bent and my feet on a raised steel bar at the end of the apparatus. I was to straighten my legs as I pulled in my stomach.

The carriage, which is set on three long springs, was difficult to slide out, then snapped back against the end of the apparatus with a loud "Bang!" that echoed through the studio. Heads turned. Alycea did not look pleased. The next time, I was told, do it smoothly, no banging. And I was told to stop arching my back. Pilates exercises are designed to protect and strengthen the back. "The more distance you put between your belly button and your spine, the more pressure you put on your back," Alycea said.

By changing the position of my feet on the steel bar and pushing, I worked different muscle groups in my legs while working my stomach muscles. "It's a real New York workout because it's really efficient," Alycea said. "You have to use all your muscles at once." And you get it all in a neat and snappy 60 minutes.

We moved on to more complex movements, my least favorite being the "hundreds." Lying face up on the reformer, I had to raise my feet six inches, suck in my stomach, squeeze my buttocks together and, holding a stirrup set on springs in each hand, keep my arms at my sides and bounce them up and down, 100 times. With so many details to focus on, you hardly feel the pain.

I was beginning to understand why Mr. Pilates called his workout contrology. For every exercise that focuses on strengthening muscle, another stretches the body and encourages balance. And each movement—whether a derivative of the sit-up with legs jutting in the air, or lying flat and pulling on leather harnesses attached to springs—involves stabilizing the core of the body, the torso and buttocks, while moving the arms or legs. (This is the part that appeals to women: The movements are small and repetitions are short, so you tone muscle without bulking up.)

After about a half hour on the reformer, Alycea introduced me to "the Cadillac," which looked a lot like a gurney with harnesses and pulleys. After more stomach exercises, including sit-ups and leg lifts, Alycea had me lie on my back and put my feet into the harnesses. With my feet above my head and my back raised off of the mat, I was hung like a side of beef. Then, using my stomach muscles, I had to pull my body down to the mat against the resistance of the springs, curling my spine, vertebra by vertebra. It felt as if I was stretching every bone in my back. But there was no pain. Instead, I felt stress ebbing until it was gone. I could have done it all day.

But that was not the best part. Alycea had me sit up and stretch to touch my toes while she pushed and rubbed my back. I was forgetting about the $65.

I left my first session with my stomach muscles dazed and confused, but I was still troubled that I had not broken a sweat. But when I arrived for my second session, Alycea reminded me that the reformer workout did not get longer, it got faster. "And that's where the aerobics come in," she said. And did they ever. I was more relaxed with the machines and my movements became smoother and faster. But when I slowed down, I heard about it.

At most Pilates gyms, you do individual sessions with a personal trainer to learn the movements—there are more than 500—until you get up to pace. After about 30 sessions, you can advance to what is called a duet—two people with a trainer—then to groups of three and four.

I had never employed a personal trainer, but I found that having one by my side was surprisingly comforting. I liked having someone there to coddle me while I suffered through the workout. Besides, it is far too easy and tempting to cheat with Pilates.

What is extraordinary about Pilates is its broad appeal. Some professional dancers do it to maintain flexibility and stay fit without adding excess stress to their bodies. And unlike running or aerobics, Pilates is good for the elderly, people with injuries, and even pregnant women. "They do it right up to delivery," Alycea said.

As for me, Pilates was a revelation. I had not realized how tight my muscles had become working in an office, slouching over a computer keyboard. By the third session, I was a convert. I was getting the aerobic workout I wanted while regaining some of the flexibility I had lost. But if I start to get that 12-year-old boy look, I just may have to ease off. For a while, anyway.

[AH, November 1998]

## Medicine Ball Pops Back Into Vogue

The medicine ball, darling of the trimming and toning crowd before its exile to six decades of exercise Elba, has bounced back. Embraced in the 1930s as the epitome of exercise chic, the medicine ball—shaped like a ball but filled with paper or cotton and covered in leather—dropped out of fashion, abandoned for the next new things to come along: vibrating belts, amphetamines and *The Jack LaLanne Show*. So old-fashioned, the medicine ball was even a punch line on *Seinfeld*, with Jerry sarcastically asking his very elderly trainer, played by Lloyd Bridges, if they were going to use a medicine ball. Had *Seinfeld* returned for another season, they may well have, and happily.

Like the martini and other long-ago icons, the medicine ball is back, its workout sometimes going under the name "plyometrics," to describe a system of measured increases in an exerciser's performance. Around the nation, the medicine ball is popping up in exercise classes and in sessions with personal trainers, winning a new generation of fans.

"I love it," said Jason White, a trainer at Equinox in Manhattan. "My clients, both men and women, get very excited about it. Other people are seeing them use it, and they just have to try it. It's a very explosive workout, a very effective addition to free weights and cardiovascular work. Because it's weighted, it makes the body work harder."

These days, the 2- to 20-pound balls are filled with gel, polyurethane chips, sand and sawdust, or occasionally water, and covered with polyurethane or rubber. "They're fantastic: you can do a million different things with them and incorporate them into any exercise," said Larry Krug, a trainer at Crunch Fitness in Los Angeles.

A medicine ball user lies on his back with knees bent and feet flat on the floor. The ball is positioned just above the head and the arms are bent. Elbows are pointed up. The ball is pulled over the top of the head and the exerciser raises his head and shoulders as the ball is moved to the top of his knees. The exerciser then returns to the starting position by bringing the ball over his head and reclining his body. In another exercise, two exercisers can face each other three feet apart and toss the ball back and forth, each aiming at a spot just above the other's head.

Or, an exerciser can kneel six feet from a wall and throw a medicine ball with both hands by bringing the ball from behind the head and releasing it in front of her head and catching it immediately on the rebound. New, true believers contend that the medicine ball is soft, easy to grip and, dare one say it, fun. "Clients completely forget that they're working out," Mr. Krug said.

One of them is Alex Meneses, 28, who stars in the movie *The Flintstones in Viva Rock Vegas*, a prequel to *The Flintstones*. She won the role of the sexy secretary, which was played by Halle Berry in the original film, and had to get in terrific shape. Quickly.

"My costumes are teeny," said Ms. Meneses, who lives in West Hollywood. "They were so small, I couldn't breathe. Working out with the medicine ball, I lost 10 pounds since April and I've kept it off. Even though I'm a runner and good at cardio, this shaped my body better, sculpting my arms, waist and hips. I've been using it three or four times a week, and I'm probably in the best shape I've ever been in."

Also, she said, "It's like playing."

Michael Blum, 43, a concert pianist in Manhattan, relies on the medicine ball "to play catch and as a weight between my legs and arms to add stress."

"A pianist has to be as internally strong as a gymnast," he said. "Emotionally and physically."

As comebacks go, this rebirth is happening quickly. "I think it's gaining popularity too because boxing is hot, and medicine balls have always been used in boxing training," Mr. Krug said. "People love boxing, and a lot of women these days are boxing, which used to be socially unacceptable. So it carries connotations of self-defense, and that's hot. Everyone at the gym sees the boxers using it and everyone else using it, and they just have to try it also because it's new."

Tony Swain, personal training coordinator at the East Bank Club in Chicago, says he is seeing members use the medicine ball "in different exercises for different muscle groups, for strength training and sports-related exercises." Maeve McCaffrey, a spokeswoman for the International Health, Racquet and Sports Club Association of Boston, a trade organization for gyms, has taken note of the ball's return. "I do think the medicine ball is experiencing a resurgence," Ms. McCaffrey said. "This might be attributed to the popularity of sports-based athletic classes."

In the 1930s, the medicine ball exercise system was prescribed by doctors to promote health for their patients through exercise. Athletes began using it to build resistance, and exercisers of the day soon took to it. But it did not take long for its vogue to pass: when the ball got wet or full of sweat, as it inevitably would, the paper and cotton inside grew moldy and smelly. The ball would change weight easily and unevenly, making it unstable, and the seams of the leather cover ruptured. The ball's unpleasant metamorphosis made the notion of exercise even less appealing than usual.

But the medicine ball found a new champion in Dr. Donald A. Chu. Dr. Chu, a former professor of kinesiology at California State University at Hayward who is the director of the physical therapist assistant program at Ohlone College in Newark, California, as well as the strength and conditioning consultant to the United States synchronized swim team and Olympic team, had observed East European track and field athletes using the medicine ball with much success in the late 1960s and early '70s to build speed and movement.

In the '80s he began working with a plastics manufacturer to build a better ball, he said, which he did, with gel, sand, sawdust, urethane or rubber shavings inside. He had intended to use it only with athletes, but then trainers started noticing. Dr. Chu, who lives in Alameda, quietly began building the medicine ball's return, even naming his Jack Russell terrier puppy Plyo.

"Most machines tend to isolate a joint or area. This does not. It sculpts the body, especially the abdomen," said Dr. Chu, who added that he exercised with his medicine ball, "but not every single day." Dr. Chu owns the trademark on his Plyoball and many users look to Dr. Chu's handbook, *Plyometric Exercises With the Medicine Ball*, which describes more than 120 movements and explanations of ways to adapt the plyoball for workouts at home or in gyms.

Another medicine ball, the Ooof Ball—"the medicine ball that bounces"—has the endorsement of Al Vermeil, strength and conditioning coach for the Chicago Bulls.

The Ooof Ball is made of polyurethane throughout (hence, the bounce) and is available at weights from 1.75 pounds to 9 pounds along with videos and booklets.

The name plyometrics was coined in the 1960s by Fred Wilt, track coach at the University of Iowa, to describe the East European athletes' "jump training." But more recently it has won wider recognition with the medicine ball's new popularity.

Of course, the essence of fashion, whether for clothing, politics or exercise, is change, and so the medicine ball's popularity may, yet again, dribble off into the sunset. "At Crunch L.A., at least, everyone is in really good shape so they really love any change that comes along," said Mr. Krug, the trainer. Next in line, the vibrating belt?

[AHi, October 1999]

# Some Shape Up by Surfing the Internet

For various reasons, including a busy schedule and two herniated discs in my neck, I got out of shape. Or, more specifically, I got into another shape altogether. While doing Internet research for an article about women's bodybuilding, I stumbled onto a site, www.trulyhuge.com. What this site was selling seemed highly unlikely: on-line training.

Sure, you can get anything on the Internet. But fit? I didn't think so.

These are the words of a changed woman. Seventeen pounds lighter, sleeping through the night for the first time in my life, energetic, fit and strong, I am the worst kind of proselytizer—worse, by far, than the reformed smoker, recovering carbo-loader or even politician. I know on-line fitness when I see it. And I've seen it.

Trulyhuge had a questionnaire that required measuring my height and the size of my body everywhere from my ankles to my wrists. It asked about injuries, access to a gym, pool, weights or any other athletic equipment. I started filling in the boxes on the screen and noticed that I hadn't been tempted to lie. Not for my weight, height, bad habits or goals.

There was something about not being seen by the recipient of these statistics that allowed me to tell the full-sized truth. I think that's when I became intrigued. Already this was a step up from my last personal training experience: no pep talks, no pitches for products I wouldn't feed my septic system and, especially, no welterweight endomorph lashing my middleweight self with tape measures. That means no on-site humiliation. As for on-line humiliation, who cares?

I wrote that my goals were to lose 15 pounds, increase my aerobic stamina, get back into my clothes (that is, get smaller, not bulk up with muscle), feel better and get a little more energy. I didn't ask about sleep. As a lifelong insomniac, it never occurred to me to include it in my goals.

I wrote that my dream workout would be portable, allowing me to keep up my routine at the gym, at my home in the country (where I have nothing but a few hand weights) and on the road. Being a writer, wife and mother, I have a haphazard schedule, one prone to constant interruption. This had helped me to fail with personal trainers before: keeping those appointments was hard, though paying for them when I canceled was even harder. After I moved upstate, I discovered that the going rate for a personal trainer was only $20 an hour, much less than what I had been paying in Manhattan. But that's still hefty enough if you train three times a week for the length of time it takes to get in shape, which I figured in my case would be a minimum of eight weeks.

So I signed up for Trulyhuge for 12 weeks, hoping that at the end of it I might be truly small. The total cost was $60, $20 a month for a diet plan, a training regimen and coaching on line. This includes unlimited questions from client and regular check-ins from the trainer.

The man on the other side of Trulyhuge is Paul Becker, who trains bodybuilders in Los Angeles along with running the Web site, which also features products, promotes his training and sells his book, *Trulyhuge*.

Within two days of my returning the questionnaire, my complete diet and exercise routine arrived by e-mail. It was portable. It accommodated gym, home and hotel room workouts. The dietary recommendations were for a higher protein-lower carbohydrate routine and included sample menus.

The advice: drink more water and less juice, and cut back on bread—not hard moves to make. His eating regimen was sensible and understandable, calling, for example, for an egg-white omelet in the morning. I don't eat eggs, so now I have a fruit shake with tofu, soy powder or skim milk every morning.

Wanting to track my progress efficiently, I waited until the first day of a new month to go back to the gym. And when it came, I went, armed with nothing more than three pieces of paper from Trulyhuge and my workout clothes.

My program required five days of 30-minute aerobic workouts each week plus three strength sessions. The aerobic exercise recommended was power walking, which I did on a treadmill at the gym. All the exercises, I was instructed, were to be done in sets of 15 repetitions unless otherwise stated.

The three strength days, each separated by a day or two of rest, broke down as follows:

▶ *Day One:* two sets of leg presses, one set of leg extensions, two sets each of leg curls and seated calf raises, and as many reverse crunches as possible.

▶ *Day Two:* two sets of bench presses, one set of incline bench presses, one set of flies, two sets of lateral raises, one set of bent-over lateral raises, one set of French presses, one set of triceps pulldowns and as many reverse crunches as possible.

▶ *Day Three:* two sets of rows and one set each of lat pulldowns, standing barbell curls, incline dumbbell curls, wrist curls, reverse wrist curls and reverse crunches.

The freehand program, or what I call the at-home/on-the-road workout, included push-ups, deep knee bends, calf raises, side leg raises and reverse crunches. By the night of day four I had the sensation that my legs were humming. Lying in bed (not sleeping, of course), I could feel my legs vibrating. Paul replied to my on-line query about this within hours. My legs, he said, were burning fat.

I was hopeful. By the end of the second week, I had lost three pounds. Was I naïve to have hoped for more?

Two and a half weeks into the program, I had dropped four pounds. I e-mailed this progress to Trulyhuge, and Paul wrote me an encouraging note saying I was doing great. I requested a more thorough explanation of the free weight routines. By the end of the day, I had received a completely understandable breakdown of the exercises.

Throughout the weeks, if I didn't e-mail, Paul did. He asked for progress reports or inquired to see if I had questions. I came to appreciate the reminder that someone out there was keeping track of my progress.

## Getting Fitness Results On-Line

More and more trainers are offering to sign up clients for on-line fitness. Here is what to expect:

**1. SIGN ON**

The first step is to find a Web site that offers training online. You will be asked to fill out a questionaire to provide personal information, like measurements, food habits and goals. After a few days, you will receive a personalized fitness regimen and nutrition plan via e-mail.

**2. WORK OUT**

A workout should include personal, detailed exercise routine focusing on your goals.

**3. DIET**

A competent trainer will assess your diet and offer suggestions and sample menus, especially if weight loss is a goal.

**4. FEEDBACK**

Expect your trainer to check in with you frequently and respond quickly to any questions.

Weight loss and training, I found out, is not something most friends and relations find terribly interesting.

After 30 days, I cut out all alcohol. Two weeks after that, I started sleeping. No, more than that: I did eight straight hours asleep, for the first time in my life. And every night since I have simply gone right to sleep—face down, face up, it makes no difference. My husband swears that once he thought I was dead. He managed to wake me, but, no matter, I went right back to sleep.

That month I lost five more pounds. But I was frustrated. I had hoped for two pounds a week. So, I tried that time-honored, weight loss motivator: I got an expensive haircut. Eight more pounds were gone by the end of the next month.

I e-mailed Paul Becker and told him how pleased I was: 17 pounds gone in less than three months. I am very pleased to be going into June without that weight. But I had to ask one more question: Why was I sleeping?

In his answer, he used an old English measure, and it was so comforting to see it in this digital age that I've kept his note tacked on my wall: "Lose a stone (14 pounds)," it said. "Sleep like a rock." He's right.

On-line trainers and coaches abound on the Web. While prices vary, expect to pay at least $20 for a one-month workout plan.

[MRo, May 1999]

# Gains and Losses: Women and Weight

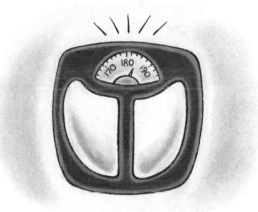

## COMMON SENSE DIET AND EXERCISE WIN OUT OVER DRUGS AND SPECIAL FOODS

America has confessed to being the fattest nation on earth. In 1998, new weight guidelines established by the National Institutes of Health declared 55 percent of the population over-weight, and 20 percent frankly obese. The problem goes far beyond the merely cosmetic: too much body fat increases the risk of illness and death from a variety of disorders, including heart disease, high blood pressure, stroke, Type 2 diabetes, gallbladder disease, osteoarthritis and some cancers. Researchers estimate that obesity may be responsible for 300,000 deaths a year in the United States. People who, as a result of genetics, tend to carry the extra weight around their midsections, as opposed to the hips and thighs, are at the greatest risk.

The reason for the national epidemic of obesity is simple: too much food, too little exercise. Anyone who takes in more calories than he or she burns off will turn them to fat. And with greasy, drive-through fast food on every corner, and a society that increasingly drives rather than walks, and spends more and more time sitting in front of one type or screen or another, the excess of calories is hard to avoid. The introduction of fat-free snacks and desserts has not helped; Americans have continued to get heavier as these foods have increased their market share. The reason is that many of the products, despite being fat free, are high in calories. And many people kid themselves, thinking that "fat-free" or "lite" is a license to eat all they want.

Diet drugs have not turned out to be the magic bullet, either. Two prescription drugs, Xenical, which blocks fat absorption, and Meridia, an appetite suppressant, bring about only modest weight losses, and both have side effects. So does the herbal product ephedra, which can raise blood pressure and has been linked to seizures and deaths from heart attack and stroke.

Perhaps the most discouraging aspect of the trend to obesity is the popular belief that it is cannot be reversed: that extra pounds are hard to lose, and, even if they are lost, impossible to keep off. But researchers say that need not always be the case, and that the impression of hopelessness is based on the histories of people who consult weight-loss clinics, and who are usually the most difficult to treat. Recent studies have identified thousands of people who have lost large amounts of weight on their own, without clinics—30, 50, and in some cases more than 100 pounds—and kept it off for five years or more. Many of the success stories are credited not to drugs or complicated trendy diets, but to a common-sense approach: exercising more and eating less, sticking to a nourishing menu rich in fruits and vegetables and moderate amounts of poultry, fish and lean meat.

# New Guide Puts Most Americans on the Fat Side

As bathing suit season approaches each year, it seems as if nearly every popular magazine touts one scheme or another for shedding that winter padding and achieving a movie-star figure in eight weeks or less. Even without the beach as an incentive, millions of Americans are perpetually struggling to lose pounds, an effort that has spawned a $33 billion diet industry.

In June 1998, the National Institutes of Health gave Americans a far better reason to be self-conscious about their bodies and to increase their efforts to lose weight, not just for summer but forever. Based on an evaluation of many big studies linking excess body fat to a long list of chronic and potentially fatal diseases, an expert panel convened by the National Heart, Lung and Blood Institute and the National Institute of Diabetes and Digestive and Kidney Disease announced a new definition of overweight, one that says 55 percent of American adults are too heavy.

In other words, according to the revised guidelines, more than half the population is too heavily larded, which makes us by far the fattest people on earth. The point at which an American would be considered overweight has been shifted downward, from a body mass index of 27 to one of 25. Those with an index of 30 or more are classified as obese. It is a guideline already established by the World Health Organization for people everywhere. If approved by the 115 health experts reviewing the guidelines, the new definition would add another 25 million adults to the 72 million who were previously considered overweight.

The National Association to Advance Fat Acceptance objected to the new guidelines, saying that changes in diet and exercise habits can improve a person's health risks even if no weight is lost. The association is concerned that the increased attention to weight will prompt even more people to try diets doomed to fail and add to the number of people who avoid going to doctors for fear of being harassed about their weight.

While the association may be correct in its belief that some people would be better off staying fat than spending their lives struggling to get their weight down to a level they simply cannot maintain, for the vast majority of overweight Americans, the problem is not genetic and not incurable. It is a consequence of eating too much, especially too much of calorically dense foods like fats and sweets, and exercising too little.

The body mass index, or B.M.I., is considered a better measure of the amount of fat on a person's body than would be indicated by the traditional height-weight charts. Though the B.M.I. is officially calculated by dividing body weight in kilograms by height in meters squared (hard for Americans who don't know their dimensions in the metric system), you can also figure your B.M.I. by multiplying your weight in pounds by 703, then dividing the result by your height in inches and dividing that result by your height a second time. (Another version involves squaring your height.)

However, even the B.M.I. is not a perfect measure of fatness. A person who is very muscular but who has a low percentage of body fat could end up with the same B.M.I. as someone who is truly fat. Therefore, the new guidelines, which were issued in 1998, also call upon physicians to measure their patients' waistlines. Fat that collects around the belly is the most serious health threat, and the guidelines say that among those with a B.M.I. of 25 to 35, men with waists of more than 40 inches and women whose waists exceed 35 inches face an increased risk of developing serious health problems.

In fact, even if your B.M.I. falls into the low-risk range of 21 to 25, if you carry too much weight around the middle you're at greater risk than someone whose weight sits on the hips or thighs. Likewise, people with an acceptable B.M.I. who gained 10 or more pounds as adults (say, after age 21) are at greater risk than those who have maintained their college weight.

The main impetus for changing the weight guidelines is the growing realization that just about any amount of excess body fat is a potential health risk. Although there is some evidence that being a little overweight when you're old is actually beneficial, this is still being debated. The most recent analysis of data from the National Health and Nutrition Examination Survey revealed that as B.M.I. rises above 25, average levels of blood pressure and artery-damaging blood cholesterol rise, average levels of protective HDL cholesterol fall and it becomes more difficult to maintain normal levels of blood sugar.

Thus, as the B.M.I. rises, the risk of developing a long list of ailments rises, too. They include coronary artery disease and resulting heart attacks, hypertension, stroke, type 2 diabetes, gallbladder disease, osteoarthritis, sleep apnea and accompanying respiratory problems and certain cancers, including cancer of the breast and endometrium. The National Institutes of Health estimates that obesity-related disease costs the nation about $100 billion a year.

Along with causing disease, of course, obesity can shorten life. In fact, the Institutes' statement on the new guidelines noted that obesity is the second leading cause (after smoking) of preventable death in the United States today.

In calculating someone's risk, the new guidelines state that more than the B.M.I. should be considered for many people in the lower ranges of overweight. Physicians will be told to look at risk factors for disease before deciding whether to urge patients to lose weight or merely avoid gaining any more. Thus, if your B.M.I. exceeds 25, before urging you to lose weight your doctor should take into account your blood cholesterol, blood sugar and blood pressure, evidence of arthritis in your knees or hips and any respiratory problems, as well as your family medical history and your own risky behaviors, like smoking, eating poorly and not exercising.

Finally, the 24-member expert panel that formulated the new guidelines recommended that normal-weight people should also remain vigilant and have their B.M.I.'s reassessed every two years. It is easier to stop encroaching weight problems early than to have to shed scores of excess pounds that have hung around your frame for years.

[JEB, June 1998]

## The Fat Get Fatter; Overweight Was Bad Enough

Bettye Travis is 5'5" and weighs 300 pounds. So when the National Institutes of Health broadened its definition of overweight in 1998 using a gauge called body mass index (B.M.I.), Ms. Travis, 47, the proprietor of a cake- and candy-making supply store in San Francisco, didn't bother to calculate hers. She said she didn't need the Government to tell her she weighs too much.

"I've been fat all my life," she said.

A lot of other people are fat, too, it turns out. By the Government's new definitions, more than one-half of all Americans aged 20 to 74 are overweight and one-fifth fall into a new category: obese.

To Ms. Travis, a board member of the National Association to Advance Fat Acceptance, the expanded definitions are another example of the way this thin-obsessed nation has turned love handles into a medical condition. But to the pharmaceutical industry, the corpulence of America means something else entirely: a booming new market for diet pills for the obese, practically served to the companies on a silver platter by the Government.

That was evident in late April 1999 when Hoffman-LaRoche, one of the world's biggest drug makers, received approval from the Food and Drug Administration to sell Xenical, the first in a new class of anti-obesity medications that work by blocking the body's absorption of dietary fat. It is the first pill to be approved since the Government recalibrated its definition of who qualifies as overweight.

The new standard relies on B.M.I., which experts say provides a better measurement of body fat than the traditional height and weight charts. Until recently, men were overweight if their B.M.I. was 27.3 or higher; for women, the cut-off was 27.8. Now, anyone with a B.M.I. of 25 or higher is overweight, by Government standards. And a new category, obese, has been added for those whose index is 30 or above. (Ms. Travis's B.M.I., for the record, is about 50.)

The Government did not pick those numbers out of a hat, nutrition experts say; studies show that people at those weights are at an increased risk of high blood pressure, high cholesterol, heart disease and other chronic disorders that contribute to premature death.

Most experts say diet and exercise—not drugs—are the best solution to a weight problem. But losing weight by dieting and exercise is not easy, and with excess body fat increasingly being viewed as a disease, the experts say, the drug industry cannot be

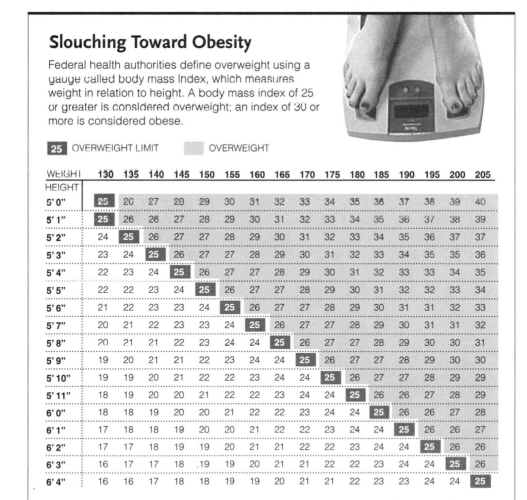

## Slouching Toward Obesity

Federal health authorities define overweight using a gauge called body mass index, which measures weight in relation to height. A body mass index of 25 or greater is considered overweight; an index of 30 or more is considered obese.

| **25** OVERWEIGHT LIMIT |  | OVERWEIGHT |

| WEIGHT | 130 | 135 | 140 | 145 | 150 | 155 | 160 | 165 | 170 | 175 | 180 | 185 | 190 | 195 | 200 | 205 |
|---|---|---|---|---|---|---|---|---|---|---|---|---|---|---|---|---|
| **HEIGHT** | | | | | | | | | | | | | | | | |
| 5'0" | **25** | 26 | 27 | 28 | 29 | 30 | 31 | 32 | 33 | 34 | 35 | 36 | 37 | 38 | 39 | 40 |
| 5'1" | **25** | 26 | 26 | 27 | 28 | 29 | 30 | 31 | 32 | 33 | 34 | 35 | 36 | 37 | 38 | 39 |
| 5'2" | 24 | **25** | 26 | 27 | 27 | 28 | 29 | 30 | 31 | 32 | 33 | 34 | 35 | 36 | 37 | 37 |
| 5'3" | 23 | 24 | **25** | 26 | 27 | 27 | 28 | 29 | 30 | 31 | 32 | 33 | 34 | 35 | 35 | 36 |
| 5'4" | 22 | 23 | 24 | **25** | 26 | 27 | 27 | 28 | 29 | 30 | 31 | 32 | 33 | 33 | 34 | 35 |
| 5'5" | 22 | 22 | 23 | 24 | **25** | 26 | 27 | 27 | 28 | 29 | 30 | 31 | 32 | 32 | 33 | 34 |
| 5'6" | 21 | 22 | 23 | 23 | 24 | **25** | 26 | 27 | 27 | 28 | 29 | 30 | 31 | 31 | 32 | 33 |
| 5'7" | 20 | 21 | 22 | 23 | 23 | 24 | **25** | 26 | 27 | 27 | 28 | 29 | 30 | 31 | 31 | 32 |
| 5'8" | 20 | 21 | 21 | 22 | 23 | 24 | 24 | **25** | 26 | 27 | 27 | 28 | 29 | 30 | 30 | 31 |
| 5'9" | 19 | 20 | 21 | 21 | 22 | 23 | 24 | 24 | **25** | 26 | 27 | 27 | 28 | 29 | 30 | 30 |
| 5'10" | 19 | 19 | 20 | 21 | 22 | 22 | 23 | 24 | 24 | **25** | 26 | 27 | 27 | 28 | 29 | 29 |
| 5'11" | 18 | 19 | 20 | 20 | 21 | 22 | 22 | 23 | 24 | 24 | **25** | 26 | 26 | 27 | 28 | 29 |
| 6'0" | 18 | 18 | 19 | 20 | 20 | 21 | 22 | 22 | 23 | 24 | 24 | **25** | 26 | 26 | 27 | 28 |
| 6'1" | 17 | 18 | 18 | 19 | 20 | 20 | 21 | 22 | 22 | 23 | 24 | 24 | **25** | 26 | 26 | 27 |
| 6'2" | 17 | 17 | 18 | 19 | 19 | 20 | 21 | 21 | 22 | 22 | 23 | 24 | 24 | **25** | 26 | 26 |
| 6'3" | 16 | 17 | 17 | 18 | 19 | 19 | 20 | 21 | 21 | 22 | 22 | 23 | 24 | 24 | **25** | 26 |
| 6'4" | 16 | 16 | 17 | 18 | 18 | 19 | 19 | 20 | 21 | 21 | 22 | 23 | 23 | 24 | 24 | **25** |

The index is calculated in kilograms and meters and can be estimated as follows. 1. Convert your weight in pounds into kilograms by multiplying it by 0.45. 2. Convert your height in inches into meters by multiplying it by 0.0254. 3. Multiply that result by itself and divide the result into your weight in kilograms.

*Sources: Shape Up America, National Institutes of Health*

blamed for putting forth a pharmacologic fix. And of course, it is lucrative: Financial analysts say the market for Xenical, which is expected to cost about $1.10 a capsule and $100 for a month's supply, could approach $1 billion a year.

Actually, Xenical is not dramatically effective; patients taking it in combination with a reduced diet lost eight pounds more, on average, than those taking dummy pills. The drug is intended for patients with a body mass index of 30, or an index of 27 if the patient also has conditions that are worsened by obesity, like high blood pressure, high cholesterol or diabetes. But doctors will be able to prescribe the drug to anyone, and Dr. David F. Williamson, who studies diabetes at the Centers for Disease Control in Atlanta, said some obesity experts worry that the Government's body mass standards will prompt interest among patients who don't really need it.

"We know that when patients advocate to their physicians that they want a drug, physicians will prescribe it," he said.

The arrival of Xenical also fits in with the broader emergence of drugs designed to enhance life rather than cure disease. The day after it was approved, the new fat-blocker took its place on Internet sites selling Viagra, the medication for impotence, and Propecia, the pill for baldness.

Unabashed promotion of Xenical comes as no surprise to Ms. Travis. But, she said: "It gives me a deep sadness. The world is a tough enough place as it is without being told that you're fat."

[SGS, May 1999]

## Scientists Unmask Diet Myth: Willpower

A thin person, the kind who has always been thin, is confronted by a chocolate cake with dark fudge icing and chopped pecans. Unmoved, he goes about his business as if nothing has happened. A fat person, the kind who has always struggled with weight, is confronted by the same cake. He feels a little surge of adrenaline. He cuts a slice and eats it. Then he eats another, and feels guilty for the rest of the day.

The simplest, and most judgmental, explanation for the difference in behavior is willpower. Some seem to have it but others do not, and the common wisdom is that they ought to get some. But to weight-loss researchers, willpower is an outdated and largely discredited concept, about as relevant to dieting as cod liver oil. And many question whether willpower even exists.

"There is no magical stuff inside of you called 'willpower' that should somehow override nature," said Dr. James C. Rosen, a professor of psychology at the University of Vermont. "It's a metaphor that most chronically overweight dieters buy into."

To attribute dieting success or failure to willpower, researchers say, is to ignore the complex interaction of brain chemicals, behavioral conditioning, hormones, heredity and the powerful influence of habits. Telling an overweight person to use willpower is, in many ways, like telling a clinically depressed person to "snap out of it."

It is possible, of course, to recover from depression and to lose weight, but neither is likely to happen simply because a person wills it, researchers say. There must be an intervention, either chemical or psychological.

The study of weight loss began in earnest in the early 1950s, when doctors and nutritionists treated overweight people by telling them to eat less. "Willpower was a kind of all-embracing theory that was used all the time to make doctors feel good and make patients feel bad," said Dr. Albert Stunkard, a professor of psychiatry at the University of Pennsylvania who has been studying weight loss for five decades.

"Most people think that willpower is just a pejorative way of describing your failures," he said. "Willpower really doesn't have any meaning." Willpower's role in weight loss was a major issue among scientists about 30 years ago, when the behavior modification movement began, Dr. Stunkard said. Until then, the existence, and importance, of willpower had been an article of faith on which most diets were founded, he said.

The behavior modification approach had its roots in a 1967 study called "Behavioral Control of Overeating," which tried to analyze the elements of "self-control" and apply them to weight loss. The study, by Richard B. Stuart of the University of Michigan, showed that eight overweight women treated with behavior modification techniques lost from 26 to 47 pounds over a year. They had frequent sessions with a therapist and recorded their food intake and moods in diaries. And the therapists helped them develop lists of alternatives to eating, like reading a newspaper or calling a friend.

"No effort is made to distinguish the historical antecedents of the problem and no assumptions are made about the personality of the overeater," Mr. Stuart wrote in his article, published in the journal *Behavioral Research and Therapy*.

After that, the focus of weight loss programs shifted toward behavioral steps a dieter takes regarding eating, said Dr. Michael R. Lowe, a professor of clinical psychology at the M.C.P. Hahnemann University in Philadelphia, and away from "something you search for within."

Behavior modification is now the most widely accepted approach to long-term weight loss. Practically, that means changing eating habits—and making new habits—by performing new behaviors. Most programs now recommend things like pausing before eating to write down what is about to be eaten, keeping a journal describing a mood just before eating and eating before a trip to the grocery store.

There is also mounting evidence that behavior affects the brain's chemical balance, and vice versa. Drugs like fenfluramine, half of the now-banned fen-phen combination, reduced a dieter's interest in eating, making willpower either irrelevant or seemingly available in pill form. And Dr. Stunkard has just com-

pleted a study that showed that people with "night-eating syndrome"—who overeat in the late evening, have trouble sleeping and get up in the middle of the night to eat—have below-normal blood levels of the hormones melatonin, leptin and cortisol.

Still, to deny the importance of willpower is to attack a fundamental notion about human character. "The concept of willpower is something that is very widely embedded in our view of ourselves," said Dr. Lowe of M.C.P. Hahnemann. "It is a major explanatory mechanism that people use to account for behavior." But Dr. Lowe said he and others viewed willpower as "essentially an explanatory fiction." Saying that someone lacks willpower "leaves people with the sense they understand why the behavior occurred, when in reality all they've done is label the behavior, not explain it." he said.

"Willpower as an independent cause of behavior is a myth," Dr. Lowe said. In his clinical practice, he takes a behavioral approach to weight control. In part, that involves counseling dieters to take a more positive attitude about their ability to lose weight. It also involves some practical steps. "Most importantly," he said, "you need to learn what behavioral steps you can take before you get in the situation where you're in the chair in front of the television with a bowl of potato chips."

It is important, he said, for dieters to keep in mind the formidable forces working against them and their so-called willpower. "We live in about the most toxic environment for weight control that you can imagine," Dr. Lowe said. "There is ready, easy availability of high-fat, high-calorie fast foods that are relatively affordable, combined with the fact that our society has become about as sedentary as a society can be."

But not all experts reject the notion of willpower. Dr. Kelly D. Brownell, director of the Yale Center for Eating and Weight Disorders, said this was the most difficult time in history for dieters, and that it would be a mistake to dismiss the willpower concept. "A person's ability to control their eating varies over time, and you cannot attribute that to biology," he said.

"There's a collective public loss of willpower because of this terrible food environment that challenges us beyond what we can tolerate," Dr. Brownell said. "One needs much more willpower now than ever before just to stay even."

All the temptations notwithstanding, thousands find a way to lose weight and keep it off, a fact demonstrated by the National Weight Control Registry, a research project that keeps tabs on people who have lost at least 30 pounds and kept the weight off for more than a year.

"A lot of times in weight loss programs, patients will say to me that they need to learn to be able to live with an apple pie in the refrigerator and not eat it," said Dr. Rena Wing, a professor of psychiatry at the University of Pittsburgh and Brown medical school, who is collaborating on the registry. Most behaviorists say dieters should instead arrange their lives so that they rarely have to confront such temptations.

"If I were to put an apple pie in front of everybody every minute of the day, I could probably break down everybody's quote-unquote willpower," she said. "We really are trying to get away from this notion of willpower. If you make certain plans, you will be able to engineer your behavior in such a way that you will look as if you have willpower."

[JF, October 1999]

## 95% Regain Lost Weight. Or Do They?

It is a depressing article of faith among the overweight and those who treat them that 95 percent of people who lose weight regain it—and sometimes more—within a few months or years. That statistic has been quoted widely over the last four decades, in Congressional hearings, diet books, research papers and seminars. And it is the reason so many people approach dieting with a sense of hopelessness.

But in fact, obesity researchers say, no one has any idea how many people can lose weight and keep it off. Now, as researchers try to determine how many people have succeeded, they are also studying the success stories for lessons that might inspire others to try. "That 95 percent figure has become clinical lore," said Dr. Thomas Wadden, a professor of psychiatry at the University of Pennsylvania. There is no basis for it, he said, "but it's part of the mythology of obesity."

Dr. Kelly D. Brownell, the director of the Yale Center for Eating and Weight Disorders, said the number was first suggested in a 1959 clinical study of only 100 people. The finding was repeated so often that it came to be regarded as fact, he said.

Since then, nearly all studies of weight-loss recidivism have followed patients in formal hospital or university programs, because they are the easiest to identify and keep track of. But people who turn to such programs may also be the most difficult cases, and may therefore have especially poor success rates.

To get a more accurate picture, two researchers are studying long-term dieters for a project called the National Weight Control Registry, and have found it surprisingly easy to collect success stories. About half the people who maintained a substantial weight loss for more than a year had done it on their own, they found. This suggests that many people have found ways to lose weight and keep it off, but have never been counted in formal studies.

"There is something very optimistic about this whole data set," said Dr. Rena Wing, a professor of psychiatry at the University of Pittsburgh and the Brown University School of Medicine. "Without much effort, we have identified 2,500 people who have succeeded."

Dr. Wing and Dr. James O. Hill of the University of Colorado are collaborating on the registry project, which they began in 1994 with financing from drug companies and other sources. They are compiling detailed histories of successful long-term dieters—people who had maintained a weight loss of at least

30 pounds for at least one year. Most of the volunteers were solicited through articles in newspapers and magazines. "It was really to convince ourselves and convince the world that there are people who are successful, and then to learn from them," Dr. Wing said. To their surprise, Dr. Wing and Dr. Hill found that on average the respondents had maintained a 67-pound weight loss for five years. Between 12 and 14 percent had maintained a loss of more than 100 pounds.

The success stories might not have been so surprising had it been clear that the 95 percent failure rate was so poorly founded. The figure comes not from any kind of random sampling, but from a study of 100 patients treated for obesity at a nutrition clinic at New York Hospital in the 1950s. In 1959, its authors, Dr. Albert Stunkard and Mavis McLaren-Hume, published a paper in which they concluded, "Most obese persons will not stay in treatment, most will not lose weight, and of those who do lose weight, most will regain it." That conclusion, Dr. Brownell of Yale said, has since become the most frequently quoted statement in obesity literature.

Dr. Stunkard, who is now a professor of psychiatry at the University of Pennsylvania, said the study was "perfectly respectable" for that period. "The paper made a big impact because everybody thought obesity was pretty easy to treat," he said. "This showed that, for whatever reason, it wasn't." But the study has little relevance to the current understanding of how to control weight, said Dr. Stunkard, who specializes in the treatment of obesity and eating disorders. The 100 patients in the study were "just given a diet and sent on their way," he said. "That was state of the art in 1959," he added. "I've been sort of surprised that people keep citing it; I know we do better these days."

The intervening years have brought significant changes to the treatment of obesity, the most important of which, Dr. Stunkard said, has been the introduction of behavior modification techniques. Since the 1959 study, though, the statistic has been reinforced by most other clinical studies, which also showed people with discouraging results.

"Unless we can prove they're typical, the data cannot be generalized," Dr. Brownell said. "The people we see in clinics tend to be more overweight and have more psychological problems. They are more likely by a factor of two to have binge-eating problems." The true failure rate could be much better, or much worse, he said. "The fact is that we just don't know."

The new research on successful dieters will disappoint those hoping for a magic-bullet solution; most had simply eaten less, and healthier, food, and exercised regularly. But judging by their accounts, it is entirely possible for people without the resources to hire personal trainers and chefs to accomplish permanent weight loss.

For inspiration, it would be difficult to surpass the story of one of the participants in the Weight Control Registry, Tammy Munson, a 32-year-old receptionist and ambulance dispatcher from Jamestown, New York, who lost 147 pounds and has kept it off for eight years.

At 5'4" tall and 185 pounds, she was overweight throughout high school, but ballooned to 253 after she graduated and got married. She knew little about nutrition, she recalled, and "didn't even realize that liquid had calories."

"I'd get up in the morning and have ice cream and cookies," Ms. Munson said. Dinner might be three or four fast-food hamburgers and candy bars. Her husband, Jeffrey, who has lost 100 pounds, was also seriously overweight. "Our wedding pictures are really funny," she said. "We broke the bed when we were first married." Ms. Munson began to face her weight problem, she said, when her blood pressure began to rise. At first she did some crash dieting, eating only about 650 calories a day.

"I read every book in the library about how to keep the weight off," she said, and eventually settled on a more balanced approach that included salads, fish, vegetable burgers, fruit and always a little dessert. And exercise. She exercises to a tape every day, jumps rope, and has begun running. In part, Ms. Munson attributes her success at least in part to the fact that she did not know success was supposedly impossible.

"You've got to find it for yourself," she said. "And don't spend money on it. You can get it for free. You can get it from reading. It's just the food pyramid, but people don't want to hear it. Slimfast, Optifast, you can't live like that forever. You eat a lot of good stuff and a little bad stuff, and you'll be fine, but you've got to have the little bad stuff, too."

The experience of Russell M. Lomando, 47, of Brooklyn, was less dramatic, but probably more typical of the people in the study. "I was 39 years old and I was walking up the train stairs in Brooklyn huffing and puffing," he said. "I could see myself going into the grave when I was 40." He used to eat, he said, "pounds of junk—doughnuts and cookies and cakes, and I'm talking boxes at a time." One day, climbing the subway stairs, Mr. Lomando made up his mind to cut out the junk, but gradually.

At first, he was able to do it only four days a week; he worked up to seven over a period of months. He took up karate for exercise, and over two years lost 50 pounds, getting his weight down to 160. "You just have to change your life-style," he said. "You just have to have the willpower to do it." But that is not necessarily easy, he conceded. "You just have to weigh the choices. Do you want to become healthier?"

[JF, May 1999]

## Just How Perilous Can 25 Extra Pounds Be?

A recent report linking moderate overweight and modest weight gain to an increased risk of death in midlife threw millions of American women into a tizzy. Even those who have accepted their ample bodies or middle-aged spread and who scoff at fashion-model thinness were alarmed to learn that those 25 pounds they put on since high school or the extra weight they had carried all their lives might kill them.

While there is no debate about the risks to health and life associated with frank obesity, defined as weighing at least 30 percent more than is desirable for one's height and frame, moderately overweight people have long assumed that their main concern was a cosmetic one. Now, it seems, they should be more worried about their health and life expectancy than about how they look.

Based on the new findings from a 16-year study of 115,000 female nurses and similar findings from a continuing study of 19,000 men who graduated from Harvard, about 300,000 deaths a year in this country can be attributed to overweight. This projection, made by the study's principal author, Dr. JoAnn E. Manson of Brigham and Women's Hospital and Harvard Medical School in Boston, may even be a conservative one, since the women and men being studied are better educated, more affluent and pre-sumably more health-aware than the average American, and are therefore likely to have lower death rates.

Furthermore, most of the women in the nurses' study have yet to reach the age when heart disease, the health problem most powerfully influenced by overweight, emerges as the leading killer. At the time the data were analyzed, the women's ages ranged from 46 to 71 and cancer was their main cause of death. Dr. Manson said she was astonished to discover that nearly one-third of the 2,586 deaths from cancer—especially cancers of the breast, colon and endometrium—could be attributed to overweight.

The new study examined two questions: the risks from gaining weight (22 pounds or more) after the age of 18 and the risks related to being heavier than the leanest women. Among women who had never smoked, those who weighed about 15 percent less than the average American woman of the same height were least likely to die during the study. For example, the average American woman is 5'5" tall and weighs 150 to 160 pounds, which the new study suggests is about 30 pounds too many to maximize one's chances of living to a healthy old age. Those who weighed less than 120 had the lowest death rates, but chances of an early death were 20 percent higher among those who weighed 120 to 150 pounds and 30 percent higher among those who weighed 150 to 160 pounds. In other words, even women of average weight and those mildly overweight have higher death rates than the leanest women.

Although previous studies have concluded that the leanest men and women have higher death risks than those slightly heavier, most of these studies did not separate former smokers from people who had never smoked and some did not take into account the possibility that an undiagnosed illness might have accounted for thinness in many of the people who died during the studies.

In the new study, which took account of those factors, at greater weights, the risks of "dying prematurely," or sooner than the leanest women, jumped more dramatically—by 60 percent among those 5'5" inches tall and weighing 161 to 175 pounds; by 110 percent among those weighing 176 to 195 pounds, and by 120 percent among those weighing more than 195 pounds.

Similar risks were found among women who gained weight as adults. Compared with those who gained less than 10 pounds after age 18, those who gained 22 to 40 pounds experienced a 70 percent increase in cardiovascular deaths and a 20 percent increase in cancer deaths. Those gaining more than 40 pounds were seven times as likely to die of heart disease during the study and 50 percent more likely to die of cancer.

What do such numbers mean to the millions of Americans whose college blazers no longer meet in the middle? First, it is helpful to realize that a woman's risk of dying in midlife is not great. Heart disease is not a common occurrence among women under 65, so even a sevenfold increase in cardiac deaths for a woman in her 50s is still a low risk of dying. Of the 4,726 deaths that occurred among the nurses, only 881 were due to cardiovascular disease. Cancer, on the other hand, is the leading killer of middle-aged women—there were 2,586 cancer deaths during the study—so even a relatively small increase in risk can be meaningful. Keep in mind, too, that the study measured deaths, not incidence of disease; far more women are likely to have been afflicted with weight-related illnesses than to have died as a result.

## Healthy Weight Ranges for Men and Women

Draft guidelines submitted by an advisory committee to the Department of Health and Human Services and the Department of Agriculture; the ranges apply to men and women of all ages and no longer allow for a 15-pound gain in middle-age. The higher weight ranges apply to people with more muscle and bone in proportion to body fat.

| HEIGHT (without shoes) | WEIGHT (without clothing) |
|---|---|
| 4'10" | 91–119 |
| 4'11" | 94–124 |
| 5'0" | 97–128 |
| 5'2" | 101–132 |
| 5'3" | 104–137 |
| 5'4" | 111–146 |
| 5'5" | 114–150 |
| 5'6" | 118–155 |
| 5'7" | 121–160 |
| 5'8" | 125–164 |
| 5'9" | 129–169 |
| 5'10" | 132–174 |
| 5'11" | 136–179 |
| 6'0" | 140–184 |
| 6'1" | 144–189 |
| 6'2" | 148–195 |
| 6'3" | 152–200 |
| 6'4" | 156–205 |
| 6'5" | 160–211 |
| 6'6" | 164–216 |

Furthermore, a small increase in the risk of disease and death among the mildly overweight is likely to mean more to society at large than to each individual. A 20 percent increase in premature deaths, and an even greater increase in nonfatal illness, occurring among more than 100 million middle-aged adults adds up to a lot of lost years of productive life and some very big medical bills for society to absorb. But to slightly pudgy individuals, a 20 percent increase in risk may not seem like much, because their risk is low to begin with.

Do not panic. If you have put on a dozen or more pounds since high school but still weigh within a desirable range (less than the equivalent of 150 pounds for a 5'5" woman or man), the increase in your risk of premature death is quite small and may not warrant any attention to the actual numbers on the scale as long as you adopt health-promoting living habits and do not smoke. Dr. Tim Byers, a preventive medicine specialist at the University of Colorado School of Medicine in Denver, said: "I would worry less about body weight and more about behaviors like food choices and physical activity. If a person is eating a diet low in fat and rich in vegetables, fruits and whole grains, being moderately overweight is less likely to have adverse consequences."

If, however, you are more than moderately overweight, even if you have not gained since age 18, your risk of an early death is substantially increased and attention to actual poundage is warranted. This does not mean going on a crash diet, swallowing formulas or taking pills and potions purported to promote weight loss. Rather, it involves adopting an eating and exercise plan that you can stay on for the rest of your life.

Scores of studies have clearly demonstrated that people are more likely to lose weight and keep it off on a diet that is low in fat, moderate in protein and high in fiber-rich foods like unrefined starches, fruits and vegetables. High-fiber foods are filling and satisfying and are less likely to lead to overeating than when people eat high-fat foods.

Add exercise to the equation and you will burn more calories during workouts and between them as well. Most long-term studies have shown that without regular exercise, few people are able to keep off lost pounds. Furthermore, even if you lose no weight through exercise, increasing your activity level can diminish your risk of developing several leading killer diseases, especially heart disease, hypertension, diabetes and some cancers.

[JEB, September 1995]

## Gaining Weight on Sugar-Free, Fat-Free Diets

Why, with the abundance of artificially sweetened, low-fat and nonfat foods now widely available, do Americans continue to get fatter and fatter? And why, with the endless stream of popular diets and weight-loss plans, do Americans repeatedly fail at losing weight and keeping it off? If you know the answers to these questions, you have already taken the first step toward permanent weight control. If you don't know, I'll tell you.

We only think we're eating carefully by choosing sugar-free or fat-free foods. Most fat-free foods have nearly as many calories as their full-fat counterparts. One-half cup of fat-free pudding, 140 calories; regular, 160. Five fat-free soda crackers, 50 calories; regular, 60. One ounce of fat-free pretzels, 110 calories; regular, 110. Furthermore, most people fail to note the portion size that supplies the specified number of calories, or they think they can have double the amount they usually eat because the food is fat-free.

Calories always count, whether they come from fat, sugar, starch or protein. Read the nutrition information on the label of all packaged foods to know what you are eating and determine the appropriate portion.

Despite the popularity of artificial sweeteners, Americans continue to increase their consumption of caloric sweeteners. Since 1970, annual per capita consumption of sugar and other caloric sweeteners has risen by nearly 30 pounds. Artificial sweeteners merely feed the desire for the real thing.

While the percentage of calories from fat we consume per person has fallen, from about 42 percent to 34 percent, we now consume about 10 pounds of added fats and oils more than we did in 1970. Consumption of cheese is also way up, thanks to our passion for pizza, cheeseburgers, tacos and the like. The percentage of calories from fat has declined only because we are consuming more calories. Will artificial fats help this picture? Judging from the effects of artificial sweeteners, I think not.

Home cooking, where the cook knows exactly what is in each dish, has fallen off sharply. More than 40 percent of the American food dollar is now spent on foods eaten out. Restaurant portions are typically two or more times larger than they should be, and they are often loaded with hidden calories. When 203 dietitians were asked to estimate the calorie and fat content of five restaurant meals, they were often way off. They guessed that a hamburger and onion rings would provide 863 calories and 44 grams of fat when the meal contained 1,550 calories and 101 grams of fat. They thought a tuna salad sandwich had 374 calories and 18 grams of fat when the displayed sandwich actually contained 720 calories and 43 grams of fat. If a trained food specialist cannot tell what's in foods eaten out, how can you?

Consumption of snack foods continues to rise, with new high-calorie snacks luring consumers away from more nutritious and lower caloric alternatives like fruit or yogurt. One Mrs. Field's oatmeal raisin walnut cookie has 240 calories; one Au Bon Pain blueberry muffin, 430 calories; one Starbucks cinnamon scone, 530 calories.

What should we eat? You know the answer: lots of fruits and vegetables and grain-based foods rich in fiber, vitamins and minerals and low in calories, fleshed out with modest amounts of animal pro-

## Is It Worth It?

Here are the minutes of exercise (or rest) needed to burn off calories in various foods.

MINUTES OF ACTIVITY NEEDED
(based on person weighing 154 pounds)

| FOOD | CALORIES SUPPLIED | RECLINING (**1.3** calories per minute) | WALKING (**5.2**) | BIKE RIDING (**8.2**) | SWIMMING (**11.2**) | RUNNING (**19.4**) |
|---|---|---|---|---|---|---|
| Chicken, TV dinner | **542** | 417 min. | 104 | 66 | 48 | 28 |
| Malted milk shake | **502** | 386 | 97 | 61 | 45 | 26 |
| Spaghetti (one serving) | **396** | 305 | 76 | 48 | 35 | 20 |
| Hamburger sandwich | **350** | 269 | 67 | 43 | 31 | 18 |
| Fried chicken (1/2 breast) | **232** | 178 | 45 | 28 | 21 | 12 |
| Doughnut | **151** | 116 | 29 | 18 | 13 | 8 |
| Pancake with syrup | **124** | 95 | 24 | 15 | 11 | 6 |
| Orange juice (8 oz.) | **120** | 92 | 23 | 15 | 11 | 6 |
| Beer (8 oz.) | **114** | 88 | 22 | 14 | 10 | 6 |
| Fried egg | **110** | 85 | 21 | 13 | 10 | 6 |
| Potato chips (10 chips) | **108** | 83 | 21 | 13 | 10 | 6 |
| Apple | **101** | 78 | 19 | 12 | 9 | 5 |
| Bacon (2 strips) | **96** | 74 | 18 | 12 | 9 | 5 |
| Raw carrot | **42** | 32 | 8 | 5 | 4 | 2 |

*Source: Journal of the American Dietetic Association*

tein—four-ounce portions of well-trimmed meat, skinless poultry or fish—and low-fat and nonfat dairy foods. Not only would such a diet reduce caloric intake, it would also significantly reduce the risk of developing a long list of chronic, often fatal diseases, including heart disease and many cancers.

Virtually every fad diet, especially those that rely on formulas, drugs, and restricted food groups or combinations of foods, ultimately fails, regardless of initial enthusiasm and weight loss. The trick is not in losing but in maintaining the loss, not for a year or two, but forever. This requires a diet that you can go on and stay on for the rest of your life.

While following a fad for two weeks may help you get started, the route to permanent weight control demands that you soon adopt an eating plan that can be followed indefinitely. That means it must be complete in essential nutrients, rich in fiber and designed to preserve your lean body mass—muscle and bone—while you lose fat. If you restrict carbohydrates, your body will use more muscle to meet its energy needs. Your eating plan should also offer variety and fit your life, whether you eat at home or in restaurants, travel a lot or entertain often.

Many people are unaware of what and how much they eat and would benefit greatly from keeping a food diary for a week or two, recording quantities of everything they eat and drink. It should soon be obvious where the extra calories are coming from and what changes are needed to lose weight. Keep in mind that all fats and oils have about the same number of calories—120 per tablespoon—and that starch-es, sugars and proteins have less than half that (a tablespoon of sugar, for example, has about 48 calories). Also, water has no calories, and every sensible weight-loss regimen urges followers to drink eight cups of water a day.

No more than a small percentage of successful dieters make it without exercise. Physical activity is crucial to preserving muscle while losing fat and to shedding health-damaging abdominal excess. Exercise also partly compensates for the metabolic slowdown that occurs when caloric intake is reduced and pounds are lost. You may expect exercise to stimulate hunger, but more often it does the opposite. Furthermore, dieters who continue to exercise after reaching their weight goal are more likely to keep the lost pounds off.

Make regular exercise a permanent part of your life. As a calorie burner, every form of exercise counts, from gardening and dog walking to strength training and jogging. To minimize boredom, it helps to have several active options.

If you've been sedentary for some time, start slowly and focus on consistency at first. Then gradually increase the duration, intensity and frequency of your activities. If possible, build up to doing one or two high-intensity workouts each week. If you are already active though overweight, try to extend your current workout or add a new activity to your routine. Last winter was the first in decades that my weight did not creep up because I added a daily three-mile walk to my other activities.

[JEB, June 1998]

## Doubts Fail to Deter "The Diet Revolution"

It was the early 1970s, the heyday of mini-skirts and quick weight-loss schemes, when fashion magazines and celebrity dieters propelled Dr. Robert C. Atkins's "diet revolution" into a national phenomenon. His book, *Dr. Atkins' Diet Revolution*, promoted a high-fat, high-protein diet spurning most carbohydrates. Many nutritionists and public health experts were dismayed, but 10 million Americans were undeterred. Their reliance on labor-saving devices and fast foods had spawned thunder thighs and rendered their waistlines a thing of the past. They made the book a bestseller.

But the Atkins scheme was neither new nor revolutionary then or in 1992 when he published his "new diet revolution"—now enjoying a resurgence of popularity among weight-conscious, meat-loving men and women seeking a quick route to a slimmer summer. More than five million copies of the paperback version are in print, and it was just ranked the second-leading best seller over the last five years by *USA Today*.

The basic diet Dr. Atkins advocated was first promulgated in the 1860s by William Banting, an English casket maker whose best-selling book, *Letter on Corpulence*, outlined a low-carbohydrate, high-protein diet. It became so popular that his countrymen began using "banting" as a synonym for losing weight, notes Laura Fraser in *Losing It: False Hopes and Fat Profits in the Diet Industry*.

There were many spinoffs—among them, Dr. Alfred Pennington's 1940 low-carbohydrate, high-fat diet, Dr. Herman Taller's 1961 *Calories Don't Count* high-fat, high-protein, low-carbohydrate diet and Dr. Irwin Stillman's strictly carnivorous *The Doctor's Quick Weight-Loss Diet*, which allowed only lean meat, poultry, eggs and low-fat cheeses.

Having been raised on shredded wheat, oatmeal, challah, Jewish rye and bagels, I was not one to be seduced by such schemes. Whenever I stop eating bagels, I dream about them. And by the time the Atkins diet surfaced, I had already shed 35 pounds and found my way to a permanent size 4 or 6 through sensible eating with occasional splurges and regular exercise.

Others I knew who succumbed to the high-fat program were less than enthralled with the results. One colleague's cholesterol level soared to over 700 milligrams after four weeks on the Atkins plan, and her doctor threatened to hospitalize her if she did not go off it immediately. Another woman told me: "No wonder you lose weight on this diet. I'm nauseous practically all the time." A third abandoned the diet when she became so weak she could hardly do her work, let alone exercise. A fourth lost 12 pounds in a month, but although he loves meat, he soon got fed up with the diet ("what's a cheeseburger without a bun?") and has since gained it back.

There has been no published study showing long-term success with the Atkins scheme. In an interview, Dr. Atkins said, "No one has ever done a study of long-term results. There has never been anyone willing or able to fund a study." He said his Center for Complementary Medicine would soon underwrite a study of 50 healthy, obese people to be conducted by a Duke University researcher who will assess the diet's effects on cholesterol and other blood lipids.

Despite any documentation of the diet's long-term results or safety, it now seems as if every third person is trying the "new" diet, having heard of people who shed 10, 20 or even 40 pounds eating all the steak, eggs, cheese, butter and cream they wanted. Since fat is the most fattening, it is reasonable to ask how a person can lose weight eating so many high-fat foods.

The answer is simple. You can lose weight on any diet that restricts the kinds or amounts of foods you can eat or the frequency with which you eat them. The Atkins diet does not allow bread, cake, ice cream, candy and cookies, or potatoes, rice, pasta, cereals, grains, milk, yogurt, fruits and many vegetables. For the first two weeks you can eat no more than 20 grams of carbohydrates a day—the amount in two-thirds of a small bagel or half a cup of rice or 12 ounces of fat-free yogurt. Because carbohydrates hold water in the body, as your body becomes depleted of stored carbohydrates, the first five pounds or so you lose on this plan is not fat weight but water, quickly regained with the first starchy food eaten.

The strict two-week "induction" diet is followed by an "ongoing weight loss" diet that includes slightly more vegetables and a few fruits like strawberries (with cream, of course), but still no starchy foods, milk or yogurt. The entire plan capitalizes on two facts:

▶ Because fats are digested more slowly than carbohydrates, dieters do not get as hungry between meals.
▶ Few people can eat endless amounts of animal protein and fat for weeks on end and so they eat less and less.

If you eat less than you did before going on a diet, you will lose weight regardless of the diet.

The Atkins plan suffers from the same limits that afflict every diet that requires people to eat in peculiar ways: a diet is something people go on to go off, and when they go off a diet, they often regain the weight they lost and then some. The late Dr. Jean Mayer, a noted nutritionist and former president of Tufts University, called the syndrome "the rhythm method of girth control."

The Atkins plan strives to put dieters into an abnormal metabolic state called ketosis, which occurs when the body burns fats for fuel in the absence of carbohydrates. Substances called ketones accumulate in the blood, and can cause bad breath, constipation, nausea and lightheadedness. Furthermore, in trying to get rid of ketones, the body excretes sodium and potassium, and that can result in dehydration and abnormal heart rhythms.

The diet is seriously short of essential nutrients, especially calcium (and its excess of protein causes the body to lose what little calcium it gets), vita-

## Dr. Atkins Responds:

Jane Brody in her Personal Health column continues to attack the Atkins diet ("Doubts Fail to Deter 'The Diet Revolution'") despite 40 years of positive clinical experience and hundreds of publications supporting the diet's safety and efficacy.

As a practicing cardiologist, my work is based on helping patients. What motivates Ms. Brody's hostility? She does a disservice to millions who lead healthier lives on my program and to many more who continue to embrace unproductive dietary programs thanks to misinformation of the sort propagated by Ms. Brody.

Typical of Ms. Brody's disregard for facts, she cites four dieters who failed on the diet, ignoring millions who have been leading healthy lives on the Atkins protocol for years.

I can appreciate the difficulty people have in understanding how a dietary philosophy dependent upon protein and fat can be healthy since our culture besieges us with the message that low-fat/high-carb foods are the key to healthy living. But, it is time for mainstream journalists and medical associations to acknowledge the truth, even if it jeopardizes advertising and financial support for "research" from food and pharmaceutical companies.

Jane Brody herself acknowledges that low-fat diets may be failing. The low-fat approach to dieting promoted by the American Heart Association and others is creating an obesity epidemic. In the decade through 1995, the per capita percentage of daily calories of fat fell from 40 to 33 percent. In that same time span, significant obesity rose from 25 to 33 percent (20 million new cases).

Furthermore, many claim that the Atkins diet is bad for the heart. Compelling evidence points in the opposite direction. In fact, the principal cause of "bad" cholesterol is excessive carbohydrate consumption.

Another criticism of the Atkins diet is that ketosis, the process by which the body burns fat for fuel, is harmful. In fact, research indicates that brain tissue may even prefer ketones to glucose, generated by carbohydrate consumption, as a source of fuel. The misconception that ketosis is dangerous stems from confusing ketosis and ketoacidosis, which occurs when a diabetic's blood sugar is out of control. Hundreds of publications on ketosis would have been readily available to Ms. Brody had she done a search of the medical literature.

She says that the Atkins diet is unbalanced when it is one of the most nutritious eating philosophies, providing a healthful level of highly nutrient-dense foods, calcium sources and vegetables.

Finally, some articles claim that the Atkins diet works because it is a low-calorie diet. If many Atkins dieters are eating fewer calories, it is only because they are less hungry and less obsessed with food. Stable blood sugar throughout the day, a cornerstone of the Atkins diet, insures fewer food cravings or false hunger pains.

Furthermore, food on the Atkins diet is less processed and more nutritious than typical pre-Atkins diets. Give the body fewer empty calories, provide it with more nutrient-dense alternatives, and the body will logically be satisfied sooner and require less food.

Dr. Robert C. Atkins
New York, June 1, 1999

mins C and D and folic acid. To combat the problem, Dr. Atkins recommends supplements, although not including a significant amount of calcium.

You may also wonder whether it is safe to be on a diet that is riddled with saturated fats and cholesterol and nearly devoid of the fruits, vegetables and whole grains which have been shown to be vital to good health. Dr. Kevin Vigilante, a public health specialist, and Dr. Mary Flynn, a nutritionist, both of Brown University, summed up the prevailing view in their new book *Low-Fat Lies, High Fat Frauds, and the Healthiest Diet in the World*. They wrote, "The Atkins diet is potentially so dangerous that the Surgeon General should probably put a warning on every book Dr. Robert Atkins sells. The diet's only salvation is that people can't tolerate it for very long—not long enough for the increase in the risk of heart disease or cancer that long-term use of such a diet could bring."

Two other currently popular schemes—the "Zone" diet and the "Sugar Busters" diet—are also hard on carbohydrates but less rigid than the Atkins plan. Dr. Barry Sears, a biotechnologist who wrote *Enter the Zone*, rightly includes just enough carbohydrates in his diet to avoid ketosis.

But the theory behind the Zone diet—that insulin insensitivity is the cause of obesity when people eat a diet relatively rich in starchy foods and sugars—has been found wanting by biochemists, who point out that it is obesity that causes insulin insensitivity, not the other way around.

The fact remains that no matter what people eat, it is calories that ultimately count. Eat more calories than your body uses and you will gain weight. Eat fewer calories and you will lose weight. The body, which is after all nothing more than a biochemical machine, knows no other arithmetic.

[JEB, May 1999]

## New Look at Dieting: Fat Can Be a Friend

Now hear this: Avocados, walnuts, salad dressings with oil, sauteed vegetables, fatty fish and some kinds of margarine may be back on the menu for health-conscious Americans, even for those trying to lose weight, if the findings of recent studies are to be believed.

For three decades now, Americans have been bombarded with advice to eat less fat for the sake of their hearts and their waistlines. One well-known expert, Dr. Dean Ornish, advocates stripping away all added fats and naturally fatty foods to achieve a diet containing no more than 10 percent of calories from fat, down from the 44 percent typically consumed by Americans in the 1960s and the 34 percent now consumed.

But now a growing number of nutrition, health and obesity specialists maintain that in trying to squeeze some of the heart-damaging grease from our high-fat diets, they have sent Americans the wrong message.

It's not fat per se that's the problem, the experts now say, but the kinds of fats Americans eat and the other kinds of foods they fill up on when they cut back on appetite-satisfying fat. For while heart disease has indeed declined as many Americans shun artery-clogging saturated fats and cholesterol, waistlines have expanded significantly and obesity has risen by 50 percent since the big push to limit fat took off in the 1970s.

The very tactic viewed as the key to weight control—stripping the diet of fat—seems to have backfired. Food companies responded to fat phobia with a plethora of fat-free, low-fat and reduced-fat products, especially the dessert and snack foods that Americans covet. The result was an overdose of carbohydrates, ranging from fat-free pretzels, crackers, cookies, cakes and frozen desserts to dinner plates piled high with pasta.

Many obesity specialists, as well as popular diet

advocates like Dr. Robert C. Atkins and Barry Sears, say these carbohydrates are the cause of the growing American girth. Even the potato, which once proclaimed "I am not fattening" in award-winning ads, now heads the hit list being circulated by carbohydrate bashers, some of whom, like Dr. Atkins, go to the opposite extreme by recommending that people can lose weight by eating all the fat they want as long as they eat few or no carbohydrates.

"The swing back to Atkins is a response to the fact that a low-fat diet hasn't worked for a lot of people because they stuff in carbohydrates," said Dr. Margo Denke, an associate professor of medicine and endocrinology at the University of Texas Southwestern Medical Center in Dallas.

Dr. Alice H. Lichtenstein, a professor of nutrition at Tufts University in Boston, agrees that "the low-fat pendulum swung too far."

"People assumed that if a food had no fat, they could eat as much of it as they wanted," she said. "But many low-fat and fat-free products have nearly as many calories as their full-fat versions. Reducing fat alone is no guarantee of weight loss. You must cut calories or increase physical activity."

Dr. Denke said, "No matter what anyone tells you, it's calories that count. Carefully controlled metabolic studies show that it doesn't matter where extra calories come from. Eat more calories than you expend and you'll gain weight."

And that is just what Americans have been doing: gaining weight on fat-free and low-fat foods consumed without regard to their caloric content. Instead of replacing some of the less desirable high-fat foods with nutrient-rich but low-calorie fruits and vegetables, they are filling up on foods loaded with added sugars and refined starches that have little to offer nutritionally besides calories, the experts lament.

"In making food choices, we must learn to eat foods that are nutritionally robust—fruits, vegetables, legumes," said Dr. Robert H. Eckel, chairman of the American Heart Association's nutrition committee and professor of medicine and physiology at the University of Colorado. "There is strong evidence that these kinds of foods help to reduce disease, not just heart disease but also cancer, diabetes, hypertension and obesity."

A survey of American consumers, however, conducted in 1997 by the Food Marketing Institute, revealed that 56 percent of shoppers who had changed their diets did so by trying to cut down on the amount of fat they consumed, but only 15 percent said they were trying to eat more fruits and vegetables.

Even people with high cholesterol levels may not need to go to fat-reduction extremes to protect their hearts. A study of 444 men with high LDL cholesterol conducted by Dr. Robert H. Knopp and colleagues at the University of Washington in Seattle showed that reducing total fat to 30 percent of calories from 35 percent and keeping saturated fats at 7 percent to 8 percent was as effective in lowering cholesterol as diets with less total fat. In fact, when fat intake dropped to about 20 percent of calories, heart-protective HDL cholesterol levels fell and heart-damaging triglyceride levels rose. Study participants had no difficulty sticking to a 30 percent fat diet, whereas more stringent diets require a dedication that most Americans lack.

There is also growing evidence that regardless of what else it may contain, a weight-loss diet devoid of fat may be counterproductive, leaving dieters perpetually hungry or unsatisfied and susceptible to overeating when their resolve fails. Dr. Mary Flynn, a nutritionist affiliated with Brown University, addresses this issue in a book written with Dr. Kevin Vigilante, also of Brown, *Low-Fat Lies, High-Fat Frauds, and the Healthiest Diet in the World*.

"A little fat helps you lose weight," the book notes. "Fat makes food taste good, and it makes you feel full. Taste is vital to the success of any diet. Without a little fat you're always going to be hungry. The key is to eat the right kind of fat, in the right amounts. You need a diet you can live with."

A study of 12 obese boys published in March 1999 in the journal *Pediatrics* showed that meals with refined carbohydrates and little fat were less effective in staving off hunger than fattier meals with the same caloric content. Dr. David Ludwig of Harvard Medical School and Children's Hospital in Boston concluded from these findings that substituting processed grains like cereals, bread and pasta for dietary fat may be making Americans fatter.

Fat in the diet also seems to play a psychological role that helps some people keep their caloric intake in check. In a study at Pennsylvania State University, normal-weight women given yogurts with various fat contents ate more at the next meal if they were told the yogurt was fat-free than if they thought they had eaten a high-fat yogurt. Likewise, people given fat-free potato chips ate less fat than those given regular chips, but over the course of a day, both groups consumed the same number of calories.

By the fall of 1999, Dr. Eckel said, the heart association is expected to issue revised dietary guidelines that will de-emphasize fat as a percent of calories in the diet, except as it figures in obesity, but will continue to recommend upper limits on saturated fats. For the last two decades, the association has recommended that healthy people limit their fat intake to 30 percent of calories, with saturated fat—the kind that is hard at room temperature—no more than 10 percent, polyunsaturates less than 10 percent and the rest from monounsaturates, which are plentiful in olive and canola oils and avocados.

"Within the current American eating pattern, it's probably wise to stay at a maximum of 30 percent of calories from fat," Dr. Lichtenstein said. "If we go above that, Americans tend to increase their consumption of saturated fats in meats. Maybe if we adopted a Mediterranean diet—rich in vegetables and fish and olive oil—we could go higher than 30 per-

## Giving Some Fats a Chance

Not all fats need be avoided, but they must be chosen wisely. Research has shown that unsaturated fats like olive oil and fish oils offer protection against heart disease and some other serious illnesses. Saturated fats, however, have long been associated with increased rates of disease, particularly heart disease.

| | SATURATED FAT | POLYUNSATURATED FAT | MONOUNSATURATED FAT |
|---|---|---|---|
| Canola Oil | 6% | 36% | 58% |
| Safflower oil | 9 | 78 | 13 |
| Sunflower oil | 11 | 69 | 20 |
| Avocado oil | 12 | 14 | 74 |
| Corn oil | 13 | 62 | 25 |
| Olive oil | 15 | 11 | 73 |
| Soybean oil | 15 | 61 | 24 |
| Peanut oil | 18 | 34 | 48 |
| Cottonseed oil | 27 | 54 | 19 |
| Lard | 41 | 12 | 47 |
| Palm oil | 51 | 10 | 39 |
| Beef tallow | 52 | 4 | 44 |
| Butter fat | 66 | 4 | 3 |
| Coconut oil | 92 | 2 | 6 |

*Source: United States Department of Agriculture*

cent fat without compromising our health, but it's important to remember that the Mediterraneans' low rate of heart disease is not just the result of a diet rich in olive oil. It's a life-style that is far more active than ours and that doesn't contain all the bizarre foods we have."

Extreme reductions in dietary fat can deprive the body of vital nutrients that play a crucial role in health. Dietary fat transports the fat-soluble vitamins A, D, E and K. Unsaturated fat from vegetable and seafood sources supplies the body with essential fatty acids needed to produce nerve cells and hormones.

There is also growing evidence that unsaturated fatty acids help protect people from serious diseases. For example, studies in Spain, Italy, Greece, Sweden and the United States linked diets rich in olive oil to a reduced risk of breast cancer. The brain, too, may benefit from monounsaturates like olive oil. A study published in May 1999 in the journal *Neurology* by Italian researchers found that a high intake of extra-virgin olive oil was associated with preservation of cognitive functions in healthy elderly people.

The ongoing Nurses Health Study revealed that among 80,000 women initially aged 34 to 59, total fat consumption did not affect coronary risk, but the kinds of fats the women ate did. Each 5 percent increase in calories from saturated fats (primarily from meats and dairy products) raised their risk of coronary disease by 17 percent.

An even greater risk was posed by trans fatty acids, which are formed when unsaturated vegetable oils are hydrogenated to make them solid at room temperature, for example, to form margarine. Each 2 percent increase in trans fat calories raised the women's coronary risk by 93 percent. A number of margarines free of harmful trans fat are now available.

Polyunsaturates and particularly omega-3 fatty acids like fish oils, on the other hand, appear to protect against heart disease, especially sudden cardiac death. Fish oils have been shown to reduce the risk of blood clots and abnormal heart rhythms and improve blood cholesterol and triglyceride levels. Studies in the Netherlands and in the United States have indicated that eating just two fish meals, or seven ounces of fish, a week can reduce a man's risk of heart attack by 50 percent.

Another type of omega-3 fatty acid called alpha-linolenic acid, found prominently in canola oil, flaxseeds, soybean oil, walnuts and many dark green leafy vegetables, also appears to offer strong protection against sudden cardiac death, according to a new study by Dr. Frank Hu and associates at Harvard School of Public Health. Among 76,000 participants in the Nurses Health Study, those with the highest intake of alpha-linolenic acid had up to a 50 percent lower risk of fatal heart attacks when compared with women who consumed the least amount of this fat.

"People who choose fat-free salad dressings are missing out on this important fatty acid," Dr. Hu said. "Fat has been perceived as the enemy, but that's not true. Some fats are good, some fats are bad. We should be substituting good fats for bad ones rather than worrying about reducing the total amount of fat."

[JEB, May 1999]

## F.D.A. Approves Fat-Blocking Anti-Obesity Drug

Until recently, Americans looking for a pill to help them lose weight have had only one option: appetite suppressants. That changed when the Food and Drug Administration approved the first in a new class of anti-obesity drugs that work by blocking the body's absorption of dietary fat, as opposed to tricking the brain into ignoring hunger.

The drug, orlistat, by Hoffman-LaRoche of Nutley, New Jersey, was approved for seriously overweight people who meet the Government's definition of obese—30 percent overweight—and for people who are 20 percent overweight and have high blood pressure, high cholesterol or diabetes, conditions that are exacerbated by obesity. At 5'5" tall, a person would weigh 180 pounds and 160 pounds, respectively, to fit those criteria.

But doctors will be able to prescribe orlistat for anyone. The midnight-blue capsules are to appear on pharmacy shelves in the next few weeks under the trade name Xenical. And despite concerns by some about its effectiveness, experts said today that the drug might soon become a familiar fixture in the medicine cabinets of millions of Americans. It will not be cheap: the drug is recommended for use three times a day, for periods of a year or longer, and the company says it expects to charge around $1.10 per capsule.

It is hard to overestimate the interest of Americans in losing weight, said Dr. David F. Williamson of the Centers for Disease Control and Prevention, an epidemiologist who studies diabetes and who has written about the drug, "I predict a brisk trade in this drug."

Experts were quick to say orlistat is hardly a panacea for obesity, and in clinical trials the drug helped obese people lose only modest amounts of weight. In one year, most patients experienced weight loss ranging from 5 percent to 10 percent of their initial body weight, the company said. And that was in combination with a reduced calorie diet. "This is not a magic bullet," said Dr. Eric Colman, the F.D.A. medical officer who reviewed the drug.

Although some weight-loss experts said that they were eager to begin prescribing orlistat, especially in combination with approved appetite suppressants, others criticized the agency's decision. "I'm sorry this drug was approved," said Dr. Jules Hirsch, an obesity expert at Rockefeller University in Manhattan.

Although the drug is on the market in 17 countries, and has been prescribed to a million people worldwide, an agency advisory panel of independent experts split 5 to 5 last year on the question of whether the drug should be marketed here. "This drug caused a 4 percent difference in body weight between placebo and the drug itself," said Dr. Hirsch, a panel member who voted against approval. "That means a 200-pound person might lose 8 pounds."

In one experiment, reported in January 1999 in the *Journal of the American Medical Association*, patients who took orlistat and followed a weight loss diet for one year lost an average of 19.3 pounds, while those who followed the same diet and took a dummy pill lost 12.8 pounds. After the year was up, some of those taking orlistat began to gain weight even as they continued to take the drug. It was not known what the long-term effects of taking the drug would be.

In seven clinical trials involving more than 7,000 patients worldwide, those who took orlistat also showed "measurable improvements" in high blood pressure, high cholesterol and diabetes, Hoffman-LaRoche said. But Dr. Hirsch said the changes "were very small, and we are not assured that such small changes are necessarily beneficial."

Orlistat works in the gastrointestinal tract, blocking an enzyme that is needed to digest fat. Instead of being digested, a third of the fat a person eats will accumulate in the intestines and be excreted in the stool. But by blocking fat absorption, the drug also blocks absorption of the fat-soluble vitamins A, D, E and K, as well as beta-carotene, and so patients must take daily vitamin supplements.

Orlistat can also cause unpleasant side effects, like bloating, flatulence, oily stool, diarrhea and fecal incontinence, that tend to discourage patients from eating fatty foods. "If patients eat a big fat meal—a pizza and a milkshake—they will pay for it in a day or two," said Dr. Richard Atkinson, professor of medicine and nutritional sciences at the University of Wisconsin.

There are also lingering fears about whether the drug might be linked to breast cancer. In data Hoffman-LaRoche submitted to the food and drug agency last year, women who took orlistat experienced slightly more breast cancer than those who did not. But the agency said today that additional data from the company showed that the risk of breast cancer was "not a real concern."

Orlistat is the second diet drug to receive the food and drug agency's imprimatur since July 1997, when fenfluramine and its close cousin, dexfenfluramine, were removed from the market. Those drugs, along with another drug, phentermine, were hailed as a diet panacea and clinics sprang up around the country to prescribe the combination, known as fen-phen. But fenfluramine and dexfenfluramine were later withdrawn from the market after concerns that they caused heart valve damage.

The other approved drug, sibutramine, sold as Meridia, is an appetite suppressant made by Knoll Pharmaceuticals of Mount Olive, New Jersey, a division of BASF. Sibutramine was approved for sale in November 1997 and became available in February 1998. It has been prescribed to more than 800,000 people in the United States, the company said.

Because orlistat and Meridia have two different mechanisms of action, some weight loss experts said today that they were likely to prescribe the drugs in combination even though they had never been tested that way.

"What was so interesting about fen-phen was that it was the first time anybody had put obesity drugs together," said Dr. Atkinson. "The problem was that both of those worked in the brain. This drug works in the gut. It's another angle from which to attack the problem."

[SGS, April 1999]

## Obesity Drug Can Lead to Modest Weight Loss, Study Finds

The largest and longest study ever of an obesity medication found that a new drug, orlistat, can help obese people lose modest amounts of weight, a recent study reports.

The study, financed by Hoffmann-LaRoche and published in the *Journal of the American Medical Association*, involved 892 healthy, but obese, adults, mostly women, who were studied at 18 medical centers across the country. Their average weight at the start of the study was about 220 pounds.

After one year, those who were randomly assigned to take orlistat and follow a weight loss diet lost an average of 19.3 pounds while those assigned to take a dummy pill and follow the weight loss diet lost about 12.8 pounds. That meant, Dr. Hauptman said, that the weight loss with orlistat was 50 percent greater than with placebo. Others pointed out that the difference was about 6½ pounds.

In the second year of the study, the orlistat group was divided, with half the participants randomly assigned to continue taking the drug and to follow a weight maintenance diet and the others randomly assigned to take a placebo and follow the weight maintenance diet. Those who took the drug regained an average of 7 pounds while those who took a place-

bo regained 12.4 pounds. Half of the study participants dropped out before the two years were up.

Dr. Steven B. Heymsfield of St. Luke's-Roosevelt Hospital Center in New York, who was the lead author of the study, said its advantage was that the study was so large and so prolonged, asking not just whether people could lose weight over a period of weeks or months but over years. "This study is the largest and longest of an obesity drug ever," he said.

Orlistat, whose brand name is Xenical, blocks an enzyme that is needed to digest fat. The fat in the food a person eats will then accumulate in the intestines and be excreted, undigested. That mechanism causes the drug's main side effect, one that Dr. David F. Williamson of the Centers for Disease Control and Prevention described as "embarrassing or inconvenient, to say the least." Most people who take orlistat complain of intestinal gas and bloating, and loose, smelly and oily stools.

The larger concern about orlistat, however, is that it is not a blockbuster drug, as even its champions admit. The average weight loss it elicits is minimal. After all, said Dr. Jules Hirsch, an obesity expert at Rockefeller University in New York, the difference in weight lost between obese people taking orlistat and those taking a placebo was fewer than seven pounds.

Dr. Heymsfield acknowledged, "It's not a magic bullet," but, he said, the people taking orlistat had other benefits that might have made them healthier by reducing their risk of heart disease. Their blood pressure was about a point lower than that of the group taking placebos; their cholesterol levels averaged 201, compared with 195 in the placebo group, and their blood sugar levels were about 2 percent lower.

And, Dr. Heymsfield said, even the disagreeable gastrointestinal side effects might be helpful. People who eat a fatty meal and then suffer the orlistat-induced consequences might think twice about indulging again. "It's like the Antabuse of weight control," he said, referring to the drug prescribed for alcoholics that makes them ill if they drink alcohol.

"The goal is not to make people reach an ideal weight," said Dr. Hauptman of Hoffmann-La Roche. Instead, he said, it is to help people "reach a more biologically acceptable weight," one where they are healthier.

Medical experts called in by the Food and Drug Administration were divided over orlistat's value. The F.D.A. usually follows its experts' advice but is not required to do so. An advisory committee to the agency split, 5 to 5, on the question of whether the drug should be marketed. Dr. Hirsch, a member of that committee who voted against approving the drug, said he considered the weight loss minimal and the improvements in heart disease risk factors so small that it was impossible to say that the drug would lead to improved health. And even if people took the drug religiously, they would start to gain back their lost weight after a year, he noted. Given

what he saw as minuscule benefits, Dr. Hirsch worried about possibly ephemeral hints of risks.

For example, the data Hoffmann-La Roche presented to the F.D.A. last year, pooled from several studies, including the current one and looking at 7,000 people, showed that 10 women taking orlistat developed breast cancer but that just one taking placebos got the disease. The company argued that there was no biological reason why orlistat would cause breast cancer, but the F.D.A. asked for a detailed analysis of the question.

That analysis, Dr. Hauptman said, was provided to the F.D.A. He said it showed that for some women the breast cancer was diagnosed within six months of starting to take orlistat—too soon for the drug to have caused the cancers. Other women already had evidence of breast cancer on mammograms when they entered the study. The company's analysis, Dr. Hauptman said, "supports our conclusion that there is no increased risk." In the study published in 1999, the women who took orlistat had the same incidence of breast cancer as those who took a placebo.

But Dr. Williamson, who wrote an editorial accompanying the orlistat article, asked whether the drug was needed. He worried about its safety when "tens of thousands or even millions of people start taking this drug." The company's studies, he added, were not designed to look at breast cancer risk and he, for one, was not satisfied that the question had been answered.

"The risk-benefit ratio for this drug is incomplete," Dr. Williamson said. "We usually don't like to buy things if we don't know what they will deliver, and we don't know what this drug will deliver."

And, he added, "someone has to pay for these drugs."

[GK, January 1999]

## History Counsels Caution on Diet Pills

The weight-loss drug Xenical, approved in April 1999, had barely reached the market when Web sites selling the drug sprang up to tap into the intense consumer demand that accompanies the debut of anything marketed to make people lose weight. But in their eagerness for pills to help them slim down, people may conveniently overlook something that doctors remember all too well: Weight-loss drugs in general have had a rather alarming history.

"There is a very checkered past," said Dr. Steven Heymsfield, deputy director of the obesity research center at St. Luke's-Roosevelt Hospital in Manhattan. Although Dr. Heymsfield does prescribe weight-loss medications for some of his patients, he said: "I believe we should use these drugs judiciously. If you forget the past you're doomed, right?"

In 1997, the popular drug combination known as fen-phen was blamed for damaged heart valves, and two drugs that had been part of it were taken off the market. (A third, the appetite suppressant phentermine, is still available.)

During the 1930s, about 100,000 Americans took a chemical, dinitrophenol, which prevented food energy from being turned into fat. "The energy is just liberated as heat," Dr. Heymsfield said. "You sort of become a firefly." Unfortunately, dinitrophenol was poisonous, causing blindness and even death.

"In days gone by, thyroid hormone was very common," said Dr. Jules Hirsch, an obesity expert and senior physician at the Rockefeller University Hospital in Manhattan. It increased metabolism, and made people lose weight. But the excess hormone disrupted heart rhythm and caused muscle weakness. "It became discredited, as it should have been," Dr. Hirsch said.

Dr. Albert Stunkard, director emeritus of the weight and eating disorders program at the University of Pennsylvania, said, "The first drugs that were used that turned out to be effective were amphetamines." These stimulants, introduced in the 1950s, suppressed appetite and may have raised metabolism.

"They were used, and then abused," Dr. Stunkard said. "But they're actually very effective, and you can lose a lot of weight. Long, continued use had bad effects, however, like making people paranoid. And when they stopped, they became depressed and regained the weight. Congressional hearings on amphetamine abuse were held in the 1960s, and after that you weren't allowed to use them for weight loss."

One of the strangest weight loss crazes was human chorionic gonadotropin, a hormone produced by pregnant women. During the 1960s, injections of the hormone were said to stimulate rapid weight loss—if they were combined with a strict, low-fat, low-calorie diet. Some patients were also told that if they cheated on the diet, the hormone would actually cause rapid weight gain. "It was a scam," said Dr. Heymsfield.

In the wake of past debacles, he said, weight loss drugs are studied longer and tested more carefully, and doctors tend to have more confidence in them. The only ones on the market besides phentermine are Xenical and Meridia.

Xenical, also called orlistat, blocks the intestine from absorbing about 30 percent of the fat that a person eats, and studies have shown that people who take it may lose from 5 percent to 10 percent of their body weight in a year. Meridia, or sibutramine, is an appetite suppressant approved in 1996. Both drugs are supposed to be used along with a reduced-calorie diet, and only by people who meet the technical definition of obese, meaning that they weigh 30 percent more than they should, or 20 percent more, with complications like diabetes or high blood pressure.

Both drugs have side effects. Meridia can raise blood pressure, and Xenical can cause diarrhea or even fecal incontinence if a person eats too much fat while taking it. But people still clamor for them, and

Dr. Heymsfield said he prescribes them if he cannot talk a patient out of the idea, or if diet and exercise have simply not worked.

"They do help people under certain circumstances," he said. But, he emphasized, the drugs do not work well without diet and exercise, and researchers do not know whether people who are helped by them will be able to keep the weight off in the long run.

[DG, May 1999]

## Weight Loss the Herbal Way: No All-Natural Silver Bullet

Deb Kuney was desperate. Through diet and exercise, she had once trimmed 90 pounds from her 260-pound frame. But Ms. Kuney, a Silverdale, Washington, resident, had gradually regained two-thirds of the weight. So she decided to take herbal weight-loss pills, which she bought at a natural-foods store. The pills contained several ingredients, including ma-huang, an ancient Chinese plant better known in this country as ephedra.

Over the next few months, Ms. Kuney, 46, says the pills helped her lose 25 pounds, though she developed dry mouth and frequent headaches. Still, she kept taking the pills. "I was afraid to get off them," she said, "or else I'd gain the weight back."

Although it's hard to say what portion of the $12 billion dietary supplement market is made up of weight-loss aids, Metabolife International, maker of the ephedra-based product Metabolife 356, is projecting sales of $900 million this year. Such herbal diet products are not only easy to obtain, but also have the appeal of natural ingredients, leading many consumers to believe that they are taking milder medicine. But are they? Are all-natural slenderizers, which are not tested in advance by the Food and Drug Administration, safe? And do they work?

Ephedra is probably the most widely used ingredient in herbal products to fight obesity. It is in most formulas promoted as "herbal phen-fen," an allusion to the now-banned phentermine-fenfluramine drug combination once prescribed for weight loss. Ephedra sinica, used in Chinese medicine for more than 5,000 years, contains alkaloids, including ephedrine, which is used in different forms in nasal decongestants and prescription asthma medications.

Scientists have known that ephedrine can act as a diet aid since the 1970s, when Danish doctors noticed that asthmatic patients taking it lost weight. Ephedrine, which is structurally similar to the drugs known as amphetamines, increases metabolism, which causes a person at rest to burn more calories. Ephedrine also appears to suppress appetite.

Dr. Steven Heymsfield, an obesity specialist at St. Luke's-Roosevelt Hospital in New York, has tested ephedra on several groups of overweight patients who were also instructed to eat a low-calorie diet. "It definitely works," he said. In Dr. Heymsfield's research, patients who took enough ephedra to consume the equivalent of 100 milligrams of ephedrine alkaloid every day for two months lost a pound or two a week. No one taking the prescribed amounts in his study became seriously ill, though reports of unpleasant side effects were common, including headaches, heart palpitations, dry mouth and insomnia.

The problem, explained Dr. Bill J. Gurley, a pharmacologist at the University of Arkansas in Little Rock, is that some ephedra users develop a tolerance to small doses and require more pills to control their appetites. "The more you take," he said, "the greater your chances of developing some type of adverse side effect," since ephedrine increases blood pressure and heart rate. The F.D.A. lists more than 1,000 people who fell ill after using ephedra; the reports included heart attacks, seizures, strokes and at least 35 deaths.

Dr. Gurley said most ephedra users who become ill can blame "their own stupidity, for going well over the recommendations on labels." But he and his colleagues have tested the potency of a dozen ephedra products and found that the amount of active ingredient in some brands varied by as much as 130 percent. Most contained less ephedrine than the labels claimed, but Dr. Gurley is still troubled. "As a consumer and a pharmaceutical scientist, it was an eye-opening experience," he said. "You can't trust what's on the label."

Although the F.D.A. says only that ephedra may be linked to the reports of adverse events it has compiled, it wants to restrict the herb's use. Agency officials have proposed a law requiring ephedra products to bear labels warning consumers to take no more than 24 milligrams of ephedrine alkaloids a day, for no more than a week.

The dietary supplements industry has opposed the F.D.A. proposal. But even supplement manufacturers concede that certain people should not use ephedra, or should speak with a doctor first. They include pregnant women, anyone with a history of high blood pressure, heart disease, diabetes or prostate problems, and those taking the antidepressants known as MAO (monoamine oxidase) inhibitors.

Dr. Heymsfield recommends starting with a daily dose of no more than 24 milligrams of ephedrine, the amount in two Metabolife pills. Blood pressure should be checked before increasing the dose, he said, adding that it's unwise to take ephedra for more than three or four months.

Some supplement sellers have begun promoting "ephedra-free" weight-loss products. One common substitute is garcinia cambogia extract, derived from a citrus fruit grown in Southeast Asia. Also known as hydroxycitric acid, or HCA, it is frequently identified as "Citrimax" on labels.

Studies on rats and dogs have shown that HCA can block an enzyme necessary to form fat in the body. But when Dr. Heymsfield gave a daily dose of 1,500 milligrams of HCA to 66 overweight men and women for three months, "we found absolutely nothing," he said.

Another widely available weight-loss nostrum, 5-hydroxy-L-tryptophan, stirred debate last year. Better

known as 5-HTP, this naturally-occurring amino acid is chemically similar to L-tryptophan, a compound found in some foods and produced by the body. Both are precursors of serotonin, a neurotransmitter involved in mood regulation and appetite. A 1992 Italian study involving 20 obese women found that 900 milligrams a day of 5-HTP helped reduce food cravings, especially for carbohydrates. The women cut their calorie intake by nearly a third.

Sales of dietary supplements containing L-tryptophan, often used to treat insomnia, were prohibited in the United States after a 1989 outbreak of eosinophilia-myalgia syndrome, or E.M.S., a potentially fatal disease of the immune system. According to the F.D.A., approximately 1,500 cases of E.M.S., including 38 deaths, were linked to L-tryptophan tainted with toxic chemicals that were byproducts of processing.

Last fall, researchers at the Mayo Clinic in Rochester, Minnesota, reported in the journal *Nature Medicine* that they had tested eight batches of 5-HTP and detected in each impurities similar to those in L-tryptophan. Stephen Naylor, an analytical chemist and a co-author of the study, conceded that some products contained only small amounts of the deadly contaminants, but added, "The issue is not how much is there, it's the fact that it's present."

After six months on ephedra pills, Deb Kuney was fed up with the side effects and worried that the supplement might damage her heart. She threw out the pills and returned to Tops, or Take Off Pounds Sensibly, a support group she had joined when she first tried to lose weight. "I feel great," she said. Ms. Kuney now weighs 200 pounds, but would like to get back to 170. She also started working for Tops, which has a nationwide network. The organization encourages its members to lose weight the old-fashioned way: through diet and exercise. A recent survey by the National Weight-Loss Registry suggests that Tops may be on to something: of 800 Americans who have kept off 30 pounds or more for at least one year, just 4 percent have used some form of diet pill.

[TG, June 1999]

# Emotional Health

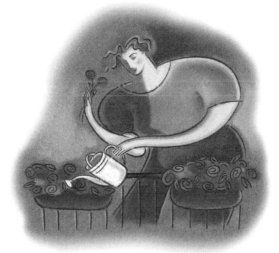

## STRESS AND DEPRESSION
## ARE WIDESPREAD

A woman rushes to finish the task she is working on, dashes out of her office and races to pick up her children before the official closing time of their day-care center. She zips into the supermarket to grab dinner on the way home, and spends the hours before bedtime cooking, helping with homework and baths, doing laundry and making lunches for the next day. If she sits down, she knows, she will fall asleep.

Women are paying a price for the strides they have made in the working world. They have never had so many professional opportunities—or so much stress. Many women find that even though they have careers, housework still belongs mostly to them. A growing number of older women are also finding themselves bringing up their grandchildren, at a time when they had expected a reprieve from homemaking and child rearing. Some juggle it all better than others.

When do emotional upsets—whether they are related to stress or not—qualify as part of life's ups and downs, and when do they signal the kind of lingering distress that needs professional help? When should a woman who suffers from melancholy or mood swings tough it out, and when should she seek psychotherapy or drug treatment, or both?

The answers are never easy. Nineteen million Americans over the age of 18, more women than men, suffer from depression, the most common form of mental illness. But they don't always know it. Clinically depressed people may see themselves and their lives in a harsh light and may not realize that depression has crept up on them and distorted their perceptions. Well-meaning friends and relatives, hoping to coax a depressed person to get help, may say the wrong thing and alienate him or her. Among those who do get help, a small but significant proportion find that no drug or any other form of therapy works. Depression is common among divorced people, and psychologists say it is often impossible to tell which came first.

Research continues to delineate the links between body and mind. Recent studies, for instance, have discovered that premenstrual syndrome has biological roots, and that in some women, the brain is unusually sensitive to cyclical changes in blood levels of the hormones estrogen and progesterone. Such research should reassure women that they have not been imagining or exaggerating their symptoms, and the discoveries may also lead to new drugs to treat premenstrual syndrome. In the meantime, the research suggests that some women suffering from severe PMS may benefit from treatment with drugs like Prozac.

Other problems have resisted scientists' efforts at solution. Research has been unable to find causes for an array of painful and debilitating disorders, like fibromyalgia and chronic fatigue syndrome, that tend to affect women more than men. The disorders are thought to have a psychological component, but the physical suffering is nonetheless real, and some researchers argue that instead of pursuing endless studies and countless tests, doctors should simply treat the symptoms as best they can.

The world of science has little to offer for life's greatest pain, the loss of a loved one, whether to death or to an illness like Alzheimer's disease that takes the mind before killing the body. For that kind of suffering, the only medicine is time. But some scars never heal.

## Human Nature: Some Fear Everything, Even Fear Itself

Not long ago, I had another episode of a recurring nightmare: the going-back-to-the-Bronx dream. In reality, my childhood apartment building on Creston Avenue has long since burned to the ground. In my dreams, though, I must get back to it, no matter how dangerous the journey. I must walk along dark streets where batterers and murderers loiter in every doorway. I must travel on subways that invariably run in the wrong direction. And when I finally arrive, the apartment is deserted, with no lock, no lights, no furniture, no family to protect me. I'm all alone in the Bronx, and I'm terrified right out of my id. At which point, I bolt awake—and the real nightmare begins.

You're up! my conscious mind brays. Good, good; you've got a lot of work to do. Forget about the Bronx and your girlish, nameless fears. You can't lie around worrying about phantoms. You need some meat behind your emotions. And so my mind offers for my inspection that fleshiest source of anxiety: work. I worry about the assignments still to be reported, the many stories that I've started but never finished, the parts of my latest book that I must have written under the influence of a J. Peterman catalogue. I review with the crack of a dominatrix's whip every craven act of procrastination that I've engaged in for the past year, for the past lifetime. I revisit some recent writing failures—clumsy sentences, idiotic metaphors—and recall verbatim snippy but searingly accurate criticisms from readers.

With my curriculum vitae beaten comatose, I move on to whipping girl Number Two: my feeble personality. I nature over my self-indulgent gloominess and failure of imagination. I worry that my daughter is doomed, that she'll blame me, or, worse, that she won't even bother blaming me. And what about my husband? Why was he putting up with me and my manufactured despair? I thought about waking him to ask that question, but then I worried he'd ask himself the same thing, and, before you know it, I'd have something new to worry about, i.e., single parenthood.

Finally, I come to the apogee of angst—that I will waste my life worrying. From the first moment of sentience, I've managed to find something to dread, something that kept me awake at night: the next day's spelling bee, the dirt under my fingernails that my teacher would surely punish me for. You see pictures of me as a little kid, and my brow is as knit as a mitten. Would it be ever thus? Was I condemned to spend my few precious decades of consciousness trapped in an Edvard Munch painting?

I'm afraid so. From what I've been able to gather through discussions with behavioral vivisectionists—also known as psychologists—I am fearful by nature. It's not a disease, they tell me, it's a temperamental flavor: call it Rocky Road.

My fearfulness can even be parsed. According to the reigning model of personality development—that is, the model accepted by at least two tenured professors who are not identical twins reared apart—one's character is constructed of some six core components, which are mixed, matched, chopped and pureed into the primordial soup we call the self. Each dimension is thought to be partly inherited, and partly formed, or deformed, by experience. The ancients knew these personality modules as the "dispositional humors," giving them zesty names like "phlegm," "choler" and "black bile." The current lingo has been castrated into proper jargon, and scientists now speak of human nature as a compendium of the traits "harm avoidance," "novelty-seeking," "self-directedness" "cooperativeness," "persistence" and "extraversion."

Noting that "tendency to wring one's hands" was not among the dirty half-dozen, I called Dr. C. Robert Cloninger of Washington University in St. Louis and asked him, "What's the recipe for a crybaby?" He took to the subject with unnerving cheerfulness. "There are two aspects of personality related to fearfulness," he said. "One is being high in the dimension of harm avoidance. This means that you're very sensitive to all sorts of potentially uncomfortable stimuli. You anticipate threats and pains, and you try to avoid them."

I shifted in my chair uncomfortably. "The other part of fearfulness is being low in self-directedness," he said. "That means you don't have much self-confidence, and you tend to think of the world as a hostile place." Just hearing him say that made me annoyed and defensive. Was he implying that I'm hostile?

"The two often go together, as you might expect," he said. "If you're sensitive to threats, it's hard to have a hopeful view of life. That negativity can end up eroding your self-esteem. On the other hand, if you are naturally high in harm avoidance, and you're raised in a supportive environment where you learn what the safe limits are, you can gain confidence and self-directedness, and avoid becoming excessively fearful."

"That's fine if you're a kid," I muttered. "But what can you do if you're a fearful adult? Can a worrywart be surgically removed?"

"It's not impossible to change," he said, "but it is difficult. One thing we've learned is that temperament tends to remain stable over the course of a lifetime."

Oh joy, I thought. So, however the depredations of time may alter my bones, heart, skin and hindquarters, I can rest assured that my inventive fretfulness will stay perky right up to the mortician's doorstep. I decided to take a different tack and explore the positive side of negativity. I called Dr. Myron Hofer of the New York State Psychiatric Institute in New York, who has studied the evolution of fear and anxiety, and asked him, "What good is fear?"

"Fear, of course, was absolutely necessary to survival in our evolutionary past," he said. "For our ancestors, the world was a dangerous place, and it paid to be nervous about it most of the time.

"Anxiety is probably the first emotion that an infant experiences, at the moment of birth and separation from the mother," he continued. "In nearly all birds and mammals, an infant that is separated from the nest will show signs of intense anxiety, particularly by vocalizing. The only species we've seen where this doesn't happen is the rabbit. For some reason, baby rabbits don't cry." So that's what I need, I thought. The world's first human-rabbit xenotransplant. Oh, wait. Hugh Hefner already tried that.

"Certain aspects of the fear response make physical sense," Dr. Hofer continued. "For example, consider the fact that your arm hairs stand on end when you're scared: that could be a holdover from a young mammal's response to separation, an attempt to stay warm in the absence of its mother by fluffing up its fur." Or take the shallow breathing and tendency toward paralysis that can accompany intense fear, he said: what better way to fool a lurking predator than to act invisible, or dead?

"A little bit of anxiety is still a good thing to have," Dr. Hofer continued. "Performance artists say they need a surge of anxiety to put on a great show. But perpetual anxiety and fearfulness are another matter. They don't make sense. Many of the threats that our forebears confronted no longer exist."

Says who? Come with me and I'll give you something to worry about. It all starts with a midnight trip—to the Bronx.

[NA, March 1999]

# Study Challenges Idea of PMS as Emotional Disorder

A study has called into question the view that premenstrual syndrome is an emotional disorder, suggesting instead that its cause is biological. The study suggests that the symptoms of PMS stem from an aberrant effect on the brain of changes in blood levels of the hormones estrogen and progesterone, which are released monthly in cyclical fashion throughout a woman's childbearing years.

The results of the study, directed by Dr. Peter J. Schmidt of the National Institute of Mental Health, were published in *The New England Journal of Medicine*. The findings could change how PMS is regarded by the medical profession and the general public, and how it is treated. For many years, it was widely considered an emotional weakness or something women made up, prompting many women with PMS to deny that they had a problem. Others viewed it as a gynecological problem even though no specific cause could be found. In 1987, PMS was listed as a psychiatric disorder.

The new study's results "demonstrate clearly a relationship between biology and behavior," Dr. Schmidt said in an interview. "In women with premenstrual syndrome," he added, "it's not that the menstrual cycle or the hormones are bad. It's that women with severe PMS respond differently to normal hormone levels. We're beginning to appreciate the complexity and relevance of hormones in human behavior. It's not a simple matter of an excess or a deficiency of hormones."

In an accompanying editorial, Dr. Joseph F. Mortola, a psychiatrist and gynecologist at Cook County Hospital in Chicago, said that if the new findings were confirmed by further studies, they could lead to the development of a "designer" chemical that would block the hormones' effects on the brain without interfering with their role in maintaining a woman's health and fertility.

The listing of PMS as a psychiatric disorder indicated that mood changes were its most prominent symptoms, said Dr. Robert Spitzer of the New York State Psychiatric Institute. Although the listing was controversial, Dr. Spitzer said, it recognized that PMS was a real and potentially disabling problem, but the listing did not address possible physical roots.

Severe symptoms of premenstrual syndrome afflict about 2.5 percent of women of childbearing age and can seriously interfere with a woman's ability to function socially and at work. The symptoms last for about a week before the onset of menstrual bleeding, then abate.

The current manual of psychiatric diagnoses, which calls the syndrome premenstrual dysphoric disorder, lists these possible symptoms:

- Feeling sad, hopeless or self-deprecating; feeling tense, anxious or "on edge"
- Marked lability of mood interspersed with frequent tearfulness; persistent irritability, anger and increased interpersonal conflicts
- Decreased interest in usual activities; difficulty concentrating
- Feeling fatigued, lethargic or lacking in energy
- Marked changes in appetite, which may be associated with binge eating or craving certain foods
- Hypersomnia or insomnia
- A subjective feeling of being overwhelmed or out of control
- Physical symptoms such as breast tenderness or swelling, headaches or sensations of "bloating" or weight gain.

Although many women of reproductive age experience one or more premenstrual symptoms to some degree, a diagnosis of PMS is based on the marked presence of at least five of the above symptoms in the last week of each menstrual cycle and their absence at other times.

That ovarian hormones are somehow the cause of premenstrual syndrome was demonstrated more than a decade ago, when several research teams eliminated the symptoms by suppressing the ovaries' ability to produce hormones. That approach, called a medical ovariectomy, usually involved the use of a drug called leuprolide, which blocks the action of messenger hormones from the hypothalamus and pituitary gland that normally prompt the ovaries to release their own hormones.

But this approach is not considered ideal for premenstrual syndrome because it interferes with fertility and causes a chemical menopause, depriving women of the benefits of estrogen to their hearts, bones, brains and other tissues.

Dr. Schmidt and his colleagues had previously shown that contrary to longstanding beliefs, mood changes and other symptoms that occur premenstrually might not result from hormones released near the end of each menstrual cycle. They demonstrated that neither the timing nor the severity of premenstrual symptoms was changed when a drug was given in the last week of the menstrual cycle to block hormonal action and abort the cycle.

The study implicates hormone action that occurs earlier in the cycle, perhaps before ovulation. In the study, Dr. Schmidt's team suppressed ovarian function in 10 women with PMS, then gave them estrogen, progesterone or an inactive placebo for four weeks. The effects in these women were compared with the responses of 10 normal women who got similar treatment.

When those with PMS received either estrogen or progesterone, their symptoms—sadness, anxiety, bloating, impaired function and irritability—increased significantly, the researchers said. But the same hormones given to normal women had no such effect. And symptoms did not develop in women with PMS who were given a placebo while their own hormones were suppressed.

Dr. Schmidt said his team would study the possibility that the difference between women with and without PMS reflected genetic differences in the brain receptors for estrogen and progesterone. The differences could result in abnormalities in how the brain handles chemical signals.

A treatment for PMS, the use of Prozac or other drugs that raise serotonin levels in the brain, suggests that in about half of the affected women, PMS may involve changes in the brain's chemistry.

[JEB, January 1998]

## Study Disputes Abortion Trauma

Abortion does not trigger lasting emotional trauma in young women who are psychologically healthy before they become pregnant, an eight-year study of nearly 5,300 women has shown, researchers report. Women who are in poor shape emotionally after an abortion are likely to have been feeling bad about their lives before terminating their pregnancies, the study found.

The findings, the researchers say, challenge the validity of laws that have been proposed in many states, and passed in several, mandating that women seeking abortions be informed of mental health risks.

The researchers, Dr. Nancy Felipe Russo, a psychologist at Arizona State University in Tempe, and Dr. Amy Dabul Marin, a psychologist at Phoenix College, examined the effects of race and religion on the well-being of 773 women who reported on sealed questionnaires that they had undergone abortions, and they compared the results with the emotional status of women who did not report abortions. The women, initially 14 to 24 years old, completed questionnaires and were interviewed each year for eight years, starting in 1979. In 1980 and in 1987, the interview also included a standardized test that measures overall well-being, the Rosenberg Self-Esteem Scale.

"Given the persistent assertion that abortion is associated with negative outcomes, the lack of any results in the context of such a large sample is noteworthy," the researchers wrote. The study took into account many factors that can influence a woman's emotional well-being, including education, employment, income, the presence of a spouse and the number of children.

Higher self-esteem was associated with being employed, having a higher income, having more years of education and bearing fewer children, but having had an abortion "did not make a difference," the researchers reported. And the women's religious affiliations and degree of involvement with religion did not have an independent effect on their long-term reaction to abortion. Rather, the women's psychological well-being before having abortions accounted for their mental state in the years after the abortion.

In considering the influence of race, the researchers again found that the women's level of self-esteem before having abortions was the strongest predictor of their well-being after an abortion.

"Although highly religious Catholic women were slightly more likely to exhibit postabortion psychological distress than other women, this fact is explained by lower pre-existing self-esteem," the researchers wrote in *Professional Psychology: Research and Practice*, a journal of the American Psychological Association.

Over all, Catholic women who attended church one or more times a week, even those who had not had abortions, had generally lower self-esteem than other women, although within the normal range, so it was hardly surprising that they also had lower self-esteem after abortions, the researchers said in interviews.

Dr. Marin said the Rosenberg scale used to measure the emotional health of the women in the study was a tool commonly used to assess overall psychological well-being. "If someone is experiencing distress of any sort, it will show up on this scale," she said.

When the researchers looked just at the aftermath of abortion, they said their results appeared to "confirm the assertions of pro-life groups and the findings in the literature that religious Catholic women are more likely to have lower levels of well-being after having an abortion than are other women."

But when the researchers considered the emotional well-being of the various groups of women before they had abortions, the women's emotional state before pregnancy accounted for their feelings after their abortions, not the abortions or their religious affiliations or involvement in religion.

Gail Quinn, executive director of pro-life activities for the United States Catholic Conference, said the findings belied the experience of post-abortion counselors. She said, "While many women express 'relief' following an abortion, the relief is transitory." In the long term, the experience prompts "hurting people to seek the help of post-abortion healing services," she said.

The president of the National Right to Life Committee, Dr. Wanda Franz, who earned her doctorate in developmental psychology, challenged the researchers' conclusions. She said that their assessment of self-esteem "does not measure if a woman is mentally healthy," adding, "This requires a specialist who performs certain tests, not a self-assessment of how the woman feels about herself." Dr. Franz said the researchers had ignored "a large amount of data about post-abortion trauma, including severe reactions like depression and post-traumatic stress syndrome."

Dr. David C. Reardon challenged the researchers' techniques. He said, among other things, that the self-esteem scale fails to measure all the characteristics of "post-abortion syndrome" and that it is not a measure of overall well-being.

Father John Vondras, former associate director of Family Life/Respect Life Activities for the Archdiocese of New York, said he could not understand why Catholic women who were frequent churchgoers would have low self-esteem since the emphasis of the church today "is to build up self-esteem." Father Vondras, who is now administrator of St. Francis of Assisi in Newburgh, New York, said that he had counseled women who have had abortions. He said, "None were churchgoers and all had post-abortion depression or guilt. Our goal is to help them heal, rebuild their self-esteem and get on with their lives."

The researchers noted that it was natural to feel stress because of an unwanted pregnancy and sad after having an abortion, but they said such sadness "is typically transitory." They expressed concern about post-abortion counseling services and self-help groups "that focus on abortion as the source of psychological trauma rather than providing a nonjudgmental therapeutic process." Such groups, they wrote, can "transform a woman's sadness into anger, contempt and disgust" and exaggerate, not ameliorate, a negative emotional impact of abortion.

Dr. Russo said further that post-abortion guilt and depression could be fostered when women were told that they could have chosen adoption or received financial support if they had kept their babies. "But what they are not told is that giving up a baby for adoption can cause lasting emotional pain or that support for unwed mothers typically lasts only one year," she said.

[JEB, February 1997]

## Hypnosis May Cause False Memories

Hypnosis, even self-hypnosis, can sometimes result in the creation of false memories— the belief that something happened even though it never did. A psychologist at Ohio State University in Lima and fellow researchers found that even when people were warned about the possibility of acquiring pseudomemories under hypnosis, more than a quarter of them did anyway.

Dr. Joseph Green, a professor of psychology at Ohio State and co-author of the study, said, "There's a cultural expectation that hypnosis will lead to more accurate and earlier memories, but that's not true."

For that reason, there is a raging controversy over the use of hypnosis to help people recall lost memories of early trauma. Many experts dispute the conclusion that such recovered memories are always real.

In the study, 48 students who had been shown to be highly susceptible to hypnosis were divided into two groups.

Before they were hypnotized, 32 of the students were warned that hypnosis could lead to false memories and could not make people remember things that they would not ordinarily remember. The remaining 16 students were not given such a warning.

Then the students were asked to select an uneventful night from the previous week—a night they had uninterrupted sleep, uninfluenced by alcohol or drugs and without any dreams that were recalled. During hypnosis, the students were asked if they had heard a loud noise at 4 A.M. during that night. After hypnosis, they were asked if they recalled hearing a loud noise at 4 A.M. during the night in question. Twenty-eight percent of the forewarned students and 44 percent of those who were not warned about false memories claimed that they had heard such a noise.

"The results suggest that warnings are helpful to some extent in discouraging pseudomemories," Dr. Green said, adding, "Warnings did not prevent pseudomemories and did not reduce the confidence subjects had in those memories." The findings were reported at the annual meeting of the American Psychological Association. The study was conducted with Dr. Steven Jay Lynn, a psychologist at the State University of New York at Binghamton and three graduate students at Ohio University in Athens.

In a separate study Dr. Green conducted with the help of three students at Ohio State—also reported at the psychology meeting—160 students were divided into three groups. One underwent self-hypnosis and another deep relaxation, while a third did counting exercises. All of them were told that the regimen would help them recall their earliest memories. Forty percent of those in the hypnosis group later recalled a memory of something that occurred on or before their first birthday. Similar recollections were reported by only 22 percent of those in the relaxation group and 13 percent in the counting group.

But Dr. Green said: "Most research supports the claim that our memories typically begin around age 3 or 4, so it seems quite unlikely that these very early memories actually happened at the stated time. Many people believe that hypnosis can lead to earlier memories, although that has never been shown to be true. People's expectations about what hypnosis can do will influence what they remember."

[JEB, September 1997]

# For Employed Moms, the Pinnacle of Stress Comes After Work Ends

Susan Reiche, a public policy manager at AT in Basking Ridge, New Jersey, can handle what work throws at her from 9 to 5. It's what life throws at her between 5 and 9 that pushes her to the limit.

After she flips off her office computer, she hurries to a day-care center to pick up her 4-year-old son and then rushes across town to fetch her 7-year-old daughter from an after-school program. She makes a quick trip to the store to buy food for dinner, then zips home, where she lets the dog out, makes dinner, referees a fight or two between the children, feeds the dog, says hello to her husband, gives her son a bath, helps her daughter with her spelling words, tosses a load of laundry into the washing machine, plays with her children, reads with them and puts them to bed.

Finally, about 9 P.M., she has a minute to sit down. Whew.

"Before that, the feeling is that if I can sit down, then I'm not doing everything I need to do," said Ms. Reiche, 37. "Most of the time, I don't even have a chance to change out of my work clothes."

For working mothers like Ms. Reiche, the evening is when all the roles they juggle—employee, mother, wife—come crashing together as they try to separate from work, spend time with their children and reconnect with their spouses. It's also a short window of time for a long list of chores, from homework to housework.

"For most working mothers, this is the most stressful part of the day," said Alice D. Domar, the director of the Mind/Body Center for Women's Health at Beth Israel Deaconess Medical Center, a Harvard University teaching hospital in Boston. As Dr. Domar's research has shown, unrelenting stress is more than just an irritation. It can take a physical toll on a woman's body, weakening her immune system, threatening her cardiovascular system and contributing to headaches, backaches, gastrointestinal distress and insomnia.

Some of the factors that make up the evening rush could be described as the duel of the deadlines, the missing co-pilot and the unpredictable audience. Just getting out of the office on time can jangle the nerves of the calmest of women, especially as the American economy has moved away from shift work. And day-care centers and baby sitters can be just as unyielding, as any mother who's been scolded by a baby sitter or charged $1 a minute in late fees at a day-care center that closes at 5:30 on the dot knows.

For Victoria Parker, 30, of Ipswich, Massachusetts, the intense pressure of having to leave work precisely at 4:30 P.M., sometimes in the middle of a meeting, to get to her baby sitter's doorstep by 5:30 contributed to her decision to quit her job as a magazine editor. "It was a frantic rush to get out of the office," Mrs. Parker said. "It was so stressful."

Even with a smooth departure, a woman can still feel stress when she gets home if her husband is unwilling or unavailable to help with child care, cooking and housework. And women whose husbands pitch in can still find themselves flying solo in the evenings.

The good news is that men in dual-income fami-

## After Work, a Full Schedule

Susan Reiche, a mother and a manager at AT, faces a long list of chores after she leaves work every day.

|  |  |
| --- | --- |
| **5:00** P.M. | Shut down office computer. |
| **5:10** P.M. | Be in the parking lot, getting into the car. |
| **5:15** P.M. | Pick up son from day care. |
| **5:45** P.M. | Pick up daughter from after-school program. |
| **6:10** P.M. | Go to grocery store. |
| **6:30** P.M. | Arrive home. Begin to cook dinner. |
| **7:00** P.M. | Eat dinner. |
| **7:20** P.M. | Finish dinner. Clean up kitchen. Start water for baths. |
| **7:45** P.M. | Son takes bath; daughter does homework. |
| **8:15** P.M. | Read with children, watch television, talk. |
| **8:30** P.M. | Put son to bed. Try not to fall asleep with him. |
| **9:00** P.M. | Daughter goes to bed. |

lies are starting to catch up with women on household chores, said Rosalind C. Barnett, a senior scientist in the Women's Studies Program at Brandeis University in Waltham, Massachusetts. Her research shows that women in dual-income couples do about 55 percent of the household chores, and men do about 45 percent.

But men who work full time put in an average of six to eight hours more a week at the office than women who work full time. Because those hours are usually tacked to the beginning or end of a man's workday, women must often take responsibility for feeding the children breakfast and dinner. "Men miss out on meal chores, and those tend to be very stressful," Dr. Barnett said.

There may be another reason husbands don't do more: their wives don't let them. In a study published in the *Journal of Marriage and Family*, researchers at Brigham Young University in Provo, Utah, concluded that about 21 percent of working mothers are "gate-keepers" who limit their husband's participation in household tasks and child care.

According to Alan Hawkins, the director of the Family Studies Center at Brigham Young University and a co-author of the study, these mothers discourage their husbands from taking on household tasks and child care for several reasons: running the household reinforces their identity as mothers; they can't or won't let go of traditional conceptions of family roles, or their standards are so high that nobody else can satisfy them.

"Sometimes what it takes is being willing to turn a job over to your husband and letting him do it his way," Dr. Hawkins said.

Even if fathers help, working mothers say that planning and organization are crucial to removing stress from evening routines. But the unpredictability of children's behavior can throw kinks into even the most carefully engineered schedules. No amount of planning can prevent a poorly timed tantrum or bitter bickering between siblings.

"Children hold together until their parents pick them up from day care, and then they fall apart," said Carol A. Seefeldt, a professor of human development at the Institute for Child Study at the University of Maryland at College Park. They fall apart for several reasons: hunger, excitement at seeing their parents, difficulty making transitions and fatigue, Dr. Seefeldt said. Fatigue may be the biggest problem.

"Many working parents keep their children up late at night so they can spend extra time with them," she said. "The child is often just physically exhausted."

Given the choice of dealing with all these stresses or making a job change, many couples opt for change. After her second child was born, Mrs. Parker, the former magazine editor, gave up her three-day-a-week job in Boston because the numbers didn't add up. After she subtracted day care costs of $4.50 an hour for each child from her part-time salary and added the stress of commuting two hours a day, she decided to stay home and squeeze in occasional writing and editing jobs during nap times and at night. "I don't regret my decision for a minute," Mrs. Parker said.

Other parents—particularly those whose high

salaries give them financial flexibility—reduce their hours and take a pay cut. Dr. Barnett said the average highly educated professional works well over 50 hours a week, not including commuting time, but would like to reduce that commitment by at least 20 hours.

But what of women who can neither cut back on work nor quit their jobs? Psychologists and others who have studied work-life issues offered these suggestions for smoothing the evening rush hours:

▶ *Learn to "compartmentalize."* When you are home, try your best to put work behind you and to focus on being a mother rather than an employee. If that is tough, keep a notebook or recorder at hand so that you can capture work-related thoughts, then move back to the home task at hand.

▶ *Take time to get reacquainted.* Many women go home and immediately start on dinner preparations. But dinner is not the most important thing on the evening's agenda; reconnecting with your family is. Offer the children a nutritious, high-protein snack, like cheese and orange juice, to stave off crankiness, then focus on them for a few minutes. Then, start dinner.

▶ *Cut corners wherever you can.* Catherine Chambliss, a psychology professor at Ursinus College, near Philadelphia, recommends looking at your typical evening and asking this: What in our routine is the most onerous task? Can it be renegotiated in some way? "As the adult, you have the freedom to define the standard," Dr. Chambliss said.

[ALK, August 1999]

## Rising Stress of Raising a Grandchild

Having grandchildren is supposed to be a storybook experience: snapshots of laughter and hugs, the license to indulge the little ones with gifts and extra helpings of dessert before returning them to Mom and Dad. But for growing numbers of grandparents, joyful dates with the grandchildren have been replaced by the responsibility of full-time child care. And doctors and other health care professionals are just now beginning to see that the demands are taking a toll on many grandparents' health.

It is not just that grandparents are exhausted from chasing after 2-year-olds and juggling after-school activities. They are suffering from problems like depression, anxiety, high blood pressure, alcoholism and strokes that doctors link in part to the stress of being parents all over again, this time under far more difficult circumstances than the first time around.

"For many, dreams of the golden years aren't so golden," said Dr. Ronald Adelman, director of the Irving Wright Center on Aging at New York Hospital-Cornell Medical Center.

The newly recognized problem of stress-related illnesses in grandparent care providers was the subject of an article in June 1998 in *Internal Medicine News*, a newspaper for doctors.

"I am amazed at the need," said Susan Silverstein, a social worker in Great Neck, New York, who counsels grandparents and the grandchildren they are raising. "A huge percentage of the grandparents describe feelings of depression and problems with eating and sleeping. Most attribute those problems to stress, but whether they are purely due to stress or to a combination of stress and physiological problems is difficult to ascertain."

Grandparents have always helped rear their grandchildren. But it is when they are bringing up their grandchildren full time that they are most likely to develop stress-related illnesses, Dr. Adelman and others say. About four million children in this country live in households headed by a grandparent, a 41 percent increase since 1992, according to the Census Bureau. Research by the American Association of Retired Persons attributes this rise mainly to high rates of substance abuse by parents; child abuse, neglect or abandonment, and divorce.

These social problems leave their mark on children in the form of depression, grief, learning disabilities and other special needs, which add to the grandparents' financial and emotional strain. In 1997, social workers at Mount Sinai Medical Center conducted a survey of the health of elementary school children in East Harlem who were struggling academically and their grandparent care providers. The survey found that 39 percent of the children suffered from depression, 36 percent had a disorder that involved excessive opposition to and defiance of authority, and 25 percent had developmental problems. Over half of the grandparents had stress-related illnesses, such as high blood pressure and depression.

Though they may be more common among the poor, such problems are by no means isolated to impoverished areas. They are prevalent among the middle-class and upper-middle-class grandparents who seek help from Grandparents Reaching Out, a support and advocacy group for those caring for children that is based in Patchogue, New York, says Mildred Horn, the founder.

A 68-year-old Long Island woman sobbed as she discussed the trouble she and her husband have had raising their 17-year-old grandson off and on since he was 3.

"My doctor says I'm on the verge of a nervous breakdown," said the woman, who requested anonymity. "My grandson's mother and father were in the Marines, and his mother used drugs and took off with another Marine when he was 2. My son took care of him for a while, but he couldn't do it, so we took him to our house."

Her grandson had been caught stealing and was in danger of failing at school, she said, attributing the problems to the physiological effects of the mother's drug abuse during pregnancy and the emotional fallout of her abandonment. "We've had him to psychiatrists," she said. "My doctor wants me to go to a psychiatrist, but I can't, moneywise."

It is common for grandparent care providers to neglect their own health when, like the Long Island woman, they are living on fixed incomes, said Margaret Hollidge, director of the Grandparents Information Center, a national resource service based in Washington. The center was established in 1993 by the A.A.R.P. in response to hundreds of calls and letters from grandparents desperate for information and emotional support on raising grandchildren, Ms. Hollidge said.

"Grandparents will often minimize their own health problems, especially when it comes down to money," she said. "Sometimes the situation is, either I go to the dentist or my grandchild does."

Even when money is not an overriding factor, many grandparents deny or play down their own symptoms for legal reasons, Ms. Horn said. Grandparents who are seeking custody of a grandchild because the parents are drug addicts often fear that if they admit to health problems they will be denied custody.

On the other hand, some grandparents are so driven to survive until their grandchildren are grown that they take better care of themselves than they did before becoming care providers.

"They take on their health problems with a new desire to get well," Ms. Silverstein said.

As a means to this end, some grandparents said they would like more help from their doctors in controlling stress. When Mildred Horn suffered two minor strokes, she said, her internist never discussed the possible connection with her home life and the difficulty of supporting the two grandchildren she has been rearing ever since her daughter was killed in a car accident 13 years ago.

But, according to Dr. Adelman, some doctors are starting to notice grandparent care providers as a group with special health risks. "This is a new phenomenon, and geriatricians and internists are just becoming aware of it," he said. "We need to ask our patients more questions about their home situations."

The biggest source of help for grandparents rearing grandchildren has come from the virtual explosion in support groups in recent years. Ms. Hollidge of the Grandparents Information Center estimated that there were 600 such groups around the country, up from virtually none five years ago. These groups provide grandparents with a wide range of information, including updates on discipline techniques ("What do you mean they don't spank anymore?" she said, was a typical question from many grandparents) and legal aspects of custody and guardianship, as well as a place to vent their feelings.

Ms. Silverstein, the Great Neck social worker, runs separate support groups for grandparents and grandchildren on Long Island through Grandparents Reaching Out. She said that the main issues that grandparents raise were their feelings of guilt at not having the energy or the knowledge to give their grandchildren all that their friends have.

"They feel a tremendous amount of incompetence," she said. "They can't help their grandkids with their homework because they don't understand computers or the type of education the kids are getting today. Along with that, a lot of grandparents struggle with a sense of isolation."

But most of the grandparents Ms. Silverstein sees are able to overcome these obstacles because they are determined to do a good job bringing up their grandchildren. She said the support groups help grandparents tap their inner strengths. "They say they feel better, stronger," she said. "I see a lot of grandparents coping effectively."

[SG, July 1998]

## When Symptoms Are Obvious, but Cause Is Not

More than a century ago, physicians encountered a syndrome they called neurasthenia, characterized by a wide variety of symptoms that variously included fatigue, weakness, muscle and joint pain, headache, memory and concentration difficulties, runny nose, disturbed sleep and palpitations. Researchers expected that a cause would soon be identified—a virus, bacterium or toxic agent—that would account for these complaints. It never happened.

Instead, through subsequent decades, a host of disorders with similar sets of symptoms were identified. They included so-called "effort syndrome" that afflicted veterans of the Civil War and World War I, chronic brucellosis, hypoglycemia, myalgic encephalomyelitis, chronic candidiasis and chronic mononucleosis.

Now the prevailing ailments go by the names of chronic fatigue syndrome, fibromyalgia, multiple chemical sensitivities, sick building syndrome, silicone-associated rheumatic disease (from breast implants) and Gulf War syndrome.

People afflicted with one or another of these syndromes are often extremely debilitated and alarmed by the limitations the ailments place on their lives. Making matters worse is a widespread but erroneous view that they are not really sick but are fakers or hypochondriacs whose symptoms are self-induced to gain attention, sympathy or relief from their usual duties.

But the professional debate is not over whether the symptoms are real—those affected are definitely sick, experts say—but rather whether there is any point in continuing a thus far fruitless search for specific causes. A more productive approach, they say, would be to treat these syndromes as one and the same and provide effective treatment regardless of the cause.

In the journal *Epidemiologic Reviews*, Capt. Kenneth C. Hyams, who heads the epidemiology division of the Naval Medical Research Center in Bethesda, Maryland, noted the remarkable similarities in the symptom complexes that are the hallmarks of these diagnoses. All are characterized by fatigue, headache, difficulty concentrating, muscle or joint pain, impaired memory and often depression and/or anxiety, with some individual variations.

The unifying fact of all these disorders is that they are defined only by their subjective symptoms. No objective criteria or consistent organic explanation can be found for any of them and, therefore, they are a challenge to study, diagnose and treat. For example, Dr. Hyams explained that some patients might be found to have an immunological deficit, but many others with the very same deficit were not sick. For others, the illness may have been preceded by a cold or flu, but there is no evidence that the infectious virus still lingers in any form.

A more probable explanation, Dr. Hyams and others suggest, is that a reaction to some physical or emotional stress triggers the symptoms that characterize these syndromes.

Faced with a lack of objective diagnostic criteria, the particular diagnosis a patient receives typically depends upon the patient's most disturbing symptom, the history of exposures the patient reports and the type of health professional seen—allergist, gastroenterologist, rheumatologist, neurologist or psychiatrist.

As Dr. Simon Wessely, professor of psychological medicine and director of the Chronic Fatigue Syndrome unit at Kings College in London, pointed out in an interview, "Each specialty goes its own way in arriving at a diagnosis." In other words, patients who see a neurologist may get a diagnosis of nerve damage whereas those who see a rheumatologist may get a diagnosis involving joint or muscle pain.

He added: "Doctors have been searching for the Holy Grail to explain these syndromes for the last 150 years without success. Neither single organic causes—viruses, immune defects, toxic agents—nor single psychological causes—childhood sexual abuse, depression or anxiety—can account for them."

Dr. Wessely said that trying to categorize these ailments as either organic or psychiatric was a disservice to patients. "If a patient is told the problem is due to a permanent deficit in the immune system or a persistent virus or chronic disability of the nerves or brain, this just generates helplessness and the patient becomes a victim," he said. "And if you say the problem is psychological, this generates anger on the part of patients who don't regard psychological ills as legitimate." Rather, Dr. Wessely insisted: "Looking for any single cause misses the point. Regardless of how or why they may have started, these syndromes are multifactorial, like heart disease."

Dr. Hyams emphasized that the lack of objective diagnostic criteria "does not mean that these people don't have problems. They're ill. There's no question." The patients are not faking their symptoms, he added.

For example, Dr. Wessely said, "Going to the Persian Gulf definitely affected the health of servicemen. We showed very considerable health effects. But that doesn't mean the disease they contracted is unique to science. They have legitimate health problems, but there is no single illness or single cause."

Viewing the problems holistically, Dr. Hyams said: "Even if these illnesses were primarily psychiatric, psychiatric illnesses have an organic basis in the mind. If a person is sick in any one place, it affects the whole body. For example, a psychiatric illness can cause changes in life-style that can have profound physiological effects."

Dr. Elaine Showalter, professor of humanities at Princeton University and author of *Hystories: Hysterical Epidemics and Modern Media*, said her analysis of the history of these disorders demonstrated that they represented "a basic human phenomenon—the way people react to various stresses, with symptoms that are not organically based.

"The symptoms are genuinely experienced, debilitating and absolutely real, but a lot of energy and money have been spent looking for organic explanations and treatments for what is basically a psychological phenomenon that is not caused by a virus, nerve gas, immune defect or any other tissue change," she said.

Dr. Hyams said, "You always find high rates of these kinds of symptoms in any population reported to have been exposed to something. People are sensitized by reported health threats if they think they've been exposed."

The most effective treatment to date for the syndromes, Dr. Wessely said, is outlined in a report on chronic fatigue syndrome issued in 1997 by the Royal Colleges of Physicians, Psychiatrists and General Practitioners. It is intended to deal with factors that perpetuate illness.

Dr. Wessely explains that the profound fatigue and muscle pain that typify these syndromes are best treated by a graded series of exercises to increase stamina. Also, patients are encouraged to shed their beliefs (for example, that any activity will make matters worse) and to restructure their approach to life through 12 weeks of behavioral therapy, intended to enhance self-confidence and a belief in a patient's ability to control his illness. If patients are suffering from serious depression or anxiety, temporary treatment with psychoactive drugs may also be offered, but as a therapeutic aid, not a cure.

[JEB, March 1999]

## Trying to Cope When a Partner or a Loved One Is Chronically Depressed

It is not at all easy to live with and love a person who is chronically depressed. Stress, conflicts, arguments and misunderstandings are far more common in close relationships with depressed people, and depression and the sexual problems that usually accompany depression are the main reasons couples seek marital counseling.

Many people living with a depressed person say they feel as though they are always walking on eggshells, constantly afraid of saying or doing something that will make matters worse, something that will prompt the depressed person to "bite your head off and make it impossible to discuss anything in a rational way," wrote Dr. Laura Epstein Rosen and Dr. Xavier Francisco Amador, authors of *When Someone You Love Is Depressed.*

Chronic depression can have devastating effects on relationships. "If your partner is depressed," Drs. Rosen and Amador said, "your marriage is nine times more likely to end in divorce than if you were married to a nondepressed person." In his new book, *Should You Leave?*, Dr. Peter Kramer states that while divorce often results in depression, "at least as often, undiagnosed depression antedates and causes divorce."

Children, too, are adversely affected by a depressed parent, who may be emotionally or physically unavailable, overly critical, impatient or easily enraged.

The problem can be even more difficult when the depressed person is a man, who may consider it unmanly to admit that he is depressed and needs professional help and may be unwilling or unable to talk about his feelings.

"When someone you love is depressed, you feel lost, afraid, confused; you long for the person who was; you don't recognize who he or she has become; you feel shut out; you feel angry and frustrated; you feel drained; you are desperate for a way to connect; you feel guilty and alone; you will do anything to help," wrote Dr. Mitch Golant and Susan K. Golant in their book, *What to Do When Someone You Love Is Depressed.*

It is a two-way problem. More than half of depressed adults report that their families and household members fail to understand their condition and do not help them cope with it, according to a study by Wyeth-Ayerst Laboratories, a subsidiary of the American Home Products Corporation and the manufacturer of the antidepressant drug Effexor.

If someone you love is depressed, the first task is to learn as much as you can about this disease and how it is likely to affect the person's thought processes, view of the world and ability to function productively and communicate rationally.

The second step is to learn how to talk to the depressed person in a helpful, empathetic way. The Golants caution against such well-intentioned but counterproductive comments as, "Snap out of it," "You'll be fine," "There, there, it's not that bad" or

"Sure, I understand—I experienced the same problems myself." Nor is it likely to be helpful or appreciated to give advice like "all you need is a vacation," "just try a little harder" or "what you really need is regular exercise."

Although such comments are meant to be reassuring, they are likely to seem patronizing and judgmental to the depressed person, equivalent to telling a kidney-disease patient that "with enough willpower, you can control your renal functioning," the Golants wrote.

Talking with a depressed loved one requires patience, fortitude and especially the ability to stand back and reflect before responding to the person's comments. Try to avoid taking things personally and answering defensively or angrily. The Golants call it adopting an "observer's mind—the ability to detach yourself so that you respond to the feelings behind your loved one's statements rather than to their literal content." The goal is to offer empathy and comfort, which cannot grow out of an angry response to a hurtful remark. Sometimes the best response is "the wisdom of silence," they say.

Cultivate the art of listening and the habit of asking the depressed person what he or she hears you saying. If you think that you have been misunderstood, say, "I don't think you're hearing me," and calmly try again, explaining yourself in a different way. Rather than blurting out angrily, "I don't understand what's wrong with you," say something like, "Help me understand what is going on with you."

Encourage a depressed loved one to seek treatment. Let the person know that you are in this together, that help is available and that getting help for depression is no more shameful than getting treatment for an ulcer or gallbladder disease. Many depressed people resist treatment because they say they are not "crazy," whatever that means. Emphasize that depression is an illness and that treatment with drugs or psychotherapy, or both, can relieve its highly distressing and life-disrupting symptoms. In a telephone survey sponsored by Family Foundation, a joint effort of the National Association for the Mentally Ill and Pfizer Inc., makers of the antidepressant Zoloft, more than 90 percent of respondents treated for depression said their families had been an important influence on their decision to start treatment.

But don't expect overnight miracles. As Drs. Rosen and Amador caution, "Do not be discouraged if you see some improvement but then continue to have some of the same communication problems." They point out that "established patterns of interaction are hard to shift." In some cases, marital or family therapy (in addition to individual therapy for the depressed person) can help the understanding of the problem and foster healthier communication patterns.

And for the partner, parent or child who is struggling to cope with a depressed loved one, it is also important to maintain as normal a routine as possible. Those who sacrifice their work, exercise or recreation to spend more time with a depressed loved one are likely to end up resentful and burned out.

The hardest thing about dealing with depression in a person you love is:

- The person is negative about everything.
- The person is often irritable and easily angered.
- The person never wants to do anything fun anymore.
- The person often misinterprets your good intentions.
- The person pays little or no attention to you.
- The person won't talk about issues that are important to you.
- The person's reactions to what you say or do are unpredictable.
- The person repeatedly rejects your suggestions for self-help.
- All of the above.

The list of choices could be a lot longer. Every spouse, parent, child or close friend of people experiencing serious depression could probably add several items to it.

[JEB, January 1998]

# Depressed Parent's Children at Risk

**D**epression is a family affair, in more ways than one. Not only does depression in one family member affect everyone else, depression in one or both parents greatly increases the risk that their children will also become depressed or develop other emotional disorders. This familial vulnerability may result from the inappropriate actions of a depressed parent or from an inherited abnormality in brain chemistry, or both. Regardless of the cause, physicians and families need to be alert to the possibility that depression and related mental illnesses will persist across generations and that failure to recognize and treat them can result in serious school, social and vocational problems.

About 2 percent of children and 5 percent of adolescents are affected by a serious depressive disorder. Although it has long been known that the children of depressed parents are at greater than average risk of becoming depressed, the extent of this risk had not been documented in a large, long-term study until Dr. Myrna M. Weissman and her colleagues at the College of Physicians and Surgeons of Columbia University published the results of a groundbreaking 10-year study in the fall of 1997.

In 65 of the 91 families studied, one or both parents had been treated for depression at the Yale University Depression Research Unit in New Haven. The other 26 were part of a long-term community study; no parents in this comparison group had a history of psychiatric illness.

The children, then aged 6 through 23, in both sets of families were interviewed initially, then 2 years later and again after 10 years by psychiatric professionals who did not know the mental health of the parents or their offspring. What they found was a frighteningly higher risk of depression and other problems in the children of depressed parents.

"The offspring of depressed parents are at high risk for depression, anxiety disorders and substance abuse," Dr. Weissman and her colleagues concluded in their report in *The Archives of General Psychiatry*. In an interview she added, "While obviously there are some children who escape, having a depressed parent is a risk factor for a child, and if both parents are depressed, the risk is even higher." Also, the children of depressed parents are likely to develop depression and anxiety disorders sooner than the children of nondepressed parents.

Compared with the children of parents who were not depressed, 10 years down the line the children of depressed parents were three times as likely to have developed major depression; had three times the risk of phobias, and five times the risk of panic disorders and alcohol or drug abuse. These children were more likely to function poorly in school, at work and in marriage.

In addition, the children of depressed parents recovered more slowly from depressed episodes and their depressions were more likely to recur. For reasons that the researchers can only guess at, the depressed children of depressed parents also were less likely than the depressed children of nondepressed parents to seek treatment for their problems.

The symptoms of depression in school-age children are not much different from those in adults. They may include: a change in appetite or weight or sleep habits (insomnia, excessive sleeping or difficulty getting up in the morning); a loss of interest in or pleasure from activities that used to be enjoyable; a loss of energy or chronic fatigue; abnormally agitated or slowed behavior; feelings of worthlessness or inappropriate guilt; indecision or difficulty concentrating; recurrent thoughts of death or suicidal thoughts or gestures. In addition, a previously normal youngster might develop antisocial behavior, violent outbursts, extreme irritability or loss of self-control. Or the child may skip school, drop out of clubs or sports or lose interest in friends or hobbies. In some youngsters, depression is expressed in physical symptoms like stomachaches and headaches.

"If such symptoms are not just a passing thing—the result, perhaps, of disliking a particular teacher or breaking up with a boyfriend—if they go on for several weeks, it's time to pay attention to them," Dr. Weissman said. "They might be an indication of depression."

Phobias and separation anxiety were also a serious and often disabling problem among the offspring of depressed parents, and they tended to develop at an earlier age in these children, especially in girls. Often these anxiety disorders are a prelude to depression. Dr. Weissman noted that a lot of children have phobias as a normal part of growing up. But she said if the phobias persist and interfere with life, they should be considered a disorder that warrants treatment. "We don't want to jump on everything and make the kid into an invalid, but we don't want to ignore problems either," she said.

In their report, Dr. Weissman and her colleagues urged pediatricians and family physicians to be alert to familial emotional problems. "When an adolescent presents with depressive symptoms, it's important to ask about the psychological status of the parents," they wrote. "Likewise, physicians should ask depressed parents about their children."

Although it has not been established that treating depressed parents has a positive effect on their children, it is reasonable to assume that a nondepressed person is likely to be better able to cope with a child's problems.

Child psychiatrists have developed effective techniques for treating childhood depression and anxiety disorders, ranging from age-appropriate psychotherapy—play therapy, behavior therapy, cognitive therapy, individual and group counseling and family therapy—to medication. For example, an excellent study last year showed that the newest class of antidepressant drugs, the so-called selective serotonin re-uptake inhibitors like Prozac, are effective against childhood depression and do not interfere with normal physical development.

For family support, guidance and educational materials, parents can contact the National Alliance for the Mentally Ill Children and Adolescents Network, 2101 Wilson Boulevard, Suite 302, Arlington, VA 22201 (telephone: 800-950-NAMI).

[JEB, March 1998]

## Some Still Despair in a Prozac Nation

Nadine McGann is thinking very hard, but she cannot remember the last time that she felt joy, or happiness, or even simple pleasure. On a good day, she drags herself out of bed after her sister's daily wake-up call, walks her dogs in Prospect Park in Brooklyn and slogs through the afternoon, fighting anxiety, inertia and fatigue. On a bad day, she mostly stays in bed. "I don't really know what it is like to feel good," she says.

Like many people who suffer from depression, Ms. McGann, who is 37, has heard the public service announcements that proclaim her condition to be eminently treatable. She has seen the advertisements for Prozac and Zoloft and Luvox and a dozen other antidepressant drugs, old and new, promotions that show smiling men and women happily going about

their lives. She can cite the studies showing that certain types of psychotherapy are effective for depression, especially when combined with antidepressants.

Ms. McGann's own experience, however, has been slightly different: In the five years since her latest battle with the illness began, she has tried virtually every treatment the mental health field has to offer—and not one of them has worked. Not drugs, either singly or in combination, not psychotherapy, not the electroshock therapy she received in 1995.

Recently, she had a device implanted under her collarbone that delivers electrical stimulation to the vagus nerve in her neck—a procedure that has proved effective for some forms of severe epilepsy, and that Columbia University researchers are trying on an experimental basis for depression. But so far that treatment, too, appears to be failing. As a last resort, she said, she may decide to undergo a cingulotomy, a form of brain surgery in which fibers deep in the frontal lobe are severed.

"It is very frustrating," she said. "I'm sort of running out of options." Ms. McGann's case is extreme: She is unable to work, and her life is severely limited by her illness. But there are many others who share her plight to some degree.

Depression, a recurrent illness that afflicts more than 19 million Americans over the age of 18, women more than men, in some cases is considerably more difficult to treat than the drug advertisements suggest. Psychiatrists estimate that 60 to 70 percent of people who can tolerate the side effects of antidepressants get better with the first drug they take. But 10 percent do not respond—even after trials on many different drugs. And still others  the estimates of how many vary—get better but do not recover completely.

"They feel somewhat improved," said Dr. Jan Fawcett, chairman of psychiatry at Rush-Presbyterian-St. Luke's Medical Center in Chicago, an expert in what doctors call "refractory" or "treatment-resistant" depression. "They might be able to function. But they don't really enjoy life."

For such people, finding help can become a full-time occupation. They wait impatiently for each new antidepressant to reach the market. They go from doctor to doctor, hoping the next physician or therapist they consult will be able to provide relief.

Ms. McGann, for example, has tried at least 20 different psychiatric drugs, and is now taking six: Effexor, an antidepressant; Clozaril and Risperdal, both antipsychotic medications; Adderall, a stimulant; and Klonipin, an antianxiety drug. She has consulted five psychotherapists from a variety of theoretical schools, as well as three experts in psychopharmacology. Her present therapist specializes in cognitive-behavioral psychotherapy, which has been shown effective in treating depression.

A 45-year-old Boston woman, who asked to remain anonymous, said she had consulted more than 40 therapists for the depressions she has experienced since childhood. Prozac was effective for a while, she said, but then stopped working—a phenomenon sometimes referred to as the "poop-out" syndrome. Other drugs and combinations of drugs failed as well. She recently decided to undergo electroshock therapy.

"I don't feel like I have a choice," she said. "This illness has taken my life away."

Many clinicians, faced with patients who do not improve, "tend to throw up their hands," said Dr. David Kupfer, chairman of psychiatry at the University of Pittsburgh School of Medicine. And even psychiatrists who specialize in treating difficult cases may resort to a hit-or-miss strategy with treatment-resistant patients, trying out any new approach they have heard about from colleagues or seen mentioned in the journals.

They may shift patients from one medicine to another, add other drugs like lithium, amphetamines, beta blockers, antipsychotics or thyroid hormone, and recommend electroshock if drugs and psychotherapy fail. Sometimes patients get better; sometimes they do not.

"Treatment-resistant depression is a continuum," said Dr. Harold Sackheim, chief of biological psychiatry at the New York State Psychiatric Institute. "Some people don't do that well with first treatment, but they respond to the second. Some will go 20 years and nothing helps them."

In the most dire and intractable cases, some physicians turn to experimental approaches like vagus nerve stimulation, which Dr. Sackheim's institute is studying as a treatment for refractory depression, or even cingulotomy, which has been found to help some people for whom nothing else works.

Researchers know little about why some people respond fully to antidepressant treatment and others do not. In some cases, the difference may lie in brain structure or brain chemistry: Different people respond differently to any type of drug. But some patients who are deemed refractory may also simply have received inadequate treatment, for example having been prescribed a drug at a dosage too low to be effective or having been taken off a drug before the four to six consecutive weeks most experts consider a reasonable trial.

Complicating things further, many patients who do not respond to antidepressant treatment are not just depressed, but have other difficulties as well: medical or neurological conditions, for example, or other psychiatric problems like substance abuse, panic attacks or personality disorders. "The frustration," Dr. Kupfer said, "is that there are a number of different factors where the final common denominator is that people are not feeling better."

And while experts agree that most types of severe or recurrent depression have their roots in biology, psychology plays a role as well. Dr. Judith Nowak, a psychopharmacologist and psychoanalyst in Washington, said that, in her experience, some people who did not respond to antidepressants or combinations of drugs had complicated life problems that could "only be understood, managed and corrected through psychological intervention."

"I've seen several people who had lifelong refractory depression and got caught in a loop of many experimental medication regimens," Dr. Nowak said, "But it really was through good psychotherapy that they were helped."

A large part of the problem is that there have been few systematic studies of refractory depression, or of how best to treat patients who do not improve after routine treatments. In particular, said Dr. Kupfer, little is known about treatment sequencing: When is it best to follow one drug with another or to add an additional drug? When is it best to add psychotherapy in addition to drugs?

Drug companies, eager to prove their products are effective for large numbers of patients, conduct short-term clinical trials to establish the efficacy of individual antidepressants, but have little interest in conducting studies of antidepressant failure, or exploring strategies for treating patients who do remain depressed or show only partial improvement.

Academic researchers have largely ignored the topic, and what research exists, said Dr. Matthew Rudorfer, associate director for treatment research at the National Institute of Mental Health, is "haphazard" at best. Many studies were conducted using older antidepressants, Dr. Rudorfer said, included only small numbers of patients or lacked rigorous scientific controls.

In the hope of stimulating more research, the institute has decided to sponsor its own clinical trial on treatments for refractory depression, and planned to award a multimillion dollar contract in the fall of 1999 to the research team with the most compelling plans for a large-scale national study.

"There is an enormous gap between a lot of people out there suffering and what we really could do about it," said Dr. Steven Hyman, director of the mental health institute. "People deserve the data." The institute's plan, Dr. Hyman said, was to include psychotherapy as well as antidepressant drugs, which most mental health experts believe are an essential component of treatment

Meanwhile, Ms. McGann, and others who suffer similarly, can only hope, and live from day to day. "I feel like I'm not a person right now," she said. "And I don't feel like I can make any decisions about my future. That's the worst part of it." For her, better answers cannot come soon enough.

[EG, July 1999]

# New Tack Promising on Winter Depression

For those plagued by winter depression, recent studies suggest that a few tiny doses of the hormone melatonin each afternoon might help to keep their demons of darkness at bay all winter.

In two preliminary studies, Dr. Alfred Lewy and his colleagues at Oregon Health Sciences University in Portland showed that properly timed doses of melatonin in amounts much smaller than are being sold could reset people's body clocks and lift their spirits. Dr. Lewy maintains that the findings strongly support the theory that winter depression is a form of jet lag in which people's daily rhythms increasingly fall out of line with clock time when dawn is delayed. By midwinter, people with winter depression feel as if they are being forced to wake up hours before their bodies are ready—as if they have just flown from California to New York.

In an interview, Dr. Lewy said the effectiveness of melatonin indicated that people with winter depression suffered more as winter darkness deepened. Their internal rhythms become adapted to darkness in the morning and do not mesh with the requirements of their lives, which force them to arise and function effectively when their body clocks say it is night. Not until spring approaches does their depression begin to lift.

Dr. Lewy, a psychiatrist and an expert on the body's 24-hour rhythms, said the preliminary findings suggested that taking melatonin in the afternoon might be nearly as effective as intense morning light in relieving winter depression. He predicted that a similar regimen could be used to help people recover faster from jet lag, adapt better to changing work shifts and adjust more quickly to daylight saving time.

Winter depression, also known as seasonal affective disorder, afflicts as many as 20 percent of the population. The disorder causes many people in northern latitudes to spend the winter beset by blues and lethargy. They tend to sleep more, eat more, crave carbohydrates, gain weight, think slower, concentrate poorly and feel fatigued, irritable and unhappy.

If the melatonin remedy holds up in larger studies, it could become the treatment of choice. Simply taking a few pills each day would greatly simplify the treatment of winter depression, which most commonly requires patients to sit in front of a light box that simulates sunlight for about an hour upon awakening every morning. For some people with winter depression, Dr. Lewy said, his studies suggest that melatonin alone might work; for others, the needed lift may come from the popular hormone and light treatment.

At the least, Dr. Lewy and others believe, melatonin might be a useful adjunct to light therapy, enabling patients to spend less time in front of a light box or enhancing the lift provided by light therapy.

Another expert on winter depression, Dr. Michael Terman, a research psychologist at New York State Psychiatric Institute, has given melatonin to a few patients who had incomplete responses to light therapy and found that the combination worked better than light alone. But Dr. Terman said the approach must be tested in large controlled studies.

Melatonin is a hormone produced only at night by the pineal gland in the brain. With sunlight, the body's primary timekeeper, melatonin helps to set the brain's biological clock, which determines all of the body's circadian rhythms, including the sleep-wake cycle, digestive functions and hormone releases.

By giving doses of melatonin equal to levels normally produced by the body in the afternoon, the Oregon researchers were able to readjust the circadian rhythms of the study subjects, convincing their bodies that night was beginning to fall in midafternoon, which meant that physiological dawn would come earlier.

Dr. Lewy and his colleagues are not sure why a disrupted circadian rhythm results in depressive symptoms in so many people. But they found that when

# Resetting the Body's Clock

The human body clock follows the rhythm of daylight, telling people to wake up after sunrise. But during the winter months in northern latitudes people often must wake up in darkness, which can cause depression and lethargy. Shown are hours of light and darkness based on latitude.

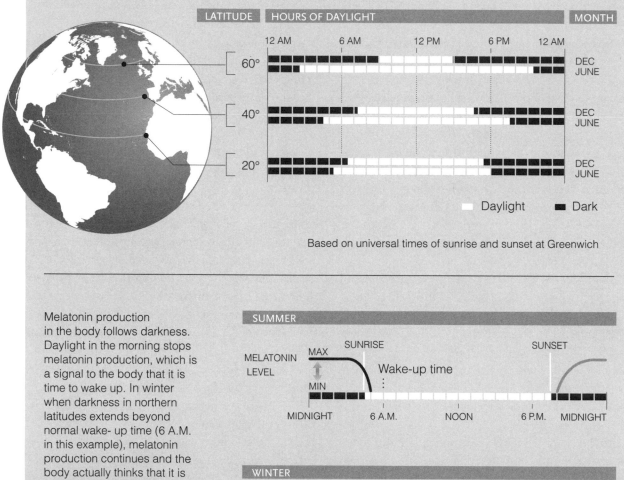

Based on universal times of sunrise and sunset at Greenwich

Melatonin production in the body follows darkness. Daylight in the morning stops melatonin production, which is a signal to the body that it is time to wake up. In winter when darkness in northern latitudes extends beyond normal wake-up time (6 A.M. in this example), melatonin production continues and the body actually thinks that it is still nighttime and resists waking up. By taking small doses of melatonin in the afternoon, the body clock and wake-up time is shifted earlier.

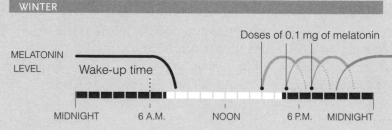

*Source: Dr. Alfred Lewy*

melatonin was used to synchronize the internal timing mechanism with the need to get up when it was still dark outside, symptoms of depression were alleviated in most of the patients studied.

The researchers published the results of a pilot study of 10 patients in January in the journal *Psychiatry Research*. During the winter that began in 1996, half the patients were given 0.125 milligrams of melatonin at 2 P.M. and 6 P.M. and the other half got a look-alike dummy medication. In three patients taking melatonin but only one on the placebo, the symptoms of depression were reversed, Dr. Lewy said. He added that he and his colleagues had also completed a second melatonin study this winter of 26 patients to determine whether the hormone, properly timed, advanced their body clocks. Nine patients took melatonin in the morning, nine took it in the afternoon and eight took a placebo.

Dr. Lewy said that the placebo and the morning melatonin, which in effect prolonged night for the patients, had virtually no antidepressant effect, but symptoms improved significantly in a substantial number of patients who took melatonin in the afternoon—this time in three doses of 0.1 milligram at 2 P.M., 4 P.M. and 6 P.M., which Dr. Lewy said better imitated the way melatonin was naturally released beginning at dusk.

Dr. Lewy and Dr. Terman emphasized the preliminary nature of these findings and cautioned against self-treatment by depressed people. There are three potential problems: possible interaction with other medications, achieving a proper dose (melatonin is sold as a "dietary supplement" without a prescription in doses no smaller than 0.3 milligrams, which is three times the amount Dr. Lewy used) and the soporific effects of melatonin. Dr. Lewy warned that some people with winter depression may become sleepy even on the very low dose he used.

Although the spring-time change to daylight saving time involves only a one-hour shift forward, it takes many people a week to adjust. This is because the increase in daylight at the end of the day works against the body's ability to advance its biological clock so that it meshes with the new clock time.

Dr. Lewy suggests that small well-timed doses of melatonin can ease the adaptation. Start with tablets containing 0.3 milligrams of melatonin. Cut each tablet into three parts. Starting on Thursday, take one-third of the tablet eight hours after your usual wake-up time, take another one-third two hours later, and the final third two hours after that. (Dr. Lewy cautioned that even these doses make some people sleepy. If this occurs, cut out one or two doses.) Get out in the morning light without sunglasses, but wear dark glasses in the late afternoon until dusk. Continue this regimen for a few days.

[JEB, March 1998]

## Coming to Terms With Grief After a Longtime Partner Dies

There are moments, such as when she hears the solemn opening chords of the second movement of Dvorak's "From the New World" symphony, when Joan Kindy feels the rush of 30 years of memories and the pain of nearly two years without her husband, Hal. It was a cherished piece of music that now, like so many things large and small, reminds Mrs. Kindy that she is a widow.

Their son, David, calls with good news about a job, and Hal is not there to share it. An osprey soars over nearby Lake Tarpon, but Hal's binoculars, which he used to bring the bird's sharp talons into focus, sit on a table. Holidays and anniversaries, sunset walks and quiet dinners at home all pass for Mrs. Kindy now without her husband.

"I actually thought I would be a lot more relieved

when he died," said Mrs. Kindy, 63, whose husband died in August 1997 of prostate cancer at age 70. "I thought, once his pain is over . . ." Her voice trailed off. "That was my prayer, that he would be out of pain and I would feel relief for him, but I didn't. It's like half my anchor is gone."

On the eve of what would have been their 32nd wedding anniversary, June 3, Mrs. Kindy said she felt better. The grief that followed his death returns at times, but more often, the memories are good. "I feel comfortable being alone without the sad feeling of being lonely," she said in her home in this suburb about 25 miles north of St. Petersburg on Florida's west coast.

Researchers say Mrs. Kindy's reaction to her husband's death is typical of many older women. Restlessness, sleep problems, feelings of depression and emptiness, of anger and guilt, even complaints of mysterious physical pain and other health problems are common responses to losing a spouse, which more than 900,000 Americans do each year, almost 65 percent of them women over age 55.

With America aging and women continuing to outlive men, many women will be widows in old age, coping with the emotional, financial and physical upheaval. Almost half the 20 million American women age 65 and over are widows; fewer than 10 percent of them are thought to remarry.

Researchers have said for decades that the loss of a spouse is one of the most wrenching events a person faces. But it is only since the 1970s that research into the psychological and physical health effects of that loss has gained momentum.

Although most older women adjust within two to four years to life as widows, a significant minority—perhaps 10 percent to 20 percent—suffer longer-term problems. These include clinical depression, abuse of alcohol and prescription drugs, increased susceptibility to diseases and even death.

Some women appear more susceptible than others to long-term problems, said Dolores Gallagher-Thompson, a clinical psychologist who studied 212 men and women for 30 months after they lost a spouse. Widows who don't recover as well include women with a previous history of depression, women whose marriages were tumultuous, those who depended on their husbands for most social contacts and those whose husbands died unexpectedly or whose deaths followed those of other close relatives and friends.

Even women without serious health problems show signs of grief long after the loss, said Dr. Gallagher-Thompson, who works at the Stanford University School of Medicine and the Veterans Administration Palo Alto Health Care System in California.

"You don't want to tell people they will get over it, that it all will be resolved with time," she said. "Healthy older adults tend to grieve for a long time," showing signs like occasional crying or yearning for or missing the spouse.

Frequently compounding the problem for widows is a drop in their standard of living. Many lose some or all of their husband's pension and face, on average, more than 15 years of supporting themselves as widows. "They might not be able to afford essentials, like prescription drugs," said Robyn I. Stone, the former United States Assistant Secretary of Aging and until recently the director of the International Longevity Center, which studies aging and longevity, in New York.

They might have seen their physical and mental health suffer in the months and years of caregiving that often precede the death of a husband when he is old, Dr. Stone said.

"For many of them, their identity was so tied to the caregiving experience that they have significant depression when their husband dies," Dr. Stone said.

Joan Kindy's story illustrates a common arc of life and death for many older women. She and Hal Kindy met in 1966 when they were graduate students in education at the University of Indiana. They married the next year, and settled into jobs in New York City—she as a teacher and administrator at New York University, he in the same positions at City College of New York.

They raised a son together. Mr. Kindy also had three daughters from a previous marriage. "Hal took retirement in 1986, when he was 60," Mrs. Kindy said. "He was tired of work. Almost immediately after he retired, we found out he had prostate cancer, and that it had spread to his spine and pelvis."

Treatment put the cancer into remission. The couple moved to Florida, settling into the comfortable rhythms of life as retirees. But among the golf and bridge playing, the volunteering and new friendships, they lived with the knowledge that the cancer could return.

In the fall of 1995 it did, and Mr. Kindy died less than two years later. After his death and the surge of activity that came with the funeral, Mrs. Kindy found herself adrift.

"I wasn't sleeping well," she recalled. "I was really restless. I would go out a lot to eat, because I didn't want to eat there alone," she said, pointing to a bare dining room table and empty chairs. "I was gaining weight because I was eating junk food."

Thoughts would trigger a rush of sadness, like the sense that she had better get home by 5 P.M. for a cocktail and dinner with Mr. Kindy, only to realize he wasn't there.

Mrs. Kindy suffered physical problems, too: pain in her neck that required massage therapy, hormone fluctuations that caused vaginal bleeding. Her doctor suspected stress was the cause, she said.

"I started to run a lot, to stay busy because then I don't have to think about things," Mrs. Kindy said. She visited relatives and friends, filling the void in her life with activity.

Six months after Mr. Kindy died, she went to a widows' support group offered through the Hospice of the Florida Suncoast, which had helped care for her husband. The group helped her see more light in a life shadowed by grief.

"It helped to talk with others," Mrs. Kindy said. "I realized my reactions to things weren't abnormal or even as intense or sad as some other widows."

It can be hard for widows to distinguish between normal grief and clinical depression, because the symptoms are similar. But depression involves more severe problems: excessive self-blame about the death; persistent hopelessness or feelings of doom about the future; thoughts of suicide; low self-esteem, and inability or refusal to accept help.

Experts say it is important for widows like Mrs.

Kindy to realize that it can take a long time to adjust to their new situation.

"People think it is going to be over in three months or a year," said Joan Gibala of the Widowed Persons Service at the American Association of Retired Persons. "They or their families think they should be better sooner. But we often hear the second year is worse," because widows pass the first anniversary of the death, the first wedding anniversary without their spouse and the first major holidays alone.

Such was the case for Mrs. Kindy. She pulls out a computer printout with an ice-blue border dotted with snowflakes. It is her Christmas letter to friends and relatives, which she mailed last year.

"My tree is up, the house is decorated for the season, and I have been through just about all the firsts since Hal's death 15-plus months ago," she wrote. "Focusing on happy memories has become easier, as has living each day in a new way."

There are friends she has made who are different from the ones she and Mr. Kindy shared as a couple. There are trips to visit family and vacations to explore new places. And there is still Mr. Kindy. He smiles out from photographs in the house and in her heart. "I feel Hal around me a lot, and now instead of feeling sad, I feel connected with good memories," Mrs. Kindy said.

But sometimes, when the music swells, or the sun sets with familiar colors that bleed across the nearby Gulf of Mexico, or that lone osprey glides above the treetops, Joan Kindy wishes Hal Kindy were at her side. "I will always miss him," Mrs. Kindy said. "I'm doing pretty well, but I miss him."

Many resources are available for widows, including books and support groups. These include:

▶ The American Association of Retired Persons Widowed Persons Service and many community groups offer publications of interest to widows. The association also sponsors support groups, including several that meet on its site on America Online. For information, visit www.aarp.org/griefandloss, E-mail griefandloss@aarp.org or write A.A.R.P. Widowed

Persons Service, 601 E Street NW, Washington, D.C. 20049.

▶ Hospices provide end-of-life care and counseling and bereavement support groups. Check the telephone book, the National Hospice Organization's Web site at www.nho.org/, or call its hospice line at (800) 658-8898.

▶ Many funeral homes provide bereavement support groups or refer people to such groups. Religious groups, health care organizations and senior centers are also good places to check.

[JAC, June 1999]

## When a Loss Remains Unresolved

Jenny and and her husband had enjoyed 15 years of an emotionally and intellectually fulfilling marriage when he suffered a stroke and Jenny's whole life suddenly screeched to a halt. Instead of gradually recovering, over the next five years her husband got progressively worse. The stroke had unmasked or hastened the onset of Alzheimer's disease, and Jenny became his permanent de facto caretaker.

Gone, she said, was the "very sweet, loving, gentle, kind human being" who had shared her interest in art, music, travel and stimulating conversation. Gone was her protector. When she collapsed one day with blood clots that had lodged in her lungs, he said, "What are you doing on the floor?" and then stepped over her to attend to his own needs. Gone was the husband she knew and loved, a husband who now doesn't even notice her presence or absence.

For the last five years, Jenny's life has been more or less frozen in time. "I can't mourn him, he's not dead, but neither is he really there," she explained.

Jenny, who spoke on the condition that her full name not be used, is suffering from what Dr. Pauline Boss calls an ambiguous loss, a loss that has left her with unresolved grief mixed with a hefty dose of guilt and anger. In the book *Ambiguous Loss: Learning to Live With Unresolved Grief,* Dr. Boss, a professor of family social science at the University of Minnesota, describes this all-too-common phenomenon as resulting from either of two circumstances: when the lost person is still physically present but emotionally absent or when the lost person is physically absent but still emotionally present.

In addition to senility, physical presence but psychological absence may result, for example, when a person is suffering from a serious mental disorder like schizophrenia or depression or debilitating neurological damage from an accident or severe stroke, when a person abuses drugs or alcohol, when a child is autistic or when a spouse is a workaholic who is not really "there" even when he or she is home.

As Dr. Lyman Wynne, professor emeritus of psychiatry at the University of Rochester Medical School, put it, "People are caught in a dilemma between experiencing their situation as a genuine loss and trying to relate to a person who doesn't respond in a normal way."

Cases of physical absence with continuing psychological presence typically occur when a soldier is missing in action, when a child disappears and is not found, when a former lover or spouse is still very much missed, when a child "loses" a parent to divorce or when people are separated from their loved ones by immigration.

Whether the ambiguously lost person is physically or psychologically absent, Dr. Boss's research has shown, it is often very difficult for people to resolve their grief and get on with their lives. "People and families become frozen, their lives grind to a near-halt, because they cannot properly mourn someone who is not completely gone," she said in an interview.

Dr. Jan Goldman, a clinical psychologist practicing

in Jenkinstown, Pennsylvania, says this kind of loss "can occur in almost any family."

"You can't escape it," Dr. Goldman said. "It's a life condition." She applauded Dr. Boss's concept of ambiguous loss because, she said, "It normalizes what people often look at as pathological." She and other professionals familiar with Dr. Boss's work emphasized that people suffering from ambiguous loss were not mentally ill, but were just stuck and needed help getting past the barrier of unresolved grief so that they could get on with their lives. Often, they are helped just by knowing there is a name for their problem.

"Putting the problem in a framework is often very therapeutic," said Dr. Evan Imber-Black, a therapist at the Ackerman Family Therapy Institute in New York and author of *The Secret Life of Families*. "It helps people to realize it's an experience that's shared with others." Also helpful, she said, is being able to talk about ambiguous losses with others in the family. "Too often the subject becomes taboo and feelings go underground, where they are much harder to deal with," she said.

Dr. John Rolland, a psychiatrist and codirector of the Center for Family Health at the University of Chicago, said Dr. Boss's work has drawn attention to a critical and underserved area of family care. He added that "families can get into unbelievable conflicts" over ambiguous losses, with different family members holding very different views of the situation.

"The moment of 'death' may not happen at the same time for every member of the family," Dr. Rolland said. "One person may be holding out hope for recovery while another is feeling 'he's died for me.'"

Mourning an ambiguous loss does not mean that memories die, Dr. Imber-Black said. "People can honor their memories of what used to be, but they must move on into the present and not remain locked in the past."

Judith Viorst, author of *Necessary Losses*, tells of a woman who "had lost her father to Alzheimer's disease more powerfully than to death." Not until the father died could his daughter wipe out the "obliter-

ating presence of the Alzheimer father and mourn the wonderful, vigorous father she had known and loved for most of her life," Ms. Viorst said.

The concept of ambiguous loss and its often wrenching consequences was brought vividly to professional attention by the many families with loved ones who were listed as missing in action in Vietnam. Dr. Wynne said, "The status of missing person left families in a precarious psychological state of neither being able to resolve their grief, as happens when someone dies, or being able to engage with the person."

Of course, not everyone gets stuck in the trap of an ambiguous loss. For example, in her book, Dr. Boss tells of a wife and mother of five whose husband was listed as missing in action after his plane was shot down in Southeast Asia. "She told me her husband had come back to talk with her twice since he was shot down," Dr. Boss recalled.

During the first "visit" the husband told his wife to sell the house and get a bigger one and a bigger car to accommodate their growing children. She followed his "instructions" and, about a year later, the husband "returned" to tell her that she had done a good job, he was proud of her, he loved her and now he was going to say goodbye.

"This is when I knew he was really dead," the wife told Dr. Boss, who concluded that the perceived conversations not only comforted the wife, but they also enabled her to move forward on her own and make needed decisions and changes that benefited her and her children.

In another instance, Dr. Boss recalled a Minnesota couple who continued to advertise for the return of their three sons 38 years after they had disappeared, as small children, from a playground. Despite numerous false alarms through the years, the parents kept alive their hope that the missing sons might one day show up. However, that hope, which Dr. Boss calls "a defense against pain, an expression of hopeful optimism rather than unconscious denial," did not prevent the parents from forging ahead like a normal family, acknowledging that their lost children were probably dead and providing love and attention for their other children.

In still another case, Dr. Boss recounts the adaptability of three sons of a woman who developed Alzheimer's disease. Instead of the sons' becoming immobilized by their mother's deteriorating condition, as she became more childlike, they played with her in a more childlike fashion and treated her distortions of language as a form of avant-garde poetry.

The best way to live with an ambiguous loss is with resilience, not denial, Dr. Boss maintains. Denial stands in the way of finding creative options, whereas resilience fosters them. When a father who normally prepared a weekly gourmet dinner was disabled by Parkinson's disease, the family preserved the Sunday night event but gave him a less demanding task of making popcorn and serving apples.

"The goal for families is to find some way to change even though the ambiguity remains," she said. With a little help, she added, people can learn to balance their grief over what was lost with a recognition of what is still possible.

[JEB, March 1999]

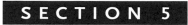

# Violence

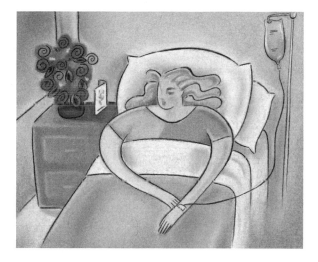

## THREATS ARISE FROM INSIDE AND OUTSIDE THE HOME

It is an ugly fact of American life that 2 million to 4 million women a year are battered by their husbands or boyfriends. Psychologists have created personality profiles of different types of batterers, but the bottom line is the same: They are dangerous men. Among female murder victims, half are killed by husbands, boyfriends or former partners, but only 6 percent of murdered men are the victims of wives or girlfriends.

Why don't women leave men who beat them? It is the first question that comes to most people's minds. But leaving is not as easy as it might seem to an outsider. It requires that the woman recognize that she does not deserve to be abused, and acknowledge that the man is unlikely to stop and that she is in danger of serious injury and maybe even death. It requires that she tap into the resources in her community to help her find a safe place to go to make a new start for herself and her children.

But outright battering is not the only threat to women. Another form of menacing behavior is stalking. A million American women a year are harassed, followed and threatened, often by ex-husbands or men they dated, but sometimes by disturbed strangers. Over the course of a lifetime, one woman in 20 will be stalked. Half of all stalkers threaten violence or damage to the woman's property; 2 percent actually do commit murder. Some victims lose their jobs as a result of the stalkers' constant pestering, and some move away to try to escape. Researchers estimate that 70 percent of stalking victims develop emotional problems as a result of the harassment, in the form of post-traumatic stress disorder, which also affects victims of rape and other forms of violence. A quarter of stalking victims consider suicide.

Experts advise women who are being bothered to reject stalkers in no uncertain terms. But, recognizing that stalkers may not be easily deterred, they also urge women to protect themselves and secure their homes.

For many women, the most troubling threats are those involving their children, and few women realize that stepfathers can pose a significant risk of violence to children not biologically related to them. Psychologists urge women with children who are thinking of remarrying to recognize that risk, and to choose new mates with the greatest care.

# Battered Women Face Pit Bulls and Cobras

The cobra is a real snake in the grass, quiet and focused before striking its victim with little or no warning. The pit bull's fury smolders and builds, and once its teeth are sunk into its victim it won't let go. Men who batter women are either like cobras or pit bulls, say two professors of psychology at the University of Washington in Seattle, who have spent a decade studying violent marriages, and the distinction can make a difference in the severity of the harm they inflict, the ability of women to escape a relationship and the risks the women face if they do leave.

"Pit bulls are great guys, until they get into an intimate relationship," said Dr. Neil Jacobson who, with his colleague, Dr. John Gottman, elaborate on their study findings in a provocative new book, *When Men Batter Women*. "O.J. Simpson is a classic pit bull. Pit bulls confine their monstrous behavior to the women they love, acting out of emotional dependence and a fear of abandonment. Pit bulls are the stalkers, the jealous husbands and boyfriends who are charming to everyone except their wives and girlfriends."

Mr. Simpson was acquitted in 1995 of charges that he murdered his former wife, Nicole Brown Simpson, and one of her friends, Ronald L. Goldman, but was found to be responsible for the deaths in a subsequent civil trial.

Pit bulls, the psychologists say, monitor the woman's every move. They tend to see betrayal at every turn and it infuriates them. And when their anger explodes into violence, they seem to lose control.

Cobras, on the other hand, are often sociopaths. They are cold and calculating con artists relatively free of the trappings of emotional dependence but with a high incidence of antisocial and criminal traits and sadistic behavior, the researchers found. Cobras' violence grows out of a pathological need to have their way, to be the boss and make sure that everyone, especially their wives and girlfriends, knows it and acts accordingly.

When they think their authority has been challenged, cobras strike swiftly and ferociously, the study revealed. Although they do not lose control like the pit bulls, they are more violent toward their wives, often threatening them with a knife or gun. They are also likely to be aggressive toward everyone in their lives, including strangers and even pets, as well as friends, relatives and co-workers. Cobras are the ones who kill the cat as a warning to wives that if they fail to toe the mark, this could happen to them.

In their study of 201 couples, including 63 couples where the wives were repeatedly beaten and emotionally abused, the Seattle based psychologists discovered an extraordinary physiological difference between the two types of batterers. They hooked up the couples to polygraphs that recorded characteristics like heart rate, blood pressure and skin resistance while the couples argued nonviolently in a laboratory setting about volatile issues in their marriages. The researchers noted that, as expected, the batterers they call pit bulls became physiologically aroused as their anger intensified, but, surprisingly, those labeled cobras calmed down internally as they became increasingly aggressive.

When the police are called in response to violence inflicted by a cobra, they are likely to find a highly agitated woman and a calm, controlled man who blames the incident on his wife, which sometimes results in the arrest of the wrong person, the researchers said.

Prof. Amy Holtzworth-Munroe, a psychologist at Indiana University in Bloomington, said that understanding the types of batterers and how they got that way should help in the development of more effective treatment programs, as well as efforts to prevent domestic violence. "Right now, we take a one-size-fits-all approach to treatment," she said. "If we increase our understanding of subtypes, we could match treatment protocols to them."

The psychologists were prompted to explore this societal scourge in detail by compelling statistics and myths about domestic violence, and frustration with the general failure of therapy and the law to deal effectively with batterers. They point to estimates that two million to four million wives are severely assaulted each year by their husbands, and half of all murdered women are the victims of their husbands, ex-husbands, boyfriends or ex-boyfriends. The comparable statistic for murdered men is only 6 percent.

Yet, in only one of six battering episodes are the police called and in only 6 percent of severely violent episodes does the batterer end up in the criminal justice system. For example, Dr. Jacobson said, when O.J. Simpson was arrested in 1989 and pleaded no contest to spousal abuse, "he was given a slap on the wrist." "If the laws were different and enforced differently, battered women would be much safer," he said. "If wife-beating was an automatic felony and the perpetrators had a mandatory jail sentence, women would have a chance to experience life without an abusive husband and an opportunity to formulate a safety plan to escape from the relationship."

Instead, Dr. Jacobson said, "batterers are often referred to treatment programs that don't work, and judges and therapists alike are conned by these men, especially by the cobras," who have little trouble convincing everyone, including their wives, that it is safe for them to return home.

Dr. Daniel Saunders at the University of Michigan School of Social Work said: "Treatment evaluation studies are still in their infancy. We're still trying to find out what works and in what types of men." The evidence thus far indicates that a combination of arrest, prosecution, fines and counseling works better than any one approach alone, he said.

In the Seattle study, the actions and responses among violent couples were compared with those of three other groups: equally unhappy but nonviolent couples, couples who exhibited some aggressive behavior but not enough to be classified as violent and happily married couples.

Participants were recruited through advertisements and were simply told the study would examine conflicts in marriage. When they joined the study, the couples completed extensive interviews and participated in laboratory-staged arguments that were videotaped and analyzed by independent observers who did not know how each couple was classified. A similar analysis was repeated two years later.

"There is occasional low-level violence in many marriages, with pushing or hitting with a pillow now and then out of frustration," Dr. Jacobson said. "This kind of behavior is found among about half of those who seek couples therapy, but it almost never devel-

## Profiles of Abuse

After a decade of research, two psychology professors have found that abusive men tend to fall into one of two categories: "cobras" and "pit bulls," each with distinct characteristics.

| PIT BULLS | COBRAS |
| --- | --- |
| • Confine violent behavior to people they love. | • Likely to be aggressive toward everyone, including pets. |
| • Jealous and fear abandonment; try to deprive partners of independence. | • Not emotionally dependent, but insist that partners cater to every desire. |
| • Prone to rage, stalking and even public attacks. | • More likely to use or threaten with knives or guns. |
| • Become physiologically aroused in an argument. | • Calm down internally as they become aggressive. |
| • Some potential for rehabilitation. | • Difficult to treat with therapy. |
| • Less likely to have criminal record; more likely to have abusive fathers. | • More likely to have criminal records and abuse drugs and/or alcohol. |

*Sources: Dr. Neil Jacobson and Dr. John Gottman*

ops into a battering relationship." Battering, the researchers insist, is not just a matter of physical aggression. Rather, Dr. Jacobson said, "it is aggression with the intent to control, subjugate or intimidate another human being, and in marriage it is almost always the man who fits this definition."

Once physical violence succeeds in intimidating the woman, it may even taper off, only to be replaced by a never-ending barrage of emotional abuse that is sufficient to remind the woman that the threat of physical violence is always present.

The two hallmarks of battering are fear and injury, Dr. Jacobson said. "Even though in 50 percent of the violent couples the wives were also violent, the men never showed fear in their voices or faces but the women virtually always were terrified and they get much more seriously injured," he noted.

Unlike the attacks by men, the violence of women is nearly always in response to battering by the man and is more self-defense than aggression, the researchers maintain. Yet, the men classified as pit bulls often profess that "they're the ones who are the victims in a violent relationship," Dr. Jacobson said. "O.J. Simpson said he felt like a battered husband. Cobras, on the other hand, know they are perpetrators and don't care."

While pit bulls may be easier to leave than cobras, in the long run they can be more dangerous. They are the ones who kill battered women on the courthouse steps when the women seek protection orders or divorces. While the psychologists found that battered women are less likely to leave cobras, those who do escape face a shorter danger period because cobras generally stop trying to pursue them and go on to new conquests.

The histories of cobras and pit bulls also tend to differ. Cobras often had violent, traumatic childhoods, criminal records and a personal history of alcohol and drug abuse. Pit bulls, on the other hand, are less likely to have a history of delinquency or criminal behavior, but they are more likely than cobras to have had fathers who battered their mothers.

Drs. Jacobson and Gottman said their research shatters many prevailing myths about domestic violence. Contrary to the claims of batterers, their wives rarely do or say anything that would provoke a vicious attack in another kind of marriage. The same words and actions in a nonviolent marriage might trigger a disagreement or argument, but not a fist in the eye. Likewise, the psychologists state emphatically, there is nothing a woman can do or say to stave off or abort a battering episode. In many cases among their study subjects, when the woman tried to end an attack by leaving, the husband pursued her and intensified the beating.

Judging from the couples studied, the researchers concluded that battering almost never stops on its own. Although the frequency of physical attacks may diminish with time, in only one case did they stop altogether. Furthermore, even when physical attacks abated, emotional abuse continued and served to keep the wives intimidated and afraid. In fact, Dr. Jacobson said, emotional abuse can be even more damaging than physical abuse because the man is "always in her face, demeaning, degrading, humiliating, harassing and robbing her of her identity."

But in another myth-shattering discovery, the researchers found that a large number—38 percent—of women managed to escape from their abusive relationships within the two-year follow-up period. None, however, were the wives of cobras, who were terrified of their husbands' propensity to use lethal weapons. But at a subsequent contact five years after they entered the study, 25 percent of the cobra wives had also left their husbands. All told, 65 percent of the wives of violent men had left them at that point.

The researchers said those who left demonstrated extraordinary courage and resourcefulness, because it is upon leaving that the women face the greatest likelihood of being killed. But, as one woman who left said, "Death would be preferable to continue in this living hell."

[JEB, March 1998]

# Planning to Escape From an Abusive Relationship

**A** common response of people who learn that a woman is being battered by the man she lives with is: "Why doesn't she leave? What kind of woman is she to stay with a man who beats her?" But experts on domestic violence and the women who are its victims say these questions, though well-meaning, reflect profound ignorance of the tenacious hold abusive men can have on their partners and the often-limited options available to women in abusive relationships.

Such a woman faces two major obstacles: fear and finances—fear for her safety and that of her children and a lack of money to support herself or them. The most dangerous time in the life of a battered woman is when she attempts to leave her abuser. Threatened by the loss of control, the batterer is likely to become even more violent and may even try to kill her. There are simply not enough shelters to protect all the women who need them.

Despite much stronger laws against domestic violence and a greater willingness of the authorities to enforce them, the risk to an abused woman's life is ever-present. Even when a batterer is served with an order of protection, he may stalk and harass the woman and taunt her with threats of further violence. More than half the women who leave violent men are hounded, badgered and forced to return, experts report.

Still, every year many women do escape, safely and permanently, gradually rebuild their tattered egos and start a new life. Sarah Buel, who had been a seriously battered wife before she finally escaped with her young son, went to college at night, then Harvard Law School and became a prosecutor and advocate for abused women, maintains that leaving a violent relationship "is all about who you know and what you know," adding, "It's about feeling empowered enough to make that break, feeling good enough about yourself to say 'I don't deserve this anymore.'"

She points out that "women are socialized to be loving, forgiving and to give one more chance," adding, "They don't want to believe that their relationship failed because they weren't willing to try harder." But according to Dr. Neil Jacobson and Dr. John Gottman, psychologists at the University of Washington in Seattle and authors of *When Men Batter Women*, "Those who stay, hoping that the violence and emotional abuse will stop, are usually disappointed."

The primary tasks of a woman trapped in a violent relationship are to learn about the resources in her community that can help her and to develop a plan that can protect her and her children while she is still in the relationship and when she is ready to get out. Possibly the single best resource is a $12 paperback book published in 1997 by Harper Perennial, *What to Do When Love Turns Violent*, written by Marian Betancourt, who spent three years preparing to escape with her children from a violent husband. She learned the hard way what resources were and were not available to help abused women and in her book provides detailed advice and helpful sources to aid in every aspect of escape.

Start with the National Domestic Violence Hotline—800-799-SAFE (7233) and, for the hearing-impaired, 800-787-3224. Through the hotline you can get a packet of helpful information (have it sent to your workplace or a trusted friend or family member) and guidance to local resources. All 50 states, the District of Columbia, Puerto Rico and the Virgin Islands now have central domestic violence coalitions that can help women find community resources, including counseling, medical clinics, shelters, safe houses, support groups, victim assistance programs, emergency funds, police domestic violence officers and mental health and legal services.

Your best resource when living with a violent partner may be the emergency number, 911. Don't hesitate to use it when you are in immediate danger. Teach your children to use it, too, and to give the operator succinct information like "My Daddy is beating my Mommy. He's drunk and he has a knife. We live at . . . Hurry."

Ms. Betancourt points out that recent laws have mandated improved police training for handling domestic violence. Laws now also call for mandatory arrests of perpetrators in most states. She urges women to report each and every violent episode to police, provide them with every conceivable bit of evidence, from photographs of bruises to torn clothing and smashed furniture, and to make sure that the police file a report and arrest the abuser. Keep several throw-away cameras in the house to easily document the abuse.

Consider wearing a pendant alarm or carrying a cellular phone to call the police when you are in danger. Have an emergency bag packed and store it outside the house, perhaps with a neighbor. It should contain keys to the car, money and copies of all important documents, including orders of protection, driver's license and car registration, birth certificate, medical insurance cards, passport and immigration papers, the children's school and immunization records and the numbers of your bank card, credit cards and Social Security cards (yours and his). You may also want to pack a few clothes for yourself and your children.

Know every way you can get out of the house, where you can go for help and how to get there. If you live in an apartment with only one door, ask the neighbors to call the police any time they hear your cries for help or suspicious loud noises coming from your apartment. Tell the children in advance that if you are forced to leave home without them because you are in danger, you will come back for them as soon as possible. Tell them, too, where they can go to be safe during a violent encounter with your partner and warn them against trying to intervene lest they get beaten or worse.

Ms. Betancourt also recommends that a woman tell her employer about her home situation and, if she has obtained an order of protection, provide the security guards at work with photos of her partner.

But even with the best of plans and most expert advice, the Seattle psychologists warn, it must never be forgotten that "all attempts to escape from abusive relationships are risky," adding, "No one can predict with anything close to certainty how a batterer will respond." They emphasize that the woman—not family, friends or professionals—is the only one who can decide if and when it is the right time to leave.

Even if you are not ready to leave a violent relationship, you may find it helpful to join a support group for abused women. These usually are available at or through local shelters. Ms. Betancourt says there you can find empathy and understanding for your plight, people who can boost your ego and offer much-needed hugs and provide useful hints on how to get the system working for you.

[JEB, March 1998]

## Places to Turn

Local police departments in most major cities now have domestic violence officers, who often can provide the help that victims need.

**NATIONAL RESOURCES INCLUDE:**

- **The National Domestic Violence Hotline.** Phone (800) 799-7233 or, from a TDD line for the hearing impaired, (800) 787-3224.

- **The National Coalition Against Domestic Violence,** which can help victims find local assistance, P.O. Box 18749, Denver, CO 80218. Phone (303) 839-1852.

- **The Family Violence Prevention Fund,** which can help people take action in their communities to end domestic violence, 383 Rhode Island Street, Suite 304, San Francisco, CA 94103. Phone (415) 252-8900.

- **The National Resource Center on Domestic Violence, Battered Women's Justice Project,** which can help abused women who have been arrested to obtain legal help, 4032 Chicago Avenue South, Minneapolis, MN 55407. Phone (800) 903-0111.

# Many Prostitutes Suffer Combat Disorder

The world's oldest profession may also be among its most traumatizing. A study has found that a serious psychiatric illness resulting from exposure to physical danger is more common among prostitutes than among troops who have weathered combat duty.

The illness, post-traumatic stress disorder, is the modern equivalent of shell shock, or combat fatigue. It leaves survivors of serious physical danger emotionally numb, and tortured by recurrent nightmares and flashbacks, often for decades.

In a study presented at the annual meeting of the American Psychological Association in San Francisco, researchers interviewed almost 500 prostitutes from around the world and discovered that two-thirds suffered from post-traumatic stress disorder. In contrast, the condition is found in less than 5 percent of the general population. Studies of veterans of combat in the Vietnam War have found that the disorder may be diagnosed in 20 percent to 30 percent, about half of whom have long-term psychiatric problems.

"Essentially, we need to view prostitution itself as a traumatic stressor," said Dr. Melissa Farley, a psychologist and researcher at the Kaiser-Permanente Medical Center in San Francisco who directed the study with colleagues from Turkey and Africa.

Dr. Farley's team interviewed male and female prostitutes ages 12 to 61 who operated on the street and in brothels in San Francisco and six large cities in Europe, Asia and Africa. The vast majority reported having sustained recurrent physical or sexual assaults in working hours.

Using a severity scale developed by scientists who study post-traumatic stress in the military, Dr. Farley's team found that the prostitutes averaged a slightly more severe form of the disease than even Vietnam veterans seeking treatment for the condition. That is an "enormously high" rating on the scale, said Dr. Matthew J. Friedman, executive director of the Department of Veterans' Affairs National Center for post-traumatic stress disorder and a professor of psychiatry at Dartmouth Medical School.

The frequency of post-traumatic stress disorder among the prostitutes appeared to be unrelated to their nationality or where they worked. It was as common in Istanbul as in San Francisco, and as common among the men and women working in three expensive brothels in Johannesburg as among those working in the streets of that city, even though less physical violence occurred in the brothels, Dr. Farley said.

Hers is the first study of post-traumatic stress in prostitutes, but other studies have shown similarly high frequencies of the disorder in other disadvantaged groups of women, including pregnant drug users, rape victims and homeless and battered women.

Dr. Farley also found that about two-thirds of the prostitutes studied complained of medical problems. Unexpectedly, few of the problems appeared to be related to sexually transmitted diseases, she said.

In contrast to the romantic vision of prostitution often presented by Hollywood, "prostitution is not just a job choice," Dr. Farley said. More than 90 percent of the prostitutes in her study said they "wanted out" of that way of life.

[AZ, August 1998]

# A Fistful of Hostility Is Found in Women

In the old Punch and Judy shows of the last century, Punch would batter Judy under the stage while the audience roared. But now it seems likely that in their private moments together Judy gave Punch back a bit of his own.

Researchers studying human aggression are discovering that, in contrast to the usual stereotypes, patterns of aggression among girls and women under some circumstances may mirror or even exaggerate those seen in boys and men. And while women's weapons are often words, fists may be used, too.

In a large-scale review of dozens of studies of physical hostility in heterosexual relationships, Dr. John Archer, a psychologist at the University of Central Lancashire in Great Britain, has found that although women sustain more serious and visible injuries than men during domestic disputes, overall they are just as likely as men to resort to physical aggression during an argument with a sexual partner.

Dr. Archer compiled interviews with tens of thousands of men and women in Canada, Great Britain, the United States and New Zealand, and discovered that women who argued with their dates or mates were actually even slightly more likely than men to use some form of physical violence, ranging from slapping, kicking and biting to choking or using a weapon. The pattern was particularly pronounced among younger women and women who were dating a partner rather than married to or living with him, he said.

"Whatever the base rate of physical aggression in the population, women tended to have a slightly higher rate than men," Dr. Archer said. In contrast, though, most instances of serious violence in his study were caused by men, as were most injuries that required medical care: Women accounted for 65 to 70 percent of those requiring medical help as a result of violence between partners. Still, "the large minority of men who got injured is fascinating," Dr. Archer said. "It counters a certain entrenched view of partner violence as being exclusively male to female."

Dr. Archer's study was reported at a meeting of the International Society for Research on Aggression held at Ramapo College in Mahwah, New Jersey, in July 1998. It is an extraordinary study, said Dr. Anne Campbell, a psychologist at the University of Durham in Great Britain, because it lends support to an emerging theory that women may respond to certain environmental stresses with physically aggressive behaviors that are analogous to men's, although often on a different scale of intensity.

For instance, she said, criminologists know that although men are more likely to commit crimes than women, crime rates in the genders are also strongly correlated. In other words, in impoverished, "high crime" areas, rates of both violent and nonviolent crimes increase proportionally among men and women.

"Unlike men, though, women tend to view crime as work rather than adventure," Dr. Campbell said. For example, women spend more of the proceeds of nonviolent crimes on staples rather than on luxuries. And women often commit violent crimes against other women with the very pragmatic purpose of attracting the protection and financial support of a "well-resourced" man.

Patterns of domestic homicide also indicate that women are capable of significant violence, although often only as a last resort. Although the vast majority of all murders are committed by men, "intimate partner" homicides were split about equally between the sexes until about 20 years ago, said Dr. Daniel Nagin, a public policy expert at Carnegie Mellon University in Pittsburgh.

In the last two decades, intimate-partner homicides have declined by about 30 percent. Dr. Nagin noted, however, that the decline has been primarily in rates of women killing men, and correlates strongly with several environmental changes. "The decline appears to be related to an improved relative economic status of females, and a decline in exposure to violent relationships," he said.

This drop also correlates with the availability of alternatives to violence for women. In an ongoing study of domestic homicides in 29 cities in the United States, the availability of resources like shelters for battered women and legal advocacy for them has correlated strongly with lower rates of domestic homicide committed by women.

"The resources for women seem to be saving the men's lives," Dr. Nagin said.

The experts in human aggression are now aware that even in childhood, similarities between male and female aggression are more substantial than is usually recognized. Until about five years ago scientists studying aggression tended to include only direct physical or verbal efforts to injure another person. Then they discovered that great damage can be done to another person so subtly that even the victim is unaware. The badmouthing, gossip and smear campaigns that can demolish an opponent as well as direct verbal or physical assaults are now formally known in psychological circles as "indirect aggression," and their patterns are tracked as carefully as punches and kicks. With indirect aggression factored in, aggression in childhood is no longer primarily a male affair.

In a large observational study of "trajectories of aggression" in children, Dr. Richard E. Tremblay of the Université de Montreal has found that physical aggression in both sexes seems to peak around age 2, then decline steadily, although it remains consistently more common in boys. Indirect aggression, however, becomes more prevalent as children grow older and is consistently more common in girls.

The effect of external stimuli on these trajectories is still under intensive speculation, but one long-term study suggests that the omnipresent influence of television violence may correlate with overall aggressive behavior in boys and girls in both the short and the long term.

In a 20-year study of more than 300 Chicago-area children, led by Dr. L. Rowell Huesmann at the University of Michigan in Ann Arbor, the more violent television a child watched at ages 6 through 8, the more aggressive behavior that child displayed, no matter what the child's sex.

And in interviews 15 years later with the grown-up study participants, the correlation between the television viewing habits of childhood and adult behavior patterns persisted, Dr. Huesmann said at the Ramapo College meeting. The more television violence the child watched, the more aggressive the man or woman became. The correlation was especially marked among those children who told researchers that they identified with the characters on the television screen, and thought the events depicted were real.

For instance, 16.7 percent of the young women who had been "high violence" television viewers as girls reported having punched, beat or choked another adult, in contrast to 3.6 percent of others. Thirty-seven percent of the "high violence" viewing women had thrown something at a spouse during an argument, in contrast to 16 percent of the others.

"The evidence is pretty compelling that there is a strong longitudinal effect," Dr. Huesmann said.

[AZ, July 1998]

## Genetic Ties May Be Factor in Violence in Stepfamilies

A woman's live-in boyfriend murders her child fathered by another man. A woman neglects her young stepsister and punishes her so viciously that she dies. A stepfather sexually abuses his wife's daughter by a former husband.

As these examples drawn from recent news articles demonstrate, the Cinderella story is hardly a fairy tale. Researchers are finding that the incidence of violence and abuse is vastly greater in stepfamilies than in traditional families in which the children are biologically related to both parents and to one another.

Of course, most stepfamilies do well, despite potential stresses. And plenty of families in which all the children are the progeny of both parents are fraught with violence and despair. But stepfamilies are at much higher risk than are traditional families. For example, Dr. Martin Daly and Dr. Margo Wilson, evolutionary psychologists at McMaster University in Hamilton, Ontario, found that the rate of infanticide was 60 times as high and sexual abuse was about eight times as high in stepfamilies as it is in biologically related families.

"We demonstrated a very large excess risk to stepchildren, an increase of thousands of percentage points," Dr. Daly said in an interview. The matter is especially pressing now when rates of divorce and remarriage are at an all-time high.

Traditional sociological explanations for abuse and conflict in stepfamilies have focused on issues like economic stress, low socioeconomic status and emotional instability. But evolutionists say these are only proximate, not ultimate, causes of the difficulties that sometimes arise in stepfamilies. The underlying trigger, the evolutionists believe, lies within inherently selfish genes, which are biologically driven to perpetuate themselves. Genetically speaking, stepparents have less of an investment in unrelated offspring and may even regard them as detrimental to their chances of passing along their own genes, through their own biological children.

Citing examples among animals—from birds and bees to lions and baboons—that share the human propensity to live in family groups, the evolutionists maintain that conflicts and incestuous relations are more common among stepparents and stepchildren and among children and their half-siblings and step-siblings because they are less closely related to one another than are parents and children in a traditional family. In fact, Drs. Daly and Wilson found that when degree of genetic relatedness is taken into account, the role that economic stress plays in problems common in stepfamilies becomes almost negligible.

"There's a lot of violence involving steprelatives that can't be explained in terms of poverty, maternal youth and other commonly cited factors," Dr. Daly said.

Dr. Stephen T. Emlen, an evolutionary biologist at Cornell University, maintains that a dearth of shared genes is the unconscious force that underlies many of the difficulties encountered in stepfamilies. These problems involve not only conflicts, violence and incest but also guilt and hurt that can result when stepparents do not form a close bond with their spouses' children, with whom they share no genes. Dr. Emlen believes that over the course of several million years, the forces of evolution have selected behaviors within families that help make sure the family genes will be passed on to future generations.

Dr. Emlen asks, for example, whether men are really so different from, say, male lions; when taking over a new family, the male will kill any offspring still present from the female's prior matings.

In a paper recently published in the journal *Social Science Information*, he wrote, "Conflicts are intensified in stepfamilies because stepparents are unrelated to offspring of the previous pairing, and extant offspring are less related to future young of the new pairing." Dr. Emlen, who has spent 20 years studying animal family systems, says this is as true of people as it is of lower animals that live in family groups, including wolves, mongooses, rodents, scrub jays, bee-eaters, wrens, ants, bees, wasps and termites.

He theorizes that through the process of natural selection, humans' genes have provided a template for certain behaviors that foster their perpetuation through biological offspring and prompt people to invest less energy in maintaining a set of genes that is less like their own.

Sociologists tend to reject such intimations of genetic determinism, citing the fact that humans have minds that can override the forces of genetics. They also note the relatively low rates of abuse or other violence in families with adopted children, who share none of their adoptive parents' genes. The evolutionists do not dispute these arguments; rather they say that an awareness of genetic forces can help people overcome them. Dr. Emlen suggested that a society cognizant of the inherent genetic risks can find ways to capitalize on the human intellect and head off trouble before it happens. Dr. Emlen emphasized that "genes confer only a predisposition, not a destiny.

"Individuals can modify undesirable tendencies once they are aware of them," he said. Modifications of hereditary "decision rules," Dr. Emlen said, "are routinely made based on who is watching, the person's social status, kinship, past experience with the individual and the relative age and dominance of the individual.

"I'm not deterministically saying you're going to have problems because you're a stepfamily," he said in an interview. "There are tons of stepfamilies who are doing absolutely fine." Still, he said it is best to head off trouble by anticipating possible flash points, adding that "it is sometimes very hard to alter things five years down the pike.

"The greatest potential value of the evolutionary perspective is that it tells us when, where and between whom conflict is most likely to occur," Dr. Emlen said.

Dr. Michael Kerr, a psychiatrist at the Georgetown Family Center in Washington, who specializes in family problems, praised Dr. Emlen's suggestions for defusing potential problems in stepfamilies. "That there should be an evolutionary base to the human family makes complete sense to me," he said, adding, "anything that moves society toward a more accurate understanding of what the problems are in families will be helpful in the long run."

Dr. Emlen suggested, for example, that single parents considering remarriage emulate female baboons, which do not accept a new male partner unless he demonstrates parenting skills. A new partner entering an existing family "may have to go an extra mile to develop a bond with a stepchild," Dr. Emlen said.

He added, "An individual with children should realize the need to look for different traits in a future mate. Qualities such as a demonstrable interest in the children, financial generosity and a willingness to become an active participant in a ready-made family come readily to mind."

A prenuptial stepfamily agreement might be signed to assure that future stepparents are aware of "the greater statistical risks of conflict, and particularly the greater challenges involved in child rearing, that are associated with reconstituted families," Dr. Emlen said. In signing such a document, they "would be acknowledging such risks and accepting their heightened responsibility for dealing with them," he said.

If stepchildren, who share at least half the genes of one parent, are at greater risk than the biological children of both parents, should not adopted children, who are genetically related to neither parent, be at even greater risk?

"Adopted children face nothing like the risk that children in stepfamilies face," Dr. Daly said. He and Dr. Emlen pointed out that unlike stepparents, both parents of an adopted child want the child and are usually screened by professionals for parental suitability.

In contrast, Dr. Daly said, "many stepparents would really prefer that their spouses' kids had not existed," adding, "What often happens in stepfamilies is that the stepparent, who is usually a man, feels exploited, pressured in a direction that his emotions and affections are not pushing him."

He suggested that stepparents "think of their investment in stepchildren as a gift, given out of love for the partner, a part of the web of reciprocity in a remarriage." He concluded that it is better to act as if you appreciate making the investment than to act as if it's your duty.

[JEB, February 1998]

# Researchers Unravel the Motives of Stalkers

Stalkers are wreaking havoc in the lives of millions of Americans. Every year, a recent national study by the Justice Department disclosed, an estimated one million women and 400,000 men are plagued by unrelenting pursuers who harass, terrorize and in some cases kill the victims or anyone else deemed to be in the way of a stalker's desired goal.

One in 20 women in the United States will be stalked at some point in their lives, various studies have suggested. In a survey last year among college students in West Virginia, 34 percent of the women and 17 percent of the men said they had been stalked. The ability of stalkers to find and harass their victims has been aided in recent years by computers, e-mail and the Internet, which has spawned a new psychiatric legal term: cyberstalking.

The extent of the stalking problem and its potential for growth through cyberstalking has astonished even the most astute researchers in the field and prompted a call for stronger laws and stricter enforcement of existing statutes to better protect the victims of stalkers, even when there is no direct threat to their physical safety.

"Stalkers simply do not fade away," said Rhonda Saunders, Deputy District Attorney in Los Angeles and head of the Stalking and Threat Assessment Team. Stronger state laws, she said, would "enable law enforcement to intervene before serious bodily injury is inflicted on the victim or those surrounding the victim."

Though stalking is centuries old, it is a relatively new crime, first rendered illegal in this country by a 1990 California statute and later by laws in every state and the District of Columbia. The legal definitions and the arrests they precipitated opened the way to detailed scientific research, which is summarized for the first time in *The Psychology of Stalking: Clinical and Forensic Perspectives*, edited by Dr. J. Reid Meloy.

Although only 2 percent of stalkers commit homicide, half of them threaten their victims with violence or say they are going to damage property or injure pets, according to studies. Even when no physical harm results, the repeated harassment commonly results in acute emotional distress and can seriously disrupt the way victims live. Some lose their jobs when stalkers plague them at work, and some are forced to move and change their identity and appearance.

Dr. Paul E. Mullen, professor of psychiatry at Monash University in Australia, who runs a clinic that treats both stalkers and their victims, said that 70 percent of the victims suffered from a form of post-traumatic stress disorder, marked by chronic anxiety, depression and sleep disturbances. Nearly one in four victims has considered suicide, he said.

Yet only about half the stalking victims ever report their problem to the police, studies indicate. Even when they do, the police may not take action until and unless the victim is physically injured or threatened with a weapon.

Movies like *The Graduate*, in which the stalking man eventually wins the resistant woman, *Fatal Attraction*, in which an unhinged woman stalks her married one-night stand and dramatic cases like John Hinckley Jr.'s attempt to woo the actress Jodie Foster by shooting President Ronald Reagan, have created many mistaken impressions about stalkers, their motives, their usual victims and how successful they are. In most cases, a man who stalks a former lover succeeds only in torturing his victim, not winning her back.

The new collection of studies reports that in addition to former boyfriends and husbands, stalkers include casual acquaintances, disgruntled employees and business associates, vengeful neighbors and total strangers, as well as former girlfriends and wives.

The studies described in the book, the first in-depth look at the psychology of stalkers, found that the underlying problems of stalkers run the gamut of psychiatric and personality disorders.

And virtually anyone can become a victim.

Although celebrities like Madonna and David Letterman, who are stalked by crazed strangers, are most likely to make the news, the vast majority of victims are ordinary people who knew their stalkers, usually as lovers or spouses.

Stalking after the break-up of a physically abusive relationship has received considerable public attention in recent years, but experts on the subject report that women are more commonly stalked by men they once dated or married who were not abusive before the relationship ended.

Dr. Doris M. Hall, a specialist in criminal justice at California State University at Bakersfield, tells of a California woman who was stalked by her former husband for 31 years. Though the woman had a hard time persuading the police to take the matter seriously, her stalker was finally arrested after being found on her block with a loaded gun.

Sometimes stalkers seem to pick their victims at random, prompted, perhaps, by the end of a relationship with someone else, by some real or imagined slight or, out of paranoia, for a reason that has no apparent connection to reality.

Dr. Kristine K. Kienlen, a psychologist in St. Peter, Minnesota, who evaluates criminals and patients who are mentally ill and dangerous, tells of a 31-year-old man who, after his divorce, began stalking a young teenage girl he knew. At first he merely attended her athletic events and wrote of his desire to date her. But after four years of failing to achieve his goal, he began breaking into her home and stealing items from her bedroom, including her photo album, the contents of which he returned to her one picture at a time.

A Minnesota woman said in an interview that she has been tormented for nearly two years by a man she had dismissed from his job for repeatedly calling her and another woman at home and at work, accusing them of "wanting his body and stealing from his home." When the man began showing up at his former boss's home with a shotgun, she got a restraining order and a gun of her own. But he has yet to be imprisoned. And only after she dismissed him did the woman learn that the "glowing recommendation" he had received from a previous employer had failed to mention that he was dismissed from that job as well for stalking two women at work.

What prompts someone to stalk need not be as traumatic as a lost love or job. A retired couple reported being stalked by a business acquaintance after a minor disagreement. And a woman in her 70s was stalked by a woman of similar age for reasons she could never discern.

Men are stalked as well, and indeed are more often victims of violence by their stalkers, Dr. Hall said. One young man, she said, sought a restraining order to end the unrelenting pursuit by his former girlfriend. The judge, who told the man he should be "flattered by all the attention," nevertheless issued mutual restraining orders, which proved useless to the man. He was killed by the woman several weeks later.

Dr. Hall said that typically, when a man sought police protection from a woman who was stalking him, the authorities did not take him seriously. In her study of 16 men who were stalking victims, 56 percent were stalked by women; 44 percent were stalked by other men. She also said that when a woman stalks after the break-up of a relationship with a man, she will often go after the man's new girlfriend, "probably because women scare more easily than men do."

*The Psychology of Stalking* includes articles by 23 experts summarizing what they have learned about this noxious behavior, its underlying psychopathology and motives and the often devastating effects it has on its victims. This is one fact on which all the researchers agree: "There is no single profile of a stalker," said Dr. Kienlen, a contributor to the book. "Stalkers exhibit a broad range of behaviors, motivations and psychological traits."

Some stalkers have psychiatric illnesses, ranging from depression and schizophrenia to erotomania—a delusional belief that the person is loved by another—and most appear to have a personality disorder like extreme narcissism or dependency or an inability to sustain close relationships.

"Stalkers tend to have both—a mental illness and a personality disorder," Dr. Meloy, a psychiatrist affiliated with the University of California at San Diego, said in an interview. "And those who stalk strangers are more likely to be psychotic than those who stalk prior sexual intimates. The latter are more likely to be drug or alcohol abusers with a dependency personality disorder."

Dr. Kienlen conducted the first preliminary study of the backgrounds and psychological profiles of stalkers. More than half of the 24 male stalkers she interviewed had evidence of what psychologists call an attachment disorder stemming from the childhood loss or absence of a caring and consistent parent or guardian, usually in the first six years of life.

Although the theory of attachment disorder has its critics, Dr. Kienlen and other experts in stalking believe it may be a "predisposing factor" for stalking behavior by making it difficult for the person to establish and maintain healthy relationships. "Their parents may have divorced and the custodial parent had little contact with the child," she said. "The parents may have had a drug or alcohol problem; the child may have been physically, sexually or emotionally abused or even totally abandoned."

Dr. Kienlen said she had encountered three kinds of attachment disorders among stalkers. The "preoccupied" stalker has a poor self-image but a positive view of others and constantly seeks their approval and validation in order to feel good about himself. When rejected by others, the person stalks to restore his sense of self.

The "fearful" stalker has a poor self-image as well but also sees others as unreliable and unsupportive. The stalker tends to get caught in a vicious cycle of wanting someone to boost his own self-image, then rejecting the person for not being trustworthy, which prompts the person to stalk because he again needs someone to boost his sagging ego.

The "dismissing" stalker thinks of other people as jerks and usually remains distant from them to maintain an inflated self-image. The stalker with dismissing attachment disorder who does form attachments becomes angry when a break-up occurs and may stalk out of revenge, to retaliate for being mistreated.

Most of the stalkers Dr. Kienlen interviewed also had extreme personality disturbances. The most frequent one encountered in stalkers was narcissistic personality disorder, which Dr. Kienlen said gave stalkers an inflated sense of self-worth and an intense need for other people to compliment and idolize them.

Other personality disorders experts frequently encounter in stalkers are extreme dependency, constantly needing the support, attention and approval of other people and borderline personality disorder, having unstable moods and an exaggerated reaction to rejection and abandonment. Only about 10 percent of stalkers have an antisocial personality disorder, with an above-it-all detachment from other people that is most often encountered in criminals.

In 80 percent of the men Dr. Kienlen interviewed, there was also a precipitating factor, such as a recent loss that seriously upset them and seemed to have brought on their stalking behavior. The losses ranged from the break-up of an intimate relationship, a lost job and death of a parent to learning that they themselves had a serious illness.

"My theory is that in these vulnerable individuals, the losses damaged their sense of self-worth," Dr. Kienlen said. "To alleviate their grief or feelings of emptiness, they compensated by focusing on stalking. Sometimes the stalker blames the victim for the loss and stalks out of anger."

[JEB, August 1998]

# Dos and Don'ts for Thwarting a Stalker

Though stalking is often glamorized in movies and sitcoms, in real life it is anything but. For most victims, it is a waking nightmare characterized by constant fear and hypervigilance that triggers lasting emotional distress and sometimes results in bodily injury or even death.

Since one in 20 women can expect to be stalked at some time during their lives, usually by men they once dated or married, it pays to know what to do if it should happen to you. Sometimes, men who have been rejected by women stalk to get revenge. These men, along with those who think "if I can't have her, no one else will," can be especially dangerous.

**Be Firm.** Experts say that in an effort to be kind and gentle, too many women give their stalkers mixed signals, leaving them with the belief that if they keep at it, they will eventually win the women they desire.

In his book *The Gift of Fear*, Gavin de Becker says that "a rejection based on any condition, say, that she wants to move to another city, just gives him something to challenge." He suggests that women should "never explain why they don't want a relationship, but simply make clear that they have thought it over, that this is their decision and that they expect the man to respect it."

Dr. Doris M. Hall, who questioned 145 victims of stalkers (83 percent of them women), also recommends firmness: "Once and only once, tell the person you want nothing to do with him. Don't try to be nice; it can only work against you."

Dr. Hall, an expert on criminology at California State University at Bakersfield, emphasizes the importance of taking any stalking behavior seriously and dealing with it aggressively from the outset. "If someone's behavior seems out of line, if it is making you uncomfortable, something's up," she said. "You have a better chance of putting a stop to it if you don't give it a chance to accelerate."

**Cut Off All Contact.** Dr. Hall compared stalkers with "naughty third graders."

"They don't care what kind of attention they get," she said, "as long as it's attention." Any kind of response on the part of the victim, no matter how negative, can be construed by the stalker as a sign that she is really interested and is trying to keep a relationship going.

Mr. de Becker, an expert on predicting violent behavior who advises stalking victims, wrote, "When a woman communicates again with someone she has explicitly rejected, her actions don't match her words."

He said that when an unwanted pursuer starts making persistent phone calls, sending messages, showing up uninvited at a woman's job, school or home, following her or trying to get her friends or family to help his cause, "it is very important that no further detectable response be given."

Mr. de Becker added: "He views any response as progress. If you call the pursuer back, or agree to meet, or send him a note or have somebody warn him off, you buy another six weeks of his unwanted pursuit."

Dr. Hall warns stalking victims to "never, ever meet with a stalker," even if he says it is only to say a final goodbye or to return the victim's belongings. It is most likely a lie and may escalate the problem. Nor is sending the police to warn him off likely to do any good, Mr. de Becker says. Unless the pursuer has committed a crime that warrants his arrest, the police can do little more than talk, which may further embolden the stalker.

Even obtaining a restraining order can sometimes backfire. Court actions infuriate some stalkers and may provoke violent behavior. Mr. de Becker has found that court orders that are introduced early carry less risk than those introduced after the stalker has made a significant emotional investment or introduced threats and other sinister behavior. "A stalker who has been at it for years and who has already ignored warnings and interventions" is not likely to be deterred by a court order, he said.

**Protect Yourself.** Under the auspices of the University of California at San Diego, the Privacy Rights Clearinghouse has developed a list of tips for self-protection against stalkers. While specific legal advice is likely to vary from state to state, the clearinghouse's practical advice can apply anywhere. Among the most important tips are these:

▶ *Keep your address private.* Use a postal box (obtained through a mail box service or the post office) instead of a residential address on everything, including your driver's license and government documents. File a change-of-address card with the post office. Give your street address only to your most trusted friends and tell them not to give it to anyone else. Do not have anything mailed or shipped to your home address. Have your name removed from any "reverse" directories that list people numerically by phone number or address.

▶ *Do not give out your telephone number.* Get an unpublished and unlisted phone number. Never print your number on checks. If asked for a phone number, give your work number. Get an answering machine that records messages on a microcassette and allows you to screen all calls. If your state has caller ID, order complete blocking on your number. If you are bothered by harassing calls, put a beep tone on your line to make callers think you are taping the call. You might even add a warning on your outgoing message, telling callers they may be taped. Also, consider getting a cellular phone and keeping it with you at all times.

▶ *Guard your e-mail.* If you are at risk of being stalked electronically, change your e-mail address to something that is hard to guess and do not enter any personal information into on-line directories.

▶ *Keep a diary.* Record every stalking incident and the names, dates and times of every contact with the authorities. Save the tapes of phone messages and anything sent by the stalker in the mail or left at your home or workplace. Do not accept packages you did not order.

▶ *Secure your home.* Trim the bushes around your house. Install a loud exterior alarm and motion-sensitive lights high enough so they cannot be removed by a person standing on the ground. Always lock your doors with dead-bolt locks. Also use window locks on basement and ground-floor windows. If you have sliding glass doors or windows, secure them with safety bars. Put locks on your fuse or circuit breaker boxes.

▶ *Secure your car, van or truck.* Always keep your garage door and car doors locked and look carefully inside before entering. Do not use parking lots where you must surrender the keys; if you must, leave only the ignition key. Get a locking gas cap and a hood-locking device that is controlled from inside. Know the locations of the police and fire departments and busy shopping centers; if you think you are being followed, head directly to one of these. When you arrive, stay in the car and blow the horn to attract attention. When traveling to and from work, vary your schedule and your route. Never stop to help a motorist in distress—phone for help.

[JEB, August 1998]

## Help for Stalking Victims

The following organizations provide assistance to people who are being stalked:

### NATIONAL RESOURCES INCLUDE:

• **The National Organization for Victim Assistance** (Nova), 1757 Park Road N.W., Washington, D.C. 20010; Phone: (202) 232-6682; Hotline: (800) 879-6682; E-mail: nova@access.digex.net.

• **National Victim Center,** 2111 Wilson Boulevard, Suite 300, Arlington, VA 22201; Phone: (800) 394-2255 or (703) 276-2880. E-mail: mail@mail.nvc.org.

• **Survivors of Stalking** provides support for stalking victims, P.O. Box 20762, Tampa, FL. 33622; Phone: (813) 889-0767 E-mail: soshelp@soshelp.org.

## Call for New Sex-Abuse Trial is
## Said to Harm Rape Shield Law

A court ruling in December 1999 ordering a new trial for a man who was convicted of sexually abusing a woman he had met on the Internet could erode protections for rape victims and discourage them from reporting attacks, women's rights groups warned.

The Appellate Division of the State Supreme Court ordered a new trial for the man, Oliver Jovanovic, a former Columbia University graduate student, after ruling that his 1998 trial was unfair because the judge kept the jury from seeing four e-mail messages his accuser sent him that expressed an interest in sado-masochism. Prosecutors have appealed the ruling.

Women's rights groups said that the e-mail messages were irrelevant because a sexual encounter should stop immediately when a woman asks, regardless of what she may have said or done earlier.

"The issue is her consent in a specific sexual circumstance," Galen Sherwin, president of the New York City chapter of the National Organization for Women, said. "Because she characterizes herself as someone who enjoys submission, that doesn't mean she means that she wants to be tied to a bed for 20 hours and tortured."

In the Jovanovic case, the woman, then a 20-year-old Barnard College student, said he used e-mail to lure her out on a date. When they met, she said, Mr. Jovanovic, 32, tied her up in his apartment for 20 hours, burned her with candle wax, bit her until he drew blood and sodomized her with a baton. Lawyers and relatives of Mr. Jovanovic bitterly denounced the judge in the case, Justice William A. Wetzel, and said the young woman lied about a consensual sado-masochistic interlude.

Mr. Jovanovic was released from prison in upstate New York after serving 20 months of a 15-year sentence.

It was not clear if the woman, who underwent six days of emotional testimony in the first trial, would testify again if the prosecutors' appeal were denied and a new trial held.

Women's rights groups said that the appellate court's ruling could extend beyond the Jovanovic case. They said it could undermine the state's rape shield law, enacted in 1975 to encourage rape victims to come forward by tightly restricting which aspects of their sex life could be brought up at a trial.

Legal experts split over the appellate court's order for a new trial. Vivian Berger, a law professor at Columbia University, said the decision was legally sound. But she said that trial judges should not apply the ruling broadly to all rape cases. She said the case was unusual because the encounter was sado-masochistic. Mr. Jovanovic, for example, might have been able to argue that he thought his accuser wanted him to continue when she asked him to stop.

The jury might not have believed him, but Mr. Jovanovic should have been able to use the barred e-mail messages as part of his defense, she said. "I think the jury should have heard them and been allowed to sort them out themselves," she said.

But Sherry Colb, a professor at Rutgers University Law School in Newark, said the issue was whether the woman consented to specific sex acts, not what she wrote in e-mail messages. She said other messages the jury saw showed her interest in sadomasochism, and the ones they were not shown were not needed.

"This evidence would have further nauseated the jury toward the victim, and have them feel this victim wasn't worth convicting someone for," she said, "which is exactly what the rape shield law was designed to avoid."

Anne Bliske, executive director of the New York State Coalition Against Sexual Assault, a lobbying group, said a two-year-old proposal from her group would end any confusion by tightening the legal standard for consent.

"Our contention is that no matter what, if a victim is clearly saying no, that's it," she said. "At that point, the act is no longer consensual."

[DR, December 1999]

# Sexuality

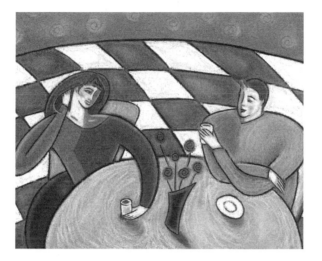

## DRUGS CAN HELP, BUT THE EMOTIONAL PART REMAINS KEY

Despite the sexual revolution of the 1960s and 1970s, much remains unknown about women's sexuality, and scientists are not even sure of the best way to go about studying it. Some people see the lack of data as a woeful state of ignorance, whereas others may rejoice in the idea that one of life's most delicious mysteries has escaped dissection.

But the introduction of Viagra, the first effective drug for male impotence, has refocused the spotlight on intimate relations. Viagra has not quite lived up to its original billing as a quick-fix miracle drug: it does not work for everyone, and it has side effects that can be unpleasant for many men and dangerous for some. When it does work, it can create, or perhaps expose, a whole new set of problems, as couples are forced to realize that there is more to lovemaking than an erection, and that intimacy cannot be recovered instantly if it has dwindled away over the years. Women who assumed that the sexual phase of their lives was over may not welcome its revival.

Then again, some embrace it, and sex researchers and drug companies are eager to provide treatments for women who complain of loss of libido. In some cases, small amounts of the male hormone testosterone, combined with estrogen replacement after menopause, may revitalize a woman's sex drive. Drug companies are busily studying Viagra and other drugs that increase blood flow to the genitals, to see if they can enhance arousal in women as they do in men.

Safer birth control pills and methods of morning-after contraception have become integral parts of the medical and pharmaceutical pleasure industry, but they, too, have their perils. Birth control pills provide no protection against sexually transmitted diseases, which remain a serious problem and a source of illness and infertility, particularly in very young women.

# Women and Sex: On This Topic, Science Blushes

Dr. Julia Heiman, a psychologist who directs the reproductive and sexual medicine clinic at the University of Washington, wanted to know whether women become sexually excited by talk of love and romance, or are they turned on by explicit talk of sex itself? So Dr. Heiman asked college students to wear a tamponlike device that detects blood flow to the vagina. While they wore it, the young women listened to romantic tape recordings and to erotic ones.

Dr. Heiman got her answer: If blood flow to the vagina is an accurate measure of sexual excitement, women, like men, are sexually excited by erotic talk, not romance.

That was in the early 1970s. Yet even now, when most fields of medicine have been transformed, Dr. Heiman's studies are still state of the art. With the recent introduction of Viagra, however, the impotence pill made by Pfizer, the world has changed.

Suddenly there is a pill for men who have trouble getting and maintaining erections. Almost as suddenly, drug-company scientists, wondering whether Viagra or something like it can enhance sex for women, are asking academic scientists what is known about women's sexual responses.

"For most medical professionals, a woman's genitals are still 'down there,'" said Dr. John Gagnon, a sociology professor at the State University of New York at Stony Brook. At their mention, Dr. Gagnon added, "Everyone averts their eyes in horror." Even worse, he said, is finding out what gives women pleasure and how to enhance their pleasure. Men worry that "if she enjoys it too much, will she do it with someone besides me?" Dr. Gagnon explained.

No one disputes the evidence that many women are unhappy with their sex lives. Dr. Sandra R. Leiblum, a psychologist at the Robert Wood Johnson Medical Center in New Brunswick, New Jersey, noted that "every survey invariably finds that many more women than men complain of sexual difficulties."

Dr. Leiblum cited a major survey in the United States that found a third of women respondents—but only a sixth of men—saying they are uninterested in sex. One-fifth of the women—but only one-tenth of the men—said sex gave them no pleasure. Dr. Leiblum said she thinks most sexual complaints in women are psychological. Most women can have orgasms easily by masturbating, she said, "when they don't feel pressured to perform, and when they don't feel concerns about how they look or how they are formed or how they smell."

But it is also much easier and more socially acceptable to study psychological problems than the physiology of sexual responses in women. "There is a huge resistance" to understanding women's sexual responses, said Dr. James H. Geer, a professor of psychology at Louisiana State University and an inventor of the tamponlike device that Dr. Heiman, his graduate student then, used in her studies. Dr. Geer and his colleagues developed that device without financing, he said, which is typically how studies of female sexuality are done.

As a result of this reluctance, the simplest questions have no answers. Half a century ago, when Dr. Alfred C. Kinsey surveyed the sex lives of Americans, he proclaimed that men and women have basically the same sexual responses, except that men are more influenced by psychological factors.

Dr. John Bancroft, the director of the Kinsey Institute at Indiana University, said that scientists now know that "Kinsey was wrong about psychological differences." Yet, Dr. Bancroft added, "Whether he was wrong about physiological similarities remains an open question."

For example, Viagra increases blood flow to the penis, enabling men to have erections. By analogy, some doctors have suggested that Viagra might also increase blood flow to the clitoris and enhance a woman's sexual response. And yet, Dr. Gagnon noted, the idea that women suffer from inadequate blood flow to the clitoris has no experimental evidence. "If there were women with inadequate clitoral swelling, how would we know that?" he asked.

Researchers who want to directly measure sexual responses in women are stymied by a lack of a good method, Dr. Heiman said. Some critics have said that her studies, involving blood flow to the vagina, focused on the wrong organ. Why did she avoid the clitoris? Because no one has figured out how to study the physiological changes in the clitoris during sexual arousal, Dr. Heiman said. It is not easy to fit the clitoris with a measuring device. "The clitoris is so sensitive that simply touching it could trigger a response," she explained.

Women often complain of having difficulty lubricating, so some researchers tried to measure the secretion of vaginal fluids while women watched erotic movies or listened to erotic tapes. The researchers used tampons, weighing them before and after the women were stimulated. But the tampons turned out to be too crude to measure the amount of vaginal secretions. So far, no one has found a reliable way to measure vaginal fluids secreted during arousal, and no one knows how much fluid is enough and how much is insufficient.

Pfizer, meanwhile, is hoping to bypass the morass of ignorance regarding women's sexual physiology and simply ask: Does Viagra improve women's sex lives? Dr. Frances Quirk, who works for Pfizer at its research center in Sandwich, England, said that the early studies of Viagra in men concentrated solely on ways to measure the drug's physical effects on erections. But the company soon redirected its efforts, Dr. Quirk said. "One of the big breakthroughs was in understanding that patient assessments and perceptions can yield valuable informa-

tion," she said. "This is probably even more important for women."

Borrowing from the same method, Dr. Quirk and her colleagues developed a questionnaire that asks women how often they have sex, how confident they are as a sexual partner and how well and how quickly they respond to sexual stimulation. They tested their survey with 1,160 women living in Britain. The results, Dr. Quirk said, appear to show a relationship between women's symptoms of sexual dysfunction and worries about the future of their sex lives.

For example, 34 percent of women who said they had difficulty becoming aroused said they worry about the future of their sex lives, whereas just 5 percent of those who had no such difficulty with arousal had this worry. And 13 percent of those who had difficulty lubricating—as compared with 8 percent who had no such problem—were anxious about their sex lives.

Now, sex researchers say, the moment of truth is looming. It was easy to justify Viagra in men because the drug, as Pfizer keeps emphasizing, does not increase desire. All it does is help a man who already has the desire for sex to achieve an erection. But the primary complaint among women is the lack of desire. For society to sanction research on sexual dysfunction in women, Dr. Heiman said, "People would have to view women's sexual desire as an important issue."

On the other hand, drug companies are not the Federal Government. They can go ahead with sex research if there is a problem that needs to be treated and a market for a drug. "One could say that having a lack of information on women's sexuality is just fine with the general culture," Dr. Heiman said, "but it may not be so fine with the drug industry."

[GK, June 1998]

# The Pill at 40: Renewed, Improved and in Its Prime

The birth control pill is pushing 40, and like many another veteran of the 1960s, it never looked so good. It is the Volkswagen Bug of drugs—a sleekly remodeled version of the 1960 prototype, housed in a box full of old associations, but completely reconfigured inside and intended for a brand-new market.

Today's pills use hormone doses that are a small fraction of what they once were. While not utterly risk-free, they are far safer than the original versions and remain among the most effective forms of birth control on the market.

Nonetheless, surveys show that even women too young to remember the 1970 Congressional hearings that widely exposed the pill's health risks continue to worry about its dangers. About one in four women who take it say they stop because of side effects, a poll commissioned by the Association of Reproductive Health Professionals found in 1997.

But doctors are now endorsing the pill with increasing enthusiasm. Side effects can be tempered by switching among some two dozen different formulations now available, they say. Further, when women are carefully screened for problems, like smoking and blood clotting disorders, that exacerbate the pill's dangers, its risks are small while its benefits extend far beyond contraception to ease a host of gynecologic conditions.

"There are so many women for whom the pill is just so wonderful," said Dr. Anita L. Nelson, an associate professor of obstetrics and gynecology at the University of California at Los Angeles and the director of a large women's clinic there. "And hopefully a woman will get some other benefit from it than just contraception."

The pill remains the most popular nonsurgical form of birth control in the country, used by about one in six women of child-bearing age. In September 1998, the Food and Drug Administration extended its contraceptive range still further, approving a four-pill emergency kit, which can help prevent pregnancy up to three days after unprotected intercourse has occurred.

The pill interferes with conception from several different angles. The estrogen and progestin that most birth control pills contain stop the pituitary gland from releasing the hormones that prompt the ovaries to release eggs. Progestin also thickens the mucus at the uterus entrance so that sperm cannot penetrate, and it thins the lining of the uterus so that an egg cannot adhere and develop there. It is quite effective with a 3 percent failure rate during the first year of use.

Despite its potency, the pill can no longer offer women the carefree sexual freedom it once symbolized: It provides no protection against sexually transmitted diseases without a condom.

But, Dr. Nelson said, the pill's long-term safety means that now it can offer women other freedoms, like freedom from the constraints of menstruation. Doctors have known for years that if a woman skips the seven dummy tablets in most 28-day pill packs—ordinarily taken to induce menstruation—and simply takes 21-day courses back to back, menstrual flow can be postponed for months, she said. This technique has been used safely for as long as a year in women with menstrual complications like migraine headaches or endometriosis, which may result in severe pelvic pain and blood loss during menstruation.

"We have to get the word out on how to do this," Dr. Nelson said. "It's perfectly safe. Athletes going to a competition, women going to meetings—there's no reason to have a period when you're midair over Frankfurt, having to try to remember the word for tampons in German."

Another newly appreciated use of the pill is its ability to free older women from the symptoms that may accompany a rocky transition to menopause. Because the early versions of the pill were most dangerous in older women, they were generally never used after age 35. In women who do not smoke, however, the new versions are often prescribed through age 50 and even beyond.

"There are several encouraging therapeutic uses of the pill in older women," said Dr. Maida Taylor, a gynecologist at the University of California at San Francisco. One is to treat a condition she calls "perimenopausal chaos" in which women who are nearing menopause become the victims of wildly erratic hormone bursts, swinging between high levels of estrogen one month and low levels the next with sweats, hot flashes, mood swings and general misery.

These women still need contraception, which the pill can provide, while it also smoothes out the fluctuating hormone levels and lets them function normally. Then, when menopause occurs, hormone doses can be tapered from those that provide contraception down to the lower doses that are used for hormone replacement in postmenopausal women.

The pill may also help older women avoid osteoporosis, Dr. Taylor said. Women lose roughly 10 percent of their bone mass between ages 35 and 50 even though they are not overtly estrogen-deficient during that time, she said. "Women who take oral contraceptives from age 35 to 50 arrive at menopause with that much more bone mass, and that translates into a significant reduction in bone fractures later in life," Dr. Taylor said. "It's like arriving at retirement with 10 percent more money in your Keogh."

Other noncontraceptive benefits that recent studies have associated with long-term use of the pill include reduced rates of ovarian cancer and malignant cancers of the lining of the uterus, and possibly also decreased rates of benign tumors of the breasts and the uterus.

But, the benefits still exact a price. The new pill is still accompanied by some old health risks, including

## Not Your Mother's Birth Control Pill

A major drop in the estrogen and progestin levels since the 1960s has made oral contraceptives safer and added several health benefits.

**SIDE EFFECTS**  Today's oral contraceptives have eliminated most of the problems caused by earlier, high-dose versions of the pill. By trying different formulations of the pill, women can avoid side effects like moodiness, bloating and weight gain associated with the old pill. In women with no risk factors, the new pill does not increase the chance of developing heart attacks or strokes. There is a small increased risk of blood clots.

**HEALTH BENEFITS**  Besides preventing pregnancy, today's pill provides significant health benefits. It is associated with reduced rates of ovarian and endometrial cancer, and possibly decreased rates of benign tumors of the breasts and uterus. It can be used to treat problems like functional ovarian cysts, endometriosis, menstrual cycle irregularities and acne. The pill can also temper hormone fluctuations and may slow bone loss in women approaching menopause.

| | 1960s | 1990s |
|---|---|---|
| **Estimated Use (U.S.):** | 1.2 million women (1962) | 15.9 million women (1997) |
| **Estrogen:** | 150 micrograms | 20-50 micrograms |
| **Progestin:** | approximately 10 milligrams | approximately 1 milligram |

*Source: American Society for Reproductive Medicine*

a danger of blood clots forming in the veins of the legs (which, if they move to the lungs, may cause serious complications or death), and an overall increased risk of heart attacks and stroke.

Heart attacks and strokes, however, now seem to be provoked exclusively in women already at risk, especially those with high blood pressure or who smoke, said Dr. Leon Speroff, a professor of obstetrics and gynecology at Oregon Health Sciences University in Portland. For women without other risks, he said, taking the pill appears to hold no added danger, although it does mandate that they be honest with their doctors about smoking and have regular check-ups.

Similarly, although women who take the pill suffer blood clots in the legs about three times more often than those who do not, the risk is greater in women who are predisposed to blood clots for other reasons, like prolonged bed rest or a family history.

Although many breast cancers are apparently nourished by estrogen, the relationship between the pill and breast cancer is complex. A study of more than 50,000 women published in the journal *Lancet* in 1996 found that breast cancer was diagnosed slightly more often in women who had used the pill during their teens and 20s. But it was diagnosed earlier and had a better prognosis than in other women, making the overall impact of the pill on their health extremely difficult to assess.

"Women who have a pre-existing tumor have an accelerated growth of that tumor because of hormone exposure. It's picked up earlier, and they actually do better," Dr. Speroff said.

In the balance, the pill of the 1990s is "very good, very safe, lots of benefits. It's a good product," he said. But veteran pill-watchers are still wary. "It is a lot safer for short-term use," said Barbara Seaman, who has been called the Ralph Nader of the pill for her 1969 book *The Doctors' Case Against the Pill*. But unanswered questions remain, she said, like the pill's long-term impact on fertility.

"It may be the most studied pill we have," Ms. Seaman said, "but that doesn't mean it doesn't need more study. There's an awful lot we still don't know. There's still a yellow light of caution. It's blinking a lot more slowly than it was, but it's still blinking."

[AZ, October 1998]

## Morning-After Contraceptive To Be Marketed

A small New Jersey company received approval from the Food and Drug Administration in September 1998, to market morning-after emergency contraceptive pills in late 1998, its chairman said. Roderick Mackenzie, the chairman of the board of Gynetics Inc., of Belle Meade, New Jersey, said his company was the first to market the pills in the United States, and that they cost about $20 a prescription.

The pills, known as Preven, are ordinary birth control pills taken at a high dose. They can prevent pregnancy if a woman takes them within 72 hours of unprotected intercourse. They work, Mr. Mackenzie said, by preventing ovulation or keeping a fertilized egg from implanting in the uterus. According to the F.D.A., they are about 75 percent effective in preventing pregnancy. The most common side effects are nausea and vomiting, which afflict 10 percent to 40 percent of those taking the pills.

Although medical experts have known for years that high doses of birth control pills taken after sex can prevent pregnancy, many doctors and women have been unaware of this method of emergency contraception.

Mr. Mackenzie said he decided to market the pills at the urging of the Food and Drug Administration. Dr. Philip Corfman, who was a medical officer at the drug agency until he left in December 1997, said that in keeping with the F.D.A.'s tradition of prompting the marketing of drugs that are needed by Americans, he had taken steps while he was at the agency to encourage the marketing of a morning-after pill.

Dr. Corfman said the F.D.A. had asked several large companies to market the pills, but they refused. So he spoke to Mr. Mackenzie, whom he knew because Mr. Mackenzie had formed a small company, GynoPharma, to bring a copper intrauterine device to the American market.

Mr. MacKenzie eventually sold GynoPharma to Johnson & Johnson. That happened on the last Friday of July 1995, Mr. Mackenzie said. "On Monday, I started Gynetics," to market morning-after pills. He expects to market a combination of two well-known birth control pills, ethinyl estradiol and levonorgestrel, both of which are off patent.

In the years since starting Gynetics, Mr. Mackenzie said he had established a partnership with a manufacturer of the pills, formulated the pills into tablets and conducted clinical studies with them.

[GK, July 1998]

## Better Loving Through Chemistry: Sure, We've Got a Pill for That

Given the national spectacle set off by a pair of runaway libidos in the White House, it might seem an odd moment in history to suggest that what Americans really need is medical help to juice up their sex drives.

But that is precisely what researchers said on the basis of a survey showing that 43 percent of women and 31 percent of men suffered from "sexual dysfunction"—a catchall diagnosis applied to troubles like lack of interest in sex, inability to have an orgasm, difficulty with erection or finding sex painful or not pleasurable. Writing in the *Journal of the American Medical Association*, the researchers called this sexual malaise "a significant public health concern" and said work was needed to develop "appropriate therapies," especially for women.

Such therapies might include counseling, hormone treatments, and, if studies now under way indicate it helps, giving the drug Viagra to women as well as men, the researchers said in interviews.

Does this mean that disappointment in the bedroom, once considered part of life's normal joys and woes, should become the next frontier in public health policy, another enemy to be conquered along with heart disease, cancer, AIDS and drug addiction? Do 43 percent of American women and a third of men really need or want professional help between the sheets?

The sex survey might be taken as an example of creeping medicalization: a trend to seize upon aches and pains that people used to live with and declare them dysfunctions that must be treated. Where it was once acceptable to leave certain conditions alone, doing so now might be considered cruel neglect. Medicalization transforms people into patients and creates new markets for specialty clinics, diagnostic tests, pills, shots, self-help books, diet plans and the ultimate cash cow—regular medical monitoring.

Industries have sprung up to cash in on menopause, prescribe psychiatric drugs for troubled dogs, diagnose the vaguest of back pains, counsel people who want sex too much and now, of course, tune up those who do not want sex enough.

The suggestion that more people need sex doctors was trumpeted nationwide on radio and television and on the front pages of newspapers. But there were problems with the study that produced this conclusion. For one thing, it was based on a new analysis of old data that had already been published in a 1994 book, *The Social Organization of Sexuality*. Moreover, two of the authors, Dr. Edward Laumann, a sociologist at the University of Chicago, and Dr. Raymond Rosen, co-director of the Center for Sexual and Marital Health at the Robert Wood Johnson Medical

School in New Brunswick, New Jersey, had served as paid consultants to Pfizer, the manufacturer of Viagra, which could see a doubling of its market for the drug if the studies in women were to pan out. The authors' financial connection was not mentioned, due to "an oversight" at the *Journal of the American Medical Association*, according to Dr. Richard Glass, an editor there.

Pfizer did not pay for the sex survey, but the authors' relationship with the company raised questions nonetheless, because drug companies have an obvious interest in research that suggests expanded uses for their products.

"We must stop ignoring female sexual dysfunction," said Dr. Raymond Rosen, one of the Pfizer consultants who wrote the article. "That's what I'm hoping will come out of this survey—accelerated research on female sexual dysfunction."

Dr. Rosen said Viagra was "being very actively studied" in women, on the theory that it might stimulate sexual response in them as it does in men, by increasing blood flow to the genitals. He said the male hormone testosterone was also being tested as a means of enhancing sex drive in women past menopause, along with estrogen, which can strengthen vaginal tissue and improve lubrication.

Before such treatments were proposed, when sexual desire waxed and waned, people were more willing to chalk it up to the passage of years or the good times and bad that characterize most lives. But drugs like Viagra and hormones that can affect sex drive have created a powerful incentive for both drug companies and doctors to find new customers. One way to do that is to label the lack of desire an abnormal condition in need of treatment, which may create a social climate in which people who are not in the mood often enough are expected to do something about it.

The trend has advantages in providing relief for conditions that people used to suffer from. Viagra, for instance, has been a boon to some impotent men and their partners. But researchers point out that providing more and more medical care for more and more ailments, particularly conditions that do not directly threaten health, can have a downside as well.

In addition to costing a lot, extra treatment exposes people to extra risks. Another paper published recently in the same journal as the sex survey noted several instances in which efforts to step up treatments actually led to harm.

In one case, pregnant women at risk for giving birth to premature babies were monitored at home for signs of early labor. The monitoring led to the use of more drugs to hold off labor, which had adverse effects like lung problems and high blood sugar in 7 percent of the women but did not lower the rate of early births.

In another case, people who had had heart attacks were given drugs to treat slight abnormalities in heart rhythm, some so mild they did not even cause symptoms. But compared to people with similar histories who were not treated, those who took the drugs had death rates two to three times higher.

People who contemplate drug therapy to resuscitate their sex lives may also risk unwanted side effects: Viagra, for instance, can cause headaches and nausea and temporarily add a bluish tinge to one's vision.

Drugs may not always be the solution to sexual woes, anyway. Despite Dr. Rosen's enthusiasm for them, the study itself acknowledged that some of the most common sexual problems had social and emotional roots that no pill could fix. Young women, for instance, tended to have more pain from sex and less satisfaction than older women, probably because they changed partners more often. They tended also to alternate between intervals of no sex and episodes of frequent activity, a pattern that may contribute to higher rates of bladder infection—a condition all but guaranteed to take the joy out of sex.

John Gagnon, an emeritus professor of sociology at the State University of New York at Stony Brook, said it was little wonder that young women felt disappointed by sex, given the ineptitude of many young men. "I sometimes wonder why young women put up with it, except that they probably don't know any better," he said.

Some women in their 60s lose interest in sex, he said. "They say, 'I had my kids, and that's why I did it, and I never really got much else out of it,'" he said.

They consider the sexual phase of their lives finished, they do not miss it, and the idea of taking a drug to create a yearning for it may not appeal to them.

Contrary to what seems to be the prevailing belief, Mr. Gagnon said, people are not necessarily un-healthy or in need of medical treatment if they do not feel like having sex all the time.

"Many people find their hobbies more interesting," he said. "Sex is a modest pleasure."

[DG, February 1999]

## Male Hormone Molds Women, Too, in Mind and Body

Try as humans may to appreciate life's complexities and half-tones, we often resort to good old-fashioned dualism, dividing the world into conservatives and liberals, rich and poor, straights and gays, somebodies and nobodies, and, of course, men and women, with their complementary genitalia and their characteristic hormones. Men have androgens, most notably testosterone, while women have estrogens.

Even the words have a binary spin: "androgen" comes from the Greek "maker of males," and "estrogen" signifies the maker of the estrus cycle, the boss of ovulation and menstruation, the essence of womanhood.

But nature abhors absolutes, and it turns out that men and women each have a fair amount of the opposite sex's hormones coursing through their blood. Scientists have known this for years, yet they have long played down the implications of that hormonal kinship, particularly when it came to studying how testosterone and other androgens work in a woman's body.

They knew estrogen to be indispensable to the growth of all embryos, regardless of sex. By contrast, testosterone has been viewed as a luxury, needed mainly to shape a male's form and sexual function, and only vestigially and irrelevantly present in women. But these dismissive assumptions were made in the absence of any research or evidence.

Now, with the explosion of interest in women's health issues generally, physicians and scientists from a broad cross-section of disciplines at last have begun to consider the role of so-called male hormones on the making of a female. They are trying to determine how closely testosterone is linked to a woman's sex drive, and whether the hormone is necessary to maintain female muscle mass and bone density into old age.

These preliminary and often conflicting investigations already have physicians sharply divided over the wisdom of giving post-menopausal women small doses of testosterone along with the estrogen-replacement therapy they may receive. Doctors in Britain and Australia are much more likely to prescribe low-dose testosterone pellets or injections for women complaining of flagging libido and depression than are their colleagues in the United States, who are hesitant to begin treating women with a potent hormone that is linked to men's comparatively early death.

With even greater trepidation, some scientists are seeking to learn the extent to which androgens influence a woman's personality, energy levels, relative aggressiveness or assertiveness, and any other traits commonly described as masculine.

"The borders between classic maleness and femaleness are much grayer than people realized," said Dr. Robert A. Wild, professor and chief of the section on research and education in women's health at the University of Oklahoma Health Sciences Center, in Oklahoma City. "We're mixed bags, all of us."

One reason researchers have neglected the study of androgens in women is a simple matter of quantity: women have, on average, much less of them than men do. There are many androgens, but the major hormone circulating freely is testosterone.

Men have between 300 and 900 nanograms of testosterone for every deciliter of blood, much of it generated by the testes, but some originating in the adrenals, the little hat-shaped glands abutting the kidneys. (A nanogram is a billionth of a gram.) In women, a high measurement of testosterone is 100 nanograms, but the average is around 40, said Dr. Geoffrey P. Redmond, president of the Foundation for Developmental Endocrinology and a physician at Mount Sinai Hospital in Cleveland.

But the testosterone level varies significantly with the menstrual cycle, as do the more stereotypically female hormones, estrogen and progesterone. That is because a woman's testosterone comes not only from her adrenal glands (which are fairly steady from week to week in their hormonal productivity), but also from her ovaries, with each organ contributing about half. And as the estrogen production in the ovaries falls and soars, so, too, does testosterone output, meaning that a woman's maximum androgen secretion corresponds with her estrogen spike and hence with her ovulation.

Thus, in women with normally high testosterone levels, the ovulatory spike may bring them into androgen ranges approaching those of a low-testosterone male.

The impact of that fluctuating testosterone on the body is not clear. Researchers have a good idea of what testosterone does to males. During fetal development, it shapes the growth of the male genitals and possibly influences brain circuitry. When a boy reaches puberty, androgen production in the testes swings into gear to sculpt the secondary sexual characteristics: the thickening of muscles and vocal cords, the widening of the shoulders, the growth of the penis and the beard and the sudden obsession with sex.

In girls? Well, scientists know testosterone contributes to their adolescent development as well. It makes pubic and underarm hair grow. It could help their muscles and bones develop, although how it interacts with estrogen—which is known to be necessary for calcium absorption and bone strength—is unclear. "I wouldn't be surprised if female athletes have higher testosterone levels than nonathletes, although that's not well defined," said Dr. Roger S.

Rittmaster, an associate professor of medicine at Dalhousie University in Halifax, Nova Scotia.

Girls with high androgen levels may also end up with comparatively small breasts, he added, for in males the presence of testosterone is known to prevent a man's circulating estrogen from prompting the breast tissue to swell. Androgens can also cause a teenage girl's skin to become oily and break out, just as the hormones do to luckless boys.

The question would be merely of titillating interest were it not for a fierce debate over the use of testosterone replacement therapy in postmenopausal women. Dr. John Studd of the department of obstetrics and gynecology at Chelsea and Westminster Hospital in London said that besides estrogen-replacement therapy, about 25 percent of his postmenopausal patients receive testosterone pellets inserted under the skin. Among those recipients are women who have had their ovaries removed, as well as non-ovariectomized women who complain that their sex drive and energy levels are not what they used to be.

The degree to which testosterone levels ordinarily decline with age in either women or men is not known, but the atrophying of the ovaries postmenopausally can, in some cases, cut down on a woman's testosterone production. Dr. Studd says the pellets clearly help his patients. "They may have their lives transformed," he said. "Their energy, their sexual interest, the intensity and frequency of orgasm, their wish to be touched and have sexual contact—all improve."

Dr. Studd insisted that the doses used in his patients are so low that they have no adverse health affects. But many American physicians remain reluctant to prescribe testosterone therapy for women. "I have not seen women who need testosterone, except those who have had their ovaries removed," Dr. Redmond said. Other American scientists said there was a strong need to do a solid clinical trial of testosterone therapy in women.

Dr. Redmond and others believe that excess androgens are a far more pressing health problem than their diminution. By far, the bulk of the new research is focused on disorders that arise when a woman's body generates too much testosterone, resulting in everything from cosmetic problems like acne, balding and the growth of facial hair so abundant that the woman must shave twice a day to more severe complications like infertility, diabetes, high blood pressure, heart disease and cancer of the uterus. Even some cases of breast cancer, a disease normally associated with too much estrogen, may in fact be the result of excess testosterone, several experts said, although the data on this remains sketchy.

Researchers said the incidence of androgen disorders in women has been grossly underestimated, and that as many as 15 to 30 percent of all women may have problems caused by the overproduction of testosterone, an excessive sensitivity to the influence of circulating androgens, or both. They suggest that doctors should be on the lookout for women—and even young girls—who may be suffering from excess androgen secretion, so that the patients can be treated early enough to prevent the onset of serious and possibly fatal complications of a lifetime of androgen overdosing.

The signs of high androgen output sometimes are obvious: a tendency to put on weight in the upper body, particularly the stomach, rather than on the thighs and buttocks, as most women do; irregular periods; and hair sprouting in great abundance on the face, the thighs, in a woolly stripe from pelvis to belly button. Doctors can also perform blood tests to check for anomalous hormone secretions.

"It's not healthy for women to have abnormalities of androgen production, and these patients ought to be identified and treated as early as possible," said Dr. Philip D. Darney, a professor of obstetrics, gynecology and reproductive medicine at the University of California at San Francisco. "We've got a lot of work ahead of us educating physicians and patients on how to identify these states."

Among the treatments used to suppress or counteract androgen production are birth control pills; spironolactone, an anti-androgen drug; and dexamethasone, a synthetic steroid hormone that suppresses adrenal activity.

But scientists concede that the line between normal and abnormal levels of androgens in women is blurry and somewhat arbitrarily assigned. The dark mustache that may be considered unacceptable on women in this country—and thus a symptom of a hormone imbalance—is often viewed as ordinary and even sexy on women in Mediterranean countries. Some critics argue that the new emphasis on androgen excess is just another attempt to pathologize variations on a theme, turning traits once considered relatively normal into diseases that must be treated with potent medications taken over a lifetime.

"What society says is normal and what is normal for women can be very different," said Dr. Rittmaster. "Women can have a full beard and still be breast-feeding."

Many of the issues surrounding androgen disorders in women were discussed at a conference in Rockville, Maryland, sponsored by the National Institute of Child Health and Human Development. The meeting was organized by Dr. Florence Haseltine, a surgeon, gynecologist and firebrand for the study of women's health.

Dr. Haseltine said she has been shown to have elevated levels of androstenedione, a precursor to testosterone. And though she admits she has no proof for her assumptions, she believes this hormonal excess explains why she becomes quite aggressive when under stress.

One common androgenic disorder in women is polycystic ovarian syndrome, when, for reasons that remain mysterious, the ovaries produce excess testosterone, resulting in infertility and problems with insulin that can prompt the onset of diabetes. Women with the disorder often are very hairy on the face and body but balding, and on an ultrasound test their ovaries may appear to be bulging in the middle, in the stromal tissue that produces androgens. The disease sometimes can be treated with anti-androgen drugs, but it must be caught early if diabetes is to be averted.

Other scientists are fascinated by a hereditary disorder called congenital adrenal hyperplasia, in which a person lacks one of the five enzymes needed to produce cortisol, an important hormone in responding to stress. As a result of the defect, precursors to cortisol released by the adrenal glands build up in a budding fetus and act like male hormones.

Girls with congenital adrenal hyperplasia may emerge from the womb looking like boys, with an enlarged clitoris and even a scrotal sac, although they have fully formed ovaries and uterus. In the worst cases, the girls may need genital surgery to give them a more characteristically female appearance.

In other instances of the disorder, said Dr. Maria I. New, chairman of pediatrics at New York Hospital-Cornell Medical Center in Manhattan, girls are born with normal genitals but masculinize later in life, becoming hairy, acned and suffering from reduced fertility. For both severe and mild cases of hyperplasia, patients are given dexamethasone to inhibit adrenal overactivity.

Dr. New and her colleagues are completing a study of the psychology, sexuality and gender identity of women who have congenital adrenal hyperplasia, to see whether the high androgen levels in the womb influenced in any measurable way the women's neurological development. Dr. New will not yet say what their results are, other than to hint that "there are definitely effects of androgens on the brain."

But whether the women are said to be more mathematical, more aggressive, more sexually active, more enamored of guns and computers, or any number of traits commonly attributed to men, the results are sure to arouse the perennial quarrel over the nature of human nature: how much is head, how much hearth and how much a few simple hormones.

[NA, May 1994]

## Facing Viagra's Emotional Ripples

With men and women extolling the virtues of Viagra, it is easy to lose sight of potential problems and limitations of the potency pill. Not the least of them is the fact that erectile dysfunction, as impotence is called medically, can often be more than just a physical matter, especially when it has persisted untreated for years.

Lovemaking involves—or should involve—far more than simply the brief union of two body parts and the release of sexual tension. Although Viagra can, in most cases, restore a man's physical ability to achieve such a union, it does nothing per se to reawaken sexual desire and foster communication and loving feelings between partners who may have long ago put these aside.

Men who are impotent often refrain from any physical or verbal expressions of tenderness and desire for fear of raising false hopes in their partners, who may do likewise to avoid inducing guilt in a man unable to perform sexually. Both may need to make changes in how they think and behave if their sexual interaction is to be anything more than physical.

Experts in human sexuality anticipate that many couples who fail to deal with the emotional aspects of sex made possible by Viagra will end up with conflicts that could seriously strain rather than solidify their relationships.

"The sexual experience goes far beyond the physical event," said Dr. Alan Bell, author of *The Mind and Heart in Human Sexual Behavior*. "Any man who thinks Viagra is the be-all and end-all of sex has another thought coming," he said in an interview. "Relationship and intimacy issues have to be faced now or there will be a terrible price to pay."

Dr. Pepper Schwartz, an author and a psychologist at the University of Washington, agreed. "A pill," she said, "cannot address interpersonal problems and feelings of anger and frustration that are common in couples who haven't had sex in a long time. A newly-restored capacity for sex needs to be accompanied by an exploration of what she wants, what he wants and what each of them expects."

Dr. Schwartz noted, "Viagra is not a desire drug. It's a capacity drug. For it to work well, couples have to deal with changes in the emotional climate of their relationship, which for some will require professional help." She offers help for such couples in her latest book, *The Great Sex Weekend*, which she wrote with Janet Lever.

Dr. Michael A. Perelman, a sex and marital therapist at New York Hospital-Cornell Medical Center, said: "There will always be some people who have a negative reaction to a spouse's desire to rekindle a sexual relationship, who find that an improvement in erectile capacity is a threat to the status quo. Although for most couples Viagra is likely to represent a very positive change, it certainly will expose marital conflicts that would otherwise have remained buried."

Resentments can fester when the man makes a unilateral decision to engage in sex and takes a pill without his wife's knowing it. "He may start getting romantic with her and she just rolls over and goes to sleep," suggested Dr. Robert Kolodny, medical director of the Behavioral Medicine Institute in New Canaan. "Or she may be sitting at the computer trying to finish a report that is due the next morning, but he keeps insisting 'I took the pill, we've got to do it now.' Many women resent doing something on a schedule that should be spontaneous, and men are likely to resent wasting the money and the opportunity provided by the pill."

Conflicts can result not only from the demands of a newly potent man on his partner but also from a partner who pressures the man to get the drug in order to resume sexual relations when the man has no interest in doing so. "The man may not like his wife or want to be close to her," Dr. Kolodny said, "or he may be withholding sexual contact to punish her or put her in her place. For various reasons he may refuse to ask the doctor to prescribe Viagra, which will upset her because she feels he's not thinking of her needs."

Dr. Kolodny urged men who take Viagra to pay more attention to the quality rather than the quantity of the sexual experience. "Some women," he said, "are already saying that the drug makes sex artificial, that the man's erection does not result from the fact that he loves her and finds her attractive. She wants more romance."

By assuring a man of a lasting erection that will not fade after a few minutes of foreplay, Viagra could give him more time to pay more attention to his partner, physically and emotionally. It also could give couples an opportunity to draw closer to one another, said Dr. Bell, a counseling psychologist in Bloomington, Indiana, and 15-year veteran of the Kinsey Institute.

"The fact that Viagra takes 30 to 60 minutes to work is an advantage," Dr. Perelman said. "This allows time for a couple to engage in foreplay, to get together in ways that pleasure both partners without them having to worry that the man will soon lose his erection."

Dr. Bell pointed out that "men with potency problems become terribly preoccupied with getting an erection, and this preoccupation is inimical to sexual intimacy.

"As long as technical competence is the major focus," Dr. Bell continued, "then anything the woman is looking for is left out. The woman begins to see the man as more concerned with erectile success than with her."

Dr. François Eid, a urologist who directs the Sexual Function Center at New York-Cornell, said: "Men who have been impotent for a while think incorrectly that getting an erection will transform them into sexual human beings. They need to communicate affection for their wives and interest them in having sex again."

Dr. Eid also emphasized the need for newly potent men to be sensitive to their partners' moods and circumstances: "A man can't just go up to his wife while she's washing the dishes and say, 'Look, I've got an erection, let's have sex' and expect a favorable response. But when he's rejected he feels diminished and the relationship suffers. The man needs to relearn how to enroll his partner into making love again."

Regardless of the method used to restore a man's potency—Viagra, a little blue pill costing about $10, is merely the newest and simplest one—the highest rate of success results when the man seeks treatment with his partner, Dr. Eid said. "This indicates that they are communicating," he added, "they've discussed it and they're committed to finding a solution acceptable to them both."

[JEB, May 1998]

# Sour Note in the Viagra Symphony

When a revolutionary new treatment is discovered for a life-limiting condition, millions of sufferers are likely to forsake caution in hope of reaping its benefits. So it seems with Viagra, the pill that can restore a man's erections even after decades of impotence.

Doctors throughout the country find themselves writing 100 or more prescriptions a day for the $10-a-pill remedy, often for men who have given little thought to its possible side effects or its chances of working well for them.

What has made Viagra so attractive is not that it is the only remedy for erectile dysfunction, as potency problems are called medically. There are half a dozen other effective treatments. But unlike the others, Viagra is a pill, making it a far simpler and more discreet remedy than its rivals, which include drugs injected or inserted into the penis and devices implanted and inflated.

But in the wave of enthusiasm surrounding this drug, many physicians and their patients have ignored its limitations and side effects—those already known and those that may become apparent after millions of men have used it.

"Whenever a new drug is introduced, pharmaceutical companies always tout it as extraordinarily effective and without side effects," said Dr. Robert Kolodny, medical director of the Behavioral Medicine Institute in New Canaan, Connecticut, and a former associate of the pioneering sex researchers, Dr. William Masters and Virginia Johnson.

"In every case, a year or two later when the drug becomes widely used, new side effects emerge that were not previously seen," Dr. Kolodny said. "This is uncharted territory. There may be interactions between Viagra and other drugs men are taking. Men may use it at higher doses than it was designed to be used. And it will undoubtedly be used by a wide range of people, not all of whom are suitable or adequately screened medically beforehand."

Dr. Kolodny noted that some women are already taking Viagra, even though no data have shown its effectiveness or hazards for women. Likewise with adolescents, who may take it because of a medical problem that causes impotence or simply as a recreational drug in hopes of enhancing their virility.

Because most men with potency problems are in the later decades of life, some Viagra users no doubt will be in very poor health, suffering from diabetes, heart disease, arthritis and other ailments. Will their hearts stand the physical demands of sexual intercourse? How will Viagra interact with other medicines they may be taking?

Men who are rendered impotent by drugs for high blood pressure or depression are likely to constitute a large share of Viagra users, but until large numbers use the potency enhancer, its possible adverse interactions with their medicines will not be fully known.

What is known so far about Viagra, also known as sildenafil, is that it cannot safely be taken by anyone using nitrate medications and, according to a report in *The New England Journal of Medicine*, about a third of men experience one or more minor side effects, including headaches, flushing, indigestion, stuffy nose and temporary changes in visual perception of color or brightness. But in tests of Viagra in hundreds of men, few dropped out because of such effects.

"Whether the promise of sildenafil will be realized after many more men have been treated and the drug has been taken repeatedly for prolonged periods remains to be seen," Dr. Robert D. Utiger cautioned in an editorial in the same issue of the journal.

In the last two decades, the causes of impotence have become clearer. Masters and Johnson, authors of the groundbreaking work *Human Sexual Inadequacy*, maintained that in four of five cases, potency problems were psychologically based, caused primarily by anxiety over being able to perform adequately. All a man needs to do, they said, is learn to relax, not worry about getting and keeping an erection, focus on the immediate pleasure of physical stimulation and all will right itself.

Masters and Johnson attributed only 20 percent of impotence cases to physical problems like nerve or blood vessel disease, hormonal deficiencies, the effects of certain drugs or the aftermath of genital surgery. But recent research has proved the statistics to be quite the opposite, with about 80 percent of impotence now attributed to physical factors and 20 percent to emotional ones.

A man experiencing impotence would be unwise to assume that he knows the cause and that only a treatment like Viagra will help. If performance anxiety is the problem, a Masters-and-Johnson approach to treatment can be effective, risk-free and, in the long run, less expensive. If the cause is loss of interest in one's partner, couple's counseling may be effective, or perhaps nothing short of changing partners will help.

If impotence stems from a physical problem, correcting or treating the disorder can sometimes reverse it. For example, an impotent man with little or no sexual desire may be producing too little testos-

terone; treatment with the hormone, not Viagra, is in most cases the proper approach. An early-morning blood test is all that is needed to measure a man's testosterone.

Viagra can treat impotence whether the condition is physical, emotional or a combination of the two. It works with sexual arousal by increasing blood flow into the penis and holding it there, resulting in an erection that can be maintained until orgasm and sometimes longer. However, it is not a sure thing. Depending on the health of the penile tissue, Viagra may or may not result in an erection sufficient for penetration.

About one-third of men who take the drug and become sexually aroused will not get an erection rigid enough to achieve intercourse, according to Dr. François Eid, a urologist and the director of the Sexual Function Center at New York-Cornell Medical Center and a researcher in the Viagra trials.

The highest failure rate occurs among men who have had radical prostate surgery. At best, half respond adequately. Figures are similar among men

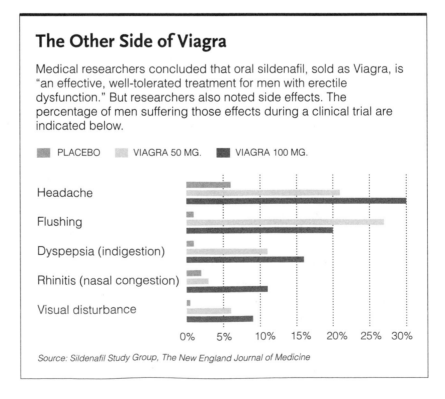

## The Other Side of Viagra

Medical researchers concluded that oral sildenafil, sold as Viagra, is "an effective, well-tolerated treatment for men with erectile dysfunction." But researchers also noted side effects. The percentage of men suffering those effects during a clinical trial are indicated below.

PLACEBO    VIAGRA 50 MG.    VIAGRA 100 MG.

Headache

Flushing

Dyspepsia (indigestion)

Rhinitis (nasal congestion)

Visual disturbance

0%   5%   10%   15%   20%   25%   30%

*Source: Sildenafil Study Group, The New England Journal of Medicine*

with long-standing insulin-dependent diabetes, 50 percent to 60 percent of whom are helped by Viagra.

Nor can Viagra compensate for a loss of nerve connections between the brain and the penis. If certain nerve pathways have been severely damaged or severed, a man may be able to obtain a drug-assisted erection but not orgasm and ejaculation.

[JEB, May 1998]

# In the History of Gynecology, a Surprising Chapter

Electricity has given so much comfort to womankind, such surcease to her life of drudgery. It gave her the vacuum cleaner, the pop-up toaster and the ice dispenser.

And perhaps above all, it gave her the vibrator. In the annals of Victorian medicine, a time of "Goetze's device for producing dimples" and "Merrell's strengthening cordial, liver invigorator and purifier of the blood," the debut of the electromechanical vibrator in the early 1880s was one medical event that truly worked wonders—safely, reliably, repeatedly.

As historian Rachel P. Maines describes in her exhaustively researched if decidedly offbeat work, *The Technology of Orgasm: "Hysteria," the Vibrator, and Women's Sexual Satisfaction*, the vibrator was developed to perfect and automate a function that doctors had long performed for women: the relief of physical, emotional and sexual tension through external pelvic massage, culminating in orgasm.

For doctors, the routine had about as much erotic content as a Kenneth Starr document. "Most of them did it because they felt it was their duty," Dr. Maines said in an interview. "It wasn't sexual at all." The vibrator, she argues, made that job easy, quick and clean. With a vibrator in the office, a doctor could ameliorate in minutes any number of symptoms labeled "hysterical" or "neurasthenic"—and guarantee habitual patronage.

"I'm sure the women felt much better afterwards, slept better, smiled more," Dr. Maines said. Besides, she added, hysteria was considered an incurable disease. "The patient had to go to the doctor regularly," Dr. Maines said. "She didn't die. She was a cash cow."

Nowadays, it is hard to fathom doctors giving their patients what Dr. Maines calls regular "vulvular" massage, either manually or electromechanically. But the 1899 edition of the *Merck Manual*, a reference guide for physicians, lists massage as a treatment for hysteria (as well as sulfuric acid for nymphomania). And in a 1903 commentary on treatments for hysterical patients, Dr. Samuel Howard Monell wrote that "pelvic massage (in gynecology) has its brilliant advocates and they report wonderful results."

But he noted that many doctors had difficulty treating patients "with their own fingers," and hailed the vibrator as a godsend: "Special applicators (motor driven) give practical value and office convenience to what otherwise is impractical."

Small wonder that by the turn of the 20th century, about 20 years after Dr. Joseph Mortimer Granville patented the first electromechanical vibrator, there were at least two dozen models available to the medical profession. There were musical vibrators, counterweighted vibrators, vibratory forks, undulating wire coils called vibratiles, vibrators that hung from the ceiling, vibrators attached to tables, floor models on rollers and portable devices that fit in the palm of the hand.

They were powered by electric current, battery, foot pedal, water turbine, gas engine or air pressure, and they shimmied at speeds ranging from 1,000 to 7,000 pulses per minute. They were priced to move, ranging from a low of $15 to what Dr. Maines calls the "Cadillac of vibrators," the Chattanooga, which cost $200 plus freight charges in 1904 and which, in its aggressive multi-cantilevered design, is more evocative of the Tower of London than the Pink Pussycat boutique.

Doctors used vibrators for many nonorgasmic purposes: to treat constipation, arthritis, muscle fatigue, inflammation laryngitis and tumors; men as well as women were the recipients of vibratory physic. But that a big selling point for the devices was their usefulness in treating female distress can be gleaned from catalogue copy and medical textbooks at the time, which spoke of the vibrator's particular effectiveness against "pelvic hyperemia," or congestion of the genitalia.

Vibrators were also marketed to women as home appliances. In fact, the vibrator was only the fifth household device to be electrified, after the sewing machine, fan, teakettle and toaster, and preceding by about a decade the vacuum cleaner and electric iron—perhaps, Dr. Maines suggests, "reflecting consumer priorities."

Advertised in such respectable periodicals as *Needlecraft*, *Woman's Home Companion*, *Modern Priscilla* and the Sears, Roebuck catalogue, vibrators were pitched as "aids that every woman appreciates," with the delicious promise that "all the pleasures of youth . . . will throb within you."

Significantly, the vibrators were almost always designed to be used externally. As a result, medically indicated massage therapy could be pitched as upstanding and asexual—and less risque than the gynecologist's speculum, which came under heavy ethical fire when it was first introduced in the late 19th century.

Dr. Maines, head of Maines and Associates, a firm that offers cataloguing and research services to museums and archives, first stumbled on her piquant subject while researching the history of needlework. Thumbing through a 1906 needlepoint magazine, she found, to her astonishment, an advertisement for a vibrator. When she realized there was no scholarly history of the device, she decided to take on the topic.

Her investigations led her to conclude that doctors became the keepers of the female orgasm for several related reasons. To begin with, women have been presumed since Hippocrates' day, if not earlier, to suffer from some sort of "womb furie"—the word "hysteria," after all, derives from the Greek word for uterus. The result was thought to be a spectacular assortment of symptoms, including lassitude, irritability, depression, confusion, palpitations of the heart, headaches, forgetfulness, insomnia, muscle spasms, stomach upsets, writing cramps, ticklishness and weepiness.

Who better to treat the wayward female plaint than a physician, and where better to address his ministrations than toward the general area of her rebellious female parts?

Dr. Maines also proposes that women have historically suffered from a lack of sexual satisfaction. By the tenets of what she calls the "androcentric" model of sex, women were supposed to be satisfied by the motions of heterosexual intercourse—the missionary position and its close proxies.

Yet as many studies have shown, about two-thirds of women fail to reach orgasm through coitus alone, Dr. Maines said. As a result, she said, many women may have spent their lives in an orgasm deficit, without necessarily identifying it as such. At the same time, religious edicts against masturbation discouraged women from self-exploration. "In effect," she writes, "doctors inherited the task of producing orgasm in women because it was a job nobody else wanted."

The vibrator was not the first therapeutic approach to treating feminine "pelvic hyperemia." Dr. Maines and other historians have described the practice of hydrotherapy, the taking to the baths or spas, as an ancient means to a sometimes climactic end. A century ago, spas like Saratoga Springs were a favorite destination of the well-to-do, who enjoyed the diversity of aqua-regimens: the warm baths, the bracing baths, the mineral baths, the gas-infused bubbly baths, the swirling proto-Jacuzzi baths.

A young woman named Abigail May, who traveled to Ballston Springs, New York, in 1800 to seek relief from the pain of her cancer, found happiness, if not a cure, in the water treatments, Dr. Maines writes, using information from a journal she found during her research. At first nervous at the sight of the douche hoses, Miss May made sure to "have laudanum handy" and then took the plunge. "I screamed merrily—so says Mama," Miss May wrote in her journal. "For my own part I do not remember much about it—I felt finely for two hours after bathing" and was "so much pleased with the Bath" that she went again not long afterwards.

The vibrator remained a staple of the doctor's armamentarium and the proper wife's boudoir until the 1920s, Dr. Maines said, when it began showing up in stag films and quickly lost its patina of gentility.

Vibrators are still widely available, of course— unless you happen to live in Alabama, Georgia or Texas, where state legislatures have banned the sale of vibrators and other "sex toys." The American Civil Liberties Union is now vigorously challenging the Alabama statute. If Alabama permits the prescribing of the anti-impotence drug Viagra, the A.C.L.U. argues, how dare it tell women that they can't have their own electromechanical prescription for joy?

[NA, February 1999]

## Issues of Gender, From Pronouns to Murder

There is no really right, widely accepted pronoun for Riki Anne Wilchins. Nor is there the right honorific. For the sake of convenience, let it be "she," and "Ms.," since she is a post-operative, male-to-female transsexual. But that's with apologies to Ms. Wilchins, for in her world view, such binary, he-she, Mr.-Ms. gender pigeon-holing oppresses.

"I would describe myself as a Riki-to-Riki transsexual," she said. "People say I transgress gender. I don't. I'm just being Riki. It's the gender system that transgresses all over me."

Ms. Wilchins, 47, is also one of the most prominent advocates in the country for "gender rights," a young movement that has begun to make measurable progress. Its members agitated with others, for example, to get crimes based on gender included in the Hate Crimes Prevention Act introduced in Congress in 1999 and reintroduced in 2000.

Ms. Wilchins, who lives in Greenwich Village, writes books: a pithy and impassioned tract called *Read My Lips* published in 1997 by Firebrand Books, a feminist press in Ithaca, New York, and, in progress, a transgender anthology and a "tranny" murder mystery. She is executive director of Gender PAC, a group based in Washington that annually takes more than 100 cross-dressers, transsexuals, gay men and lesbians to Capitol Hill to advocate on gender-rights issues.

Every time a transsexual or cross-dresser or some-one otherwise "gender-different" is reported murdered in the United States, her group posts the news at its Web site and sends it out over its on-line news service, seeking—usually unsuccessfully—the same kind of attention that the anti-homosexual murders of Matthew Shepherd and Billy Jack Gaither received.

The group has also organized vigils after each murder, but lately, she said, the killings have been coming too frequently, about one a month, to mark each one. Whether the reported rate is up because of improved information or increased violence, she does not know. Probably both, she said, theorizing that as homosexuality becomes more accepted, society is shifting more anger to the "differently gendered."

Ms. Wilchins also fights small personal battles every day: the battles of someone who looks different enough to draw stares, who, at a willowy six feet, gets strangers asking her, "Just how tall are you?" and who, with a horizontal scar on her neck from surgery to reduce her Adam's apple, gets strangers' pointing and asking, "What's that?"

"My throat," she tends to answer.

She began an interview in her walk-up apartment by saying amiably but firmly: "I'm not going to talk about when I got my surgery, you know," adding later, "It's a civil rights movement; it's not about what's between my legs."

Other life details were all right, though. Ms. Wilchins grew up as Richard in Cincinnati, her father was a surgeon, she was valedictorian of her high school class, she dropped out of several colleges beginning with Indiana University but eventually came close to earning a doctorate in psychology. She moved to New York in 1981 and works as a computer consultant on Wall Street.

But those life details were also not all right, each one edged with pain. Her late father brutalized her verbally and she is estranged from her family, she said, forbidden to see her nieces and nephews; when she began to "transition," many years ago, her girlfriend of seven years in Cleveland left her—"She wanted Richard," Ms. Wilchins said.

In high school, she said, though she lettered in sports and chased girls, "the boys in the locker room knew they were supposed to beat me up," though they couldn't have said why. While she considers herself a lesbian, gay and feminist groups long rejected her as not a "real woman" and thus not a "real lesbian." And when she starts a new job, colleagues often stare at her unabashedly.

Being different is like a tax she pays at every turn, Ms. Wilchins said; but she is also acutely aware that she has it easier than many gender-crossers. She's white, she's educated, she's tall, and, with her delicate features and slim build, she can move fluidly from commanding respect on a subway platform as a man in cap and jeans to stopping South Beach traffic as a roller-blading woman.

Many of the murder victims have been poor and black or Hispanic; and "the man who is 6'4" with chest hair and also likes to wear a dress is perhaps the most hated person in our country," she said. "To my way of thinking, he's the bravest person."

After an hour or two of talking with Ms. Wilchins, you feel something creakily dislodge in your mind. As Ms. Wilchins describes it, "You get on a trajectory where you feel, like, I may not be a 'real woman,' but God knows I'm not a real man, and you start looking around and realize how ridiculous it is for people to be stuck in gender roles."

It suddenly does not seem so strange that Ms. Wilchins would prefer the sex-neutral honorific of "M.," and to be referred to as "s/he," with the possessive not his or her but "hir."

One of Ms. Wilchins's fondest dreams, she said, "is that a straight married man can decide to wear a dress into work and the worst thing anyone will say is: 'Nice outfit. Is that report done?'"

[CG, June 1999]

## Group Sends Book on Gay Tolerance to Schools

In a move likely to fuel debate, a coalition of mainstream health and education groups sent the nation's school superintendents a booklet saying there is "no support among health and mental health professional organizations" for the idea that homosexuality is abnormal or mentally unhealthy.

The Just the Facts Coalition, representing the American Academy of Pediatrics, the National Education Association, the American Psychological Association and seven other groups, said the 12-page booklet would be mailed today to the heads of all 14,700 public school districts in the United States. The coalition said the booklet "provides information that will help school administrators and educators to create safe and healthy environments in which all students can achieve to the best of their ability."

The publication also expresses concerns about the potential harm to gay students posed by "reparative therapy" and other techniques intended to change sexual orientation.

"I think this is a history-changing moment," said Kevin Jennings, executive director of the Gay, Lesbian and Straight Education Network, a New York organization devoted to ending anti-gay bias in the schools. "The entire mainstream education and mental health establishment has said that it isn't lesbian, gay and bisexual students who need to change, it is the conditions in our schools that need to change."

But conservative groups attacked the booklet, saying that it was based on politics, not science.

"They're saying they want to present factual information on homosexuality, but we believe that they're presenting propaganda," said John Paulk, a homosexuality and gender analyst for Focus on the Family, a Colorado Christian group that holds Love Won Out conferences where reparative therapy is endorsed and participants are taught how to combat what they say are pro-gay messages children receive in schools.

Janet Parshall, chief spokeswoman for the conservative Family Research Council, also condemned the coalition's mailing. "If they're going to talk about 'the facts,' here's a fact: All the major religions of the world consider homosexuality wrong," she said.

Deanna Duby of the National Education Association, a leading union of school teachers, said the coalition was formed after members heard about the Love Won Out conferences and decided a response was needed. Ms. Duby, who helped create the booklet, said the publication was approved by the education association's leadership, including its president, Bob Chase.

Most of the organizations represented by the coalition, Ms. Duby said, had already passed resolutions on their own condemning reparative therapy and endorsing the need for "safe environments" for gay students.

The booklet, "Just the Facts About Sexual Orientation & Youth," is divided into chapters, including sections on how sexual orientation develops; reparative therapy, "transformational ministries" and other religion-based efforts that try to help homosexuals change their sexual orientation; and laws protecting gay men and lesbians from discrimination.

"Because of the religious nature of 'transformational ministry,' " the booklet advises, "endorsement or promotion of such ministry by officials or employees of a public school district in a school-related context could raise constitutional problems."

The publication states that "therapy directed specifically at changing sexual orientation is contraindicated, since it can provoke guilt and anxiety while having little or no potential for achieving changes in orientation."

Five of the organizations in the coalition contributed money to print and distribute the booklet, as did Michael Dively, a philanthropist and former member of the Michigan Legislature who is gay.

Responding to the booklet, Mr. Paulk, of Focus on the Family, said that no scientific studies had been done on reparative therapy, and that organizations that have "debunked" the technique were acting on the basis of political motives, not scientific evidence.

But Bruce Hunter, director of public affairs for the American Association of School Administrators, which represents public school superintendents and is a member of the coalition, said his organization agreed with the message of the booklet. Still, he said, the publication is likely to be used by school administrators "based on community values."

"There are many communities in this country that are just too conservative for that, and I trust superintendents to know their communities," Mr. Hunter said. "On the other hand, when push comes to shove, occasionally you have to stand up, and we would hope they would stand up for tolerance."

Other members of the coalition that endorsed the booklet are the American Federation of Teachers, the National Association of Social Workers, the National Association of School Psychologists and the Interfaith Alliance Foundation.

Copies of the booklet can be obtained by calling any of the organizations that are participating in the effort, a spokesman said.

[EG, November 1999]

# U.S. Awakes to Epidemic of Sexual Diseases

The burly man from the city Health Department who showed up at Gina G.'s apartment brought unpleasant news: A blood test had revealed that Gina, a soft-spoken, bookish woman of 38, had been swept up in a raging local epidemic of a sometimes forgotten disease, syphilis.

"I just froze," she recalled tearfully, dabbing a crumpled tissue behind thick red-framed glasses. "I said, 'Syphilis?' And he said, 'Yes, ma'am. Make sure you come in as soon as you can.' And I closed my door, and went in my room and cried."

Gina, who spoke on condition that her full name not be used, is being treated at a dilapidated city clinic, where doctors say penicillin shots, once a week for three weeks, should cure her. Her condition, which could cause serious heart or brain damage if left untreated, came as a shock; she has never had symptoms and has no idea how long she has been infected. But Federal and local public health officials are hardly surprised.

These experts say the United States is in the throes of an epidemic of sexually transmitted diseases that in poor, underserved areas like Baltimore's inner city rivals that of some developing nations. For the last 17 years, AIDS, the deadliest sexually transmitted disease the world has ever faced, has preoccupied the public and the medical community, drawing time, money and attention away from other sexually transmitted infections. Yet as these other infections spread, researchers say, they are fueling the AIDS epidemic.

Alarmed by high rates of some of the most common sexually transmitted infections—human papilloma virus, chlamydia and herpes—as well as by local outbreaks of syphilis and gonorrhea, which are less prevalent, the Centers for Disease Control and Prevention in Atlanta is starting a far-reaching campaign to curb sexually transmitted diseases, known as S.T.D.s. Outside experts describe it as the most intense Federal effort of its kind since World War II.

"It is a national disgrace that we do not have in place in this country an effective S.T.D. prevention system," said Dr. Judith N. Wasserheit, who directs the center's Division of S.T.D. Prevention. "The notion that we have a safety net of clinical and public health services to deal with the S.T.D. epidemic is a myth. In fact, much of the American public is not even aware that there is an epidemic."

Gina certainly was not. A former housekeeper who now attends college full time, she has been tested several times for H.I.V., the virus that causes AIDS. Her knowledge of syphilis came from watching a television special on the notorious Tuskegee experiment, in which poor black men in rural Alabama were left untreated for the disease. She did not realize it was still around. "It's a real wake-up call," she said.

Officials at the disease control centers hope to extend that wake-up call beyond Baltimore. Beginning in 1999, the agency instituted a radical change in the way it distributed prevention dollars to the states; each health department that applies must enlist community partners, like school boards and managed care organizations, in its prevention campaign. The idea is not only to broaden the campaigns' reach, but to break what Dr. King K. Holmes, professor of medicine at the University of Washington, calls the "conspiracy of silence" that has allowed these infections to flourish.

The centers are also pressing to rid the nation of all new cases of syphilis; in 1996 there were 52,995. In his budget for the fiscal year 1999, President Clinton asked Congress to appropriate $10 million for the elimination effort, which Dr. Wasserheit estimated would take at least 10 years. And in March 1998, 30 leaders in education, health, religion and entertainment met in Washington to advise the C.D.C. on how to get its message out, in much the same way AIDS activists have.

"There is a wellspring of public and policy debate now about sexually transmitted diseases," said the

Rev. Beth Meyerson, who directs Missouri's prevention program and attended the session. "It is really unprecedented."

Much of the debate was spawned by a 1996 report by the Institute of Medicine, the research branch of the National Academy of Sciences, titled "The Hidden Epidemic." The report, which concluded that "an effective national system for S.T.D. prevention currently does not exist," offered a blueprint for how to create one, from increasing medical research to the politically-charged issue of offering condoms in schools.

An estimated 10 million to 12 million new cases of sexually transmitted infections are reported each year to the disease control centers; that is roughly 80 times the new cases of tuberculosis, H.I.V. infection and AIDS combined. According to the institute, the Government spent $230.8 million in 1995 on programs to prevent sexually transmitted infections other than H.I.V. But the direct cost of treating these infections was $7.5 billion.

While experts have long known that sexually transmitted diseases contribute to cervical cancer, infertility and infant mortality, a pressing reason to curb them is that doing so could help to curb AIDS.

People with syphilis, gonorrhea, chlamydia or herpes are two to five times as likely as others to become infected with the AIDS virus, in part because they may have open sores that provide H.I.V. an easy route of entry to the body, Dr. Wasserheit said. In addition, those who have both H.I.V. and another sexually transmitted infection are more likely to spread the AIDS virus during sexual contact and are thus more infectious, she said.

This is one reason the C.D.C. is so worried about Baltimore's syphilis epidemic. In May 1997, the Federal agency took the unusual step of sending one of its employees, Dr. Noreen Hynes, on a long-term assignment to lead the city's fight against the epidemic.

"Baltimore has very high rates of H.I.V. mortality, which we believe this epidemic is contributing to," Dr. Hynes said. "Now people are beginning to realize that separating out H.I.V. from other S.T.D.'s is not appropriate."

While each of these diseases follows its own pattern, the picture as a whole is bleak. National rates of syphilis and gonorrhea, which are easily cured with antibiotics, have dropped steadily over the last decade, but still far exceed those of any other industrialized nation. The rates are particularly high in rural and inner-city areas where access to health care is poor; Dr. Wasserheit said 4 percent of African-American girls ages 15 to 19 were infected with gonorrhea.

The risk is hardly limited to African-Americans or people of low income. While data are incomplete for human papilloma virus and chlamydia, experts agree they are becoming increasingly common among teenagers, including those who are middle class. A three-year survey at Rutgers University found that 60 percent of female students had been infected with the human papilloma virus.

Herpes, meanwhile, is spreading at a surprising pace. A study released in October 1997 by the disease control centers found that one in five Americans older than 12 was infected with the genital herpes virus, a 30 percent increase from two decades ago. Rates among white teenagers quintupled.

In New York City, officials say chlamydia is the most pressing problem; teenagers account for about 40 percent of the 25,000 cases reported each year. "A large amount of chlamydia in a city with a large amount of H.I.V. is a dangerous combination," said Dr. Isaac Weisfuse, the assistant commissioner of the city Health Department.

Unlike breast cancer or Parkinson's disease or AIDS, sexually transmitted diseases have no natural constituency; patients and politicians do not go to Washington to fight for money to prevent them. Moreover, experts say, doctors are not on the lookout for these infections. A 1994 nationwide survey of 450 doctors and 514 other health care professionals, cited in the Institute of Medicine report, found that 60 percent of the doctors and 51 percent of the other providers did not routinely evaluate their new patients for sexually transmitted diseases.

"Sexually transmitted diseases are not on anybody's radar screen," complained Dorothy Mann, executive director of the Family Planning Council in

Philadelphia. "They are seen by mainstream medicine as relegated to some other kind of people, not the kind of people they see. And that is just not true."

In Baltimore, city officials said that 115 infants were born infected with syphilis during 1996 and 1997, in part because doctors failed to screen the mothers. Some were stillborn, said Dr. Peter Bielenson, the city Commissioner of Health; others have suffered mental retardation and other complications.

"It's outrageous," Dr. Bielenson said. "In the county surrounding us, in a nice hospital, we had two moms who tested positive. But the doctor did not believe the moms tested positive and the babies were born, with bad outcomes."

Different people offer different explanations for the Baltimore epidemic, which began in 1994 and has earned the city what Dr. Hynes called "the dubious distinction" of having syphilis rates that are 18 times the national average, the highest in the country. For every 100,000 people in Baltimore, 80 are infected; the rate is three to four times higher in areas where the epidemic is most concentrated.

Dr. Bielenson blames a wave of crack use that fueled the inner-city drugs-for-sex trade. Others, including some at the C.D.C., point to urban redevelopment; when public housing projects were torn down, they say, "sexual networks" were broken up as carriers were scattered to other parts of the city, where they found new partners.

In any event, the epidemic has moved out of the inner city—not to the suburbs, but to less impoverished areas that ring the inner city, said Dr. Jonathan Zenilman, an associate professor of medicine at Johns Hopkins University, who has been keeping detailed case maps. "Saying that this is a drug-related epidemic is a disservice," he said.

Gina is typical; she said she does not use drugs and does not associate with anyone who does. "Many of our patients are innocent victims," said Jackie Miller, the physician's assistant who administered Gina's penicillin shot on a recent morning. "They are totally freaked out."

However it began, experts agree that syphilis got out of hand when, just as the epidemic began to skyrocket, local and Federal budget cuts prompted the city to scale back its two sexually transmitted disease clinics, which together diagnose and treat half the reported infections in Baltimore.

The number of nurse practitioners and physician's assistants, Dr. Bielenson said, dwindled from 16 to 10. Patients were turned away; the number of annual visits to the clinics dropped from 36,000 in 1990 to 22,000 in 1996. In addition, the city lost some workers who were responsible for tracking down the sexual partners of those who were infected and bringing them in for treatment.

In many cities, Dr. Wasserheit said, the story has been the same. "There are over 3,000 local health departments in this country," she said. "Only half even provide S.T.D. services."

Baltimore, she said, "is an excellent example of what happens when people are not paying attention."

In late 1997 and early 1998, city officials took great pains to turn the epidemic around. Dr. Bielenson, the health commissioner, said he had drummed up more than $400,000 in help from the city, state and Federal governments; the money is being used to hire more clinic workers and case trackers.

Among these gumshoes is Sheridan Johnson, the burly man who knocked on Gina's door. His colleagues call him "Super-Epi," as in epidemiologist, for his ability to find patients and bring them in for treatment. He says he is successful more than half the time; in 1997, he and his colleagues found and examined 48 percent of the people they were looking for.

Theirs is a challenging task, requiring persistence and a gift for smooth talking. On a recent Friday afternoon, Mr. Johnson had five potential syphilis patients on his call list; after knocking on five doors, he found only one, who insisted she had already been tested and that the test proved negative.

Another had given his address as a homeless shelter, and Mr. Johnson left yellow cards that declared, "This is Urgent!" at the homes of the other three. "Hopefully," he said, "they'll call me."

[SGS, March 1998]

# Pregnancy, Childbirth and Matters of the Womb

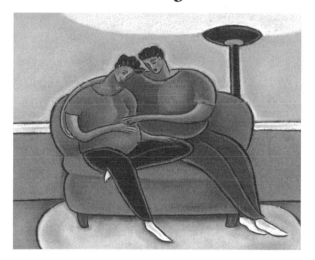

## MYSTERIES REMAIN AMID TECHNOLOGICAL ADVANCES

Why do human pregnancies last nine months? Why is labor so long, hard and painful? Why are human infants, compared to other mammals, so helpless and dependent for such a long time? The reasons are not known for sure, but researchers have speculated prolifically about them and continue to study them, with most of their ideas revolving around the notion of compromise, between a mother who needs a pelvis narrow enough to let her walk upright, but wide enough to let her give birth to a baby with an advanced brain and a big skull.

Short of performing a caesarean section, doctors can do little to alter or shorten the arduous course of labor and delivery. But today, as never before, they can do a great deal to ease the pain, while leaving the mother perfectly alert so that she can experience the birth, and strong enough to push the baby out. Although public sentiment during the 1970s and 1980s favored drug-free "natural childbirth," during the 1990s the pendulum began to swing the other way, with more and more women deciding labor pains were a rite of passage they could do without and asking for spinal and epidural anesthesia.

Many still prefer to let nature take its course, however, and birth assistants, or doulas, who stay with a woman in labor and help her get through it, are becoming increasingly popular.

The greatest technological progress, however, has taken place not in childbirth, but a step earlier: conception. Few areas of medicine have seen the kind of extraordinary advances that have occurred in the brave new field that has come to be known as "assisted reproduction" or "reproductive technology." Couples who might have been considered hopelessly infertile just 20 years ago are today becoming parents, with the help of fertility drugs, in vitro fertilization, donor eggs and sperm, and techniques that inject a single sperm cell into an egg to fertilize it. Parents can even choose their baby's sex and screen out embryos with certain genetic disorders before pregnancy begins. In the future, women about to undergo chemotherapy for cancer, which often causes sterility, may be able to have ovarian tissue removed and frozen, and returned to their bodies later so that they have a chance of becoming pregnant. And improved treatment of fibroid tumors promises to help women avoid hysterectomy and preserve their ability to have children. But, what to tell the children who owe their existence to some of the more imaginative feats of reproductive technology? Children born as a result of sperm or egg donation—and thus not related biologically to one or both of the parents who brought them up—have been compared to adoptees, most of whom nowadays are told the truth about their backgrounds as soon as they are old enough to talk. Later in life, many adopted children seek out their biological parents. But few people find it easy to explain egg or sperm donors to a small child—and so it is an explanation that many parents who have had this kind of help choose to forego.

# $50,000 Offered to Tall, Smart Egg Donor

The advertisements appeared in newspapers at the nation's top schools—Ivy League colleges, Stanford University, the Massachusetts Institute of Technology, the California Institute of Technology.

"Egg Donor Needed," the advertisements said, adding, "Large Financial Incentive." The advertisements called for a 5'10", athletic woman who had scored at least 1400 on her Scholastic Achievement Test and who had no major family medical problems. In return for providing eggs, she would receive $50,000.

Within weeks, more than 200 women responded to what is believed to be the largest amount of money offered for a woman's eggs. Darlene Pinkerton, who with her lawyer-husband Thomas Pinkerton, placed the advertisement on behalf of an infertile couple, said that most respondents were from Ivy League institutions and that she was starting to get calls from women in countries as far away as Finland and New Zealand. Women from state colleges and universities are calling, Ms. Pinkerton said, as are women who are too short or whose S.A.T. scores are too low.

When she ran the same advertisement four months earlier, without mentioning the price the couple would pay, Ms. Pinkerton said, she got only six responses.

Until recently, ethicists argued whether $50,000 was too much to pay for an egg donor. They debated whether it was coercive for couples to ask for S.A.T. scores or height or favorite books when they sought egg donors. But, some ethicists say, a $50,000 price, in a donor market that in early 1998 was reeling from offers of $7,500 for donors, makes them wonder whether the business is getting out of control.

The couple offering $50,000 wants to remain anonymous, Ms. Pinkerton said. But, she said, they decided to offer $50,000 "because they can."

The couple also realized that it might be hard to find a donor who met their criteria. They are "highly educated," Ms. Pinkerton said, and want a child who can be highly educated as well. They are tall, so they want a child who is tall.

"We have heard that only one percent of the college population is over 5'10" with over 1400 S.A.T. scores," Ms. Pinkerton said.

Lori Andrews, a professor at Chicago-Kent College of Law, is taken aback by the heights that payments are reaching. "I think we are moving to children as consumer products," Ms. Andrews said. "When prices for donors reach $50,000, it gets to be a meaningful, life-altering sum," she said.

Dr. Mark V. Sauer, who directs the assisted-reproduction program at Columbia University's College of Physicians and Surgeons in New York, said he found women, even Ivy League women, who were willing to donate their eggs for $5,000. And so, Dr. Sauer asks, why would a couple want to pay $50,000? "I can understand the motive for the donor—it's like winning the lottery," Dr. Sauer said.

After all, he said, it takes just three to four weeks to produce eggs. The donor takes fertility drugs to stimulate her ovaries to produce more than a dozen eggs, has regular ultrasound exams so a doctor can follow the eggs' development, and then is anesthetized while a doctor aspirates the eggs from her ovaries through a needle.

But, Dr. Sauer asked, what are the egg recipients thinking when they offer to pay so much for a donor with such specific traits?

"What genetic textbook did they read," he asks, that would tell them that they could order up a tall, smart, athletic child by paying $50,000 for a donor?

But other experts say they fail to see what is so wrong with looking for specific traits in a donor and paying $50,000 for them. Dr. Norman Fost, who directs the program in medical ethics at the University of Wisconsin in Madison, said it was not so crazy to ask for height and S.A.T. scores.

Dr. Fost said he worried more about parents who tried to engineer their children after they were born, pushing them to get perfect grades and to take endless S.A.T. tutoring courses. "I don't think that genetic engineering is any more pernicious," he said.

As for the $50,000 payment to the egg donor, why not? "It's like offering someone a million dollars to play professional football," Dr. Fost said. "You are perfectly free to walk away from it. People make these choices all their lives."

In the end, he said, "whether children are valued and how they are treated has very little to do with how they are conceived."

[GK, March 1999]

## Quandary on Donor Eggs: What to Tell the Children

In the quiet moments they share with their 5-year-old, when they are brushing her hair or tucking her in for the night, Lynn and Peter G. like to tell their daughter the story of her birth. Children love such tales, and theirs is typical—loving parents, a wanted pregnancy, an adorable baby.

Typical, that is, except for "the nice lady who helped Mommy," an egg donor named Sarah.

"I tell her Mommy was having trouble with, I call them ovums, not eggs," explains Mrs. G., a 50-year-old Los Angeles therapist who spoke on the condition that her surname, and her daughter's name, be withheld to protect the child's privacy. "I say that I needed these to have a baby, and there was this wonderful woman and she was willing to give me some, and that was how she helped us. I want to be honest that we got pregnant in a special way."

Over the last decade, as reproductive scientists have perfected the use of donated eggs to help infertile couples conceive, an estimated 6,000 women in the United States have given birth in this fashion, according to the American Society for Reproductive Medicine. Though much has been made of their age—many are entering motherhood in their 40s, and some in their 50s and even 60s—there has been little discussion of what may be the most divisive question within the growing "donor egg" community: Should the children be told?

The issue of children having genetic roots different from their parents, of course, is not entirely new; it has been around for decades both in the form of adoption and of sperm donation. But while some might regard donated eggs as the female equivalent of donated sperm, experts say that for a variety of reasons, the two cannot be equated.

Egg donation, which requires surgical intervention, is much more invasive than sperm donation, both for the donor and the recipient. And men, who tend to equate fertility with virility, are likely to keep their use of donor sperm a secret. Women are more inclined to talk about infertility. As a result, said Dr. Andrea Braverman, director of psychological services at Pennsylvania Reproductive Associates in Philadelphia, questions of privacy and disclosure have suddenly become urgent.

"Donor egg quite frankly blew the lid off the whole decision to tell or not to tell," Dr. Braverman said.

The G. family, it appears, is atypical. Though no one has kept a tally, experts say most couples do not reveal that mother and child have different genetic roots. Pediatricians, friends and even grandparents are kept in the dark. There are, however, regional differences. In California, where women are more likely to know their donors, the trend is toward openness. On the East Coast, where donation is often anonymous, disclosure is less likely.

"Despite the popular genre of psychology books that say all the different ways you can do your disclosure, I'm not finding too many people who are actually doing it," said Dr. Mark V. Sauer, director of reproductive endocrinology at Columbia-Presbyterian Medical Center in New York. "The great majority are keeping it a secret."

This has provoked a deep rift among mental

health professionals who counsel infertility patients. On the one side are those who argue that withholding the information is immoral, in part because family secrets can be devastating and in part because genetic histories are becoming increasingly important as scientists explore the hereditary aspects of disease.

Dr. Susan Cooper, a psychologist at Reproductive Science Center-Boston, is in that camp. "Secrets in families go sour," she said, citing the experience of adoptees, who as recently as 15 years ago were not routinely told about their backgrounds.

"Everybody has a right to know the truth about where they come from and how they got to be who they are," Dr. Cooper said. "People are curious about where they come from. Who are they genetically connected to? I cannot imagine that some donor children will not want to find out who the donor mother was."

On the other side are those like Dr. Susan Klock, a psychologist at Northwestern University School of Medicine who says that the decision is deeply personal and that families must do what is best for them. Though egg donation is too new to have been studied thoroughly, Dr. Klock's research tracked 35 sperm donor families and found that 86 percent had not told their children and did not plan to.

"They didn't think it was relevant," she said, "and of the couples who had told other people, many regret having done so, because now they feel compelled to tell the child."

The debate is taking on increasing intensity as the first wave of donor egg children reaches an age where, experts say, they can begin to comprehend the rudimentary facts of reproduction. The technique is used in infertile women who do not produce eggs, or whose eggs are damaged, typically by chromosomal abnormalities that come with age.

The first baby conceived with donated eggs was born in 1984, and demand for the procedure exploded around 1990, amid news reports that it was available for post-menopausal women. Those children are now in elementary school, a time of inevitable questions about where babies come from and of classroom assignments to draw family trees.

"We don't have it all worked out," said Peter G., a 45-year-old social worker. His wife said she was not inclined to "pull all of Sarah's family into this." Though she wants her daughter to know her history, she does not want to overemphasize it. "It's so complicated," she said with a sigh. "I try to balance."

It was precisely to avoid this kind of complex balancing act that one of Dr. Braverman's clients, a 42-year-old woman who spoke on condition that she not be identified, has decided not to tell her 5-year-old twins that they were conceived with donated eggs. She and her husband are longtime friends of the egg donor and the donor's husband. Their children—who are genetic half-siblings—are playmates. But the four parents have made a pact to keep their collaboration quiet, though they may revisit the issue when the children are adults.

"What, truly, is there to be gained?" the woman asked. "I can only think of things that would be confusing, overwhelming, create curiosities and bring up other issues for my donor's family."

She never feels burdened by her secret, she said, although there are moments of "small, wry humor" that she and her husband share when people comment about how much the twins resemble her. When the pediatrician asks for a medical history, she added, "I have to stop. I think, 'Don't put your health history. Focus on the donor's history.'"

Couples who adopt have always faced this dilemma. But as with sperm donation, there are crucial differences between babies who are adopted and those conceived through donated eggs.

"In donor egg, nobody gave up a child; somebody shared their eggs," said Patricia Mendell, who directs a telephone support line for the New York chapter of Resolve, an advocacy group for infertility patients. Lynn G.'s sentiments are similar: "She's not the mother," she said of Sarah, her donor. "I carried her. I nurtured her. I'm the mother."

Some say that, on the issue of disclosure, reproductive science today is where adoption was 20 or 30 years ago. It was not until the early 1980s that experts reached a consensus that adopted children should be told that they are adopted, said Bill Pierce, president of the National Council for Adoption, a Washington-based advocacy group.

Despite a growing movement toward openness,

Mr. Pierce said, there remains bitter controversy about whether adoptees should be permitted to track down their biological parents. Two states, Alaska and Kansas, have laws allowing adopted children to obtain their original birth certificates. Mr. Pierce's group, which opposes that, is challenging a similar Tennessee statute in court.

Only three states—Oklahoma, Texas and Florida—have enacted legislation regarding egg donation, but that was only to clarify that the donors have no rights or duties with respect to raising the child. Policy makers have yet to tackle the issue of whether children have a right to track down their genetic roots, although some think they should.

"I think there is a morally suspect asymmetry between what goes on in reproductive technology and what we have agreed are emerging rights for adoptees," said Dr. Arthur Caplan, director of the Center for Bioethics at the University of Pennsylvania. "I think you owe people you make in new ways some stable base of security about their identity."

The majority of egg donors remain anonymous. Although fertility clinics keep records that match donors to recipients, access is restricted. The rules vary from state to state.

"In New York, we have coded records with anonymous donors," said Dr. James A. Grifo, director of reproductive endocrinology at New York University Medical Center. "We are required by law to keep them in separate locked quarters, so that no one can walk into our office and link Mrs. So-and-So with Donor X."

Asked how long he must keep the records, Dr. Grifo paused. "That's not clear," he finally said. "I guess forever."

Dr. Grifo said that many of his patients agonized over what they would tell their children, some so much that they backed out of the process entirely. "But," he said, "I have never seen someone who brings in their 1- or 2- or 3-year-old and is unhappy with what they have done. They are some of the most grateful patients I have ever seen."

Of course, finding the right language to talk to a child about sophisticated matters of reproduction and infertility is hardly easy, and the self-help shelves of bookstores are notably thin on the topic. Carole Lieber Wilkins, a Los Angeles therapist and mother of a 10-year-old son by egg donation, has written a small pamphlet, *Talking to Children About Their Conception: It's Easier Than You Think*. She suggests that parents begin telling their children as soon as they are born.

"Parents need to practice doing this when children are nonverbal, so they can get accustomed to the sound of words that are very awkward and uncomfortable to use, like donor or infertility," she said. "That way, we can make all our mistakes before our kids have a clue."

But as the G. family has discovered, that is easier said than done. There is a natural grieving process that accompanies egg donation, as couples mourn their inability to conceive a child to whom they are both genetically linked. Talking about it inevitably brings up painful memories of infertility, and there are times, Lynn G. said, when she would rather forget. "Sometimes," she said, "I just want to push it away."

Although the couple decided when Lynn was pregnant that they would be open with their daughter, it was not until her birth that, Peter G. said, the proportions of the decision hit him.

"It's easy to be in denial when you are caught up in the joy of the moment," he said. "Then you realize that at some age, depending on when she starts talking or what she understands, you are going to have to make some decisions about what you are going to say."

The couple have tried to introduce the concept naturally. When their daughter, whose light brown hair is straight as straw, looks admiringly at her mother's curly dark locks, Lynn reminds her that Sarah, the egg donor, has straight hair. "And she would say, 'Sarah?' And then I would tell her the story."

At the same time, as their child grows older, the couple find themselves becoming less open with outsiders. They do not want her to resent them someday for revealing information she might want to keep private. They are bracing themselves, as well, for the tumultuous teenage years, when they expect that she will want to delve into her genetic roots. Although Lynn G. said that would be difficult for her, she does not intend to stand in the way.

"I made a choice," the mother said. "I wouldn't give up what I chose, but with all choices, there are consequences."

[SGS, January 1998]

# Researchers Report Success in Method to Pick Baby's Sex

With an announcement that produced applause and handwringing, doctors at a fertility center near Washington reported that they can substantially stack the odds that a couple can have a baby of the sex they choose. The method, developed by the Genetics & IVF Institute in Fairfax, Virginia, involves sorting sperm by the amount of DNA they contain and then using them for artificial insemination.

It capitalizes on the fact that there is only one difference between sperm that carry the Y chromosome, which produces males, and those with an X chromosome, which produces females: sperm with a Y chromosome have about 2.8 percent less genetic material. The investigators report that if they select for X-bearing sperm, they end up with sperm samples in which 85 percent of the cells have an X chromosome. If they select for Y-bearing sperm, the result is a sperm sample in which 65 percent of the cells contain a Y chromosome.

In a paper published in the journal *Human Reproduction*, the investigators, led by Dr. Edward F. Fugger, report results for couples who wanted girls. Of 14 pregnancies that progressed far enough for doctors to determine the fetus's sex, 13 fetuses were female. Ten out of the 11 babies born so far were girls. Dr. Fugger said that the group had produced about the same number of pregnancies for couples who wanted boys and that the results were consistent with what the sperm sorting would predict. But, he said, the investigators are not releasing the results of those pregnancies until they are published in a medical journal.

Of course, sex selection techniques have been promoted and marketed for decades. But, said Dr. Alan DeCherney, the chairman of obstetrics and gynecology at the University of California at Los Angeles and the editor of the journal *Fertility and Sterility*, "Nothing worked until now." The Genetics & IVF Institute, a private, for-profit medical center, is a leader in fertility research and prides itself in being among the first to offer new reproductive techniques. Dr. Fugger noted that hundreds of animals of a variety of species had been born after sperm sorting before his group began using the method and that there was no evidence that sperm sorting caused birth defects. But other fertility experts raised questions about the ethical quandaries opened up with a decision to provide sex selection and about whether the animal tests were adequate to show safety in humans.

Sex selection has been used for millennia, with folk remedies that supposedly guaranteed a baby of a particular sex, female infanticide and, more recently, the abortion of fetuses because of their sex. Decade after decade, so many groups have claimed that they had a method for sex selection that the entire field became tainted, said Dr. Richard Rawlins, the director of the in vitro fertilization laboratories at Rush University in Chicago. Most recently, claims that male sperm could be separated because they swim faster were found to be without scientific basis. To sift sperm, researchers at the Genetics & IVF Institute stained the DNA and then used a cell sorter that lined up sperm individually in a stream, where each sperm's DNA content was measured and the X-containing sperm separated from those with a Y chromosome. The scientists said it took most of a day to sort the approximately 200 million wriggling sperm of a single ejaculate as they pass single file through the machine's DNA detector.

Dr. Joseph Schulman, director of the Genetics & IVF Institute, said most of the couples wanted to choose their baby's sex for "family balancing." A few wanted sex selection because they were at risk of having babies with genetic diseases that afflict boys almost exclusively, he said. Dr. Schulman said that, so far, the institute was not offering the method to couples who have no children and want a first child of a particular sex, but he did not rule out that use.

Monique Collins of Gainesville, Virginia, was one of the first to have sperm sorting, in March 1995. She had two sons, who were aged 2 and 6, and urgently wanted a daughter. "Having a daughter for me was like having a baby for some people; that's how important it was," she said. She and her husband, Scott Collins, had a girl on August 13, 1996, after Mr. Collins's sperm was sorted at the institute.

The Virginia researchers are using a technique whose development began 16 years ago, when Dr. Lawrence A. Johnson, a scientist at the Department of Agriculture's research service in Beltsville, Maryland, began working on a sperm separation method. His goal was to do sex selection for farm animals. Dr. Johnson labeled the DNA in sperm cells with a temporary, nontoxic, fluorescent chemical. Once that chemical was in the sperm cells, they would glow blue under a laser light. The more light that was emitted when the laser shined on a sperm cell, the more DNA the cell contained. That gave Dr. Johnson a way to detect small differences in DNA content. He modified a cell sorting machine so that it would detect it.

Commercial interests soon stepped in. In 1996, the Colorado State Research Foundation and Cytomation Inc. of Fort Collins formed a company,

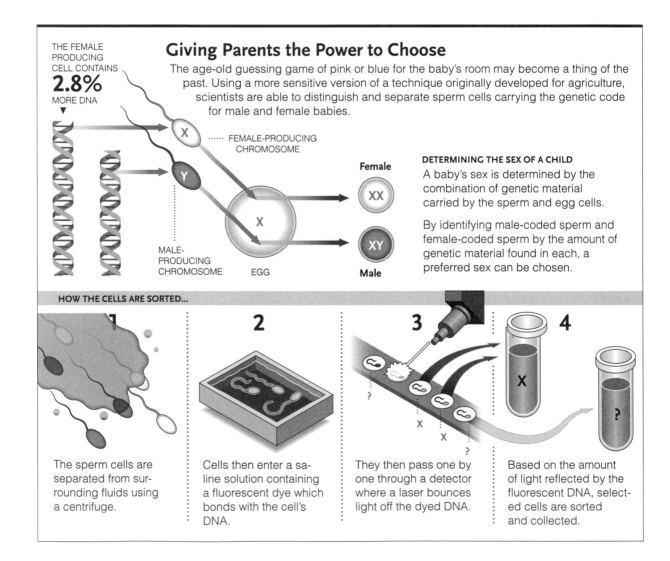

**THE FEMALE PRODUCING CELL CONTAINS**

**2.8%** MORE DNA

## Giving Parents the Power to Choose

The age-old guessing game of pink or blue for the baby's room may become a thing of the past. Using a more sensitive version of a technique originally developed for agriculture, scientists are able to distinguish and separate sperm cells carrying the genetic code for male and female babies.

X ······ FEMALE-PRODUCING CHROMOSOME

Y

MALE-PRODUCING CHROMOSOME

X

EGG

**Female**

XX

**Male**

XY

**DETERMINING THE SEX OF A CHILD**

A baby's sex is determined by the combination of genetic material carried by the sperm and egg cells.

By identifying male-coded sperm and female-coded sperm by the amount of genetic material found in each, a preferred sex can be chosen.

**HOW THE CELLS ARE SORTED...**

**1**

The sperm cells are separated from surrounding fluids using a centrifuge.

**2**

Cells then enter a saline solution containing a fluorescent dye which bonds with the cell's DNA.

**3**

They then pass one by one through a detector where a laser bounces light off the dyed DNA.

**4**

Based on the amount of light reflected by the fluorescent DNA, selected cells are sorted and collected.

XY Inc., and appointed Dr. George Seidel, a professor of physiology at Colorado State University, as scientific director. They plan to use the sperm selection method for breeding animals, starting with cows and horses. It is easier to sort cow and horse sperm than human sperm, Dr. Seidel said, because the DNA difference between X and Y sperm is more marked. In cows, X-bearing sperm have 3.8 percent more DNA than Y-bearing sperm, and in horses, X-bearing sperm have 4.1 percent more DNA, whereas the difference in human sperm is just 2.8 percent.

"There's no question that it works," Dr. Seidel said. Molecular biological studies indicate that more than 90 percent of the X- and Y-bearing animal sperm are sorted correctly, he said. "We just checked the pregnancies on 30 animals and just one was the wrong sex," Dr. Seidel said. Researchers at the Genetics & IVF Institute began their program five years ago, licensing the method and modifying the machine to sort human sperm. The first couple they assisted wanted a daughter because the woman carried a gene for a rare disease, X-linked hydrocephalus, that strikes boys almost exclusively. Two of her brothers had died of the disease and so had two of her sons. Using sperm sorting, she and her husband had a healthy girl who is now almost 3, said Dr. Susan Black, a geneticist and infertility specialist at the institute.

But despite the encouraging results so far with human sperm sorting, the reactions of some fertility experts indicated that the Genetics & IVF Institute might be stepping into an ethical minefield. When it comes to sex selection, Dr. DeCherney said, "most people feel this is tampering with nature," and find it abhorrent. And unexpected ethical issues can arise, said Dr. Rawlins, the in vitro fertilization laboratory director at Rush Medical College. In the early 1990s, Dr. Rawlins and his colleagues offered couples a method of sex selection, which did not turn out to efficiently sort sperm. Dr. Rawlins said he and his colleagues saw sex selection as a way to help couples who had genes that could cause sex-linked diseases to have normal children. In addition, Dr. Rawlins said, he and his colleagues thought it would be acceptable to offer sex selection to couples who had already had two or three children of one sex and who wanted a baby of the other sex.

But, Dr. Rawlins said, he learned that some couples in whom the method failed were aborting their fetuses. He ended his program. None of the Genetics & IVF patients who wanted girls have aborted fetuses of the undesired sex, although one couple who wanted a boy aborted a female fetus, Dr. Black said. Dr. Barry Zirkin, who heads the division of reproductive biology at Johns Hopkins University's School of Hygiene and Public Health in Baltimore, Maryland, said he remained to be convinced about the safety of the method, which involves staining sperm's DNA and piercing the sperm with a laser. Dr. Fugger said that when the institute began offering the treatment to people "there had been more than 300 animals born. Now there are more than 400 animals in five different species and there are no adverse effects in any of them." And, he added, "we currently have normal, healthy babies. Our experience is the same as the experience in animals." But Dr. Zirkin said several hundred animals was not enough to pick up a rare or subtle defect. It is one thing, he said, to use experimental methods for infertile couples who could not have babies any other way. But, he said, "to me, sex selection is another category.

"This is not curing a disease and it's not curing a societal problem," Dr. Zirkin said. "There is no reason for haste and every reason to be cautious."

[GK, September 1998]

## Dancer's Ovarian Tissue Transplant Gives Hope to Other Young Women Facing Infertility

An operation that appears to have restored ovarian function to a young woman whose ovaries had been removed has offered hope to thousands of other young women facing infertility brought on by cancer treatment or benign conditions like ovarian cysts.

The procedure has also touched off speculation—some of it farfetched, scientists say—about whether ovarian transplants might one day be used to help women ward off menopause indefinitely and have babies well into their golden years.

In September 1999, researchers revealed for the first time that ovarian tissue worked normally after being removed from a young woman, frozen and returned to her body two years later. The woman is Margaret Lloyd-Hart, a 30-year-old dancer from Arizona whose ovaries had been removed because of cysts and other noncancerous medical problems.

Ms. Lloyd-Hart, who had the tissue re-implanted in February 1999, has ovulated and had a menstrual period, which means that she may be able to become pregnant, said her surgeon, Dr. Kutluk Oktay of New York Methodist Hospital in Brooklyn.

Her case is the first known success of an eagerly awaited procedure that holds out the hope of restoring fertility to young women who must have their ovaries removed because of noncancerous disorders like cysts or endometriosis, or who face infertility as a side effect of chemotherapy for cancer.

Women at a few other medical centers have also had ovaries removed and frozen, but Dr. Oktay's report is the first case in which the tissue was given back to the patient and found to work.

"This is great news, and important information," said Dr. Jairo Garcia, director of the in vitro fertilization program at Johns Hopkins Hospital in Baltimore. "The application of this is of tremendous value for younger patients who had malignancies and are scheduled for radiation or chemotherapy, which jeopardize their reproductive potential."

But the procedure cannot stop menopause in older women, and it cannot be done for women with ovarian cancer, Dr. Oktay said, adding that he was disturbed by press reports, particularly in British tabloids, proclaiming that menopause could now be reversed and women with ovarian cancer could give birth.

The research was first reported in England because one of Dr. Oktay's co-authors on a paper about the technique disclosed the information to the British press. "We've been swamped with people who are menopausal or perimenopausal calling us, thinking they can freeze an ovary and have it returned," Dr. Oktay said. "This is not a procedure for menopausal women. It's for women under age 30. It's meant for preserving ovarian function in women who are otherwise going to lose it, mostly because of cancer treatment or the ovaries coming out for benign conditions. It's not meant for somebody with ovarian cancer."

Women close to menopause are not candidates for the procedure because their ovaries do not have enough eggs to restore fertility after freezing and thawing, he said. And, he added, no doctor would put a cancerous ovary back into a patient.

Asked if a young woman could have one ovary removed at, say, age 25 and given back later at 50 to ward off menopause and extend her childbearing years, Dr. Oktay said that for now he would not perform such an operation on a healthy woman. First of all, he said, it is not known whether removing an ovary might harm her health or fertility. Second, doctors do not yet know how long or well the transplanted tissue will survive and function.

But other experts said Dr. Oktay's report suggested *Brave New World* possibilities. Dr. Arthur Caplan, director of the center for bioethics at the University of Pennsylvania, said: "If you could freeze ovaries, you could give them back to other people. It's when the ovary doesn't go back to the place where it started that it gets very interesting."

Dr. Oktay said that transplanting ovaries from one

woman to another was not practical at present. Women who lack ovaries but want to become pregnant can do so with eggs donated by another woman, he said. They do not need an entire ovary. "If you put in somebody else's ovary, the body would reject it," he said. The immunosuppressive drugs needed to prevent rejection cannot be taken during pregnancy, said Dr. Garcia. But, he added, that could change.

Dr. Oktay said he did not see much point in an older woman having an ovary transplant just to prevent menopause, when she could more easily take estrogen. "Taking immunosuppressive drugs to keep an ovary just so you don't have to take hormone replacement doesn't make sense," he said.

Ms. Lloyd-Hart had had one ovary removed at age 17 because of benign cysts. The other, thought to be diseased, was removed when she was 28. But that ovary turned out to be healthy, and Ms. Lloyd-Hart, hoping to have children some day, had segments of it frozen at the University of Arizona. Two years later, she was referred to Dr. Oktay.

Researchers in his laboratory, Dr. Guvenc Karlikaya and Dr. Vulent Aydin, sewed bits of the tissue to a scaffold made of surgical foam. Then, Dr. Oktay and Dr. Shavi Shapira implanted the tissue into Ms. Lloyd-Hart's pelvis, where it soon began producing hormones.

A few months later, she took hormones to stimulate eggs to mature. The treatment worked: she ovulated, and then had a menstrual period, like any fertile woman. If she wants to become pregnant, doctors will have to stimulate the ovarian tissue again, retrieve eggs and perform in vitro fertilization.

Dr. Garcia said he thought that the freezing and re-implanting technique had great potential. But, he cautioned, doctors need to study it to find out how much of the grafted tissue survives and how many eggs it can produce. "We have a long way to go to make sure it's working and really is therapeutic for the patient," he said.

[DG, September 1999]

## Big Study Finds No Link in Abortion and Cancer

In a study that may put to rest a longstanding concern, Danish researchers who reviewed the fates of more than 1.5 million women found no overall increased risk of breast cancer among those who had had induced abortions.

The Danish study, published in *The New England Journal of Medicine*, is far larger, more comprehensive and based on more reliable data than any investigation conducted in the United States of a possible link between breast cancer and abortion, said experts who reviewed the data.

The study showed that even women who had two or more abortions were no more likely than those who never had an abortion to develop breast cancer later, strongly suggesting that abortion has no biological effect on the risk of developing the disease.

A debate on the issue has raged since 1980, when a theoretical concern was raised that interrupting a pregnancy could leave many cells in the breast vulnerable to cancer because the hormones of late pregnancy had not caused them to mature. Dozens of studies had produced inconsistent results, with some showing a small increase in the risk, some showing a slightly decreased risk and others showing no effect.

Despite the conflicting evidence, about 10 states had considered legislation requiring that women seeking an abortion be informed that the procedure could increase the risk of developing breast cancer. Montana enacted such a law.

In an editorial accompanying the report, Dr. Patricia Hartge of the National Cancer Institute wrote that the Danish study "provides important new evidence to resolve a controversy that previous investigations have been unable to settle."

By using data from mandatory registries of births, cancer cases and abortions maintained by the Danish Government, the researchers were able to eliminate a serious potential reporting bias inherent in nearly all previous studies of a possible link.

Most earlier studies, some of which suggested that having an abortion raised a woman's risk of breast cancer by as much as 50 percent, relied on interviews with breast cancer patients and comparable groups of healthy women. These reports, called case-control studies, were subject to bias introduced by women's well-known unwillingness to admit to having had an abortion.

Researchers had long suspected that cancer patients were more likely than healthy people to be forthcoming about potentially embarrassing factors that might have contributed to their illness. Then in 1991 a Swedish study confirmed that women with breast cancer were 50 percent more likely than healthy women to disclose a prior abortion. And surveys in this country have shown that women generally admit to only about half the abortions performed.

"This study overcomes this problem of reporting bias that has plagued so many studies in the past," said Karin Michels, an epidemiologist at the Harvard School of Public Health. "The Danish study used registries rather than asking the women if they had had abortions. This is the major strength of this very important study, apart from its size."

In September 1996, Ms. Michels published a review of all evidence of the breast cancer-abortion issue available up to that point—nearly 50 studies in all—and concluded that "the quality of the studies was inadequate to permit any conclusion about the relationship between induced abortion and breast cancer."

A month later, Dr. Joel Brind, a biochemist at Baruch College in New York who is opposed to abortion, published a combined analysis of 23 studies that he said showed that abortion increased the risk of breast cancer by 30 percent.

Also in 1996, a large case-control study involving 6,888 women with breast cancer and 9,529 healthy women, directed by Dr. Polly A. Newcomb of the University of Wisconsin Comprehensive Cancer Center in Madison, indicated "a weak positive association" between abortion—whether induced or spontaneous—and the risk of breast cancer. The study indicated that the risk was slightly higher for induced abortions than for spontaneous ones, prompting the researchers to suggest that "reporting bias" may have influenced the finding.

While most previous studies in the United States described as "large" involved only 200 to 300 breast cancer patients, the Danish study analyzed the abortion histories of 10,246 women with breast cancer among all the 1,529,512 Danish women born from April 1, 1935, to March 31, 1978. The analysis included all births to these women and whether they had had an abortion and, if so, at what stage of pregnancy.

A total of 370,715 abortions had occurred among 280,965 women. Over all, the study found, these women were not any more likely to develop breast cancer in the ensuing years than were women who had never had an abortion.

Among the 2.3 percent of women who had abortions after the first trimester, however, the researchers found a gradually increasing risk of breast cancer as the term of the aborted pregnancy advanced. Thus, for women whose pregnancies were terminated after 18 weeks, the risk found was nearly twice that of women who had had abortions from 7 to 10 weeks of a pregnancy.

The researchers, headed by Dr. Mads Melbye, an epidemiologist at Statens Serum Institut in Copenhagen, concluded that although the data were statistically significant, the number of women with second-trimester abortions was too small to warrant a firm conclusion and that further studies should be done to determine whether late abortions raised a woman's risk of cancer.

[JEB, January 1997]

# Drugs, Safe and Not Safe, in Pregnancy

T he thalidomide tragedy of the 1960s, in which thousands of women who took the drug for morning sickness gave birth to babies with deformed limbs, touched off intense concern and a vast amount of research about the safety of drugs taken during pregnancy. Many drugs (and druglike substances, including coffee, alcohol and tobacco) were tested in laboratory animals or studied in pregnant women. Some were found to be potential hazards to developing fetuses, usually only at the beginning of pregnancy but in some cases only near the time of birth and in others throughout gestation.

Now most pregnant women are cautioned to avoid any and all medications that are not absolutely essential, as well as "pleasure drugs" like alcohol and tobacco and sometimes coffee and caffeine. But while this is sound advice in general, it can often result in needless discomfort for women who avoid taking a harmless drug that could help them. It also causes undue anxiety among those women who must take medication or who inadvertently took one or more drugs before they knew they were pregnant.

In December 1968, for example, I got the Hong Kong flu the day I was expecting the start of menses. Frequent doses of aspirin kept me from burning up, but 10 days later I remained seriously ill and still had not gotten my period. Now I was coughing so hard I cracked a rib. This time the diagnosis was double pneumonia, for which antibiotics and codeine cough medicine were prescribed. Two weeks later, my gynecologist informed me that I was pregnant. When I asked the doctor about the harm that might have been done by the drugs I had taken, he replied reassuringly, "If you had not taken them and had died of pneumonia, you would not be having any baby."

Still, I spent the next eight months fretting about the harm that might have resulted to my unborn child. But by what seemed at the time to be a miracle, 36 weeks after contracting the flu I gave birth to perfectly healthy, full-term identical twin boys.

I have since learned that it is reasonably safe for pregnant women to take a number of drugs in common use, though they should consult their doctors before taking any drug. Even some vaccines, including the flu vaccine, are safe to administer to pregnant women. Furthermore, most medications pose no hazard to a nursing infant because the amount that gets into breast milk is usually too small to have a noticeable effect on the baby.

Regarding what is safe, let's start with a general recommendation from Dr. Jennifer R. Niebyl, head of obstetrics and gynecology at the University of Iowa College of Medicine, who says, "Pregnant women should be discouraged from using over-the-counter drugs for trivial indications."

Thus, a common cold is best treated with rest, fluids, a humidifier and, if needed, a saltwater (saline) nasal spray like Ocean. Topical medications, like a decongestant nasal spray, are safer than oral ones, and if any cold remedy is used, combination drugs are best avoided. Cough remedies containing iodide should be avoided because they may cause a large goiter in an unborn child.

For aches and pains, try local applications of heat and rest. But if, say, you have a headache you can't shake and it's interfering with your life, acetaminophen (like Tylenol) is safer than aspirin near the end of pregnancy because it does not prolong bleeding and is not toxic to newborns.

To reduce the risk of vaginal yeast infections, a common problem among pregnant women, antibiotics should be used only when needed to control a known bacterial infection. Safe antibiotics include penicillin and its derivatives, erythromycin and the cephalosporins. On the other hand, sulfonamides are best avoided in the third trimester, and tetracyclines, which cause discoloration of babies' teeth, should not be used beyond 25 weeks of gestation.

The drug metronidazole, commonly used to treat intestinal parasites, is best avoided in the first trimester. Lindane (as in Kwell), formerly widely used to treat lice infestations, should be avoided entirely during pregnancy, and pregnant women should wear rubber gloves when treating children for head lice; safer alternatives are the pyrethroids with piperonyl butoxide (Rid and R, for example) or a fine-toothed comb.

The new nonsedating antihistamines used to treat allergies have not been tested for safety in pregnancy. But women who have been receiving desensitization shots can continue to do so at a maintenance dose during pregnancy. Women with asthma can safely use theophylline, aminophylline, terbutaline and cromolyn sodium. And it may surprise you to learn that the potent immune-suppressing drugs prednisone and prednisolone are considered drugs of choice during pregnancy because they are nearly completely inactivated by the placenta.

Also safe are alphamethyldopa and propranolol to treat chronic hypertension. For women plagued by heartburn, antacids are safe for use in any trimester, but bicarbonate of soda, magnesium trisilicate and the new H2 blockers and proton pump inhibitors are potentially toxic to the fetus.

Reports on the safety of the new antidepressants called selective serotonin reuptake inhibitors (S.S.R.I.s) have been mixed. One large study of Prozac found no increase in miscarriage or major birth defects, but infants exposed in the womb were more likely to have minor defects. The latest report, based on 524 pregnancies, half of which involved the use of an S.S.R.I., found no increase in major malformations, miscarriage, stillbirth or premature birth associated with the either S.S.R.I.s or tricyclic antidepressant drugs taken in recommended doses during pregnancy.

Although most medications taken in normal doses by a nursing mother are safe for infants, a few are definitely too toxic for a baby. These include chemotherapy drugs to treat cancer; lithium to treat bipolar disorder and drugs like cyclosporine that suppress the immune system. Even when taking a safe drug, a nursing mother would be wise to coordinate the dosages with the baby's schedule, just after the baby has been fed or before the baby's longest sleep.

For more information about the safety of over-the-counter drugs during pregnancy, see *I'm Pregnant and I Have a Cold* by Dr. Craig V. Towers, a perinatologist at Long Beach Memorial Medical Center in California.

Barbara K. Hackley, a nurse-midwife at the Yale School of Nursing, recently reviewed the safety of immunizations during pregnancy in *The Journal of Nurse-Midwifery*. She approves of the toxoid and inactivated vaccines—tetanus, diphtheria, hepatitis B, influenza and pneumococcal vaccines—although she advises that even these vaccines are best given in the second and third trimesters in case they may have some effect yet unrecognized on a young fetus. Flu vaccine (taken each fall to include the latest strains) is now recommended for all pregnant women. To be avoided are live virus and bacterial vaccines, including those for measles, mumps, rubella and chicken pox.

Legal recreational drugs like alcohol, nicotine and caffeine are also common concerns among pregnant women. Cigarette smoking during pregnancy can compromise fetal growth, resulting in babies that are smaller than they should be at birth, and may also cause long-lasting intellectual deficits. Heavy consumption of alcohol during pregnancy causes fetal alcohol syndrome marked by subnormal growth, muscle and heart damage, and low intelligence or mental retardation. Although an occasional drink is highly unlikely to have any adverse effect on a developing fetus, the Food and Drug Administration advises pregnant women to refrain from drinking any alcohol.

Caffeine and coffee, on the other hand, have been pretty much cleared of earlier suspicions of fetal harm, at least when consumed in moderation: no more than three cups of coffee a day. In 1980, after reports of birth defects in mice induced by caffeine, the F.D.A. warned pregnant women to limit their intake of coffee. But considerable evidence accumulated since has not implicated coffee as a cause of birth defects in humans. Still, there is some evidence that consuming more than three cups of coffee a day may slightly reduce birth weights.

[JEB, November 1999]

# Herbal Remedies Tied to Pregnancy Risks

Many women trying to become pregnant are careful to avoid ingesting any substance that might impair their fertility or damage a developing embryo. According to a study in March 1999, several popular herbal remedies should be added to the list of substances that could have detrimental effects on men as well as women and could interfere with conception or a healthy pregnancy.

Despite the widespread belief, often fostered by advertising copy, that herbal preparations are "natural" and "drug free," those that have druglike effects in the body do in fact contain potent chemicals that act like drugs.

And, like many prescription and over-the-counter drugs that are known to be unsafe before or during pregnancy, some herbal remedies may also be expected to interfere with normal reproductive function. This expectation prompted researchers at Loma Linda University School of Medicine in Loma Linda, California, to explore the effects of four popular herbs on eggs and sperm. Their findings were published in *Fertility and Sterility*, the journal of the American Society for Reproductive Medicine.

Three of the herbs, St. John's wort, Echinacea purpura and Ginkgo biloba, had ill effects on either eggs or sperm or both. The damage, the researchers said, included a reduced ability of sperm to penetrate an egg, changes to the genetic material in sperm, poor sperm viability and, in the case of St. John's wort, mutation of the tumor suppressor gene, BRCA1, a change that can increase the risk of breast and ovarian cancers in women who inherit the mutated gene.

Of the herbs tested, only saw palmetto, which is commonly taken by men to relieve the symptoms of an enlarged prostate, did not damage eggs or sperm in the doses tested. But even saw palmetto reduced the viability of sperm that were exposed to the herbal preparation for seven days.

The journal's editor, Dr. Alan H. DeCherney, said, "This is a very important study that could provide important information to patients suffering from infertility." He added, "The growing popularity of these herbal products means we must examine all their possible effects."

The researchers emphasized that their study, which was conducted in the laboratory on both human sperm and hamster eggs, indicated only a potential risk to those who take the herbs in question. They said it was possible that no untoward effects would occur in people who used the herbs in the usual recommended doses.

"To our knowledge, no data exist on concentrations of these herbs in semen or serum," the team, headed by Dr. Richard R. Ondrizek, noted. Thus, it is not possible to say whether the herbal doses tested represented an amount that may actually reach the eggs or sperm in people who use these preparations. Also, the remedies, which are sold over the counter as dietary supplements, are not required to undergo premarket tests for safety or accuracy of dosage.

In the studies, the researchers examined the effects of two concentrations of herbs, one high and one low, but in both cases the amounts that eggs and sperm were exposed to represented a tiny fraction of the recommended dosages on product labels.

For echinacea, ginkgo and saw palmetto, the researchers examined amounts that represented one-thousandth and one-hundredth of the recommended daily doses. For St. John's wort, they also looked at a concentration of one-millionth of the recommended dose.

Two types of studies were conducted. In one, hamster eggs that were prepared for fertilization were exposed to various concentrations of the herbs and then inseminated with sperm. Sperm were unable to penetrate the eggs exposed to higher doses of St. John's wort and penetration was impaired by the higher doses of both echinacea and ginkgo.

In the second study, human sperm were exposed for seven days to different herbal concentrations. This long-term exposure to St. John's wort and echinacea resulted in significant changes to the sperm and reduced their viability. In addition, the prolonged

exposure to St. John's wort caused some mutations.

[JEB, March 1999]

## A Study Finds Link Between Birth Defects and Solvents

Canadian scientists report in a study that women who were exposed to organic solvents like phenol, xylene and acetone during pregnancy had a greatly increased chance of having a baby with a birth defect.

But leading experts on birth defects said the study had serious methodological problems. They said they feared that the paper, published in the *Journal of the American Medical Association*, would needlessly frighten pregnant women.

The research, by Dr. Sohail Khattak, a pediatrician and a clinical pharmacologist, Dr. Gideon Koren, a clinical pharmacologist, and their colleagues at the Hospital for Sick Children in Toronto, involved women who had contacted the hospital's program, Motherisk, for pregnant women who are worried that they have been exposed to something that might harm their fetuses.

The investigators focused on organic solvents that caused birth defects in animals when they were administered in high doses. They compared 125 women who said they were exposed to such chemicals, usually at work, with 125 women who said they were exposed to other chemicals or drugs that had not been known to cause birth defects. As a rough gauge of the exposure, the investigators asked the women if their eyes had watered or if they had had a headache or trouble breathing.

Thirteen of the babies born to mothers who said they had been exposed to organic solvents had major birth defects, including congenital deafness, club foot and spina bifida; almost all of the women whose babies had these more serious birth defects had reported symptoms of exposure. Just one woman in the control group had a baby with a major birth defect.

Dr. Khattak said that the findings offered strong evidence that these chemicals cause birth defects. Because his group knew the women's professions, how long they had worked with chemicals, and what precautions they had taken, he said, the researchers had "a unique advantage" in assessing exposures.

But other scientists were unconvinced. "They've added to the suspicion that there might be an association," said Dr. David Erickson, the chief of the birth defects and genetic disease branch at the Centers for Disease Control and Prevention in Atlanta. But, Dr. Erickson said, "I don't think this nails it down in any firm way." To do so, he said, would require a much larger and more expensive study involving meticulous measurements of chemicals and notation of the time that women are exposed.

In animal studies of chemicals that cause birth defects, timing and dose are critical, and scientists believe the same is true for humans. Asking women to recall the time of their exposure and then asking if they had had a headache when they thought they were exposed is not sufficient, said Dr. Lewis Holmes, chief of the unit that studies genetics and birth defects at Massachusetts General Hospital in Boston.

Dr. Holmes and Dr. Allen Mitchell, who directs the Slone Epidemiology Unit at the Boston University School of Public Health, noted that the women in the study were not randomly selected. Half who said they had been exposed to organic solvents had had previous miscarriages—compared to a fifth of the women in the control group—which could mean that it was the genetic makeup of the parents, and not the workplace, that caused the high rate of birth defects, Dr. Holmes and Dr. Mitchell said.

The control group of women had far fewer birth

defects than usual, Dr. Erickson said, one baby rather than the expected four to six, which made the comparison even more dramatic.

Dr. Khattak said not every chemical that causes birth defects causes only one specific kind of defect and that the women were exposed to a wide variety of chemicals, which could account for the diverse group of birth defects in their babies. He added that the extraordinarily high numbers of birth defects in the group that was exposed to the chemicals could not be dismissed.

But Dr. Mitchell said, "Think of all the women of childbearing age who will be scared to death."

[GK, March 1999]

## No Benefit Found for Fetal Monitors

A large study has found that the use of home fetal monitors fails at its intended purpose: to prevent women at high risk of premature labor from giving birth too early.

Each year, doctors prescribe such monitors to thousands of pregnant women to detect uterine contractions, which are often signs of early labor. The devices, which are strapped around the abdomen, are used daily for up to 10 weeks at a cost of about $30 to $100 a day. Women believed to be in early labor are then admitted to the hospital and given medicine to stop the contractions.

The goal of monitoring is to avoid premature delivery, a leading cause of disability and death in newborns. Studies of home monitoring have been conflicting, with some showing that it lowers the rate of preterm births and others finding that it is no more effective than daily telephone conversations with a nurse to discuss labor symptoms.

In the study, doctors from Kaiser Permanente Medical Center in Santa Clara, California, sought to settle the issue by comparing daily monitoring with daily and weekly phone contact with nurses. They followed 2,422 women who, for various reasons, were considered to be at high risk of delivering prematurely.

All of the women met with a nurse for intensive education on the symptoms of early labor, such as cramping and backache. Then they were randomly assigned to one of three groups: one group got a phone call from a nurse once a week, another group was called once a day and the third group was called daily and used home monitoring machines. The women with the monitors used them twice a day, then transmitted the results to the hospital electronically over the telephone.

The study showed that neither the monitoring nor the daily calls were better than weekly calls in preventing preterm births. In each group about 14 percent of the women delivered prematurely, at less than 35 weeks' gestation. The study also cast doubt on the use of drugs to stop contractions, since these drugs were given most often to the women who had daily monitoring.

"I hope that this study will convince doctors that they shouldn't routinely use monitors," said Dr. Donald C. Dyson, the lead author of the study, published in *The New England Journal of Medicine.*

Dr. Frederic D. Frigoletto Jr., chairman of obstetrics at Massachusetts General Hospital in Boston, said, "This well done, well controlled, large trial is for me personally definitive."

Dr. Dyson's findings contradict one of his previous studies, which suggested that home monitors could prevent preterm delivery in women carrying twins. The newer study, which included 844 women pregnant with twins, found no such effect. "We couldn't identify a subgroup for whom this worked," Dr. Dyson said.

If early detection and treatment of contractions do not prevent preterm births, the question is: what does? The rate of preterm deliveries—those occurring earlier than 37 weeks' gestation—has remained about 8 or 9 percent for about 30 years, despite efforts to prevent them and an abundance of new knowledge about their causes, said Dr. Jay Iams, a professor of obstetrics and gynecology at Ohio State College of Medicine in Columbus. And the 1 percent to 2 percent of preterm deliveries before 32 weeks account for half of all deaths just before, during or soon after birth.

"We're in a transition phase," said Dr. Iams, who wrote a commentary accompanying the study. "We know a lot of facts; we just haven't figured out how to put them together to reduce prematurity."

[SG, January 1998]

## Ultrasound and Fury: One Mother's Ordeal

If I had been paying more attention, I might have noticed the plaque outside the room that the obstetrician was ushering us into: Patient Education. And had I noticed, I almost surely would have been alarmed. I was 20 weeks pregnant with my first child and had just had a "routine" ultrasound examination. What did I need to be educated about?

But I did not notice, and I was not anxious or on guard. I had enjoyed the sonogram. Expectant parents do. It is a bonding opportunity. It is baby's first video. I had already had amniocentesis several weeks earlier, to check for chromosomal abnormalities associated with so-called elderly gravidas like my 38-year-old self.

I knew that my baby had 23 neatly matching pairs of chromosomes, that her spinal tube had closed and that she did not have a gruesome defect like anencephaly—no brain—that would propel me to have an abortion despite having struggled for years to get pregnant.

In sum, I knew my baby was healthy and magnificent, and had gone into the ultrasound expecting added proof of her splendor.

The obstetrician began discussing the scan results. Her tone was hesitant, clipped, distinctly not the voice of reassurance. A siren of panic began wailing in my skull. She said this was fine, that was fine, blah, blah, blah. Come on! I thought angrily. Get to the point! What's wrong with my baby?

Finally, the doctor came to the problem. The left foot. She said the results were difficult to interpret.

The foot was in a funny position in the uterus, crammed down deep in the pelvis, so it could be simply a matter of its position at the moment. But the sonographer had not been able to see the profile of the foot, no matter what angle she came at it from, and that is what happens when you have a clubfoot. My husband and I looked at each other in dumb, grim shock. Clubfoot? Neither of us was sure what a clubfoot was, what it looked like or how bad a defect it was. The term was so thuddingly ugly and Dickensian that we could not help imagining the condition must be ugly and severe.

The obstetrician told us we had a couple of choices. We could go to a university facility for a more in-depth sonogram, or we could just do nothing and go on with the pregnancy. A clubfoot would not affect the course of the pregnancy, she said, and any effort to correct it would have to wait until after the baby was born.

Oh, sure, do nothing and forget all about it—that is a realistic option, I thought bitterly. Thus we started down a rutted path trudged by so many tens of thousands of people each year, that of medical testing and retesting, the contemporary version of consulting the Oracle of Delphi or a platter of entrails. It is a path that is getting bumpier and more perilous by the month, as ever more high-tech assays are added to the list of prognostic options.

And while genetic testing in particular has generated a squall of debate over its ethical, legal and psychic implications, many of the same questions are raised by more widespread technologies like ultrasound. Among them: How do you interpret equivocal or confusing results, and how does a patient react to a test's inherent uncertainty? What do you do—what can you do—with bad news once you have received it? Most important is the taint of eugenics surrounding many of these screens: How perfect must a person be to deserve health insurance, a job, a parent's love, or life itself?

Leaving the obstetrician's office, my husband and I headed for a medical library to do research on clubfoot. The pictures in textbooks were devastating. Some of the feet were extremely deformed, bent in and up at the ankle to form the letter J. Toes and heels were bunched and twisted. The feet were often stunted, and the calves of the clubfoot leg were comparatively underdeveloped. We knew, intellectually, that textbooks use worst-case scenarios to make their point, and we read that clubfeet can vary enormously, from mild and flexible to severe and rigid; but we still felt sick with sorrow to think her foot could be as distorted as some of the pictures before us.

That night, my husband and I did not sleep at all. We wept and wept. Privately, we each pleaded with the universe to make the follow-up sonogram come out normal. We offered up our own body parts in exchange: eyes, arms, feet.

The universe was deaf. The next day, a doctor at a nearby university hospital concurred with the preliminary diagnosis of clubfoot, subtle though the evidence was. "Good catch!" he said admiringly of the previous sonographer's work.

In the car ride home, I howled so hard I thought the sky would crack; but the sky stayed whole and calm and blue.

A week later, we met with a genetics counselor at a different university to discuss the odds that the clubfoot might not be an isolated defect, but part of a larger genetic syndrome. We had yet another sonogram, performed by doctors with extensive expertise in ultrasound diagnosis. Happily, they were able to rule out larger genetic anomalies, but of the clubfoot they were certain. "There is a varus deformity of the left foot," they said bluntly.

I became obsessed with clubfoot, medically and culturally. I learned that for several months to a year our daughter would have to wear a thigh-high cast designed to twist her foot gradually into a normal, usable position. I learned that the cast would have to be changed every week, that casting alone might not work, and she might require one or more operations. As for the asymmetry of her calves, that would be untreatable and permanent.

I read of famous clubfooted figures in history and literature: Lord Byron, Goebbels, the town simpleton in *Madame Bovary* whose leg had to be amputated after Dr. Bovary tried unsuccessfully to treat the deformity. But I also spoke to mothers of children with clubfeet and was inspired by their stories. They assured me the casts in no way slowed their children down or interfered with motor milestones like crawling. They said that with their feet fixed, the children could walk and run with the best of the nonclubbed masses. Finally, toward the end of my pregnancy, I began to relax.

In late August of 1996 I gave birth to a healthy daughter with a lusty set of lungs, a full head of black hair—and no clubfoot at all.

The use of ultrasound scanning during pregnancy is now so widespread it seems almost as banal as taking a patient's blood pressure. Unlike amniocentesis, it is considered safe, noninvasive and painless for both mother and child. Formal studies indicate that 70 percent of all pregnant women get at least one scan, and the true number is probably higher, said Dr. E. O. Horger 3d, chairman of obstetrics and gynecology at the University of South Carolina School of Medicine in Columbia. If a woman does not request ultrasound, many obstetricians will recommend it, as mine did, "just to see how things are going." They make that suggestion even though the American College of Obstetricians and Gynecologists, the American Academy of Family Physicians and other medical organizations advise against the routine use of ultrasound in pregnancy.

These groups emphatically favor ultrasound when there is medical justification, for example, if the woman begins bleeding or may be carrying twins. But they see no benefit in laissez-faire scanning when the pregnancy is going fine.

Behind that position are the results of a large clinical trial called the Routine Antenatal Diagnostic Imaging with Ultrasound, or Radius, study, published in *The New England Journal of Medicine* and elsewhere in 1993. In that study, 15,151 women with low-risk pregnancies were randomly assigned to one of two groups. The first received routine ultrasound examinations in the second and third trimesters, while the other group received no sonograms unless there was a problem, like bleeding.

The study found no benefit from routine screening. Ultrasound did not reduce the number of infant deaths during delivery, nor did it in any way lead to an improvement in the newborn's health. More fetal anomalies were picked up in the screened group, but that early detection had no tangible effect, like an increase in abortions, or better care for the newborns. The researchers concluded that universal ultrasound would add millions of dollars to the cost of prenatal care with no payback in better babies.

The response to the study was immediate and furious, and continues resonating. "Among practitioners, those who did not believe in routine ultrasound now feel justified, while the majority of those who did believe in it have attempted to ignore or discredit the study," said Dr. Bernard G. Ewigman of the University of Missouri School of Medicine in Columbia, the first author of the report.

Much of the harshest censure of the study has come from doctors who excel in ultrasound diagnosis. They criticize the criteria used in selecting the women. "They excluded those cases that would automatically warrant a scan, like a patient who's not sure how far along the pregnancy is," said Dr. John C. Hobbins, director of obstetrics at the University of Colorado Health Sciences Center in Denver. "By design they narrowed down the study population to the point where it doesn't represent the real world."

They also criticize the skills of those who did the scans in the study, complaining that too many birth defects were missed and thus many chances to make a difference in outcome were likewise missed. For example, if a fetus is found to have gastroschisis, in which the bowels protrude through a hole in the abdomen, the newborn has a much better chance of surviving and thriving if it is delivered in the same hospital where the corrective surgery will be performed, rather than having to being moved.

But Dr. Ewigman and others respond that such defects are too rare to justify automatic screening policies, and that the happy stories are more than countered by drawbacks. False positives like mine are said to be very rare, yet without trying I learned of three other women whose fetuses were incorrectly diagnosed as having clubfeet. And while these mistakes were joyfully resolved, false positives can have devastating outcomes. Dr. Horger cited the case of a woman who received an ultrasound diagnosis that her fetus had no kidneys, a fatal condition. She aborted the fetus at 18 weeks, and an autopsy revealed apparently normal kidneys.

More often women receive murky results that are difficult to interpret, but that offer just enough substance to nourish anxiety. During several scans performed in her third pregnancy, a neighbor of mine was told that her baby might have a serious kidney defect. There was nothing to do but wait and worry. Months later, she gave birth to a healthy daughter.

Dr. Sheryl Burt Ruzek, a professor of health education at Temple University, said the rampant use of ultrasound "has created false expectations that by having repeated screenings we can improve the likelihood of a good outcome of pregnancy." It gives the illusion of perfectability, but like most medical assays, ultrasound is imperfect. It can find problems where none exist, and, more often, it misses defects that exist. More than half of all defects have been shown to go unnoticed by ultrasound. "The search for the perfect child is making women very anxious about reproducing," Dr. Ruzek said. An unfortunate byproduct of expecting perfection is the urge to sue upon arrival of an imperfect baby. Dr. Horger said one of the most common causes of obstetrical lawsuits is the failure of a doctor to pick up a birth defect on ultrasound. Although the Radius study indicates that early detection of most abnormalities does not do much good anyway, doctors end up screening just to cover themselves.

A particular problem with ultrasound is that while women know that amniocentesis and most prenatal tests are designed to look for defects, they approach their sonogram with optimism. "They're persuaded they'll be reassured, and will get their first picture of the baby," said Dr. Gail Geller, a bioethicist at Johns Hopkins University. "But the physician's training is to find something that might be wrong. There's a cognitive dissonance between practitioners and patients." Indeed, she said, "physicians can sound almost excited when they find something." That happened to us, with the doctor who murmured appreciatively, "Good catch."

In the end, many researchers said that women should be entitled to have ultrasound and other prenatal tests, but that the process of informed consent must be taken far more seriously than it currently is. Women should be told in detail of the limitations of screening, and of the fact that clinical studies show no benefit to scanning during a normal pregnancy, Dr. Geller said. Nor is it clear that doctors should

bother ferreting out every minor aberration—every cleft lip, every excess finger.

We still do not know why our daughter's foot appeared clubbed on three sonograms when it was not. The ultrasound specialists who gave us the final, definitive diagnosis said they stood by their original call and suggested the foot may have corrected itself during the later stages of pregnancy.

I am skeptical. I think this is a case of ambiguity prematurely corseted into certainty, and of insufficient data on all the possible variations of a normal fetal foot (not to mention any other body part) at 20 weeks gestation. I think my child has inherited her mother's unusually supple feet, which can point and twist in many directions and even mimic a clublike contortion. Perhaps my daughter was dreaming that she was a ballerina, flexing her foot into en pointe position, and preparing to dance the dance.

[NA, November 1996]

## Why Babies Are Born Facing Backward, Helpless and Chubby

Childbirth: it's a miracle, right? One minute you're standing there, an awkward, frightened and comically proportioned woman, face twisted with the first contractions of labor, uterus lurching to your epiglottis, mind suddenly skeptical that it's feasible to do the pelvic equivalent of expelling a Crenshaw melon through your nostril, and the next minute . . .

Oh, sorry, 23 hours later, you're sitting peacefully in bed, face now suffused with a Botticellian glow, body significantly lightened, a pointy-headed, purplish newborn at your breast. It's magic, it's sacred, it's among a woman's greatest triumphs—but, holy epidural, the author of Genesis sure said it all by socking Eve with the curse of childbirth right after making her mortal.

As anybody who has ever experienced or witnessed a baby being born will readily attest, the pain

of labor and delivery deserves its legendary status, ranking as it often does somewhere above, say, a root canal and below an unanesthetized amputation. Human births are thought to be so difficult because we are pushing the envelope of evolution: the baby's large cranium is nearly too big to fit through the woman's pelvis, which must remain narrow to accommodate bipedal locomotion. We are, the assumption goes, too brainy for our poor, upstanding mothers' good. All told, human births were thought to be among the most troublesome in nature, resulting in greater rates of stillborn young and maternal deaths than seen in other mammals.

But as researchers have discovered in a series of recent studies, human birth is not the most difficult in the animal kingdom by any stretch, nor is it as unusual as biologists and anthropologists long believed. Dr. Melissa Stoller of the University of

Chicago has carried out the first detailed analysis of the birth process in nonhuman primates, in this case, baboons and squirrel monkeys. Her findings overturn the long-held assumption that most primates plop straight down through the mother's pelvis and that only human babies are forced during birth to turn their way through a harrowing corkscrew bend to take advantage of the widest possible points in the woman's birth canal. Instead, Dr. Stoller discovered that baby monkeys must also twist their way through the birth tunnel with contortionist efforts, although they rotate in different directions than humans do as they struggle toward the world.

Moreover, the ratio between the size of the infant's head and the diameter of the mother's pelvis turns out not to be as miserably incompatible for humans as it is for some other monkey species.

Nevertheless, humans do retain a few singular elements in their style of giving birth. Dr. Wenda Trevathan, an evolutionary anthropologist at New Mexico State University in Las Cruces and the author of the classic text *Human Birth: An Evolutionary Perspective*, argues that much of the pain and anxiety surrounding human birth is cognitive in nature and that it is not necessarily a bad thing.

Unlike other mammals, women know they will

## Short but Hard Trip Into the World

In these diagrams of the birth process from a midwife's point of view, the newborn's head passes through the inlet (1), midpoint (2) and outlet (3) of the birth canal; the maternal spine is at the bottom. It was once thought that among primates, only human infants had to turn sideways to navigate the canal; however, in monkeys and apes that undergo such twists, the newborns still normally emerge head first and facing the mother.

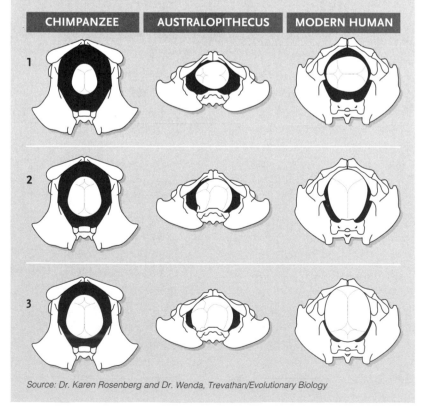

*Source: Dr. Karen Rosenberg and Dr. Wenda, Trevathan/Evolutionary Biology*

have a bloody difficult time in labor and delivery. They've seen it, they've heard about it, and they've been warned since girlhood to expect it. That knowledge of impending misery, Dr. Trevathan argues, leads women to seek assistance during birth, a practice that is extremely unusual among mammals. Most expectant animals do the opposite, finding a quiet spot away from the group and giving birth in unobtrusive solitude, a practice that incidentally makes it quite hard for field researchers to witness births of the species they study. But humans almost universally solicit help: whether of a midwife; an elder female relative; on occasion, a male partner; and today, of course, an obstetrician.

Reporting in a recent issue of the journal *Evolutionary Anthropology*, Dr. Trevathan and Dr. Karen Rosenberg of the University of Delaware said that in a survey of 296 cultural groups around the world, only 24 offered instances of women sometimes giving birth unattended, and those cases almost always involved experienced mothers. First-timers, it seems, universally have someone in attendance.

Women are not seeking aid just for the companionship, Dr. Trevathan said. For mechanical reasons, women need help getting the infants out safely. Here is where humans differ dramatically from other primates. Among monkeys and apes, newborns normally emerge from the birth canal head first and facing their mother. Indeed, some of the twists and turns that Dr. Stoller reported seeing among baby baboons and squirrel monkeys as they passed along the canal put them into just such an advantageous presentation.

With the baby facing her, the mother primate can easily perform several critical maneuvers. She can pull the baby up out of the tight squeeze, and sometimes the infant will even start hoisting itself up once its arms are free of the canal, for many primates are born with highly-developed motor skills. She can unwind the umbilical cord from the baby's neck should that be necessary, as it frequently is. And she can wipe the mucus from the baby's mouth to allow it to begin breathing.

Within minutes after birth, the newborn is clinging to her hairy chest and nuzzling for a nipple.

Dr. Trevathan explains that women cannot perform these essential tasks on their own, and for that we can blame bipedalism. The demands of standing upright have resulted in a pelvis that, for complex anatomical reasons, is best exited by the infant in a rear-facing position, rather than looking up at the mother. Because of this awkward presentation, the mother cannot guide the baby out without bending its spine backward, risking spinal cord injury and death. She cannot unwind the umbilical cord, nor can she clear her baby's mouth of mucus. For all these operations, any one of which can spell the difference between life or death for her child, she needs a helping hand. Thus was born the practice of midwifery, or its ancestral equivalent.

Dr. Trevathan dates the use of birth attendants to the onset of bipedalism, about five million years ago or so—considerably before human brain size began reaching its current considerable proportions. She views obstetrical intervention as perhaps the oldest medical specialty.

She also proposes that the emotions surrounding childbirth—the fear, the uncertainty, the desperate desire to not be left alone—are deep-seated sensations, the spurs to insure that women do not try to go it alone.

"I argue that the fear and anxiety we have may be deeply rooted in our psyche and that they served an important function in the past," Dr. Trevathan said. "They're natural instincts, as basic to us as love or anger, and they're not going to go away with education, or being told, 'Don't worry, you can always have a C-section.'"

Human childbirth can also be viewed as one of the early examples of need-driven cooperative behavior, with one woman agreeing to help with another's birth in return for similar assistance when she is in labor. "What we see here is a prime example of a cultural solution to a biological problem," Dr. Rosenberg said. That obstetrical give-and-take can even be seen as a driving force in the evolution of intelligence, just as the needs of cooperative hunting have traditionally been.

The use of birth assistants has very likely accounted for the relatively low rate of maternal deaths and stillbirths seen historically in normal deliveries. Serious problems can arise when babies attempt to come out feet first, or breech, but the condition is equally common, and dangerous, among nonhuman primates and other mammals.

What counts as a backward birth differs from one species to another, though. Dr. Lawrence G. Barnes, curator of vertebrate paleontology at the Natural History Museum of Los Angeles County and a researcher who studies the evolution of whales, said that whale calves sometimes come out of the birth canal head first, rather than the proper tail-first presentation. That is fatal for the neonate because its face is exposed to the water as the rest of its body is still emerging, so it cannot get to the surface before drowning.

Danger also arises for human mothers when they give birth under severely unhygienic conditions, as they frequently did in the 18th and 19th centuries. At that point, male doctors had taken over the business of birth assistance from midwives, and they often brought to the mother's bedside infectious microbes from their nonpregnant sick and dying patients elsewhere.

Today, septic conditions and poor medical care plague pregnant women in many underdeveloped nations, resulting in huge numbers of unnecessary deaths. In 1996, Unicef reported that 1 in 13 women in sub-Saharan Africa, and 1 in 35 in South Asia, dies of causes related to pregnancy and childbirth each year, compared with 1 in 3,200 in Europe, 1 in 3,300 in the United States and 1 in 7,300 in Canada.

The rapid growth of the human brain, or encephalization, in the last two million years or so has added to women's birth trauma. Yet the near-mismatch between the human pelvis and infant head is not the unique and severe problem that many imagine. It is true that among the great apes—chimpanzees, orangutans and gorillas—the female pelvis is quite roomy, and birth is far easier than it is for humans. But that is not the case for small species of monkeys, which have comparatively large brains without the bulk of adulthood seen in the apes. Among squirrel monkeys, for example, the fit of the birth canal is so tight relative to the baby that, as Dr.

Stoller notes in her doctoral dissertation, labor obstruction is quite common. In one colony in Alabama, 16 percent of the infants are stillborn, and 34 percent of the young born alive die soon after birth, often of birth-inflicted injuries.

In shaping birth patterns, evolution seems to push to the limits of viability when there is a difficult problem to solve. Miles Roberts, head of the zoological research department at the National Zoological Park in Washington, said the most extreme ratio in primates of large infant size to narrow maternal birth passage was among the tarsiers, a small, insect-eating monkey found in Indonesia and the Philippines.

In this case, the fetus must grow a very large brain during gestation because it will have to start foraging for itself within a month. Insects are simply too energy-poor a food source to allow the mother to nurse the infant at length, as many primates do. "The infant has to get to work quickly in the three-dimensional space of an arboreal habitat," Mr. Roberts said. "That means it needs extensive motor coordination, which means it has to start out with a big brain." Tarsier birth is so difficult and improbable, Mr. Roberts said, that once the baby is out, "you can't imagine how the mother ever gave birth to such a huge thing."

The young tarsier is said to be born at a precocial, or relatively mature, stage, with much of its brain development complete. Most animals that gestate for a long time are precocial. In the elephant, for example, pregnancy lasts 21½ months, said John Lehnhardt, assistant curator of mammals at the National Zoological Park. When the calf emerges from the womb, the mother gives it a kick, shaking the mucus from its trunk, and within minutes the animal is on its feet, ready to move. If it were helpless at birth, it would immediately fall prey to predators.

The spotted hyena, which surely deserves the Eve Memorial Medal of Honor for Withstanding Childbirth Hell, offers another striking example of a highly precocial species. In that animal, gestation lasts 120 days, extremely long for a predator, and the infant comes out comparatively large, mature and ready to kill, its jaws snapping, its teeth fully erupted. But the mother must give birth to those killers through an extraordinary organ the size and shape of a penis; the genitals are masculinized because the females are sculpted in the womb by high levels of androgens, or male hormones. First births are often deadly, as the penis-like organ rips open as best it can yet nonetheless leaves many fetuses lethally trapped within the tube.

Dr. Laurence G. Frank of the University of California at Berkeley has estimated that the cost of this bizarre system is enormous: 65 to 70 percent of firstborn young and up to 18 percent of first-time mothers die. Yet the benefits of giving birth to extremely aggressive young outweigh the drawbacks. Mothers that survive have an easier time from then on, and their infants can thrive: spotted hyenas are among the most successful African carnivores.

Mammals with large litters usually have short gestation times and give birth to quite helpless, unformed looking creatures. Such species are said to be altricial, and they include cats, dogs and many rodents.

Humans are unusual in having a very long pregnancy time, comparable to that of the great apes, yet they give birth to infants that are far more immature, helpless and mewling than an infant chimp or orang-utan. This system is evolution's solution to the big brain-small pelvis dilemma. The baby's head and brain grows as much as it can in the womb, and then it continues developing long after birth. Human babies are thus believed to be secondarily altricial: our early hominid ancestors probably gave birth to more precocial young, but an extended period of altricial helplessness was superimposed over that to permit a burst of post-utero brain growth. Newborn humans are essentially fetuses for another nine months after birth.

Given the infant's protracted period of total helplessness, human parents must diligently attend to their needs far longer than any other primate parents. Some evolutionary biologists propose that some of the last touches made to infants in the womb are essentially cosmetic, turning the baby into something so cute the parents will feel compelled to care for it.

Dr. Sarah Blaffer Hrdy of the University of California at Davis suggests that the adorable factor accounts for why the human infant puts on layers of fat right before birth, while the fetuses of great apes remain quite trim for their odyssey through the pelvis. "You have to ask why the baby doesn't wait until it's out of birth canal to plump up like that," she said. Perhaps a pinched and scrawny infant would lack the esthetic appeal needed to seduce its parents irrevocably. And once the mother has fallen in love, she forgets the pain, she forgets the hassle, and she gladly accepts indentured servitude for the next 18 years.

[NA, July 1996]

## What's Missing in Childbirth These Days? Often, the Pain

**M**ore and more women are deciding that labor pain is a rite of passage they can do without and are gratefully accepting pain medicine during childbirth, doctors reported at a 1999 meeting of the American Society of Anesthesiologists in Dallas.

It is a development that pleases many doctors, who say women should not suffer needlessly during labor. But the trend troubles some childbirth educators, midwives and other advocates of natural childbirth, who say young women who pass up the opportunity to overcome labor pain on their own are missing out on one of life's great transforming experiences and needlessly exposing themselves and their babies to the side effects of anesthetic drugs.

In part, the doctors said, the change is a result of improvements that allow effective pain relief with much smaller doses of anesthetic drugs and fewer side effects. There also appears to be a relaxing of attitudes among women: The use of anesthesia in labor is no longer judged a sign of weakness or selfishness.

From 1981 to 1997, there was a tripling of the percentage of women in labor at large hospitals who had regional anesthesia—spinal or epidural injections—to 66 percent from 22 percent. At smaller hospitals, the percentage doubled from 1992 to 1997, to 42 percent from 21 percent. Regional anesthesia numbs the pelvic region but does not affect the mind, so patients remain fully aware and in control.

The findings, from a survey of 750 hospitals around the nation, were presented by Dr. Joy L. Hawkins, director of obstetric anesthesia at the University of Colorado School of Medicine in Denver.

"The change," Dr. Hawkins said, "comes from women going to childbirth education classes, reading about the birth process, talking to anesthesiologists and obstetricians and exploring their options so they can make a decision about what they want. And I think obstetricians are very comfortable now recommending epidurals."

In the past, she said, many hesitated, out of fear that the drugs would slow down a woman's labor, decrease her ability to push and increase the likelihood that she would need a Caesarean. "That is clearly not the case," Dr. Hawkins said. "The techniques we have are so safe and effective that it should come down to what a woman needs to give herself the ideal birth experience."

Dr. David Birnbach, director of obstetric anesthesiology at St. Luke's-Roosevelt Hospital Center in Manhattan, said a major change occurred in the mid-1990s when doctors began to offer patients "walking epidurals," an injection of anesthetic into a space near the spinal column that relieves pain but does not take away sensation or the woman's ability to walk. The walking epidurals use much less medication than earlier epidurals, which did numb the legs and made it impossible to move them.

"Our satisfaction rates are sky high," Dr. Birnbach said. "Doctors and patients are both asking for it. Patients can enjoy the birth experience. They can fully participate." In 1990, Dr. Birnbach said, only 10 percent of women giving birth at St. Luke's-Roosevelt Hospital had epidurals. In 1999, he said, more than 90 percent did.

"In New York City, most of the hospitals now have 60 to 80 percent epidural rates," he said, adding that this was typical of most large cities. But rates tend to be lower in smaller communities, where there may be fewer anesthesiologists.

"Thirty years ago, we said drugs were dangerous and may be bad for the baby," Dr. Birnbach said, adding that patients were told to use breathing techniques and self-hypnosis to help them deal with the pain, without drugs. "The vast majority of women were in extreme pain." Now that anesthesia is safer, he said, women are telling their doctors that they do not want to suffer the pain unnecessarily.

Although some critics still say the use of epidurals can lead to an increase in Caesareans, Dr. Birnbach said that at his hospital, as the use of epidurals continued to grow, the Caesarean rate dropped every year in the past five years, to about 20 percent. "Our obstetrician with the highest epidural rate has the lowest Caesarean rate," he said.

Epidural anesthesia for childbirth costs $500 to $1,000, and is covered by most insurers. "Epidurals sell themselves," Dr. Birnbach said.

But what doctors call progress saddens those who favor natural childbirth or childbirth without anesthesia. Ina May Gaskin, president of the Midwives Alliance of North America, in Summertown, Tennessee, said: "If you tap into the popular culture, there's a huge fear of birth. Women are saying, 'I've got to get my epidural.' It's more acceptable, I think to the dismay of nurse-midwives."

Natural childbirth is "hugely empowering," Ms. Gaskin said. "It's hard, yes, but we do things in life that are hard. We don't shrink from them. After a natural birth, you have so much power you feel you could do anything. Women go on being grateful for that birth and will go on remembering it as a signal event in their lives that changed them. If you cancel out the awareness of the body in labor, you miss a lot of the ecstasy."

Ms. Gaskin also said she did not think that women were fully informed about the risks of epidurals. She said there were not enough data about the newer, low-dose versions to determine whether or not they impeded labor. In addition, she said, some women had adverse reactions to the drugs or developed fevers from them that led doctors to fear infection and to put newborn babies through invasive tests to rule out infection.

Dr. Hawkins said the main complications from epidurals were soreness at the injection site, a drop in blood pressure and a 1 in 200 chance of a headache. Other problems were "incredibly rare," she said.

Not all women are caught up in the trend. Caledonia Kearns, a book editor in Brooklyn, had her baby at a birthing center, after 14 hours of labor with-out any drugs whatsoever. She eased some of her pain with warm baths and showers, and was allowed to walk about and eat and drink during labor. Her husband, both grandmothers and other family members saw her daughter being born.

"Natural childbirth was very important to me," she said. "I felt like I had done this tremendous thing. But it's a very personal choice. I think people deliver how they need to deliver."

[DG, October 1999]

## Doctors Report Rise in Elective Caesareans

The Manhattan woman was in the first trimester of pregnancy with her first child when she decided how she wanted the baby delivered. She had read about childbirth in pregnancy books, heard war stories from friends and relatives and feared that she could not endure whatever labor pain she might have before the epidural kicked in. She told her doctor that when her pregnancy was full term, she wanted a Caesarean section.

"I spent a long time counseling her," said Dr. Andrei Rebarber, her obstetrician at New York University Medical Center. He told her that she had a greater chance for complications, including hemorrhage, infection and death, from a Caesarean section than from vaginal delivery. "I told her I won't do a Caesarean section without a medical indication. I feel that it's unethical."

But the woman, a 46-year-old credit manager who spoke on the condition that her name not be published, saw the situation differently. "I was surprised it wasn't my choice," she said. "It's my body." She said that she was willing to pay the extra cost of a surgical delivery if her insurance company did not cover it. At five months pregnant, the woman was still trying to decide once and for all whether to stay with Dr. Rebarber, whom she respects, or switch to a doctor who will honor her choice.

Needless to say, this woman's request is unusual.

For years, pregnant women's choice has been synonymous with the most natural childbirth possible. And it has been a consensus among medical professionals that many Caesareans are unnecessary, with a rate of about 21 percent of all births in this country in 1998, down slightly from a record high of nearly 25 percent in 1988 and far higher than the 5 percent of 1965. Hospitals and medical groups pressure doctors to avoid doing Caesareans unless there is medical justification, like failure of labor to progress or signs of distress in the fetus. The Department of Health and Human Services has the goal of lowering the rate to 15 percent by 2000.

But the pendulum is beginning to swing, slightly, in the other direction. Though no figures exist for elective Caesareans, some doctors say that more women are asking for C-sections, even when they are not necessary. And doctors are sharply divided on how to respond.

Several recent reports that question the safety of vaginal deliveries in certain circumstances are driving this turnaround. For example, in May 1998, the Food and Drug Administration issued a public health advisory on vacuum-assisted delivery devices, tools that are sometimes used for difficult vaginal births. Each year from 1994 to 1997 in the United States, according to the advisory, five newborns have died or been seriously injured after delivery with these devices.

Another report concerned the safety of vaginal delivery for women who previously had Caesareans. Though doctors have encouraged such women to try to deliver vaginally, a large Canadian study published in 1996 found that the chance of major complications to the mother were greater than previously shown: nearly twice as great as from a Caesarean section that was scheduled before labor.

In general, childbirth is considered extremely safe for both mother and child. Still, the findings on vaginal deliveries have left some doctors questioning whether the Caesarean section rate really is too high and some women wondering whether it is worth the pain and uncertainty of going through labor when scheduled surgery is so convenient.

"The assumption that our C-section rate is too high is based on zero data," said Dr. Charles Lockwood, an obstetrician at New York University Medical Center and a member of the committee of obstetrical practice of the American College of Obstetricians and Gynecologists. Lowering the C-section rate to 15 percent, he said, "may be dangerous."

In England, there has been a marked increase in the number of women asking for Caesareans when they are not medically necessary, according to two recent commentaries in the *British Medical Journal*. The authors offered several reasons: medical advances like local anesthesia that have made Caesarean sections safer, and evidence that long, difficult vaginal deliveries can cause "substantial morbidity," like stress incontinence and other pelvic damage to the mother, and cerebral palsy or even death to the baby.

"We are at a turning point in obstetric thinking," said Dr. Sara Paterson-Brown, an obstetrician and gynecologist at Queen Charlotte's and Chelsea Hospital in London and an author of one commentary. "I'm not saying that Caesarean section is good and vaginal delivery is bad, but there's increased evidence that the picture is no longer black and white."

Elective Caesareans in England have increased to 6.5 percent of C-sections in 1995 from 4 percent in 1980, said Dr. Robert Kyffin, a research fellow with the Royal College of Obstetricians and Gynecologists in Manchester. Overall, England's Caesarean rate has increased to 16 percent, up from 10.4 percent in 1985.

From late 1997 to late 1998 at Diana Princess of Wales Hospital in Grimsby, staff members have had 10 requests for Caesarean sections, half for no medical reason, said Dr. Ibrahim I. Bolaji, author of the other commentary and an obstetrician and gynecologist at the hospital. "For one woman, convenience was the reason," he said. "Her husband works with the service and she wanted to schedule her delivery before he had to leave the country. Two other patients didn't want to go through labor pain, and one wanted a C-section because one of her relations had a problem with normal labor."

Dr. Bolaji said each request was granted. Some doctors, he said, agree to do elective Caesarean sections to avoid malpractice lawsuits in the event that something goes wrong in a vaginal birth, long a concern of obstetricians. "Doctors have little to gain and a lot to lose by not doing a Caesarean," he said.

## The Delivery Debate

Small but growing numbers of expectant mothers are asking to choose their methods of delivery. Here are some of the factors they consider.

### VAGINAL DELIVERY

**Benefits:** A more natural experience in the eyes of some.

**Risks:** Urinary and fecal incontinence, sexual dysfunction and, for mothers who have had a previous Caesarean, a ruptured uterus.

### CAESAREAN SECTION

**Benefits:** Women don't have to endure labor pains and in some cases can choose time of delivery.

**Risks:** Urinary tract infection, inflammation of the uterus wall, blood clots, hemorrhaging and a higher risk of death.

*Source:* New England Journal of Medicine; *American College of Obstetricians and Gynecologists*

But fear of litigation is not the only factor. The commentaries cited a survey published in 1997 in which 31 percent of female obstetricians in London said that they would choose a Caesarean for themselves in an uncomplicated pregnancy. The main reason given was fear of damage to the pelvic organs from a vaginal delivery. Doctors say that a small percentage of women who give birth vaginally suffer long-term pelvic damage, like urinary incontinence and loss of muscle tone in the vagina that can interfere with sexual satisfaction. Such complications are most common after several vaginal deliveries.

A number of American doctors criticized the British commentaries for playing down the risks of Caesarean sections. "I'm astonished that any woman would want to have a Caesarean unless there's a problem with the pregnancy or the labor," said Dr. Vicki L. Seltzer, past president of the American College of Obstetricians and Gynecologists and chairwoman of obstetrics and gynecology at Long Island Jewish Medical Center in New Hyde Park, New York.

It is unclear whether Caesarean section is safer for the baby in an uncomplicated pregnancy and whether it is safer than using a vacuum extraction for some difficult deliveries, Dr. Lockwood said. "That's a hot area of debate," he said.

Physicians like Dr. Michael Brodman, vice chairman of obstetrics and gynecology at Mount Sinai Medical Center in New York, have received more requests for elective C-sections in the last few years but not in the numbers reported in England. "My sense in the community that you're a better mother if you deliver vaginally isn't holding water anymore," he said.

Dr. Jennie A. Freiman, a gynecologist in New York City's Upper East Side, was so convinced that her two children would be better off with a Caesarean delivery that she scheduled one for each of them. "The minute I found out I was pregnant, I told my obstetrician I wanted a Caesarean section," she said.

Doctors are divided in how they handle a request for an unnecessary Caesarean. Dr. Lockwood and Dr. Rebarber will not perform one on a woman with an uncomplicated first pregnancy but will consider doing it if she has had a vaginal delivery that was harmful or extremely difficult. Others, like Dr. William Ledger, chairman of obstetrics and gynecology at New York Presbyterian Hospital, Cornell campus, will perform Caesareans on first-time mothers with no medical need, but only after trying to change their minds. All doctors emphasized the need to tell patients the risks involved.

As for the pregnant credit manager, her husband and her friends have tried to talk her out of having an elective Caesarean section, arguing that it was not worth switching doctors and risking medical complications. She resolved to conquer her fear of labor. But she said her desire for a Caesarean was so strong that she changed her mind many times in the remaining four months of her pregnancy.

[SG, September 1998]

## Benefits of Assistant for Childbirth Go Far Beyond the Birthing Room

As a physician's assistant, Marcia Gaddy has delivered many babies, but the first time she went into labor, she panicked. "I didn't know what to do," she said. "I was very scared and I felt very alone, even though my husband was there to hold my hand."

So, to make childbirth easier the second time around, she hired a doula, a person who is trained to work as an adjunct to doctors and midwives, giving women in labor the continuous emotional and physical support that these practitioners seldom provide. "She helped me redirect my fear into a challenge," Ms. Gaddy said. "Labor went much more quickly and was much easier."

Ms. Gaddy, of North Brunswick, New Jersey, is among the small but growing number of women—they include Elle Macpherson, the model, and Ricki Lake, the talk show host—who have used labor doulas. The term (pronounced (DOO-la) is derived from a Greek word meaning servant or handmaiden.

Research shows that childbirth does go more smoothly with a doula: Labor is 25 percent shorter, the need for epidural pain relief is 60 percent less and the Caesarean section rate is reduced by half.

Now a study has reported that the benefits extend beyond the birthing room. Women in the study who had doulas during labor were assessed as more sensitive, loving and responsive to their infants two months later. Since doulas were assigned to the women at random, the study eliminated the possibility that women who chose doulas were innately more nurturing than the others in the study group, said Dr. Susan H. Landry, a psychologist at the University of Texas at Houston Medical Center who conducted the study. It was presented at a meeting of the Pediatric Academic Societies in New Orleans.

"I was surprised and really thrilled by the long-term findings," Dr. Landry said. "It's very exciting that such a brief intervention could have such striking effects."

Doulas do not deliver babies. Rather, they suggest different positions and breathing techniques to help ease labor pain and they comfort women who are anxious, frightened or feel overwhelmed. Right after delivery, they give advice on breast feeding and many assist mothers at home with their newborns.

Doula training consists of a three-day course that covers the anatomy and process of labor, as well as techniques for providing emotional and physical comfort to women in labor, said Kathie Lindstron, president-elect of Doulas of North America, an international organization that trains and certifies doulas. In addition, a doula must also attend at least three deliveries to be certified.

Doulas attend just 1 percent of all births in this country, but they are gaining wider acceptance by doctors, hospitals and insurance companies, said Debra Pascali-Bonaro, a doula in River Vale, New Jersey, and spokeswoman for Doulas of North America.

"Doulas complement the work that midwives do," said Jane Arnold, director of midwifery services at University Hospital and Medical Center in Stony Brook, New York. "We usually can't be with a woman throughout her labor because we have more than one woman in labor at once. But a doula can be there all the time."

Ms. Pascali-Bonaro said that doulas can be helpful even when a midwife or doctor is present. "At moments when a woman in labor needs medical care, a doctor or midwife is busy providing medical support but a doula can offer emotional support," she said.

"We are trying to find innovative ways of lowering the Caesarean section rate," said Dr. David M. Roth, chief of obstetrics and gynecology for Kaiser Permanente in White Plains, New York. Kaiser feels the use of doulas "will be well received by patients and will probably be cost-effective," he said.

The University of Texas study included 104 pregnant women who were delivering their first babies at Ben Taub Hospital, a county hospital in Houston.

The women were randomly assigned to three groups: 33 women had a doula with them during labor and childbirth, 35 women served as a control group, receiving mainly narcotic pain medicine on request, and 36 women got epidurals, which provide stronger pain relief, on request.

Dr. Landry wanted to see if the degree of pain control during labor correlated with a woman's ability to nurture her child. Two months later, researchers visited each woman at home to observe her with her baby and rate the quality of mother-child interaction with the Bayle Scales of Infant Development, a series of standard measurements.

The researchers did not know which women had had doulas. But the women in the doula group scored about 5½ on a scale of 1 to 7, with 7 being the highest, whereas the women in the other groups scored about 4½. "A one-point difference on these scales is significant," Dr. Landry said.

She sees two reasons why the doula group scored higher. This study, like others, found that women with doulas had shorter labors, fewer labor and delivery complications and fewer Caesareans, and since the women themselves felt better after delivery, they may have been better able to cope with the demands of new motherhood. But she thinks a stronger factor was that the mothers wanted to do unto their babies as the doulas had done to them. "The doula was modeling for the women how to nurture," Dr. Landry said.

Only half of the women in Dr. Landry's study were married, raising the question of whether a woman with a supportive partner by her side would benefit from a doula. But research by Dr. John H. Kennell, a pediatrician at Case Western Reserve University School of Medicine in Cleveland, reports that the answer, at least as far as the labor outcomes are concerned, is yes.

Dr. Kennell's latest study involved 42 married women who were at high risk for Caesarean sections because their labor was being induced. Twenty of these women were assigned a doula in the hospital and the other 22 were not. The Caesarean rate for the doula group was 20 percent, compared with 62 percent for the others, Dr. Kennell said.

"In all of our studies, it's clear that it's important for a father to be present," he said. "But even when a father has been to childbirth classes, he can get frantic, distressed and exhausted. A doula is trained in the labor and delivery experience."

When Ms. Gaddy was in labor in December 1997, the duties of her husband and her doula broke down this way. "I leaned on my husband between contractions," she said, "but my doula worked with me during contractions."

[SG, May 1998]

## Deaths Linked to Sex After Childbirth

Doctors routinely advise women to refrain from sexual activity for several weeks after childbirth, and for most women postpartum pain and exhaustion are incentives enough to comply. But for those who do not follow doctors' orders, the consequences can be serious and, in rare cases, even fatal.

In *The Postgraduate Medical Journal*, a publication of the British Medical Association, doctors describe two young women who died while having intercourse within eight days of giving birth. Both had had normal vaginal deliveries and died of air embolisms, air bubbles in the major arteries to the heart and brain.

Death during intercourse is rare and occurs mainly in middle-aged men with heart disease, said Dr. Philip Batman, the lead author, who is a pathologist at Bradford Hospitals National Health Service Trust in Bradford, England. What led him to investigate such deaths in pregnant women and new mothers, he said, "was the coincidence of seeing two women in the same small town in Yorkshire die of embolisms during intercourse in the last three years."

He said women were more vulnerable to air embolisms soon after childbirth than at other times, because air forced into the uterus during sex can enter the bloodstream through blood vessels that were torn during delivery. Earlier research found that pregnant women are also at increased risk because air can become trapped between the sac containing the fetus and the uterus wall, then escape through blood vessels on the surface of the uterus.

In reviewing the records of more than 20 million pregnant women from 1967 to 1993, Dr. Batman and colleagues found that 18 had died from air embolisms during pregnancy or soon after childbirth. At least four of these women died while having sex, though Dr. Batman said they could not determine the exact number. One of the four had taken amphetamines, which could have contributed to her death, he said.

Though there are no statistics on maternal deaths during sex in the United States, there are a handful of recent reports in the medical literature, all involving pregnant women. But since the risk is extremely slim, most doctors sanction intercourse during pregnancy, said Dr. Sharon Phelan, a spokeswoman for the American College of Obstetricians and Gynecologists and an associate professor of obstetrics and gynecology at the University of Alabama School of Medicine in Birmingham. "The only time a doctor might tell a woman not to have intercourse is if she's had a number of preterm births," she said, explaining that intercourse can touch off contractions and then premature labor.

Doctors used to recommend that women avoid sex for six weeks after childbirth, but the rules have been relaxed in recent years with the realization that six weeks is an arbitrary time frame and that many women probably disregard the advice anyway, said

Dr. Joshua A. Copel, chief of the high-risk obstetrics group at the Yale School of Medicine.

Literature from the American College of Obstetricians and Gynecologists states that women can usually have sexual intercourse "in about three or four weeks," or when they feel comfortable, a sign that the uterus has healed. Obstetricians say that it also takes about this long for incisions outside the vagina or from a Caesarean section to heal.

The biggest risks of having sex too soon are not fatal complications but tears in the incisions or infections in the uterus caused by bacteria on the sperm, doctors say.

[SG, October 1998]

# Breast Is Best for Babies, but Sometimes Mom Needs Help

A gay New York pediatrician enlisted 30 nursing mothers to supply breast milk for the baby he and his partner have adopted. The baby, at five months of age, was thriving on the donated milk. In another part of town, a 19-year-old Bronx woman was prosecuted for the death from starvation of the 7-week-old baby she had been faithfully nursing but inadequately nourishing.

Each case dramatically illustrates well-known but little-heeded facts about breast-feeding.

*Fact one*: As good as infant formulas are, breast milk is still universally recognized as superior food for the first six months of life, which is what prompted the pediatrician to go to great lengths to get breast milk for his baby.

*Fact two*: As the young Bronx woman so tragically learned, nursing does not necessarily come naturally to either mothers or babies, who often need help in mastering this skill.

Corollaries to these facts are two problems.

*Problem one*: American employers make few accommodations for new mothers, most of whom get no or only brief paid maternity leave. In Norway,

mothers may get full pay for 42 weeks of maternity leave or four-fifths pay for 52 weeks, but American law stipulates only 12 weeks of unpaid leave. Nor do most American employers provide child care at the workplace so that mothers can nurse their babies during the workday, or private areas where nursing mothers can pump and refrigerate breast milk for later use.

*Problem two*: Although most hospitals that deliver babies employ a lactation specialist, new mothers generally leave the hospital within two days of childbirth, before most problems with nursing are likely to surface. Many mothers could benefit greatly from a home visit from a lactation specialist within the first two weeks of a birth. Experts say that the first few weeks of nursing are pivotal, and this is the time that many struggling mothers give up. They rarely get the kind of practical guidance on nursing from pediatricians that they would get from lactation specialists trained in solving breast-feeding problems.

Breast-feeding has enjoyed a well-deserved burst in popularity in recent decades, when pediatric specialists finally succeeded in overcoming the commercial pressures on modern women to feed their babies formula. Lately, however, the numbers have been dropping from their peak in the 1980s. In the spring of 1999, only about 60 percent of mothers were nursing their babies when they left the hospital and only 30 percent were still nursing six months later. By the end of 1999, according to the goals set in a report "Healthy People 2000" by the Surgeon General, Government health officials had hoped that three-fourths of all new mothers would be nursing when they took their babies home.

And while well-educated women have the highest initial breast-feeding rates, they are also the women most likely to run into career conflicts should they wish to continue nursing for the full first year of their babies' lives, as recommended by the American Academy of Pediatrics.

Even before a new mother's milk comes in, the colostrom her breasts secrete helps her baby's development. Colostrum contains substances that promote maturation of the infant's gut and that facilitate digestion. It also contains immune substances that protect against infection.

The protein in human milk is well absorbed and used, especially by the infant's brain. Fats in breast milk are more digestible than those in formula, and breast milk calories are used more efficiently. Breast milk also contains growth factors, enzymes, hormones and other substances that may aid an infant's development.

Studies have shown that breast milk enhances the development of the immune system. All other things being equal, babies who are breast-fed suffer fewer bacterial and viral illnesses and are better protected against allergies, diarrhea, ear infections, diabetes and possibly cancer as well. They also respond better to immunizations.

But there are health disadvantages to breast-feeding as well. Infection with H.I.V., the virus that causes AIDS, can be transmitted from mother to baby through breast milk. So can antibiotics and other drugs a mother may have to take. Also, infants who inherit a condition called galactosemia, an inability to process one of the sugars in breast milk, should not be breast-fed.

Mothers may have physical problems that interfere with nursing. The Bronx teenager whose nursing infant died, for example, had undergone breast reduction surgery, which greatly reduced her milk supply. Her baby seemed to be nursing properly but, unbeknown to her, got little nourishment. Lacking medical guidance and thinking she was doing the best for her baby, the young, inexperienced mother never realized that the infant was starving.

Every new mother needs and deserves some help

---

## Breast-Feeding Help

New mothers may be worried that they are not doing it correctly or that their baby is not getting enough to eat.

### WHAT TO EXPECT

- Baby is feeding well 8 to 12 times every 24 hours.
- Urine is pale in color, and baby wets at least six diapers every 24 hours after the third day.
- Bowel movements are soft and mustard-colored after a week.
- If any weight is lost after birth, it is regained by the second to third week and continues to rise steadily.

### CALL THE DOCTOR IF

- Baby fights the breast, will not stay latched or cries after one to two minutes.
- Baby cannot be kept awake long enough to take much milk.
- Diapers are damp rather than soaked, and baby has fewer than six wet diapers per day.
- Baby passes very little stool or has dark green, mucous stools.
- Skin color is pale, blue or yellow.
- Rectal temperature is higher than 100.5° F.

For help or to find a lactation consultant in your area, call La Leche League at (800) LA-LECHE. On the Web: www.nursingmother.com.

with breast-feeding. Even those with nursing experience may need help since babies differ in their ability to nurse. Sometimes, too, a mother's milk does not come in fully by the third day after delivery—stress, for example, can delay milk production—and the baby may need supplemental formula for nutrition or at least water to prevent dehydration.

Help should start well before the baby is born, with information about the benefits and risks of breast-feeding and general guidance on technique. A woman with inverted or flat nipples can correct their shape by wearing a special shield in her bra during the last months of pregnancy. Those who will have to return to work soon after giving birth may want to work out a plan for part-time nursing, supplementing with formula or perhaps breast milk that is pumped during the workday.

Even a mother who is determined to nurse can become discouraged if her nipples get very sore or cracked. This can be avoided or alleviated by learning how to remove the baby from the breast by first sliding a finger into the corner of the infant's mouth to break the suction. Soreness can be relieved by warm or cold compresses or by blowing warm (not hot) air from a hair dryer on the nipples.

Nursing mothers also have to pay careful attention to their own diets. This is no time to try to lose those extra pounds that accumulated during pregnancy. A healthy diet can be achieved by each day following the recommendations of the Food Guide Pyramid: 6 to 11 servings of grain-based foods, 3 to 5 servings of vegetables, 2 to 3 servings of fruits, 2 to 3 servings of a high-protein food and 2 to 3 servings of dairy products plus at least eight 8-ounce glasses of water a day. Many doctors also recommend that nursing mothers continue to take their prenatal vitamins. In general, experts recommend avoiding caffeinated drinks. In addition, mothers often find that certain foods they consume upset a nursing baby's digestion and are best avoided.

As for medications, although most do get into breast milk, only a relative few should be avoided when nursing. These include doxorubicin, ergotamine preparations, lithium, methotrexate, cyclosporin and bromocriptine.

[JEB, March 1999]

# Estrogen Patch Appears to Lift Severe Depression in New Mothers

No one says new mothers have it easy. Nights spent waking up every two hours and days spent trying to figure out just why the baby is crying so much leave about 80 percent of new mothers physically exhausted, emotionally drained and despondent over their seeming inability to do anything well. Call it the baby blues.

Most of these women feel better after two weeks, but 10 percent have a form of clinical depression that can last for many months. Mothers with so-called postpartum depression feel so sad, anxious and helpless that they have trouble taking care of the baby and themselves. In the most severe cases, they are suicidal.

Despite the prevalence of the condition, doctors disagree on the best way to treat it and there is little research to guide them. But in 1996 British doctors reported rapid improvement in postpartum depression in women who were treated with a skin patch that delivered estrogen into their bloodstreams.

The results of the six-month study, published in *The Lancet,* a medical journal published in Britain, involved 61 women with severe postpartum depression. Thirty-four of them used an estrogen patch for three months and 27 used a patch with a dummy medication. Although all the women improved over time, those receiving estrogen improved faster and to a greater extent than did those in the comparison group, the researchers found. They said that 80 percent of the women in the treatment group were no longer clinically depressed after three months, while most of those in the comparison group remained depressed for at least four months.

"This is a very important development and very logical treatment," said Dr. John W. W. Studd, an obstetrician and gynecologist at Chelsea and Westminster Hospital in London who was one of the researchers.

His enthusiasm was shared by some experts on postpartum depression in this country. "This looks very hopeful," said Dr. Joan R. Youchah, an obstetrician and gynecologist and a psychiatrist at Albert Einstein Medical College in the Bronx. "This is a method of treatment that people have thought about but not studied. It's a good new direction to look in."

Dr. Michael W. O'Hara, chairman of psychology at the University of Iowa in Iowa City and a leading authority on postpartum depression, said, "This may be an alternative for women who don't respond to antidepressants."

Doctors have long thought that postpartum depression is related at least in part to the sharp decline in estrogen that occurs immediately after childbirth. Estrogen levels normally fluctuate from 80 to 200 picograms per liter of blood in women of reproductive age who are not pregnant, Dr. Studd said. During pregnancy, the levels shoot up to 5,000 picograms and immediately after childbirth they plummet to the range of 80 to 100 picograms, he said. The amount of estrogen used in the study elevated the women's estrogen to a normal prepregnancy level, he said.

Precisely how a drop in estrogen might set off depression is unknown, but studies show a relationship between the hormone and several neurotransmitters that influence mood, including serotonin. Dr. Studd believes it is no coincidence that many women become depressed during the various times when their estrogen levels ebb. "Depression is twice as common in women as men and it tends to occur at times of hormonal change—premenstrual, postnatal and menopausal," he said.

But he said it was too early to recommend estrogen as a treatment for postpartum depression until more studies were done. Perhaps the biggest unanswered question is whether estrogen is more effective than the standard treatments for postpartum depression, namely antidepressants and psychotherapy. Despite their widespread use, even those treatments have not been well studied against postpartum depression. Which of the treatments is used first depends largely on whether a woman seeks help from a psychotherapist or from a medical doctor.

A small study conducted by Dr. O'Hara found that two-thirds of women with mild to moderate postpartum depression were cured after three months of interpersonal psychotherapy, which focuses on people's relationships. But many women with severe postpartum depression need antidepressants in addition to psychotherapy, he said. Doctors estimate that this combination helps about 90 percent of women with the problem.

But there are drawbacks to those treatments. "Psychotherapy is a lot more work than taking a drug," Dr. O'Hara said. "Many women find it easier to take a pill."

On the other hand, doctors say, many women must try several antidepressants before they find one that works for them. Another disadvantage of antidepressants is that they pass into breast milk, and their effect on infants is unknown. "As a result, we advise women to stop breast-feeding when they take antidepressants," Dr. Youchah said.

The estrogen patch may also prove to be a problem for nursing mothers, since estrogen can interfere with milk production, said Dr. Joseph F. Mortola, an associate professor of obstetrics and gynecology and of psychiatry at Harvard Medical School. But Dr. Studd, who has used the estrogen patch in his clinical practice for 10 years, said the patch did not suppress milk production once breast-feeding was established.

Although Dr. Studd's study did not compare the effectiveness of the estrogen patch with other therapies, it did find that several women who had not responded to antidepressants before the study were helped by the estrogen. While it appears that estrogen comes closer than antidepressants to treating the underlying cause of postpartum depression, experts say it is too early to call it the magic bullet. "Other hormones also decline after childbirth," Dr. Mortola said. "Whether estrogen is an effective treatment for postpartum depression by itself is debatable, but it could add to the treatments that we already have."

[SG, May 1996]

# Diagnosing Fibroids Is Simple; Deciding What to Do Is Hard

When Susan H., age 40, began experiencing excessive menstrual bleeding and almost constant pelvic pain and cramping, her doctor's diagnosis was straightforward and certain: She had multiple uterine fibroids, benign tumors that grow within the smooth muscle of the uterine wall or on the uterine surface.

Susan's response was equally sure: "I did not want a hysterectomy. I hadn't ruled out having children, and even if I never had a child, I did not want to lose my uterus."

Instead, she had an abdominal myomectomy, in which individual fibroids are surgically removed through a pelvic incision. Susan was up and walking in six hours, and fully recovered after two weeks. Now, a year after the surgery, she is free of symptoms and pleased to have preserved her child-bearing potential.

Victoria L., 50, was not contemplating more children. Yet even though her fibroids were numerous enough and large enough to distend her abdomen and cause backaches, "I was dead set against a hysterectomy," she said. Instead, Victoria underwent embolization, a procedure in which a catheter is threaded into the uterine artery, and tiny plastic particles are injected into the blood vessels that feed the fibroids, cutting off their blood supply and causing them to shrink. In a week, Victoria was back at work and feeling fine.

"The result was amazing," she said of the procedure. "The symptoms are all gone, and my stomach is no longer bloated."

These women, both New York City residents who spoke on the condition that their full names not be used, are not unusual in insisting on alternatives to hysterectomy to treat fibroids. Nor are they unusual in having the tumors. At least 25 percent of women suffer from uterine fibroids at some point, medical experts say. These benign growths are most common between the ages of 30 and 40, but can develop at any time, according to the American College of Obstetricians and Gynecologists.

Although no one knows exactly what causes fibroids to develop, they seem to occur more often in blacks than in whites. Some scientists suspect a genetic link, as they can run in families. The female hormone estrogen fuels the growth of fibroids, which tend to shrink after menopause. There is no known correlation, however, between the use of low-dose birth control pills and the development of the tumors.

While not cancerous, fibroids can cause considerable problems, including heavy menstrual bleeding, pelvic and back pain, bladder pressure, constipation and, depending on their size and location, infertility, miscarriage and premature labor and birth.

Historically, hysterectomy has been the treatment of choice for fibroids that cause severe symptoms. Indeed, fibroids are the most common reason for the procedure, accounting for approximately a third of the hysterectomies performed in the United States, according to the Center for Uterine Fibroids at Brigham and Women's Hospital in Boston. That is more than 200,000 hysterectomies annually, which many women and doctors now regard as too many.

"I foresee that in the next few years, any doctor that does a complete hysterectomy for fibroids will have a lot of explaining to do," said Dr. Ernst Bartsich, a clinical associate professor of obstetrics and gynecology at New York Presbyterian Hospital. Dr. Bartsich prefers myomectomy, which leaves the uterus intact.

One of three types of myomectomy may be performed, depending on the fibroids' size and location. For larger fibroids on the outside of the uterus or ones that have penetrated the uterine wall, an abdominal myomectomy is generally considered best. It is major surgery, involving two to three days in the hospital and at least a week's rest at home. The results can be dramatic, however, especially for women with multiple and very large fibroids.

For smaller fibroids on the outside of the uterus, a surgeon may choose to perform a laparoscopic myomectomy, in which a tiny incision is made in the abdomen to accommodate a laparoscope, a thin, telescopelike instrument. While viewing the uterus and surrounding organs through the laparoscope, the surgeon uses thin tubes fitted with surgical instruments to remove the fibroids.

Easiest of all is a hysteroscopic myomectomy, in which a hysteroscope, an instrument similar to a laparoscope, is inserted through the vagina and into the uterine cavity to remove fibroids just beneath, or protruding from, the lining of the uterus. An outpatient procedure, this involves, on average, a 24-hour recovery period. It is especially effective in treating fibroids that cause heavy bleeding, Dr. Bartsich said.

The downside to myomectomy is that fibroids may recur. Studies show that about 10 percent of women who undergo the procedure need further surgery because their tumors grow back. Also, "myomectomy can be difficult when the uterus is so distorted, and the tumors so many and so large that you wouldn't know where to start," said Dr. Brad Quade, the clinical co-director for the Center for Uterine Fibroids at Brigham and Women's Hospital.

For tumors that are hard to reach through myomectomy, there is fibroid embolization, the new, less invasive technique used to treat Victoria L.'s fibroids. No longer strictly experimental but not yet a standard procedure, embolization is performed by interventional radiologists, specialists who use X-ray guidance to carry out minimally invasive procedures.

Through a tiny incision in the groin, a catheter is inserted into the femoral artery and then into the uterine artery. The catheter is used to inject the plastic sand-sized particles that block the blood vessels feeding the fibroids.

"The shrinking starts immediately, because fibroids are very vascular and dependent on their blood supply," said Dr. Alan Boykin, the director of vascular and interventional radiology at Maimonides Medical Center in Brooklyn. Dr. Boykin added: "It is painful at first—it almost feels like you're in labor for about 24 hours. But after a day in the hospital, a woman can go home, and after about three days, she can resume normal activities."

Embolization seems to be effective, though the procedure's long-term results are not known. And women like the fact that it is minimally invasive, with a brief recovery time. But, Dr. Quade said: "There are concerns about damage to the ovaries and about the integrity of the uterus itself, because of cutting off the blood flow. There is also the same issue as for myomectomy—the recurrence of fibroids. We don't yet know about recurrence risk and how it compares to myomectomy."

Because of the risk of damage to the ovaries, Dr. Boykin and most other doctors who perform embolization restrict it to women who are not planning a pregnancy. "The risk of ovarian failure is only about 1 percent," Dr. Boykin said. "Still, that is enough that I recommend embolization only to women who are not going to have children. And because the procedure is still new, I am limiting it to patients who have significant pain or bleeding from fibroids."

Women considering embolization should check with their health insurers, because many insurance plans still classify the procedure as experimental and do not cover it.

Other treatments, some new and some time-tested, are available for fibroids. Myolysis is an innovative laparoscopic procedure in which needles transmit electricity to shrink the blood vessels feeding the fibroids. Cryomyolysis is a similar procedure, involving a freezing probe.

Endometrial ablation does not treat the fibroids themselves, but the symptom of heavy bleeding. In a new version of this procedure, a balloon is placed in the uterine cavity via a catheter. The balloon is then inflated with a hot liquid. The heat thins the endometrial lining, which reduces the bleeding. (Because the uterine lining becomes too thin to support a pregnancy, this procedure is also recommended only for women who have no plans to conceive.)

Drug treatment with synthetic hormones called GnRH agonists is sometimes used to shrink fibroids before surgery. They temporarily induce a menopausal state, and should not be used for more than three to six months.

Finally, there is hysterectomy, which many doctors and patients now see as a treatment of last resort. The advantage is that it gets rid of fibroids permanently and prevents other diseases of the uterus. The disadvantage of the invasive procedure, which can be performed abdominally or vaginally, is that many post-hysterectomy patients experience bladder problems, bowel problems or sexual dysfunction, which can occur even if their ovaries are left intact.

Dr. Bartsich avoids hysterectomy whenever possible for the treatment of fibroids. But if the tumors are too numerous or too large, or if the patient insists on a hysterectomy, he sometimes recommends a supra-cervical hysterectomy, in which the cervix is left intact. "That is important for pelvic function, pelvic support and sexual function," he said.

Women must be told about their options and must take charge of their own treatment, the physicians say. "There is a belief that after the last pregnancy, the uterus is useless," Dr. Bartsich said. "The consumer has to know about alternatives and demand them. It's the only way we will get past this idea that losing her uterus is part of a woman's destiny."

[TH, June 1999]

## A Less Invasive Alternative for Fibroids

For Kristie Wolek, the trouble started in the spring of 1998, when her periods became so heavy that the blood loss made her severely anemic. She was exhausted all the time.

The problem was caused by four fibroids, benign tumors in her uterus that had been tiny and harmless for more than a decade but had recently begun growing rapidly. Two doctors recommended a hysterectomy, an operation to remove the uterus and the only sure cure for fibroids. Though Ms. Wolek, 43, did not want to have more children, she did not want a hysterectomy, either. But she thought she had no choice.

Shortly before she was to have the operation, however, a friend called to tell her about a television news report about a clinic near her home in Chicago that was offering a new, minimally invasive alternative. In August, 1998, Ms. Wolek had the operation, called fibroid embolization, which shrinks the fibroids by blocking their blood supply.

Instead of enduring major surgery and several weeks of recuperation, she felt fine in two days and has had no problems since.

Ms. Wolek is fairly typical of the hundreds of women around the country who have had the operation in that she learned of it not from her doctor but from the news. Though the same can be said for many treatments, fibroid embolization has attracted exceptional attention.

And some experts are concerned that its heavy promotion by doctors and medical groups on news programs and the Internet makes women think that it is an established treatment when it is not. "I think it's an interesting procedure," said Dr. Bryan Cowan, director of reproductive endocrinology at the University of Mississippi Medical Center in Jackson, "but, unfortunately, there are people who have run out and grabbed the banner and are touting this, with no evidence that it represents the standard of care."

## Shrinking Fibroids

Fibroids affect 20 to 40 percent of women. Fibroid embolization, which reduces the size of tumors by blocking their blood supply, is an alternative to major surgery for some women.

1 A catheter is inserted into the femoral artery through a tiny incision in the thigh.

2 The catheter is moved into the uterine artery.

3 Tiny plastic or sponge particles are injected into the artery.

4 The particles flow to the fibroids. Within minutes the blood flow is almost completely cut off.

Catheter    Fibroid
Femoral
artery
Uterine
artery

Fibroid    Particles
Catheter
Uterine
artery

*Source: Society of Cardiovascular and Interventional Radiology*

Other hysterectomy alternatives have been developed, but recent studies have shown that this one requires minimal recovery time and reduces symptoms of those fibroids that resist other treatments.

"I get 20 e-mails a day from women in all 50 states and even from as far away as Japan, Hong Kong, Egypt and Nairobi," said Dr. Carlos Forcade, an interventional radiologist at New York United Hospital Medical Center in Port Chester, New York, who performs fibroid embolization.

Dr. Gaylene Pron, an epidemiologist at the University of Toronto and coordinator of a multicenter study on fibroid embolization, called it "a women-driven technology," saying, "Women want this, or, rather, they don't want surgery."

Any woman of reproductive age can get fibroids, but they are most common in women over 35. According to the Society of Cardiovascular and Interventional Radiology, about 20 to 40 percent of these women have fibroids of significant size, and among African-American women, the incidence is about 50 percent. Fibroids run in families, though the cause is unknown.

In most cases, fibroids cause no symptoms and require no treatment. But if they grow large enough or appear in sensitive areas of the uterus, they can cause several problems, like dangerously heavy menstrual bleeding, severe pelvic pain and possibly infertility and miscarriage.

At first, doctors try to control fibroid-related symptoms with nonsteroidal anti-inflammatory drugs or birth control pills, but when medicine is not sufficient, women need surgery. More than 200,000 women in the United States have hysterectomies each year because of fibroids.

There are less invasive kinds of surgery to get rid of small fibroids, like hysteroscopy, in which a fiber optic scope is inserted into the vagina to remove them. But for women with relatively large ones who hope to become pregnant, the only surgical option is myomectomy, abdominal surgery to remove the individual fibroids. But with myomectomy, about 10 percent of women need further surgery because the fibroids grow back, the American College of Obstetricians and Gynecologists reports. And doctors have found that myomectomy is least effective for women with multiple fibroids or individual fibroids that are deeply embedded in the uterus.

Embolization seems to work on fibroids that myomectomy cannot eliminate, according to doctors who have studied them. The procedure is usually done in a hospital with the patient under local anesthesia. The patient can go home the next day.

At the 1999 annual meeting of the Society of Cardiovascular and Interventional Radiology in Orlando, Florida, Dr. James B. Spies, vice chairman of radiology at Georgetown University Medical Center in Washington, said that 89 percent of his 61 patients had less menstrual bleeding and that 96 had less pelvic pain. The tumor sizes shrank by half, on average, he said. In the six years that patients have been followed, he said, none have had new fibroids grow. Dr. Spies said that 3 percent of women suffered complications, like injury to the uterus and infertility. He also said that the treatment failed in fewer than 1 percent of the women, who then needed to have hysterectomies.

One of the biggest questions about the treatment is its effect on a woman's fertility. Though Dr. Spies and other doctors have had patients go on to have normal pregnancies, most of their patients are in their 40s and are not interested in pregnancy. About 1 percent to 2 percent of women go into premature menopause after the procedure, said Dr. Scott Goodwin, the first doctor to do fibroid embolization in this country.

"Some women may be suffering ovarian damage because the embolism material migrates to the ovaries," said Dr. Goodwin, chief of cardiovascular radiology at University of California, Los Angeles Medical Center.

Because of the risk of infertility, Dr. Goodwin and Dr. Spies do not recommend fibroid embolization to women who hope to become pregnant unless they are poor candidates for myomectomy and therefore would face infertility with any other fibroid surgery.

Dr. Susan Haas, chairwoman of the Massachusetts section of the American College of Obstetricians and Gynecologists and an assistant professor at Harvard Medical School, said she considered it "on the cusp between experimental and standard practice" because it looked promising in the short term. But she was at a recent meeting when doctors discussed technical problems. "I heard there were arteries that couldn't be catheterized," she said.

Because it is new, most insurance plans do not cover the embolization, but doctors say they can often persuade insurance companies to pay for it for individual patients by showing them research about the outcomes. But they say that some women want the operation so badly that they pay for it on their own, at a cost of as much as $15,000.

[SG, April 1999]

# The Teenage Years: Raising Healthy Daughters

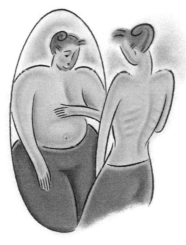

## PHYSICAL AND EMOTIONAL CHALLENGES DURING LIFE'S SECOND DECADE

Sometime during the tumultuous years between puberty and adulthood, too many teenage girls in America seem to lose their way. Studies have shown that self-esteem drops and school work suffers during the teen years, as girls seem to lose sight of educational and career opportunities and become increasingly focused on superficial frills like hairstyles, weight, manicures and makeup.

Our culture is assaulted by images from television, advertising and movies of glamorously got-up, rail-thin young women that few mothers would hold up as role models for their daughters but that many teenage girls find irresistible. A telling example of the power of the media occurred in Fiji during the 1990s, a culture in which plumpness had been prized. Once television arrived, complete with programs featuring waif-like women and girls, the girls in Fiji began to idolize them, and their own concept of what was attractive changed. Many began dieting, and for the first time in Fijian history, girls began to develop eating disorders.

It is during the teenage years that girls are most likely to take up smoking, experiment with alcohol, drugs and sex and become prone to eating disorders: the deliberate starvation of anorexia nervosa, and the bingeing and vomiting of bulimia.

How can parents help? One way, experts say, is to reevaluate the values that are communicated at home. Parents are sometimes shocked to realize how much emphasis they themselves place on appearance, criticizing their daughters' choice of clothing or hairdo, picking on the girls for gaining weight, encouraging them to consider nose jobs or liposuction or validating teenage obsessions with fashion and looks by spending inordinate amounts of time, money and energy on buying clothes.

Girls need to be recognized for their abilities and achievements in a way that makes it clear that those things are far more important than looks. Like adults, children need success, and praise when it is due. And vulnerable girls need protection from environments that may ultimately prove destructive to them. A girl with a weight problem may never make it as a ballerina or gymnast, but, doctors point out, she may starve herself to death trying. Parents need to help girls set more realistic goals and find pursuits in which they can succeed.

But families must also be aware that sometimes the best of intentions can backfire, including peer counseling programs in which the counselors are young women who have recovered from anorexia or bulimia. One such program, at Stanford University, did not help and may have even been associated with an increase in eating disorders. One reason, researchers suggest, might be that the counselors were so poised, thin and attractive that they may have inspired some young women in their audience to emulate them—right down to their eating disorders.

# A Sex Guide for Girls, Minus Homilies

It is a Darwinian law of nature that adults believe everything was better when they were young: music, books, movies, clothes, bagels and, of course, young people. But once in a while, adults are humbled. Something comes along that they look at wistfully, or maybe petulantly, and say: "Hey! Where was that when I was a teenager?"

Such is the response of many a mature woman to a new wave of books and computer Web sites aimed at adolescent girls, on the ever-daunting topic of being a girl. Being a teenage girl has always meant confronting a whole new set of crises and paradoxes: breasts that grow too slowly or too fast, periods, pimples, sexual urges, boys with their flim-flam hands and virgin/whore complexes. But until recently, girls mostly navigated their swelling, captious seas on their own, sometimes not even aware of the facts of menstruation until the day they started bleeding and went screaming to their mothers for a Band-Aid.

Now, girls need not go it alone, naïve or humorless. There are sources where they can learn about their bodies, minus the medicalese and pious homilies. At the forefront of this female informist movement is a book, *Deal With It! A Whole New Approach to Your Body, Brain and Life as a Gurl*, written—or, more accurately, choreographed, produced and emceed—by Esther Drill, Heather McDonald and Rebecca Odes. Based on a Web site, gURL.com, that the three women started in 1996, the book offers a frank, detailed and zealously nonjudgmental take on all aspects of girlhood.

It is a funny book, vividly designed in today's *de rigueur* style of bold colors, cartoon icons and choppy text blocks. The cover is a two-parter, showing a young woman on the front standing with her back to the reader, throwing open her yellow raincoat in the manner of a flasher. Flip to the inside cover, and the flasher is turned frontward in fetching bra and panties. Inside the book, tampons are drawn with grinning faces; an emotional "crush" is shown as a sneaker squashing a bug underfoot.

Yet the book's purpose is serious. It addresses virtually everything a young woman might want to know about herself, and herself in relation to others. Some of the text is written by the three authors, based on information screened by a variety of experts, and some consists of the comments and asides of girls.

Girls talk about their pubic hair and the hair around their nipples. To one alarmed query, a girl-commentator replies: "Relax! This is normal! It's called vaginal discharge." Girls talk about the even more "gross" realization that their parents have sex and sometimes even enjoy it.

The most incendiary topics are presented in clear, nonincendiary language. If a girl is pregnant, *Deal With It!* lays out her options, from the considerable challenges of life as a teenage mother to what an abortion involves and which states require parental notification or consent. The entire pharmacopeia of recreational drugs is described in detail, each one's effects and risks outlined without hellfire, brimstone or fearmongering.

"We wanted to give girls resources and information, but not be preachy about anything one way or another," Ms. McDonald said in an interview. "In our way of thinking, girls are smart; they can make choices; and what they need most is accurate information."

The intended audience for the book is girls from "the edge of their teens" to those "who are way past them but still reeling from the trauma." As such, the book covers topics that while arguably fine for a high school senior to encounter, may be a bit much for a reader of, say, 14. For example, one section discusses fellatio in language far too graphic to quote here, as girls give each other hints on how to do it well, and how to gracefully handle the aftermath.

The authors argue that knowledge is power, and that even young girls are smart enough to metabolize and store away information for future use, or to simply bypass those sections that do not apply. "We're trying to frame things so that girls can understand them and not be afraid of them," Ms. Odes said. "We think it's always better to know what you might encounter. Not telling a girl the name of something isn't going to keep her from doing it." Besides, Ms. Drill said, "if they pick up *Cosmo* magazine, or *Playboy*, they'll see the same thing." She added, "At least we're trying to contextualize it in a responsible way."

The specificity and wisecracking tolerance of *Deal With It!* demonstrate how radically the sexual education of young girls has changed over the years. Until this century, in fact, girls were on their own when it came to coping with their changing bodies and desires.

"They may have been given facts about childbirth, and many young women might have seen it for themselves, in their homes," said Joan Jacobs Brumberg, a professor of history at Cornell University and author of *The Body Project: An Intimate History of American Girls.* "But personal material in letters, autobiographies and memoirs of the time suggest that mothers were incredibly silent when it came to talking to their daughters about sexuality."

Formal sex education was introduced about 1905, and with an unambiguous intent, according to Jeffrey P. Moran, an assistant professor of history at the University of Kansas and author of *Teaching Sex: Shaping Adolescence in the 20th Century.*

"It was part of a moral movement to prevent young people from having sex outside of marriage," he said. "The idea, which has continued throughout this century, was that sex education could influence and change youthful behavior." Sex education courses often culminated with a slide show of suffering from tertiary syphilis: skin covered in carbuncles, noses eaten away by ulcers. "The idea was to put the fear of God in young people if they should stray," Dr. Moran said. And today, he said, with the risk of AIDS still looming, sex education classes continue to emphasize the negatives of indulgence.

"Insofar as Web sites and books are now laying out all the information that young people might need to know, and letting them make their own decisions," Dr. Moran said, "that's quite different from having the information carefully selected and handed down to them by authorities."

It was their discontent with the voices of authority that initially drove the three young women to start gURL.com, when they were graduate students at New York University. They had disliked the teenagers' and women's magazines they read as young girls, with their emphasis on boyfriends, thigh size and eye shadow. "It would be absurd to say that girls don't care about what they look like or what's in style," Ms. Drill said. "But it's insulting to think that that's all girls care about."

They devoted a highly caffeinated year of their lives putting the Web site together, and now it is visited by about 800,000 people a month. Other sites aimed at young girls are beginning to crop up, some under the aegis of groups like Planned Parenthood or Rutgers University, but none with nearly as keen an ear for teenage sensibilities.

Not everybody approves of gURL and its ilk. Coleen Kelly Mast, an educational consultant with Respect Inc. in Bradley, Illinois, which believes in saving sex for marriage, argues that many proponents of giving young girls the "whole truth" and "complete information" about their bodies often present a narrow and one-sided story of human sexuality.

"The information they give focuses on passion and pleasure, but it leaves the heart out of it," she said. "Girls and women are not told that all this playing with various forms of sexual pleasure, whether with themselves or a partner, can be a hindrance rather than a help to eventual satisfaction in marriage."

Sarah Brown, director of the National Campaign to Prevent Teen Pregnancy, said that as a general matter, she had "always felt that lots of information is better than no information." But she worries that too much information, too much peer-based schmoozing, can raise anxieties rather than lower them.

"The magic combination is not only lots of information, but lots of adults, and parents most of all," she said. "Adults are well positioned to provide context. Despite the stereotype of inevitable conflict between teenagers and their parents, all our research and experience show that parents remain very powerful influences in kids' lives. A mother shouldn't feel that she can give a book about the body and sexuality to her daughter and be done with it."

No, the mother can sit down with her daughter, with book or computer keyboard in hand, all the while muttering how much better kids have it today.

[NA, November 1999]

# Eating Disorders Haunt Ballerinas

In the early 1990s, Michelle Warren and Linda Hamilton, two specialists in eating disorders, began a three-year "intervention" survey of 40 beginning students at the School of American Ballet, affiliated with the New York City Ballet.

"We were trying to see which girls developed or were predisposed to problems," said Dr. Warren, a professor of obstetrics and gynecology at Columbia Presbyterian Medical Center and the director of its Menopause and Hormonal Disorders Center. But 60 to 70 percent of the students dropped out of the survey, and the study was canceled after a year. "Some dropped out because of injury," Dr. Warren said. "But basically when the girls started getting into trouble, they didn't want to answer questions."

Denial, Dr. Hamilton said, is a large part of the problem of eating disorders, a problem that affects a large number of young ballerinas. Determined intervention might have helped avert the sudden death on June 30, 1997 of Heidi Guenther, no longer a student but a 22-year-old member of the Boston Ballet. Ms. Guenther died of heart failure, thought to have been brought on by eating problems. She had lost weight and had complained to her family of a racing, pounding heart, but she refused to see a doctor.

Dance is a highly competitive, high-pressure and physically demanding profession. In classical ballet, there is popularly believed to be an ideal "Balanchine" body type for women, with the jobs going to tall, slender women with long necks, long legs and short torsos. The problem of eating disorders has created a minor industry of nutritionists and therapists specializing in dancers' emotional and physical problems. Despite increasingly sophisticated methods, however, eating disorders in ballet remain extremely difficult to treat.

At a news conference in Boston, company officials said that in 1995, Ms. Guenther, then a member of the Boston Ballet's junior ensemble, had been encouraged by Anna-Marie Holmes, now the company's director, to lose five pounds. She lost the weight over a summer break and was then told not to lose more weight, they said.

Ms. Guenther was promoted to the senior company in September 1996. Some two months later, she again began to lose weight, and she was told to "be careful not to get too thin," company officials said. A spokeswoman for Ms. Guenther's family said that she had planned to relax and gain weight in the summer. At her death, she weighed about 100 pounds, which is low but normal for a ballet dancer of Ms. Guenther's height, 5'3".

"She was smiley, bubbly," Bruce Marks, director emeritus of Boston Ballet, said. "That didn't change. She was full of beans, full of life." But there was recognition that she might be having problems, he said, at a traditionally difficult time when young dancers make the jump into a major company.

Eating disorders range from anorexia nervosa (deliberate self-starvation) and bulimia (recurring binge eating and self-induced vomiting) to "disordered eating," a term coined by the women's task force of the American College of Sports Medicine for any chronic restrictive and ritualistic compulsive eating problems. Men are not immune to eating disorders. But they are much more prevalent in women, in part because society and the world of ballet place a higher value on women's looks.

"The problem is much more common in middle- and upper-class women, particularly white women and young women under 25," Dr. Warren said.

"Dance is one of the worst areas. The average incidence of eating disorders in the white middle-class population is 1 in 100. In classical ballet, it is 1 in 5."

Most are female students and the youngest female professionals, particularly those with less physical facility and less-than-perfect bodies. Older women tend to suffer from less serious eating problems, like yo-yo dieting and the age-old dancers' regimen of diet soda and cigarettes, which affect about 46 percent of professional ballet dancers, according to Dr. Hamilton.

Men tend to start their dance training later. With fewer in the field, they experience less competition. And a part of their work, partnering, requires solid muscles and strength.

Women begin their ballet training at around age 7, and the crucial point in that training, when they are judged to have the talent and perseverance to become a professional, generally occurs during the already troubled years of puberty. Dancers are reluctant to talk about the problem, the older ones dismissing it as no longer so serious in an era when more information is available about nutrition for dancers.

Ms. Guenther's case may be an isolated incident. But the pressured world of ballet encourages driven personalities, offering a life that is largely confined to the studio and its mirrored reflections, a life that is determined by the orders of authority figures like teachers, choreographers and company directors.

"People attracted to dance may be looking for that kind of structure," said Marijeanne Liederbach, director of research and education at the Harkness Center for Dance Injuries in Manhattan. "Achieving a triple pirouette or 105 on the scale are tangible goals in a difficult world."

Dancers who negotiate the psychological and physical pressures of ballet training and of performing in some companies tend to be eager to please, she said, and may believe they are disciplined and passionate enough about their art to be able to disregard their need for food. What makes the problem even more serious for women is that physiologically, as reproductive mammals, their bodies fight to preserve a minimum amount of body fat.

Women dancers must also deal with the reality or perception of the ideal ballet body. In that respect, the pendulum seems to be swinging back toward greater diversity.

"If people can convince me they can move and they can dance, I hire them," said Heinz Poll, director of the Ohio Ballet. One outstanding ballerina in the company had "the most unballetic body in the world," Mr. Poll recalled. "Everything about her was wrong. But the moment she lit up dancing, you forgot that. It was very simple." But Dr. Hamilton pointed out that dancers often get eliminated in auditions before they dance a step because their bodies are not what the director is looking for.

Thinness was not always prized in ballet. Louise Fitzjames, a French ballerina of the mid-19th century, was depicted in a famous caricature as a dancing asparagus in a "Ballet of the Vegetables" and was described by one French critic as "having no body at all" and being "as skinny as a lizard or a silkworm." A century later, Edward M. M. Warburg, who helped found a precursor to City Ballet, teasingly described George Balanchine's first ballerinas as "field hockey girls."

Balanchine is credited with, or accused of, creating the concept of the ideal ballet body. Gelsey Kirkland has written that as a troubled young dancer at City Ballet in the late 1960s, she was told by Balanchine that he wanted to "see the bones."

Though the type has been predominant in City Ballet, there has always been physical variety in the company. "I like mountains, I like valleys," Balanchine commented when someone complained to him about the ridiculous look of a line of swans with the very tall, voluptuous Gloria Govrin at one end and the tiny Suki Schorer at the other.

Dr. Hamilton, the specialist in dancers' eating disorders, performed with City Ballet from 1969 to 1988. "Balanchine was interested in tall, thin women who looked like models when I was there," she said. "And a lot of his dancers run companies today." But dance, she said, has gone along with societal pressures to look a certain way.

Peter Martins, director of City Ballet, said that the company "does not currently, nor has it ever, required a specific body type, but rather engages its dancers based on their ability." He described today's dancers as "fundamentally very responsible about their own health."

Spokesmen for the major ballet troupes in New York City said that they offered informal, confidential help to dancers with problems. Dr. Hamilton writes regularly in *Dance Magazine* about these and other issues, though most of her mail is about eating problems. Workshops on nutrition and health are conducted regularly in the major ballet schools. "But do you think they listen?" asked Edith d'Addario, director of the Joffrey school. "They sit there eating yogurt all day."

Even the gentlest and most private intervention can backfire. "You need to take charge without pushing them off the deep end," said Laveen Naidu, a former member of Dance Theater of Harlem and a long-time teacher at its school. "Yes, this is a visual art form with certain esthetics. We have to fit in. But everyone is different. We tell the students that they don't have to look like someone else. But it's 'mirror, mirror,' all the time."

A student who seems to be losing too much weight is questioned quietly about what she is eating, he said. "But you may in fact be unintentionally doing more damage. The most important thing is to know when to turn it over to a professional."

Ultimately, Dr. Warren suggested, parents must face the fact that their daughters may not have a chance at becoming ballet professionals. Parents must watch for signs of potential eating disorders, among them recurrent problems with weight, menstruation and stress fractures of the bones. "The key thing is to catch them before they get into a situation where they have such a distorted view of their bodies that they don't realize they are skinny," she said.

"If the individual goes through puberty and has a lot of problems with her weight, it is very unlikely she is going to make it as a dancer. People have to realize that the child is not going to make it if they are not thin. Mothers must start thinking twice. Is it worth the risk?"

[JD, July 1997]

## Efforts to Fight Eating Disorders May Backfire

What better way to prevent eating disorders among young women in college than to let them hear firsthand the harrowing tales of others who have had those conditions? It is an approach used on many campuses in this country.

But one such program, designed by students at Stanford University, turned out to be a case of good intentions gone awry, researchers have found. It did not prevent eating disorders, and may have even made them worse. Because the program was similar to those offered at many colleges and universities, the researchers have recommended that all those plans be evaluated to determine whether they should be continued.

Eating disorders have become more common in the United States and other developed countries in the last 30 years. Ten percent of American college stu-

dents are affected, more than 90 percent of them women. The reason for the increase is not known, though social pressures to be thin are assumed to play a role. The disorders are most likely to follow efforts to diet, and teenage girls who are slightly overweight have the highest risk.

Some become binge eaters, wolfing down huge amounts of food and becoming overweight. Others develop bulimia, bingeing and then "purging" with laxatives, vomiting or using other drastic actions to lose weight. Those with a rarer disorder, anorexia nervosa, shun food in a compulsive drive to lose weight, becoming emaciated but nonetheless thinking they look fat. Treatment for anorexia, consisting of psychotherapy and sometimes antidepressant drugs, works for only about a quarter of patients. In 10 to 18 percent of cases, the disorder is fatal.

The analysis of the program at Stanford, published in the May 1997 issue of the journal *Health Psychology*, began in 1993 when Dr. Traci Mann, the lead author of the study, observed two undergraduates making a presentation about eating disorders to a psychology class. The two young women, one recovered from anorexia and the other from bulimia, were members of a student group called Body Image, Food and Self-Esteem. The group was independent of the university administration, which offered counseling and treatment for eating disorders, but no prevention programs. The students provided objective information about eating disorders and also talked about their own experiences.

As Dr. Mann watched, several things struck her. The two students were slim, attractive, poised and healthy looking, the kind of young women that others might admire and even try to emulate. It also seemed to Dr. Mann that the reality of eating disorders was harsher than these students let on. "My college roommate had been bulimic," she recalled, "and the most salient thing to me was that she was suffering. She suffered all the time."

But Dr. Mann did not think the Stanford students communicated that, or made it clear that people with eating disorders had lost control. "They made it look too easy, as if you could get anorexia, get over it and then be thin and a leader like them," she said. "The presentation separated the behavior from its mental illness aspect."

Dr. Mann decided to study the program. She had 597 female students fill out a questionnaire about their eating and dieting habits and behaviors related to eating disorders. Next, she randomly divided the group and invited only half to hear the students' 90-minute presentation. Then, four and twelve weeks later, she asked both those who had heard the presentation and those who had not to answer the survey again.

On the first questionnaire, 20 percent of the students reported binge-eating, and 21 percent reported fasting. Three percent had induced vomiting to lose weight, and 2 percent had used laxatives. When she compared the responses on the later questionnaires of those who had attended the presentation with those who had not, she found that hearing the information did not lower the rate of abnormal behaviors.

In fact, it was associated with a small increase in some of them in the second questionnaire, which then disappeared by the third one.

Dr. Mann offered several explanations for the failure of the program. First, the attractiveness of the speakers might have sent out a different message from the one they were trying to present. "Some people might want to be like them for the wrong reason," she said.

In addition, because the presentation was directed to both healthy women and those who already had eating disorders, it might have reached neither. The messages for those two groups should be different, Dr. Mann said. For instance, healthy women should be warned that eating disorders are chronic and hard to treat and are considered a form of mental illness. But women who already have symptoms may feel so stigmatized by such dire pronouncements that they might avoid treatment. They may be more likely to seek help if the disorders are described less harshly.

Dr. Katherine Halmi, director of the Eating Disorders Program at Cornell Medical Center in White Plains, New York, said Dr. Mann's findings matched those of other researchers. "The evidence is there that merely going into classrooms and having groups and giving information and having recovered people come and talk is not going to be effective," she said. "We ought to stop pouring money into it. We need to think of other strategies."

Dr. C. Barr Taylor, a professor of psychiatry at Stanford who was not involved with Dr. Mann's study, has also studied programs aimed at preventing eating disorders in college students as well as sixth- and seventh-grade girls. Although he questioned Dr. Mann's conclusion that her data showed a harmful effect from the program, he agreed that one-shot presentations by recovered patients did not help and might be detrimental.

"The kids may identify with those peers in exactly the way you don't want," Dr. Taylor said. But he added that long-term education programs could help by changing girls' attitudes about weight. The benefits, though, are not large, he cautioned.

"We have not solved the problem of preventing eating disorders," Dr. Taylor said.

[DG, May 1997]

# Girls and Puberty: the Crisis Years

The teenage years have never been easy. They can be especially difficult for girls, who experience hormonal influences that wreck their prepubescent physical equality with boys, cause radical changes in body shape and weight and sometimes touch off emotional and reproductive upheavals. But for many reasons, the challenges facing adolescent girls have never been greater than they are today. An unprecedented number of girls fall from the grace of childhood innocence to discover cigarettes, drugs, alcohol, depression, eating disorders and unwanted pregnancies.

Several studies, including a survey of 2,400 girls and 600 boys 9 through 15 years old, conducted by the American Association of University Women in 1991, and an even larger survey in 1997 by the Commonwealth Fund among 3,586 girls and 3,162 boys in grades 5 through 12, have documented that more often than not, young girls entering puberty experience a crisis in confidence that renders them vulnerable to risky health behaviors that they may not have the strength or will to resist.

Dr. Emily Hancock, a psychologist in Berkeley, California, and author of *The Girl Within*, said the various studies and her own interviews with dozens of high school girls and college women had revealed that self-esteem in girls peaked at the age of 9, then began to plummet.

She found that girls gradually lost their prepubescent "strength, independence, spirit and lucidity and become riveted to the issue of how they look." They begin to think they cannot measure up to the competition, especially the stereotypical waiflike image of the ideal American woman with a tiny waistline.

"They look great—the facade is really wonderful—but the foundation is very shaky and many fall into depression, eating disorders and drug abuse," Dr. Hancock said in an interview. At one Ivy League university, she found that "the girls compete with each other about wearing size 2 or size 4 pants, and 50 percent have eating disorders."

The Commonwealth Fund survey revealed that by high school age, only 39 percent of girls were highly self-confident and that older girls had less self-esteem than the younger ones. "In contrast," the fund reported, "older boys were more likely to be highly self-confident than younger boys, with more than half of all boys in high school indicating high self-confidence." Not surprisingly, the survey revealed, "girls were particularly likely to be critical of themselves, and one-quarter of older girls reported that they did not like or hated themselves. In contrast, only 14 percent of boys said they felt this way."

Hand in hand with a loss of self-esteem in girls comes depression. The fund reported, "An alarming 29 percent of girls reported suicidal thoughts, 27 percent said they were sad 'many times' or 'all the time,' and one-third of older girls said they felt like crying 'many days' or 'every day.' Yet few who reported symptoms of depression had consulted a mental health professional, and many said they had no one to turn to when they felt depressed or stressed. Instead, the girls often turned to cigarettes, alcohol and drugs for relief.

Cigarette smoking among teenagers is once again on the rise, particularly among girls, despite overwhelming evidence that smoking can cause their skin to wrinkle prematurely, impair their breathing capacity and ruin their health, not to mention making them smell like an ashtray. In the new survey, 14 percent of high school girls said they smoked between several cigarettes to a pack or more a week. Two-thirds of the smokers said they used cigarettes to relieve stress; half said they were influenced by other smokers.

Drinking by young girls also now rivals that by boys. In the new survey, 15 percent of teenage girls reported drinking alcohol weekly or monthly and 20 percent said they had used an illegal drug in the past month. All told, 39 percent of girls in grades 5 through 12 reported either smoking, drinking or using drugs in the past month.

Sex for many teenagers has become almost a rite of passage, often devoid of caring, romance and pleasure. More than two-thirds of high school seniors have had sexual intercourse, and each year there are almost one million teenage pregnancies, 85 percent unplanned.

The Commonwealth Fund survey also found "a disturbingly high incidence of violence, with 18 percent of girls in grades 5 through 12 reporting some form of physical or sexual abuse," more than half of which was perpetrated by a family member. Such abuse, the survey showed, frequently leads teenage girls into risky health behaviors, with those reporting abuse being twice as likely to drink alcohol, smoke cigarettes or use drugs and three times as likely to have eating disorders as girls who did not report abuse.

A frequent trigger of eating disorders is repeated dieting. It starts frighteningly early. Many 9-year-olds report that they are dieting to lose weight. Up to 25 percent of adolescents—90 percent of them girls—regularly purge themselves to control their weight. In the Commonwealth Fund survey, nearly one girl in five in the ninth grade admitted to having binged and purged, and the incidence of bulimia was twice that among high school seniors.

In her new book *The Body Project*, Dr. Joan Jacobs Brumberg, a professor of women's studies at Cornell University, wrote, "Girls today make the body into an all-consuming project." This emphasis on the body, she and others maintain, has shifted the focus of adolescent girls from developing their interests and talents, internal character and contributions to society to fretting over their shape and appearance—their weight, hair, clothes and makeup. And Dr. Sharlene Hesse-Biber, an associate professor of sociology at Boston College and author of *Am I Thin Enough Yet?* pointed out, "Binding self-esteem so closely to weight and physical appearance may set the stage for psychologically damaging cycles of weight gain and self-hatred."

Dr. Brumberg noted that adolescent girls now faced a new tyranny: the "lean, taut, female body with visible musculature." She wrote, "Our national infatuation with 'hard bodies,' combined with the idea that bodies are perfectible, heightens the pressure on adolescents and complicates the business of adjusting to a new, sexually mature body. The fitness craze can aggravate adolescent self-consciousness and make girls desperately unhappy—if not neurotic—about their own bodies."

[JEB, November 1997]

## Yesterday's Precocious Puberty Is Norm Today

A friend who runs the child care program at a Brooklyn high school reports that one of the newly enrolled mothers, a freshman, is 13. Her baby's father is 14. While children having children is not a new phenomenon, the ever-dropping age of puberty is.

Many parents become worried when their 7- or 8-year-old daughters begin to develop breasts or grow pubic hair. They wonder, is this normal? Will the surge of sex hormones adversely affect the girls' behavior, moods or physical growth? Can girls who are still emotionally and socially immature adjust well to early physical maturation? And when should more explicit sex education and cautions about birth control begin?

In 1997, Dr. Marcia E. Herman-Giddens and colleagues described the results of physical examinations of 17,077 American girls, which revealed that white girls were showing bodily signs of sexual maturity an average of one year earlier than previous studies had indicated, and black girls two years earlier.

The findings, she and others suggest, should prompt a redefinition of the ages at which puberty is considered precocious. Current medical textbooks state that just 1 percent of girls younger than 8 show signs of puberty. In a review in the October 4, 1999 issue of the journal *Pediatrics*, Dr. Paul B. Kaplowitz, Dr. Sharon E. Oberfield and members of the Lawson Wilkins Pediatric Endocrine Society, concluded that "the onset of breast development between 7 and 8 years of age in white girls and between 6 and 8 years in African-American girls may be part of the normal broad variation in the timing of puberty and not, in most cases, a pathological state."

Breast development is stimulated by estrogen, which is released from the ovaries upon a hormonal signal from the pituitary gland. The growth of pubic hair, however, is a result of stimulation by androgen, the so-called male sex hormone, also produced by the ovaries.

There has been much speculation about why earlier maturation may be occurring in girls, especially because there has been no apparent advance (and no racial difference) in the onset of puberty in boys. For girls, better nutrition over all and fewer infectious diseases no doubt play a role, because these trends result in more consistent growth. The increase in childhood obesity may also be a factor, because fatty tissue is a source of the sex hormone estrogen. Another suggested possibility is increased exposure to certain plastics and insecticides that degrade into substances that have estrogenlike effects.

But whatever the reasons, the phenomenon is real and, to many parents, worrisome. The report by Dr. Kaplowitz of the Medical College of Virginia and Virginia Commonwealth University, Dr. Oberfield of Columbia University College of Physicians and Surgeons and members of the endocrine society should prove reassuring.

A common concern involves the ability of girls as young as 7 or 8 to cope with menstruation. Dr. Kaplowitz and his colleagues point out that a 7-year-old who is developing breasts will not undergo the start of menstrual cycles, or menarche, for another two years. That time gap should give par-

ents and pediatricians enough time to prepare. Also, once a girl starts menstruating, she is potentially able to become pregnant and needs explicit sex education.

But the main concern for pediatricians and for some parents is the effect that hormones might have on the child's growth. Estrogen is known to cause the growth plates in long bones to close, which can slow or shut down growth.

Here, the new evidence is most reassuring. Dr. Kaplowitz and his co-authors point out that "the younger the age at onset of puberty, the longer the duration of puberty," meaning that the adolescent growth spurt occurs for a longer time in early-maturing girls. This in part offsets the loss of adult height that might occur when the skeleton matures earlier. Indeed, girls who undergo early menarche tend to grow somewhat more than girls whose menarche occurs later. The end result is little if any difference in adult height.

Who should undergo evaluation for early puberty? The authors recommend that white girls younger than 7 and black girls younger than 6 who show breast or pubic hair development should be examined to be sure they have no disorder that involves an excess production of hormones that could distort their development. Girls who have any of the following conditions should be fully evaluated:

▶ An unusually rapid progression of puberty that would cause rapid skeletal maturation and a predicted height four inches less than their genes might dictate or less than 4'11".
▶ The presence of any newly developed problem involving the central nervous system, including headaches, seizures or neurological deficits.
▶ Behaviors suggesting that the girl's emotional state, or the family's emotional state, is being adversely affected by the progression of puberty.

[JEB, November 1999]

# Parents Can Bolster Girls' Fragile Self-Esteem

Although opportunities for girls and young women to develop to their fullest potential as human beings have never been greater than they are today in the United States, several studies in recent years have documented that far more girls than boys founder en route.

Girls are more likely than boys to experience a crisis in self-confidence as they enter puberty. Too many girls turn their attention from what they can do to what they look like and seek to bolster their egos and counter their uncertainties by smoking, drinking, using drugs and getting pregnant.

Schools and society—especially the mass media—have received most of the blame for the decline in self-esteem and rise in health-damaging behaviors among teenage girls, and to be sure, schools and the media play an important role in undermining girls' self-confidence and ambitions and focusing their attention on superficial issues like makeup, hairstyles, clothing and weight.

But there is also reason to believe that a very large part of the problem starts in the home, sometimes even before a girl is born. It starts with parents who wish for a boy, as some prospective parents do. A girl born to such parents has one strike against her.

Parents play the largest and most important role in shaping their children's sense of themselves and supporting them through the barrage of cultural and peer pressures that do so much to distract them from what is truly important: the kinds of people they are and the contributions they can make to family, friends and the world.

Too many parents think they fulfill their parental responsibilities by supplying children with material objects, from crib toys to computers to automobiles. Too many parents put their own needs and pleasures above those of their children, and the children end up shortchanged emotionally, nutritionally and physically. Parents sometimes forget that children never asked to be born, and that once they are born it is the parents' responsibility to love and nurture them and help them grow up healthy and strong, mentally and physically, within their biological limits.

Every girl—every child—needs and deserves to be held, cuddled, kissed and told repeatedly that she is loved and valued. Every girl needs and deserves parental attention to her developmental progress. She should be read to and played with, encouraged to test her mettle against ever more challenging tasks and praised for her efforts, not just her successes.

Short of being protected from physical harm, she should never be discouraged from trying to do something that might be mentally or physically beyond her, whether it is climbing a tree, doing a puzzle or building something fantastic with toys or tools.

To develop a healthy ego, every child, boy or girl, must have a sense of autonomy. Children need the right to make decisions for themselves and the opportunity to learn from their mistakes. The parents' job is to make sure the child considers all the relevant facts before plunging ahead. Dr. Sharlene Hesse-Biber in her book *Am I Thin Enough Yet?*, quotes an unhappy woman named Anna: "I was raised by a domineering mother and also a strong father who didn't give me very much personal space to develop, so I was really used to being told what to do. I learned from a very young age to surrender myself to other people's will, desire, and wants—to really set myself aside."

Parents should encourage girls to pursue their dream, whether it is to become a large-animal veterinarian, corporate executive, astronaut, architect or baseball player. Girls should no longer be channeled into safe, feminine professions, unless that is their dream. When at age 4 I told my father I wanted to be a veterinarian, he didn't say girls don't become veterinarians (which was true in 1945). He said, "Cornell has a College of Veterinary Medicine." And I grew up thinking I would go to Cornell and become a vet.

Girls should be encouraged to pursue all manner

of activities, physical and otherwise. It was my father who taught me to swim at age 3 and roller-skate at 4, who took me bicycle riding and hiking, who bought me an Erector set and a chemistry set and who supported my interest in nature and baseball. Girls, like boys, need physical outlets to release their pent-up energies and help dissipate their emotional turmoils.

And all children need adult attention to their nutritional well-being. Children reared on take-out and fast food by parents who are "too busy" to cook nutritious meals are not likely to develop respect for the kind of fuel they put in their bodies when parents are not looking.

Girls with shaky egos who despise their bodies or suffer from eating disorders often report that their parents, usually the father, frequently commented on their appearance. As a woman named Donna, who suffered lasting harm to her self-esteem, told Dr. Hesse-Biber: "My dad used to call me fat. I wouldn't have noticed on my own. It was hard for me, growing up, being a fat kid. Dad hated it. He wanted me to be thin."

A college woman named Jane told Dr. Hesse-Biber: "My parents were always complimenting me on how I looked. It was such a big deal. I remember my father would say 'you look good, you lost weight.'"

Although there may be little a girl can do to change her parents' behavior, Dr. Mary Pipher, author of *Reviving Ophelia: Saving the Selves of Adolescent Girls*, has suggested a number of things girls can do for themselves. She urges girls to stop talking about weight and appearance, their own or that of others, and cautions against teasing other girls about how they look or dress or do their hair or makeup.

Dr. Pipher suggests that girls concentrate on goals that they can control—how they spend their time and with whom—and focus on developing their own interests and talents. If their friends continue to dwell on superficial concerns, Dr. Pipher suggests changing friends to ones they can respect. She also suggests making friends with older people to gain different perspectives on life and events. Further perspectives, as well as an enhanced sense of self-worth, can be gained from doing volunteer work, for example, helping to improve a local park or aiding people who are elderly or handicapped.

Finally, Dr. Pipher suggests avoiding magazines, films and television shows that emphasize looks over behavior. The most effective way to change the cultural norm that now promotes sylph-like bodies is to boycott the vehicles that promote it. I applaud whoever wrote the scene in the movie *In and Out* in which a super-thin supermodel is told by her boyfriend (played by Matt Dillon): "Go get something to eat. You look like a swizzle stick!"

[JEB, November 1997]

## Emotional Ills Tied to Stunted Growth in Girls

Adding to the accumulation of evidence of a connection between the mind and physical health, a large study has found a link between emotional problems in girls and stunted growth. The study, published in a June 1996 issue of *Pediatrics*, found that adolescent and pre-adolescent girls who were overly anxious grew up to be roughly one to two inches shorter, on average, than other girls.

The association was not found for boys, possibly because emotional disorders are less common and more transient for them, the researchers said. But the finding about girls builds on previous research that showed that children and adults of both sexes with anxiety or depression have lower-than-normal amounts of growth hormone, the chemical that stimulates the growth of muscle and bone in children and teenagers.

The height difference found in the study is less important than what it implies about the power of the mind over the body, said the lead author, Dr. Daniel S. Pine, a child psychiatrist at the New York State

Psychiatric Institute and Columbia University in New York.

"Our study raises the question: What are the many biological things that are going on in children with anxiety?" he said. "What are the many ways, besides stature, that anxiety affects children?"

Dr. Martin T. Stein, chairman of the American Academy of Pediatrics committee on psychosocial health, said: "This article is fascinating because of the connection it shows between emotional disorders and the neuroendocrine systems. We know that growth hormone release is controlled by the brain, so it's understandable that it would be influenced by emotional disorders."

The findings were but one aspect of a large study that has documented the rates of psychiatric problems among children and identified the medical and social problems associated with them. The study focused on 716 children, approximately half boys and half girls, who were randomly selected from two counties in upstate New York. For nine years, from adolescence or pre-adolescence until adulthood, participants were assessed for symptoms of depression as well as two anxiety disorders. One was separation anxiety, characterized by excessive uneasiness about leaving home, even to go to school or sleep overnight at a friend's house. The other was overanxious disorder, defined as pervasive worrying about things like appearance or academic performance.

The researchers found that anxiety in particular was relatively common, with 226 of the girls and 149 of the boys initially showing some symptoms of overanxious disorder, and 168 of the girls and 124 of the boys initially having signs of separation anxiety.

But nine years later, anxiety was associated with shorter adult stature only for the girls. After taking into account various factors known to influence adult height, like socioeconomic status, the researchers found that the girls who had had anxiety at any point in the study were shorter than those who had been emotionally healthy throughout.

The older the children were when a diagnosis was made, the stronger its influence was on stature, the researchers found. The strongest association was seen in girls who were 11 to 20 when separation anxiety was diagnosed; they were 1.7 inches shorter than the girls in whom no emotional problems had been found. Girls who had been depressed also turned out to be shorter than other girls, but the effect was marginal, Dr. Pine said.

The researchers offer several possible explanations for why the mind-body link was not found in the boys in the study. For one thing, depression and anxiety disorders are relatively rare in boys after puberty, the period when the connection with height appears to be most significant.

"Before puberty the rate of depression among boys and girls is roughly equal, but after puberty it's twice as common among girls," Dr. Pine said. "The findings on anxiety are less clear, but it looks like girls who are anxious are anxious longer than boys."

[SG, June 1996]

## Study Finds TV Alters Fiji Girls' View of Body

"You've gained weight" is a traditional compliment in Fiji, anthropologists say. In accordance with traditional culture in the South Pacific nation, dinner guests are expected to eat as much as possible. A robust, nicely rounded body is the norm for men and women. "Skinny legs" is a major insult. And "going thin," the Fijian term for losing a noticeable amount of weight, is considered a worrisome condition.

But all that may be changing, now that Heather Locklear has arrived. Just a few years after the introduction of television to a province of Fiji's main island, Viti Levu, eating disorders—once virtually unheard of there—are on the rise among girls, according to a study presented at the American Psychiatric Association meeting in Washington. Young girls dream of looking not like their mothers and aunts, but like the slender stars of *Melrose Place* and *Beverly Hills 90210.*

"I'm very heavy," one Fijian adolescent lamented during an interview with researchers led by Dr. Anne E. Becker, director of research at the Harvard Eating Disorders Center of Harvard Medical School, who investigated shifts in body image and eating practices in Fiji over a three-year period. The Fijian girl said her friends also tell her that she is too fat, "and sometimes I'm depressed because I always want to lose weight."

Epidemiological studies have shown that eating disorders are more prevalent in industrialized coun tries, suggesting that cultural factors play a role. But few studies have examined the effects of long-term cultural shifts on disordered eating in traditional societies.

Dr. Becker and her colleagues surveyed 63 Fijian secondary school girls, whose average age was 17. The work began in 1995, one month after satellites began beaming television signals to the region. In 1998, the researchers surveyed another group of 65 girls from the same schools, who were matched in age, weight and other characteristics with the subjects in the earlier group. Fifteen percent in the 1998 survey reported that they had induced vomiting to control their weight, the researchers said, compared with 3 percent in the 1995 survey. And 29 percent scored highly on a test of eating-disorder risk, compared with 13 percent three years before.

Girls who said they watched television three or more nights a week in the 1998 survey were 50 percent more likely to describe themselves as "too big or fat" and 30 percent more likely to diet than girls who watched television less frequently. Before 1995, Dr. Becker said, there was little talk of dieting in Fiji. "The idea of calories was very foreign to them." But in the 1998 survey, 69 percent said that at some time they had been on a diet. In fact, preliminary data suggest more teenage girls in Fiji diet than their American counterparts.

The results of the study have not been published, but were reviewed by the psychiatric association's scientific program committee before being accepted for presentation at the meetings.

Several of the students told Dr. Becker and her colleagues that they wanted to look like the Western women they saw on television shows like *Beverly Hills 90210.* One girl said that her friends "change their mood, their hairstyles, so that they can be like those characters. So in order to be like them, I have to work on myself, exercising and my eating habits should change," she said.

But Dr. Marshall Sahlins, Charles F. Grey professor emeritus of Anthropology at the University of Chicago, said that he doubts that television was the only factor in the changes. "I think that television is a kind of metaphor of something more profound," he said. In contrast to the solitary couch-potato viewing style displayed by many Americans, watching television is a communal activity in Fiji, Dr. Becker said. Fijians often gather in households with television sets, and sit together, drinking kava and talking about their day's activities, with the TV on in the background. "What we noticed in 1995 is that people had a sort of curiosity, but it was a dismissive curiosity," Dr. Becker said. "But over the years they have come to accept it as a form of entertainment."

Fiji residents have access to only one television channel, she said, which broadcasts a selection of programs from the United States, Britain and Australia. Among the most popular are *Seinfeld, Melrose Place,* which features Ms. Locklear, *E.R., Xena, Warrior Princess,* and *Beverly Hills 90210.*

Dr. Becker said that the increase in eating disorders like bulimia may be a signal that the culture is changing so quickly that Fijians are having difficulty keeping up. Island teenagers, she said, "are acutely aware that the traditional culture doesn't equip them well to negotiate the kinds of conflicts" presented by a 1990s global economy. In other Pacific societies, Dr. Becker said, similar cultural shifts have been accompanied by an increase in psychological problems among adolescents. Researchers speculated, for example, that rapid social change played a role in a rash of adolescent suicides in Micronesia in the 1980s.

[EG, May 1999]

# In Quest for the Perfect Look,
# More Girls Choose the Scalpel

Standing in front of the full-length mirror, the girl fights back tears. Her thighs are too big, her breasts too small and her nose bumpy. Or so this 16-year-old thinks, comparing herself with *Baywatch* babes and Victoria's Secret models.

To make matters worse, boys never call, and getting undressed for gym is a mortification. But such problems have quick fixes, the magazine ads promise.

"If I can look better, why not?" the girl asked during a recent consultation with a plastic surgeon. Her parents are living proof, she said, since her mother was rejuvenated by a face lift and her father's brow was smoothed of its furrows. The doctor was not persuaded. He said later that he had stalled by scheduling another appointment, and that he hoped the family did not look elsewhere in the meantime.

The girl's 40-something parents are part of a tide of baby boomers who are being tucked, peeled and augmented as never before. But it is the teenage girls now flocking to the suites of plastic surgeons from Park Avenue to Beverly Hills who pose an ethical problem for doctors, who must decide whether to operate on patients who are too young to vote, but old enough to feel social pressures to be physically perfect.

"We are capable of doing awful things to these kids," said Dr. Mark Sultan, chief of plastic surgery at Beth Israel Medical Center and one of two dozen doctors who said they were seeing more teenagers than ever before who are eager to change their looks and willing to go through often painful surgery to do so.

The surgeon's task, Dr. Sultan and others said, is to weed out youngsters with true deformities from those responding to media messages and peer or parental pressure. "We have to decide what is real, what is imagined and what is exaggerated," he said.

Although a relatively small number of young people have had plastic surgery, the numbers are growing, and many more who approach doctors are turned away. At least 14,000 adolescents nationwide had such procedures in 1996, a slight increase from 1992, when the boom began, according to data from the American Society of Plastic and Reconstructive Surgeons. In all age groups, 700,000 procedures were done in 1997, up 70 percent in four years.

But professionals agree that those numbers are a vast understatement, perhaps by as much as half, since they do not include the many procedures now done by dermatologists, ophthalmologists, ear, nose and throat specialists, dentists and others.

And the makeovers of choice are changing for teenagers. A generation ago, it was not unusual for youngsters to have their noses straightened or ears pinned back, procedures that doctors say are appropriate for those with ungainly features. But these days, more controversial procedures, like breast augmentation, liposuction and tummy tucks, are gaining popularity in this impressionable age group. In the New York area, these procedures, among two dozen available, range in cost from $2,000 for liposuction to $5,000 for a tummy tuck.

Nationwide in 1992, there were 5,519 nose jobs among teenagers, 3,024 ear operations, 978 breast implants, 472 liposuctions and no tummy tucks. Four years later, nose jobs were down to 4,313 and ear pinnings to 2,470. But breast augmentations were up to 1,172, liposuctions increased to 788 and tummy tucks to 130.

Stalling is a popular tactic among doctors, who count on the fact that teenagers are by definition mercurial. Dr. Christopher Nanni, for one, set out to dissuade an overweight girl from Bay Ridge, Brooklyn, who came to him recently after many failed attempts at diet and exercise. She was 16 years old, 5'3" tall and weighed 185 pounds. Her mother, divorced and struggling on a secretary's salary, was not enthusiastic about either the costs or risks of liposuction.

Dr. Nanni put the girl on a sensible diet and encouraged her mother to buy her a treadmill. Come back in a year or two, he told them. If liposuction seemed appropriate then, he would do the procedure, at a big discount. "I was kind of disappointed, but it made sense," the girl said grudgingly, still preferring the quick fix to the ordeal of losing weight.

Her mother was thrilled. "As a parent you want your children to be happy, so I went along with it," she said, describing her daughter's misery each time they went shopping or attended a big family gathering. But when Dr. Nanni resisted, she was relieved. "I respect him immensely for not just taking my money," she said.

The availability of new procedures can be a relief to adolescents overwhelmed by an otherwise intractable physical disfigurement. One New Jersey teenager, 5'4" tall and weighing 220 pounds, doggedly set out to lose 100 pounds, succeeded, and kept the weight off for more than a year. Left behind, however, was an apron of excess skin that brought her to the office of Dr. Gerald H. Pitman, who had never before treated a girl so young.

Impressed by the girl's resolve and her mother's silence during their first meeting, signals that the child was mature and self-motivated, Dr. Pitman agreed to operate. When the girl was between the ages of 15 and 18, Dr. Pitman did a series of surgeries on her abdomen, thighs, upper arms and breasts.

"Not only did he make me look beautiful, he made me feel beautiful," said the girl, who once wore men's size 38 jeans and is now a sleek women's size 6. Like most of the youngsters interviewed, she spoke on the condition, set by her parents, that she not be identified.

The New Jersey girl, who is now 19, rarely looks at photographs from the time when she had fat rippling from her knees. But she still recalls being "tortured" by classmates, who called her names and shunned her during games of spin the bottle. "Who would want to be with a fat disgusting girl who can't get out of her own way?" she said now, her hair pulled back to reveal fine cheekbones.

All the doctors interviewed spoke of the need to distinguish a child's wishes from a parent's, which often requires chasing the adult from the examining room during the initial meeting. Dr. James L. Baker,

a surgeon in a suburb of Orlando, Florida, the state that is second to California in the number of plastic surgery procedures done each year, described one such consultation recently. The mother announced that her daughter was miserable about her nose. The girl sat silent, staring at the floor.

"Why don't you like your nose?" the doctor asked the child.

"My mother thinks it's too big."

"Then why don't we do your mother's nose?"

He rejected the case.

In extreme situations, doctors say, a child abuse complaint is filed against a parent who insists on a needless operation, since no surgery is without medical risk.

---

**A CLOSER LOOK**

## Teenage Surgery

Most adolescent cosmetic operations are still nose jobs, but other procedures are increasing.

| COSMETIC PROCEDURES PERFORMED ON PEOPLE 18 AND YOUNGER* | 1992 | 1996 |
|---|---|---|
| **Breast augmentation** | 978 | 1,172 |
| **Collagen injection** | 0 | 135 |
| **Eyelid surgery** | 0 | 267 |
| **Liposuction** | 472 | 788 |
| **Nose reshaping** | 5,519 | 4,313 |
| **Tummy tuck** | 0 | 130 |

*By plastic and reconstructive surgeons. But other specialists, including dermatologists and dentists, are also legally permitted to perform cosmetic surgery.

*Source: American Society of Plastic and Reconstructive Surgeons*

The general surge in cosmetic surgery has its roots in demographics, medical technology and health care economics. As baby boomers of financial means hit 50, they are doing anything and everything to arrest the ravages of age. Meanwhile, new procedures are invented and old ones become safer and less stigmatized. And plastic surgeons, doing elective procedures not covered by insurance, are aggressively marketing themselves with slogans like: "No Ifs, Ands or Butts: You Can Change Your Bottom Line in Hours."

"This is a huge problem for the public," said Dr. Jane Petro, a Westchester plastic surgeon. "There is enormous pressure to do things the patient isn't going to be helped by, because someone shows up with a check."

Consultation with a teenage patient is a distinct art. It generally involves repeat visits, over several months, to mitigate impulsiveness. The negatives—for example, scarring and loss of sensation after breast enlargement—are stressed. Sometimes, meetings with a therapist are required, especially when an eating disorder is suspected.

The doctors say they look for red flags in body language. Does the child smile? Interact easily with the mother? Cringe after disrobing? Does the patient's perception of the defect match the evidence in the mirror? Has the youngster, or the parent, had repeated plastic surgeries? "They have to be able to tell me what they don't like," Dr. Baker said. "And if the answer is, 'I'm just ugly,' that's not good enough."

At heart, the doctors are trying to determine whether the youngster's complaint is a realistic cry for help, a frivolous attempt at perfection or a symptom of a more serious psychological problem. A 12-year-old stooping from the weight of triple-D cup breasts, for instance, "qualifies as a medical emergency," said Dr. George Beraka, a Park Avenue surgeon. By contrast, a girl "who hates her nose one day and her ears the next," he said, "maybe needs a psychiatrist."

Doctors disagree about whether they ought to function as therapists as well as surgeons. "With adolescents, their ideas about their bodies change as fast as their bodies do," said Dr. Nicholas Perricone, a professor of dermatology at Yale University. "They are facing so many issues, so many forces from the outside. We see more neuroses than psychiatrists."

Dr. H. George Brennan, a plastic surgeon in Newport Beach, California, balks at what seems to him psychobabble. "I'm not suggesting you operate on every kid who walks in the door," he said. "But it's no different than orthodontia. We didn't do psychotherapy before we straightened a teenager's teeth."

Some surgeons regularly include psychologists or psychiatrists in their consultations, to weed out patients with psychological problems, like distorted body images. But even girls without serious mental health problems are often at war with their flesh in many ways. "The body is a screen on which they project negative feelings about themselves," said Dr. Ann Kearney-Cooke, a Cincinnati psychologist and author of a curriculum to teach girls skills to improve body image. "If they don't know how to handle attention from boys they want a breast reduction. We need to spend time teaching them to set boundaries."

The majority of young patients are girls. When boys have a procedure done, they usually want their ears pinned back or enlarged breasts reduced, a condition caused by hormone imbalance.

Beyond body image issues, some doctors say that refusing plastic surgery for the young may toughen them for the stings and disappointments that lie ahead. "To teach them to deal with adversity, they have to bump into some things in life," said Dr. Susan Craig Scott, a plastic surgeon and mother of a teenage girl. "There is definitely something to be said for learning to deal with the hand life gives you."

Moreover, sometimes the passage of time enables a cosmetic surgery patient to realize that the desire for such drastic change was an immature mistake. One young woman, for instance, went to Dr. Richard Ellenbogen in Los Angeles a few years ago when she was a teenager because she hated her crooked nose, she said. Before she knew it, seduced by the glossy brochures in the waiting room, she was on a self-improvement treadmill that included surgery on her chin, ears and breasts, along with liposuction and hair extensions. Now, just a few sobering years later, she sees that it was a mistake to "get so caught up in it" and said she would caution a daughter to think twice. "I'd want her not so set on her looks," she said.

Even when they go along with the idea of surgery, many parents try to caution children that it is not a panacea. One father in Greenwich, Connecticut, reluctantly let his 10th-grade daughter get a nose job before she left for boarding school. Even after the surgery, he still asks himself whether the girl's unhappiness was a "reflection of something deeper."

"Did she want to change her nose, or did she want to be a different person?" he asked. "I don't think we'll ever be sure." He drummed his concern into the girl beforehand. "He pounded it into my head that I'd still be the same person," she said. "If you're a loser on the inside, you'll still be a loser on the inside. I just thought I'd be happier, that it would make me feel better."

And what has changed? "I'm not thinking about how I look all the time and looking in the mirror constantly," she said. "But I still have the same personality. I'm pretty much myself."

[JG, November 1998]

## Birth Rate at New Low as Teenage Pregnancy Declines

The teenage birth rate, which has been dropping steadily for six years, has dipped so sharply that it has helped push the nation's overall birth rate to the lowest point since the Government began keeping records in 1909, according to data made public in 1999 by the National Center for Health Statistics.

The birth rate, calculated as the number of births per 1,000 people in a given group, is one measure of how the native-born population grows. The rate among girls ages 15 to 19 dropped 16 percent from 1991 to 1997, the most recent year for which figures are available. In one year alone, from 1996 to 1997, the rate dropped 4 percent.

In absolute numbers, there were fewer babies born in 1997—3.88 million, nearly 500,000 of them to teenagers—than in any year since 1987, the center said. It cited the declining teenage birth rates, coupled with the aging of the general population, as the reasons the overall birth rate in 1997 dropped to a low of 14.5 births per 1,000 Americans. The previous low of 14.6 per 1,000 was recorded in 1975 and 1976, said Stephanie Ventura, a demographer with the health statistics center. By comparison, Ms. Ventura said, the birth rate in 1957, at the height of the baby boom, was 25.3 per 1,000.

The dip does not forecast a decline in population, demographers say, because it does not account for the influx of immigrants and because American women are still having enough babies, about two per couple, to replenish the population. "What this means is that births will make a smaller contribution to our annual growth rate than they have in the past," said Carl Haub, a demographer at the Population Reference Bureau, a nonprofit research institution.

The sustained declines in teenage births were seen as good news by the Clinton Administration, which cited the new figures as evidence that teenage pregnancy prevention programs are working. "Communities and parents all across America have joined with us to help our young people understand that they should delay parenthood until they are ready to nurture and support a child of their own," said Donna E. Shalala, the Secretary of Health and Human Services.

Vice President Al Gore said, "This good news shows us that when Americans come together in support of our basic values, we can send a clear message that our children should not be having children."

But experts say teenagers, themselves, as much as their parents or other adults, are responsible for the drop. Studies show young people are delaying sex until they are older, having sex less frequently and using birth control more often, and more responsibly. The Alan Guttmacher Institute, a nonprofit research organization that has analyzed the trends, cited teenagers' use of Norplant, the contraceptive implant, and Depo-Provera, an injectable contraceptive that became available in the early 1990s, as important reasons for the decline. "Many groups want to take credit for the drop in teenage pregnancy, but the credit truly goes to the teenagers," said Jacqueline E. Darroch, the institute's vice president. "About 20 percent of the decrease since the late 1980s is because of decreased sexual activity, and 80 percent of the decrease is because of more effective contraceptive practice."

The teenage birth rates dropped in all 50 states, although they vary considerably from state to state, with Vermont having the lowest rate, 26.9 births per 1,000, and Mississippi the highest, 73.7 per 1,000. There were declines in all racial and ethnic groups, but the greatest dips were recorded among Puerto Rican and non-Hispanic black teenagers, for whom the rate dropped about 25 percent during the six-year period. "The teen birth rate is the only age group where we have seen a sustained decline in the birth rate since the early 1990s," said Ms. Ventura, who is the co-author of the center's latest analysis of state-by-state birth data, from which the statistics made public are drawn. "The rates for women in their 20s have been flat, and for women in their 30s, the rates are increasing."

Out-of-wedlock births also declined for the third year in a row, and the birth rate for unmarried black women is lower now than in any year since 1969, when it was first calculated, the center found. Births to unmarried women declined slightly in 1997 but still accounted for 32 percent of overall births. Among teenagers, 78 percent of new mothers were unwed.

[SGS, April 1999]

## Teenagers and Sex: Younger and More at Risk

The American public is ignoring a serious sexual scandal—the young ages at which boys and girls now engage in sexual intercourse, often risking pregnancy and sexually transmitted diseases, including infection with the virus that causes AIDS. Millions of American children are at risk of having unsafe sex, and it is critical that they learn, first, how to resist pressures to have sexual intercourse at such young ages and, second, how to protect themselves from unwanted consequences if and when they decide to go all the way.

While there has been a decline in the teenage pregnancy rate resulting from the increased use of contraception and a leveling off of sexual activity among teenagers, there are still too many girls and boys engaging in reckless sexual activity. Teenage pregnancy rates are much higher in the United States than in many other developed countries—twice as high as in England and in Canada and nine times as high as in Japan.

American teenagers, their parents and teachers should be aware of the findings of a study conducted in New Zealand among more than 900 21-year-old men and women. As studies have found in the United States and Britain, the New Zealand study reported that half the men questioned reported having intercourse for the first time by age 17 and half the women by age 16. In New Zealand, nearly a third of the women and 28 percent of the men were 15 or younger when they first had sex. But looking back, many who became sexually active in their early or mid-teens had regrets about starting so young.

Now older and wiser, 54 percent of the women and 16 percent of the men said they should have waited longer before engaging in sexual intercourse, and among the women whose first sexual experiences occurred before age 16, 70 percent said they wished they had waited.

According to the study's findings, which were published in January 1998 in the *British Medical Journal,* 13 percent of the men who first had intercourse before age 16 contracted a sexually transmitted disease, compared with 6 percent of those who waited longer to initiate sexual activity. Among the women, the comparable figures were 28 percent and 12 percent.

Although the New Zealand researchers did not ask about the use of contraception and unwanted pregnancies, studies in this country have shown that 22 percent of girls ages 15 through 19 fail to use contraception the first time they have sex. And among 1,510 Americans ages 12 through 18 questioned in 1996, fewer than half reported consistently using contraception.

As might be predicted, each year in the United States, about three million teenagers acquire a sexually transmitted disease, according to the Alan Guttmacher Institute. One-fifth of the people diagnosed with AIDS are in their 20s, and most were infected as teenagers. The Guttmacher Institute, a nonprofit group that studies reproductive health, also reports that each year nearly one million teenage girls, including 20 percent of the sexually active girls ages 15 through 19, get pregnant.

## Beyond Saying "No"

Too often young women are pressured into unwanted sex. To give teen girls the language to resist having sex before they're ready, the Girls Inc., Will Power/Won't Power program offers sample responses to pressure lines.

### HE SAID, SHE SAID

**Line:** Everybody's doing it.
**Response:** Well, I'm not everybody. I'm me. Besides, I know it's not true that everybody's doing it.

**Line:** If you love me, you'll have sex with me.
**Response:** If you love me, you'll respect my feelings and not push me into something I'm not ready for.

**Line:** I know you want to do it, too. You're just afraid of what people will say.
**Response:** You can't read my mind. Besides, if I wanted to do it, I wouldn't be arguing with you.

**Line:** We've had sex before, so what's the problem now?
**Response:** I have a right to change my mind. I've decided to wait until I'm older to have sex again.

**Line:** If you won't have sex with me, I won't see you anymore.
**Response:** Too bad. I'll miss you.

**Line:** Let's do it. You know I want to marry you.
**Response:** Marriage is a long way off for me. I want to wait to have sex.

**Line:** Don't you want to try it to see what it's like?
**Response:** That's a stupid reason to have sex.

**Line:** But I have to have it.
**Response:** No you don't. If I can wait, you can wait.

**Line:** Come on, have a drink. It'll get you in the mood.
**Response:** No thanks. I don't want to get drunk and not know what I'm doing.

One-fifth of the unmarried teenagers who get pregnant do so within the first month of first intercourse and one-half within the first six months. With little instruction at home or at school on how to resist the pressures to have sex and with even more erratic access to effective contraception, such consequences are hardly surprising.

The New Zealand researchers, from the University of Otago Medical School in Dunedin, cited familiar reasons for the falling age at which first intercourse occurs. "Children are exposed to sexual images through the media," they wrote. "Social and peer pressure may arise from the portrayal of sex as glamorous, pleasurable and adult, while negative consequences and the responsibilities involved in sexual relationships are seldom portrayed." That's putting it mildly. In the 1998 movie, *Slums of Beverly Hills*, a precocious 13-year-old decides to have sex with an older boy "just to get it over with."

Is this the message we want to convey to American youth—that sex is something you try, like rollerblading or water skiing, to see what it's like or to add to your roster of achievements? Dr. Ann Davis, an adolescent gynecologist formerly at the Floating Hospital in Boston, said, "Often when I ask a young teen whether she is sexually active, she will seem ashamed to admit that she is not." Virginity may no longer be the prize it once was. Nor does having an abortion or bearing a child out of wedlock carry the stigma it used to. Still, these are hardly desirable options for young people, whose primary goals should be to get an education and acquire skills to be able to support themselves.

Lest you think that girls who have sex do so because they find it irresistible, in a 1992 national survey, 25 percent of them said that their first experience was "voluntary but unwanted." The percentage of unwanted sexual activity, as well as the failure to use contraception, rises with the gap in age between the boy and the girl. Experts in the field say that age 9 is none too soon to teach girls how and why to say "no" and what to do should they say "yes."

The problem admittedly is not easy to tackle. A study published in 1998 in the journal *Family Planning Perspectives* disclosed that girls who have intercourse at an early age, as well as those who fail to use contraceptives and those who have children, tend to be depressed, have low self-esteem and possess little sense of control over their lives. Thus, reducing the incidence of early and risky sexual activity may involve much more than instruction about sex and contraception. It may require giving girls a reason to be hopeful and an opportunity to believe in themselves and their ability to make something of their lives. When a girl's home life fails to instill such hope, it falls on the shoulders of schools and after-school activities to fill in the gaps.

Programs like the two developed by Girls Inc.—Growing Together and Will Power/Won't Power—have proved effective in delaying sexual activity among young girls. Growing Together involves five two-hour mother-daughter workshops designed to foster communications about sexuality and other sensitive issues. Will Power/Won't Power is an assertiveness training program to help teenagers refuse to become sexually active without jeopardizing their friendships with peers of both sexes. Both programs explore the opportunities life holds and help girls realize what they may lose by becoming pregnant. The programs' techniques could be adopted in communities and intermediate and high schools. For details, contact Girls Inc. at (212) 509-2000 or on the Web at www.girlsinc.org.

[JEB, September 1998]

# Coping with Cold, Hard Facts on Teenage Drinking

The latest statistics on teenage drinking are startling:

▶ A 1997 national study of teenage students revealed that 54 percent of eighth graders, 72 percent of 10th graders and 82 percent of 12th graders had consumed alcohol, and more than a third of 12th graders had been drunk at least once.

▶ More than one-third of high school seniors see no great risk in consuming four to five drinks a day. Yet 16 percent of teenagers have had "black-outs" where heavy drinking erased their memories of what happened the previous evening. And alcohol is the single biggest factor behind the leading cause of death among teenagers—traffic accidents.

▶ Teenagers who start drinking before age 15 are four times as likely to become alcohol dependent as those who begin drinking at age 21, the legal drinking age.

▶ An American Academy of Pediatrics survey found that teenagers who drink one day a month typically consume nearly three drinks at a time, and those who drink six or more days a month average more than five drinks at a time.

▶ A Harvard study of college drinking showed that more than two-fifths of students indulge in binge drinking, defined as consuming five drinks at one sitting by men or four drinks by women. Of college students who drink, one-third drink to get drunk.

▶ According to the Federal Office of Substance Abuse Prevention, college students spend more money on alcohol than on soft drinks, coffee, tea, milk, juice and books combined.

▶ The highest rate of binge drinking—greater than 80 percent—occurs among college students who live in fraternity and sorority houses, and the second highest rate is found among athletes who participate in intercollegiate sports.

▶ Alcohol is involved in 95 percent of violent and property crimes on campuses, including date rape, and 40 percent of students' academic problems are alcohol-related.

As with most health problems, the best way to deal with them is to prevent them from occurring in the first place. Alcohol abuse by teenagers, college students or anyone else is a preventable disorder. Colleges around the country have undertaken a concerted effort to curb excessive drinking by students, both on and off campus. But long before youngsters reach college age, parents play the largest role in fostering a healthy respect for alcohol in their children.

First and foremost, parents must set a good example by using alcohol only in moderation, preferably with meals, and never suggesting it as a solution to stress or other emotional problems. Although parents tend to think that peer pressure is the primary influence on drinking by teenagers, youngsters say otherwise. According to a survey released last year by the National Institute on Drug Abuse, the leading reasons given by high school seniors for drinking are to have a good time with friends, to see what it's like, to feel good, to relax or relieve tension, to relieve boredom, to get away from problems and to cope with anger or frustration. Only 8 percent gave "to fit in with a group I like" as their reason for drinking.

"Parents should emphasize that getting drunk is always to be avoided," said Dr. Henry Wechsler, director of College Alcohol Studies at the Harvard School of Public Health. "Most parents aren't teaching their kids anything about alcohol, especially not that alcohol in large quantities has many dangerous effects. Too many kids think that as long as they don't drive, it's okay to get drunk."

Of course, parents should always pay attention to their children's behavior and the friends they hang out with, be consistent about discipline and be clear but realistic about their expectations for academic achievement. Students about to go off to college should be cautioned about checking out the drinking practices in various sororities and fraternities before they consider joining one.

Dr. Wechsler said parents also could help by monitoring the activities of their state and municipal alcohol control boards with regard to enforcement of the minimum drinking age, sales of alcohol around college campuses and bars that offer students "specials"—high volumes of alcohol (usually beer) for a low price—which he said encouraged binge drinking.

Dr. Tim Marchell, director of substance abuse services at Cornell University, suggested that parents discuss social life at college with their college-bound children and review all the things there are to do there besides partying and drinking.

Under a grant from the Center for Science in the Public Interest, Cornell and the University of North Carolina are testing an education program aimed at changing attitudes about alcohol and campus drinking practices. Jan Talbot, community health educator at Cornell University, said a university survey revealed that the drinking norm was much lower than most students believed. The survey showed that 62 percent of Cornell students consumed zero to three drinks when they partied, not five or six, as many students believed.

The program also emphasizes the secondary effects of excessive drinking on other students, including unwanted sexual advances to women, destructive behavior, routines that disrupt sleep and

studying and vomiting in the street or communal bathrooms. "We're trying to reshape the environment in which students make choices," Dr. Marchell said. "We're trying to increase student awareness of and intolerance for the second-hand effects of other people's drinking by drawing attention to the problems excessive drinking inflicts on the entire community."

Because members of fraternities and sororities drink two to three times as much as other students on the same campus, Cornell has instituted such regulations as having all parties in Greek houses catered and regulated to prevent excessive drinking and insisting that all new fraternity and sorority members attend an alcohol education workshop. And because athletes are the second largest group of excessive drinkers, Cornell is also working with athletic coaches to foster a change in student drinking behavior.

Cornell has also increased the availability of alcohol-free social activities during the hours that students typically engage in drinking. The idea is to show students they can have a good time without indulging in alcohol. The activities, under the rubric of "Up All Night," are scheduled between 11 P.M. and 2 A.M. and include movies, food and various forms of recreation.

Finally, colleges have to work with local businesses to get bars accessible to students to refrain from offering alcohol specials that encourage excessive drinking.

[JEB, April 1999]

## Steroid Use by Teenage Girls Is Rising

Whether trying to reach stardom in high school sports, working to achieve a fashionable lean-but-muscular look or suffering from a deep psychological disorder, teenage girls are using illegal anabolic steroids in sharply increasing numbers, health authorities say.

The increased usage among girls, which some

researchers attribute in part to a kind of reverse anorexia, has caught up to levels that began to be established by boys in the 1980s. And steroid use, researchers say, exposes girls to the same severe health risks, but with the added potential of destroying their ability to bear children.

The National Institute on Drug Abuse says about

175,000 teenage girls in the United States have reported taking anabolic steroids at least once within a year of the time surveyed—a rise of 100 percent since 1991. The surveys, by the University of Michigan's Institute for Social Research, the National Household Survey of Drug Abuse and the Youth Risk and Behavior Survey System, were done in schools or the home through anonymous self-reported questionnaires.

Dr. Lloyd D. Johnston, director of the Michigan project, which has been conducting annual youth surveys since 1975, said the actual number of users may actually be higher than the most recent surveys show, since people tend to underreport drug use. The rate among teenage boys has also continued to rise, to the current estimated level of 325,000.

Other indications, including the results of a small study in Oregon, are that steroid use among both girls and boys is increasing unabated. The three national surveys were conducted before Mark McGwire set baseball's single-season home run record in 1998, acknowledging that he used androstenedione, a precursor of testosterone, to help him build muscle. Whether androstenedione, which is allowed in professional baseball but banned in other sports, does in fact build muscles remains a matter of medical dispute, though the perception of many athletes, both adult and adolescent, is that it does. In any case, sports medicine doctors generally agree that its potential for inducing serious side effects is similar to that of anabolic steroids.

"I get calls every day from the coaches and parents of girls as well as boys," said Dr. Linn Goldberg, a physician at Oregon Health Sciences University in Portland and a United States Olympic Committee drug testing official. "Some are concerned and some want to know whether their children should use androstenedione." His answer is an unequivocal no, either to use of steroids or androstenedione.

Anabolic steroids are synthetic substitutes for testosterone, the hormone that directs the body to produce or add male characteristics like increased muscle mass, facial hair and a deep voice. The hormone exists in females as well, though in much smaller amounts. Liver cancer, heart disease and uncontrollable aggressiveness are among other serious side effects that can occur in both males and females of all ages.

The health damages might not appear for years or decades after the steroids are taken, said Dr. Gary I. Wadler, a professor of clinical medicine at New York University School of Medicine.

Dr. Charles E. Yesalis, a steroid authority at Pennsylvania State University, was among the first to analyze the 1997 female-adolescent data in December of that year in the *Archives of Pediatrics and Adolescent Medicine* and to sound the alarm. Most prevention programs, he said recently, have not been effective. "I am asked to speak in schools and other institutions," Dr. Yesalis said, "but you don't get anywhere with speeches or charts or film clips or posters. We know one-shot messages don't work."

Dr. Goldberg said teenage boys and girls generally obtain illegal steroids from people who congregate at commercial gyms. "That's where most people say they obtain them," Dr. Goldberg said. "Someone, in this part of the country, will go down to Mexico, where it is easy to get the stuff, and bring it back, either in pill form or injectables." And then one young person will buy some and distribute them to his or her schoolmates, he said.

The new interest among teenage girls, these and other health experts say, reflect a gradual change in attitude, and fashion, or teenage peer pressure, away from a preoccupation with thinness. Some teenage girls now desire to look more healthy and somewhat more muscular, but this has led some girls toward an unhealthy compulsion to be ever fitter with larger muscles.

"We've gone from the overweight beauty of the Rubens women, to the thin rail of the Twiggy types and now back to something in between, the lean but muscular type," Dr. Wadler said. "These are people who are virtually addicted to the mirror. But they will never be satisfied with what they see, and this is now happening to teenage girls who want bigger muscles no matter how much bigger their muscles have become."

Dr. Harrison G. Pope Jr., chief of the Biological Psychiatry Laboratory of Harvard Medical School's

McLean Hospital, and colleagues referred to a similar disorder in male weight lifters as "reverse anorexia" after it was observed in 1993. The researchers recently updated the work with a study of 32 women bodybuilders, 17 of whom showed signs of an emotional disorder called body dysmorphism, which is the excessive preoccupation with a trait or traits of the body viewed as ugly or defective whether they are or not.

Several women in the study were so addicted to working out that they cut off job opportunities and close personal relationships. But Dr. Pope said too little research had been done on this emerging obsession among teenage girls to draw specific conclusions about its complex causes.

The case of one of the worst known adverse reactions to steroid use, reported by Dr. Goldberg, is that of a 19-year-old West Coast woman who was preparing to enter her first bodybuilding contest, lifting weights and eating a high-protein diet. She then switched to a drastically reduced intake of food and water. Obsessed with her goal, she began taking anabolic steroids and a diuretic. The steroid would add muscle and the diuretic would drain the body of fluid and make the muscle stand out more.

She won the contest, but it will probably be her last. After she collected her trophy, she resumed drinking water and eating normally, and her weight shot up by 25 pounds in three days. It turned out that the diuretic had masked the actual amount of muscle she had built up, said Dr. Goldberg, who was one of a group of health experts who reviewed the case. When she drank more fluids, he said, her muscles pushed out to the full over-developed size and crushed blood vessels in her legs. Called compartment syndrome, the condition put her limbs, if not her life, in danger, and surgeons had to cut open both legs to protect her vascular system and remove significant amounts of the new muscle tissue.

Dr. Goldberg and Dr. Diane L. Elliot hope to educate girls about the dangers of steroid use as they have done with boys. They recently completed a program, called Atlas, that is supported by the National Institute on Drug Abuse and is aimed at reducing steroid use among young male athletes. A main element of the program, involving 3,200 male athletes at 31 high schools in Oregon and Washington, was to teach the students to educate one another on the problems. The number of male students that reported having used steroids within a year was cut by 50 percent. Under another National Institute on Drug Abuse grant, they are developing a similar program for girls.

Dr. Yesalis said the Goldberg-Elliot program was the only one he knew of that worked. "Unless young people are taught to know where and how to draw the line, to know that it's not right to try to win at all costs, they're not going to listen when you tell them steroids put their lives at risk for the glory of winning," he said.

[HBN, June 1999]

# Menopause and Aging

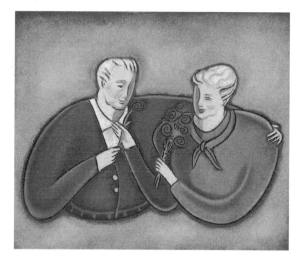

## BALANCING THE BODY'S CHEMISTRY
## LATER IN LIFE

Menopause, in biological terms, is not a mystery. A woman is born with only so many follicles in her ovaries, which produce both eggs and sex hormones like estrogen. When she runs out of follicles and eggs, there it is: menopause.

But why do the follicles run out? Why aren't women born with more, so that they can go on bearing children until late in life?

Theories abound. One school of thought holds that menopause is a sort of accident, a luxury of our extended life spans, because we were not designed to live as long as we do. Not that long ago—certainly not long enough for evolution to have caught up—women did not live long enough to reach menopause. Today, they do. Or so that theory goes.

But another theory says that menopause has advantages that have caused evolution to preserve it. A woman who stops having children in middle age no longer risks dying in childbirth, and thereby increases her chances of sticking around to raise the children she did have—which increases their chances of reaching adulthood, reproducing and passing on their genes (and hers, of course). Still another idea is that in some societies, menopausal women, acting as aunts and grandmothers, play an essential role in helping to care for the children of younger relatives.

Whatever the reasons for menopause, and despite the apparent simplicity of what actually brings it on, the effects of plunging estrogen levels can be profound, and sometimes devastating. After menopause, women face significant increases in their risk of heart disease, Alzheimer's disease and broken bones, along with more benign but troubling symptoms like hot flashes, mood swings, vaginal dryness and, sometimes, loss of libido.

Estrogen replacement therapy can forestall those consequences, and among women who take the hormone for five years, the overall death rate while they are on the drug is 37 percent lower than in those who do not take it. Nonetheless, many women are wary of estrogen, and particularly fearful of evidence that it may cause a small increase in their risk of breast cancer. Several alternative drugs do exist to prevent bone loss, though none works as well as estrogen.

Whether to take the hormone or not, and when to take it, are individual decisions to be made by women and their doctors, taking into account the woman's medical history and her risk factors, especially her risk for heart disease, osteoporosis and breast cancer. But whatever a woman decides, she can always change her mind later.

# Theorists See Evolutionary Advantages in Menopause

The Hadza people of northern Tanzania are a small group of hunter-gatherers who share a language, a culture and a distaste for gardening. Time and again, government and church agencies have sought to transmute them into full-time farmers, but the Hazda have always returned to the bush, where they subsist on wild goods like fruits, honey, tubers and game. The terrain is hard and hilly, and so is the life, but on one incomparable resource the foragers can always rely: a pack of old ladies with hearts like young horses.

As Dr. Kristen Hawkes of the University of Utah and her colleagues have found in their extensive studies of the Hadza, women in their 50s, 60s, 70s and beyond are among the most industrious members of the group. They are out in the woods for seven or eight hours a day, gathering more food than virtually any of their comrades.

When a young woman is burdened with a suckling infant and cannot fend for her family, she turns for support, not to her mate, but to a senior female relative—her mother, an aunt, an elder cousin. It is Grandma, or Grandma-proxy, who keeps the woman's other children in baobab and berries; Grandma keeps them alive. She is not a sentiment, she is a requirement. As Dr. Hawkes, Dr. James O'Connell of the University of Utah and Dr. Nicholas Blurton Jones of the University of California at Los Angeles reported in *Current Anthropology*, a nursing Hadza woman always has a postmenopausal helper.

There are only about 750 Hadza, and they are contemporary hunter-gatherers, not pristine relics of prelapsarian humanity. Nevertheless, the centrality of elder women to their group's survival has thrown fresh kindling on the spirited debate over the origins and purpose of human menopause.

As doctors and women thrash out the best way to "treat" menopause, pitting the benefits of estrogen therapy to the heart and bones against the risks the hormone poses to the breast and possibly the ovaries, evolutionary scientists address the menopause mystery from a more high-flown, though no less quarrel-prone, perspective. They ask whether menopause is an ancient adaptation or a contemporary artifact. Is it the well-wrought product of natural selection, or the incidental byproduct of an unnaturally prolonged life span?

Proponents of the adaptationist camp generally see menopause as the thriftiest solution to the problem of exorbitant offspring. By this view, the ludicrous amount of time required for a mother to rear children to maturity led to the need for so-called premature reproductive senescence, an early retirement program for the ovaries. Through the mechanism of menopause, an ancestral woman theoretically was spared the risks of childbirth, and thus had a heightened chance of living long enough to see her existing children out the door. Dr. Jared Diamond, a physiologist at the University of California at Los Angeles Medical School has said that menopause, like big brains and upright posture, is "among the biological traits essential for making us human."

The artifactualists insist that prehistoric women almost never survived past the age of 30, let alone long enough to experience the thrill of hot flashes. By their reckoning, menopause is a modern luxury, the result of women now outlasting an egg supply that more than sufficed for the cameo appearances that their Stone Age foremothers called lives. "For most of our existence, we simply didn't live very long," said Dr. Alison Galloway, an anthropologist at the University of California at Santa Cruz. "Menopause happens because, through technology, we've extended our lives to the point where we run out of egg follicles. There's nothing beneficial about it."

Dr. Hawkes lends a new spin to the debate, combining elements of each camp and adding a few bold spirals of her own. She agrees with the artifactualists that menopause per se is not an adaptation—it is not the product of selective design. A woman's ovaries do not shut down "prematurely," she says. They last 40 or 45 years, the same time as the ovaries of our close relatives, chimpanzees and gorillas. In a sense, she says, women do outlive their egg supply, which is fixed before birth and cannot be added to, as men continuously generate new sperm.

On the other hand, Dr. Hawkes concurs with the adaptationists that prehistoric women very likely often survived past menopause, and that they were instrumental to the survival of their families. She goes further. Only with the ascent of the grandmother, she says, were human ancestors freed to exploit new habitats, to go where no other hominid or primate had gone before, and to become the species we know so well.

"The Grandmother Hypothesis gives us a whole new way of understanding why modern humans suddenly were able to go everywhere and do everything," Dr. Hawkes said. "It may explain why we took over the planet."

In another new study that touches on the evolutionary basis of menopause and maternal longevity, Dr. Thomas Perls of Harvard Medical School and his colleagues describe in the journal *Nature* their finding that women who lived to be at least 100 years of age were much likelier to have remained fruitful well into middle age than a comparable group of women who died at the age of 73. Looking at two sets of women born in 1896 who were equivalent in race, religion and other factors but who differed in their life spans, the researchers found that among the 54 women who died in 1969 at the age of 73, only 5.5 percent had given birth in their 40s. By comparison, 19.5 percent of the centenarians had children after 40, one of them at age 53.

Because the women in Dr. Perls's analysis all had their families before the rise of fertility-enhancing technology, the researchers see the stark discrepancy in maternal stamina between the two groups as evidence of innate selective drives at work. They propose that the genes allowing the centenarians to stay fruitful for an exceptionally long time continued working long after menopause to lengthen the women's life spans, supporting the view that a woman's extended survival is indeed crucial to her offsprings' prospects.

The older a woman is at last birth, the more years she must stick around to keep her family afloat. (The researchers also believe that menopause, the complete cessation of fertility, evolved to prevent aging women from dying in childbirth while they still had dependent young, but their analysis of the centenarians offers no direct proof of that.)

The notion that menopause has adaptive value for women and their offspring is itself getting a bit long in tooth. Dr. George C. Williams, a renowned evolutionary biologist, first proposed it in 1957 to explain the seemingly anomalous nature of human menopause. Other female primates, and even species like fin whales and elephants that live into their 80s, can continue bearing young to the bitter end, he pointed out.

Why are humans different? And why does menopause occur universally among women, and during a short window of time—at the half-century mark, give or take four years—while other depradations of age, like gray hair or presbyopia, occur gradually and randomly? Dr. Williams saw in menopause the thumbprint of natural selection, and suggested that the early cessation of reproduction paradoxically enhanced a woman's reproductive "fitness," by assuring that she lived long enough to see her children bear children themselves—that she became a grandmother.

Others have picked up and expanded on the rudimentary Grandmother Hypothesis. Dr. Diamond has proposed that aging women, and men, were repositories of essential information in preliterate times, living libraries for their clans, able to distinguish edible from poisonous plants and to recall events of long ago that remained pertinent to survival.

In traditional societies, clan members are often related, and so by aiding the tribe the elders help themselves. Only women need protection from the hazards of advanced maternity, Dr. Diamond says, and so only women need to undergo premature reproductive senescence to keep them around for the benefit of their kin.

Yet efforts to demonstrate the adaptive value of menopause have proved elusive. Dr. Kim Hill and Dr. Magdalena Hurtado, anthropologists at the University of New Mexico, spent years studying the Ache, a group of hunter-gatherers living in eastern Paraguay.

They tried to estimate the impact of postmenopausal women on the welfare of their children and grandchildren, to see if the presence of a grandmother had a measurable effect, for example by reducing the mortality of grandchildren. The anthropologists concluded that the Ache grandmothers did not make enough of a cumulative difference to their families to justify, in Darwinian terms, the loss through menopause of their own reproductive capacity.

Using mathematical models, Dr. Alan Rogers of the University of Utah estimated that a postmenopausal woman would have to double the number of children her children bore, and eliminate infant mortality among those grandchildren, to make menopause look like a sound strategy for propagating one's genes. That is not a grandmother—that is Neutron Nana.

"Adaptive menopause is an interesting idea, and I'm trying to keep an open mind," said Dr. Steven N. Austad, a professor of zoology at the University of Idaho in Moscow and author of *Why We Age*. "But I just don't see evidence to support it."

Before anybody consigns the Grandmother Hypothesis to a conceptual nursing home, however, Dr. Hawkes and her colleagues offer evidence in the Hadza study that elder women can make an enormous, and quantifiable, difference to their kin. The researchers found that whenever the mother of young children gave birth to a new baby and was absorbed by the rigors of breast-feeding, it was only through the intervention of a senior female relative that the older children's weight stayed up. And the harder the elders foraged, the higher the numbers on the researchers' bathroom scale.

Importantly, the elder Hadza women were flexible in how they apportioned their assistance. If a woman could help her nursing daughter, she did. If she had no daughter, she helped a niece, or a cousin once removed.

Dr. Hawkes pointed out that in the Ache study showing little benefit from grandma, the researchers had focused on the relationships between mothers, their children and their children's children. Dr. Hawkes and her colleagues were more inclusive in their analysis. "If we restricted ourselves to counting the reproductive success only of women whose moms were still alive, we'd underestimate the effect of help from senior women by a huge amount," Dr. Hawkes said. "And you expect, with strategic critters like ourselves, that natural selection would favor adjusting help to where it was needed most."

Dr. Hawkes proposes that what distinguishes a human female from her chimpanzee or gorilla cousins is not that the woman goes through menopause and the chimpanzee does not, but rather that the chimpanzee, at 45 and with ovaries failing, is globally decrepit and close to death, while a woman can live decades after follicular fadeout.

But young chimpanzees do not need elder females to help them. Once they are weaned, they feed themselves, and so there are no selective pressures to keep Aunt Chimsky alive. Only human children are fed for years after leaving the breast, and a senior female can serve up nuts and berries as well as can a mother, and better when mother is lactating.

Dr. Hawkes and her co-workers suggest that the extension of life past menopause was a watershed event in human prehistory. With a labor force of elder females available to help provision the young, adults were then free to colonize new territories unavailable to those primates that did not provision their weaned young, and that were thus restricted to feeding grounds where the pickings were easy enough for juvenile fingers. Suddenly humans could migrate to places where it required full adult strength and cunning to extract food. They could go wherever they pleased. After all, there were older women around to help.

Supporting this proposition are the foraging patterns of the Hadza. Very young children find much of their food themselves, but they depend on adults for half their calories, and those calories come from foods, like deeply buried tubers, that only an adult can obtain. Growing old, then, may be nothing new, and the postmenopausal years worthy of celebration and gratitude. Grandma is great, she is strong, and she baby-sits for free.

[NA, September 1997]

# Menopause Begins Silently, Before Its Symptoms

I was in my mid-40s and still menstruating regularly when my gynecologist suggested that I start taking estrogen. But I thought he was jumping the gun since I would probably not enter menopause for five more years.

Now that I have a better understanding of the perimenopause, the years leading up to a near-shutdown of ovarian function, I can see his point, albeit belatedly. Menopause is a process, not a discrete event. Ovaries do not stop working abruptly unless they are shut down by chemotherapy or surgical removal. Rather, there is a gradual decline in hormone production over about 15 years, a decline that can produce sometimes mystifying symptoms and set the stage for serious health problems later on.

Millions of American women, those between the ages of 35 and the early 50s, are now in their perimenopause, and a better understanding of its common symptoms and ways to cope with them can make a tremendous difference in the quality of these women's lives and their future health.

Estrogen production usually starts declining gradually when a woman is in her mid-30s; by the mid-40s, she may begin to experience clear symptoms of estrogen deficiency. Her menstrual periods may become somewhat irregular—shorter or longer, lighter or heavier—or she may experience premenstrual syndrome, menstrual cramps or headaches that are showing up for the first time or worse than in the past. Hot flashes may become bothersome during the day, and night sweats may disrupt her sleep, resulting in increased irritability, fatigue and difficulty concentrating.

But the symptoms of perimenopause are often more subtle. According to Dr. Nancy Lee Teaff and Kim Wright Wiley, authors of *Perimenopause: Preparing for the Change*, "When they first begin to appear, perimenopausal symptoms may seem unrelated to each other, and women often treat each problem individually, not seeing the connection until years later." Among the possible symptoms are insomnia, difficulty concentrating, poor memory, reduced stamina, itchy or dry skin, wrinkling, urinary incontinence or frequency, vaginal dryness, headaches, declining libido and mood swings.

"A woman may say, 'I'm falling apart,' failing to recognize that she has only one condition, perimenopause, that is manifesting itself in many ways," Dr. Teaff and Ms. Wiley wrote.

At the same time, other hidden changes may be taking place that can increase a woman's risk of future health problems. High levels of estrogen during a woman's childbearing years protect against heart disease, which is why women rarely develop it before they turn 50. Estrogen helps raise the blood levels of the "good" cholesterol, HDL, which counters arterial clogging. It also maintains the elasticity of blood vessels and diminishes the tendency of the blood to form clots.

In the book *Perimenopause: Changes in a Woman's Health After 35*, Drs. James E. Huston and L. Darlene Lanka point out that heart disease is the leading killer of women 50 to 75 years old, claiming five times as many lives as breast cancer.

Estrogen also helps maintain bone density and ward off the later development of osteoporosis. Few women realize that they begin to lose bone in their 30s; the loss merely accelerates at menopause if estrogen is not taken along with an adequate amount of calcium through food or supplements.

"During the approximately 15 years of perimenopause, you have a good shot at averting the adverse changes these two conditions can wreak on your body later in life," Drs. Huston and Lanka said.

Dr. Teaff recommends that perimenopausal women who are experiencing symptoms have their estrogen level tested during the second, third or fourth days of the menstrual cycle. If symptoms include changes in menstrual patterns or hot flashes, another test, for FSH (follicle-stimulating hormone, produced by the pituitary), should be done on blood drawn during the first six days of the menstrual cycle and repeated the next month.

It would also be a good idea at this time to have a base-line bone density test, as well as a test for total cholesterol and its various fractions. In fact, while you are at it, the perimenopause is a good time to undergo a complete physical, including a mammogram and electrocardiogram. The results may prompt you to take a greater interest in your future well-being. That entails paying more attention to your diet and exercise habits.

As ovarian function slowly declines, muscle mass may begin to wane, accompanied by a rise in body fat and a gradual thickening around the waist and abdomen. You can minimize these changes by adhering to a diet low in fat and rich in vegetables, fruit and whole grain foods, along with moderate amounts of lean protein. Do not forget low-fat and nonfat dairy products; they are your best sources of calcium. A quart of skim milk or its equivalent can supply a perimenopausal woman's daily calcium requirement.

Regular exercise, including aerobic, muscle-building and flexibility-enhancing activities, are vital to countering the physical and emotional effects of declining levels of estrogen. That holds true even if you take hormone replacement, which is not nearly so effective in protecting the health of a sedentary woman as it is in a woman who remains physically active through menopause and beyond.

Then there is hormone replacement, which a growing number of gynecologists believe should begin years before a woman ceases to have regular menstrual periods. The most common, estrogen and progestin in a pill, is not the only regimen. If you are troubled by a loss of sexual desire, a testosterone supplement may restore your libido (testosterone is the libido hormone for both men and women). If vaginal or urinary problems are your only symptoms, estrogen cream inserted daily into the vagina may do the trick, although the amount of estrogen that would reach the bloodstream is not adequate to protect your heart and bones.

You can increase your body's overall estrogen supply naturally by eating flaxseed (two or three tablespoons a day) and more soy-based foods, including tofu, soy milk, soybeans and soy nuts. Consult *Estrogen: The Natural Way* by Nina Shandler for amounts and recipes using foods rich in plant estrogens. But eating large amounts of estrogen-rich foods exposes you to unopposed estrogen, which, without the balancing effects of progestin, may result in overstimulation of the uterine lining and heavier menstrual bleeding. When hormone replacement is given in pill form to a woman who still has a uterus, estrogen is combined with a progestin to diminish the risk of uterine overstimulation and prevent uterine cancer. Even if you are still menstruating regularly, hormone replacement can help to reduce perimenopausal symptoms.

[JEB, January 1998]

## Scientists Now Envision Life Without Menopause

No need to stockpile Tampax and O.B.s in anticipation of a great increase in tampon demand. But the prospect has arisen—well, more like the hint of a promise of a prospect—that perhaps, some distant day, scientists will be able to delay the onset of menopause until well into a woman's old age. For they have recently done something much like it in mice.

Researchers based at Massachusetts General Hospital's Vincent Center for Reproductive Biology here genetically altered mice to remove a gene connected to cell death. In their study, published in February 1999, the animals' ovaries remained active in the mouse equivalent of 100-year-olds. And though the altered female mice did not become pregnant, some of their eggs remained viable enough to produce embryos if fertilized in vitro.

Now, stop, just stop, before the futuristic scenarios

of 85-year-olds giving birth come to mind. First, there are solid indications that far from every woman would want to delay menopause, which on average sets in at age 51. An increasingly popular school of thought sees the end of fertility as manageable and even positive. And doctors say female patients often say they are happy to give up the bleeding and the birth control.

But the primary rub is scientific, not cultural. Perhaps no one is more excited about the mouse results than the experiment's lead researcher, Dr. Jonathan L. Tilly, but even he begins with caveats, including the biggest one: "The approach that we and our collaborator, Dr. Stanley Korsmeyer of the Dana-Farber Cancer Institute, used is to silence a gene. And we know of no technique to silence genes in humans."

Other giant questions remain: Would silencing the same gene in humans, if it were possible, have the same effect? Would it be safe? Does preserving ovarian function bring the health benefits one would expect? Still, Dr. Tilly said, his team's findings amount to a dramatic and unexpected development in a growing and promising field—the study of the causes and health effects of menopause.

Scientists had good reason to hope that the "bax" gene silenced in the mice would influence menopause. Bax is known to be connected to cell death, or apoptosis, and menopause sets in when an organism's immature eggs have died through apoptosis, and the barren ovaries stop producing estrogen. "It was almost a no-brainer to ask the question: If we take the gene out of the oocyte—or immature egg—what happens to the ovary?" said Dr. Tilly, a molecular biologist. But the power of the effect of knocking it out nonetheless stunned the researchers, he said. "In my wildest dreams I never thought it could work as well as it did," he said. "It's hard to predict that one gene only would be so important, that there would be no backup system to take its place."

Though direct applications for humans are far away, the mouse finding does offer scientists the valuable chance to explore what happens to women's health when they enter menopause, hormone specialists agree. "It's a chance to make some observations on what's due to aging and what's due to the absence of estrogen," said Dr. Daniel Federman of Harvard Medical School. "You now have animals aging, but there's estrogen around—that's the biggest prospect."

It is well known that menopause tends to bring health problems: mainly increased risk for osteoporosis, heart disease and dementia. What has not been so clear is the exact connection between the hormonal changes of menopause and those problems—particularly, whether lack of estrogen alone is the culprit, or whether the ovary produces other beneficial hormones that stop after menopause. Despite those gaps in understanding, it is increasingly common for menopausal American women to take estrogen to replace what they lose. But such therapy has drawbacks, including a lack of effectiveness in some women and fears of increased cancer risk.

If scientists can better understand what triggers bone loss and cardiovascular problems in menopausal women, "We have some chance of intervening in a way that doesn't necessarily directly involve estrogen," said Dr. Frank Bellino, the endocrinology program administrator for the National Institute on Aging. Dr. Tilly said that because the mouse findings involve keeping ovaries viable and their eggs alive, they could also—eventually, perhaps—mean help for women who undergo premature menopause, or who become infertile because of chemotherapy.

Better understanding of how eggs age would also probably help women over age 40 who find their chances of becoming pregnant greatly diminished because of their old eggs, he said. Mainly, however, the mouse findings cast light on the strange life of the ovary. It used to be thought that a woman had only a small number of eggs, and after releasing one each month from the ovary, she simply ran out, bringing on menopause. Now, it is known that she begins with millions of eggs, but they die relatively quickly and are never replaced, earning the ovaries their reputation as the fastest-aging organs in the body.

Before a female fetus is born, she has up to seven million egg cells. By the time she is born, a baby girl has only one million or two million left, and their number dwindles until only about 400,000 or so are left at puberty, and virtually none by age 50. The overall goal of his research, Dr. Tilly said, "is to understand why the ovary ages, and can we regulate the process for the benefit of women's health?"

A broader question is at issue as well, one that would interest all women: Does giving a woman's ovaries greater longevity mean she will live longer? If the aging of the ovary furthers the aging of the woman, doesn't it stand to reason that younger ovaries would mean, effectively, younger women? Maybe, Dr. Tilly said, but "right now, we don't have conclusive proof that the animals will live longer; they're sitting in cages, hopefully aging well." His researchers also are awaiting results from other laboratories about whether the expected health benefits to the hearts and bones of the mice actually occurred.

It is much too early to speculate, he said. He added, however: "If you look at what happens to women when their ovaries fail, and all the health risks they face, it's quite possible the animals will live longer."

Even if the test mice do live longer, researchers cannot conclusively link their longevity to their ovarian function, because the bax gene silenced in them has been silenced in their entire bodies—their immune systems, their brains, everywhere. But Dr. Tilly is now working with bax-silenced mice whose ovaries have been removed to determine whether it is the silencing of bax in the ovaries or in the rest of the body that helps the mice age better.

"Our fingers are crossed," he said.

[CG, June 1999]

## Weighing the Pros and Cons of Hormone Therapy

Making an informed decision about whether to take replacement hormones during and after menopause is hard enough for women with no prior health problems. It is far more difficult for a woman who has had breast cancer or who has a strong family history of this most common cancer in women. Because estrogen can stimulate the growth of a breast cancer, women and their doctors are understandably reluctant to consider hormone replacement for someone at high risk of developing a new or recurrent cancer.

But this means that such women may miss important health benefits of estrogen after menopause, among them a reduced risk of heart disease, osteoporosis and Alzheimer's disease as well as diminished menopausal symptoms like hot flashes, night sweats and vaginal dryness.

The drug tamoxifen provides another, though imperfect, hormone replacement option for high-risk women to reduce the risk of developing breast cancer. Though it has drawbacks, this so-called "designer estrogen" also offers women who take it an opportunity to glean some of the benefits of estrogen replacement, such as reduced risk of cardiovascular disease.

But these questions remain: Can some former breast cancer patients safely take hormone replacements, and if so, which ones? Are there reasonable alternatives that will grant women at least some benefits of estrogen without adding to their concerns about developing a new or recurrent cancer?

The answers concern 2.4 million American women, and millions more worldwide, who have survived breast cancer, as well as those at high risk of the disease. At a consensus conference in 1997 sponsored by The Hormone Foundation, the Susan G. Komen Breast Cancer Foundation and others, experts and patient advocates concluded that treating menopausal symptoms and long-term health risks in breast cancer patients should be "tailored to individual patients' needs" and employ strategies that "would avoid the use of estrogen while providing its benefits."

Estrogen plays a critical role in the initiation and promotion of breast cancer. Many studies have shown that the longer a woman's breast is exposed to high levels of estrogen, the greater the chances of eventually getting breast cancer. The cells of most breast cancers have receptors for estrogen and respond to the hormone's growth-stimulating effects. Patients with these cancers are typically given treatments to block the effects of their own estrogens.

Recent findings strongly suggest that this increased risk extends to postmenopausal women

## Examining Breast Cancer Risk

As a woman and her doctor discuss whether or not she should use hormone replacement—and take tamoxifen—they need to make an assessment of risk for breast cancer, considering the following factors:

### HIGHEST RISK FACTORS

**Family:** One or more first-degree relatives—mother, daughters or sisters—who have had breast cancer. But only 10 percent to 15 percent of breast cancers are familial, and not all of these are hereditary.

**Genes:** An inherited alteration in the BRCA1 and BRCA2 genes, which are responsible for hereditary breast cancer. Thirty to 70 percent of cases of hereditary breast cancer have mutations in one or both of these genes. If someone with a cancer diagnosis and a family history of the disease has been tested and found to have an altered BRCA1 or BRCA2 gene, others in the family can be tested to see if they also have the mutation.

### OTHER RISK FACTORS

**Age:** Breast cancer mainly strikes older women. By age 35, a woman has a 1 in 622 chance of developing breast cancer. By age 85, the lifetime risk has risen to the familiar 1 in 8.

**Childbirth:** Having a first child at age 30 or later, or having no children, nearly doubles the risk of breast cancer in comparison with the risk faced by a woman who has her first child before reaching 20.

**Early menarche and late menopause:** Both of these factors lengthen the exposure of breast tissue to growth-stimulating estrogens. Menstruation before age 14 carries a risk 30 percent higher than when it begins by age 16. Likewise, a woman who enters menopause at age 55 or later has increased risk.

who take replacement hormones, either estrogen alone or estrogen with progestin (the latter is added to protect the uterine lining from estrogen's growth-stimulating effect). For each year that women take these hormones, the risk of developing breast cancer rises slightly, by roughly equal to the increase associated with a one-year delay in the onset of menopause. After 10 years on hormone replacement, according to the experience of 80,000 nurses, the increase in risk is about 30 percent.

Further evidence of estrogen's influence on breast tissue comes from the effects of designer estrogens like tamoxifen. These substances act as weak estrogens and block the action of natural estrogen in some tissues. Tamoxifen has been shown to help prevent a new or recurrent breast cancer apparently by blocking the stimulating effects of natural estrogen on breast tissue. Early evidence presented recently shows a similar effect by a second designer estrogen, the bone-building drug raloxifene.

Though not ideal substitutes for the real thing, designer estrogens offer high-risk women some estrogen benefits. Tamoxifen, for example, does reduce cardiac risk, but not to the extent that estrogen does. But tamoxifen, like estrogen, also stimulates cell growth in the uterus and increases the risk of uterine cancer. Raloxifene, marketed as Evista to help prevent osteoporosis, also has some of estrogen's cardiovascular benefits and, unlike tamoxifen, it does not stimulate uterine cell growth.

Ongoing research should lead to the development of better designer estrogens, perhaps one that protects the heart, bones and brain as well as the breast and uterus and diminishes menopausal symptoms. Meanwhile, what are the options for a menopausal woman who has had breast cancer or is at high risk of getting it?

First and foremost, she needs to adopt the healthy habits known to or strongly suspected of reducing the risk of heart disease, osteoporosis and Alzheimer's disease. This familiar list includes quitting smoking; achieving and maintaining a normal body weight; doing regular weight-bearing exercise like brisk walking or strength training; reducing consumption of meat and dairy fat, sugars and refined starches; and eating more vegetables, whole grains, beans and fish.

Also, a postmenopausal woman, even if she takes hormones, should consume at least 1,500 milligrams of calcium a day (from nonfat dairy products like yogurt and skim milk, calcium-rich vegetables and calcium-enriched orange juice supplemented, if needed, by calcium tablets). She might also take a daily supplement of vitamin E (200 to 800 International Units, to protect against heart disease and Alzheimer's disease) and vitamin D (to bring her daily total to 800 International Units, for proper absorption and use of calcium).

Many menopausal women have recently turned to the lowly soybean as a substitute for replacement hormones, but the jury is still out on how effective it is. Soy contains weak estrogens called isoflavones, which may mimic some of the effects of natural estrogen. Despite glowing testimonials for soy foods like tofu, tempeh, soy milk and soy-based candy bars, properly designed studies have found that soy is only slightly more effective than a look-alike placebo in controlling hot flashes, a common and easily assessed symptom of menopause. Researchers suspect that soy may help some women substantially, others slightly and still others not at all. Still, experts say soy is worth a try for women with bothersome symptoms.

But, when it comes to the long-term benefits of natural estrogen, the data on soy are preliminary, findings are inconsistent and the amount of soy needed to gain significant benefit is far more than American women are likely to consume. Dr. Mark Messina of Loma Linda University in Loma Linda, California, who consults for the soy industry, said the ability of soy to protect against breast cancer, osteoporosis and heart disease is at best speculative.

If there is an effect on breast cancer risk, it most likely operates during the teen and young adult years rather than after menopause, when a woman's own estrogen production is minimal. Most researchers believe that soy consumption is not the primary reasons Asian women have much lower rates of breast cancer than American women do.

[JEB, September 1998]

## A Study Plays Down Estrogen Link to Breast Cancers

Whether to take estrogen or not is the dilemma faced by millions of women at menopause who want the hormone's protection against heart disease and osteoporosis, and yet fear that it may also increase their risk of breast cancer.

A recent study of 37,105 women offered some reassurance, finding little evidence to link hormone replacement with the most common types of breast cancer, known as ductal carcinoma in situ or invasive ductal or lobular cancer. Ductal and lobular tumors account for 85 percent to 90 percent of all invasive breast cancers.

The researchers did find an increased risk of other, less common types of breast cancer in women who took estrogen. But they said that finding was not completely discouraging, because the types of cancer they found have a better outlook, respond well to treatment and are less likely to spread than the more common forms. The less risky types are called medullary, papillary, tubular and mucinous tumors.

Some other researchers questioned the findings, and most agreed that the new study would not resolve the vexing questions for women. It adds one more page to a catalog of earlier studies that had mixed results, with most showing no link between hormone replacement and breast cancer, and a few finding a small increased risk.

Dr. Thomas A. Sellers, an author of the study and a professor of epidemiology and associate director of the Mayo Clinic Cancer Center in Rochester, Minnesota, said the findings indicate that over all, the benefits of hormone treatment outweigh the risks. In addition to protecting against heart disease and brittle bones, estrogen prevents hot flashes and other symptoms of menopause, and may help preserve mental sharpness.

The other authors of the study were Dr. Susan M. Gapstur and Dr. Monica Morrow of the Northwestern University Medical School. Their article was published in the *Journal of the American Medical Association*.

Dr. Sellers emphasized that the study did not determine whether the benefits of treatment also outweighed risks for women who have a high risk of breast cancer because their mothers, sisters or any other relatives have the disease.

Dr. Patricia Ganz, a cancer researcher and clinician at the Jonsson Cancer Center at the University of California at Los Angeles, said the study would not change the advice that doctors give to high-risk women or those who have already had breast cancer. Dr. Ganz said it was not clear that estrogen was risk-free for those women.

Another expert not involved in the study, Dr. Kathy Helzlsouer, director of breast and ovarian surveillance at the cancer center at Johns Hopkins University in Baltimore, called the study well designed and said it suggested that if there was any risk of breast cancer from the hormones, that risk would be quite small. "From that standpoint it is reassuring," Dr. Helzlsouer said. "But it really needs to be replicated." She said that the number of the less risky cancers in the study, 82, was very small, and that further studies were needed to determine whether the finding would hold up.

Dr. Trudy Busch, an epidemiologist at the University of Maryland School of Medicine in Baltimore, wrote an editorial accompanying the journal article, noting that the most important conclusion was the lack of any connection between hormone replacement therapy and the most common forms of breast cancer. "I think we've gone kind of overboard on this estrogen-breast cancer thing," Dr. Busch said in a telephone interview. "We've been looking for a connection for 50 years, and it doesn't show up."

But Dr. Larry Norton, chief of medical oncology at the Memorial Sloan-Kettering Cancer Center in New York, said the study did not justify a blanket endorsement of estrogen replacement. The types of tumors linked to the treatment tend to be stimulated by estrogen, he said, "and it is sensible that estrogen use will increase their incidence."

The study is one of the few to break down cases of breast cancer by type, rather than grouping them together. "In the past, there have been dozens of studies looking at the risk of breast cancer associated with hormone replacement therapy," Dr. Sellers said. "If you look at all the data, there is a slight risk, perhaps 30 percent. But that's treating breast cancer as a single disease. What we have done in this study is to take what clinicians have long known about breast cancer, that it doesn't always behave the same."

The study, the Iowa Women's Health Study, conducted from 1986 to 1996, followed 37,105 women who were 55 to 69 years old in 1986. About 40 percent of the women had taken hormone replacement therapy. In the entire group, there were 1,520 cases of breast cancer. Among women who had ever taken hormone replacement therapy, the researchers found no increased risk of the more common types of breast cancer.

But the risk of the less common, less dangerous cancers was increased. Women who had taken estrogen for five or fewer years had an 81 percent increase in risk over those who had not taken it, and those who had used it five years or longer had an increase of 265 percent. The figures were adjusted to take age into account, so that the greater risk with longer use was not a reflection of higher risk among older women. The researchers said they could not explain why hormone use should be associated with some types of cancers and not others.

The findings do suggest that replacement therapy is safe for many women, Dr. Sellers said. "But it's easy for me as a scientist and a male to say that," he said. "It's really a personal decision. One in two women in this country die of heart disease, but if you ask their greatest fear, it's breast cancer. The individual's perception of risk is paramount." Recently, his mother asked his advice about starting hormone replacement, and, Dr. Sellers said, "I told her to go for it."

[DG, June 1999]

# Hormone Use Helps Women, a Study Finds

Hormone replacement after menopause can significantly reduce a woman's risk of death as long as she continues it, a large study has found. In the first decade of hormone use, the chance of dying was 37 percent lower among women in the study who were using hormones than among women who did not, primarily because of fewer deaths from heart disease among the users.

But the mortality benefit among those taking hormones dropped to 20 percent after 10 or more years of hormone use when the women's risk of death from breast cancer rose. Increased breast cancer risk is the major worry for women using hormone replacement, but the 16-year study of 60,000 postmenopausal women suggested that even women with breast cancer might benefit as a group, if they took hormones.

The director of the study, Dr. Francine Grodstein, an epidemiologist at Brigham and Women's Hospital in Boston, said that "even if a woman has breast cancer, she is probably more likely to die of heart disease than of breast cancer because the survival rate for breast cancer is high."

Dr. Grodstein said she and her fellow researchers, whose findings were published in *The New England Journal of Medicine*, hoped their results would help to clarify what has been a great source of conflict, concern and confusion among menopausal women and their doctors: how to decide for whom and for how long hormone replacement may be beneficial.

In an accompanying editorial, Dr. Louise A. Brinton and Dr. Catherine Schairer of the National Cancer Institute pointed out that "in some women at low risk for cardiovascular disease but at high risk for breast cancer, the benefits of hormone therapy may not outweigh the risks." They added that decisions about taking replacement hormones "need to be personal ones and should involve detailed discussions between a woman and her physician."

Dr. Lynn Rosenberg, professor of epidemiology at Boston University School of Medicine, said in an interview: "It's time to re-evaluate the way hormone supplements are being used. In many areas they are being prescribed across the board regardless of a woman's risk factors."

Dr. Nananda F. Col, a practicing physician and epidemiologist at New England Medical Center/Tufts University School of Medicine, said: "By looking at total mortality, the study enables us to put all the little pieces together and not just look at the effects of hormones one disease at a time. The study shows that short-term therapy provides benefits without risks in terms of survival. But for long-term therapy, a woman needs to go beyond averages and individually tailor her decision based not only on survival but also on quality of life issues," for example, mood, vaginal dryness and weight gain.

Dr. Col, who published a study on patients' decisions about hormone therapy based on their individual risks in the *Journal of the American Medical Association* in April 1997, said it would be "incorrect to interpret the new findings as saying all women should be on therapy," adding, "but it would be equally incorrect to interpret the study as saying that all women should stop taking hormones after 10 years."

The lowered mortality risk among those who took hormones lasted only a short while among the women who stopped taking them. Three years after discontinuing the hormones the women were no better off than those who never took them. The majority of the women took estrogen alone and the others took a combination of estrogen and progestin. Although cancer deaths, including deaths from breast cancer, also dropped over the first decade of hormone use, women taking replacement hormones for more than 10 years faced a 43 percent increase in their risk of death from breast cancer. Despite this increase, those who continued on hormones had a significantly lower overall mortality rate 16 years later.

Surprisingly, having a family history of breast cancer did not affect the mortality risk associated with hormone use. Among women in the study whose mothers or sisters had breast cancer, hormone replacement was not associated with a greater risk of death than among women with no such family history.

In the first 10 years of hormone use, the women who developed breast cancer had lower death rates from their disease than did women who never took hormones. This may reflect a tendency toward earlier detection of cancer among hormone users, or it may result from stopping estrogen, a known promoter of breast cancer growth, once the cancer was diagnosed, Dr. Grodstein suggested. But, she said, as the women aged the increasing rate of breast cancer overwhelmed these effects and resulted in an overall rise in deaths from breast cancer, although total mortality still remained lower among hormone users.

Dr. Rosenberg said the study showed "we really have to worry about the risk of cancer after women have been on these drugs for many years," adding, "After long-term use, we're beginning to see adverse effects on breast cancer mortality."

The study was conducted among the 121,700 women participating in the continuing Nurses' Health Study, a project that began in 1976, with researchers questioning and examining the women every two years, until 1992. The study is the largest and longest detailed examination of the mortality benefits and risks associated with long-term use of postmenopausal hormones. The participants were similar in education and health backgrounds, reducing the chances that those who chose to take hormones were healthier to begin with. When the data were analyzed taking many risk factors for disease and death into account, the outcome changed little. Previous smaller studies also found a reduction in mortality. But they asked only once about hormone use, which would not account for women who stopped its use.

The newer study showed that women with one or more risk factors for heart disease were likely to derive the greatest mortality benefit from hormone replacement. Over all, these women faced a risk of death half that of similar women who did not take postmenopausal hormones. The risk factors considered were a family history of heart disease, cigarette smoking, high blood pressure, elevated blood cholesterol and obesity. Sixty-nine percent of the study population had one or more factors.

Dr. Grodstein said in an interview that women who wished to avoid the risk of breast cancer associated with long-term hormone use would be wise to reduce their coronary risk by "stopping smoking, exercising regularly, losing weight and eating well." She said, however, that mortality risk should not be a woman's only consideration in deciding whether to take postmenopausal hormones and for how long. "There are also quality-of-life issues, how taking hormones affects a woman's day-to-day life, for good or bad," she said.

Furthermore, she said, "women should recognize that hormone replacement is not a single decision made at menopause. Women and their doctors should re-evaluate that decision every five years or so because the risks and benefits change with time." For example, in the first decade or so after menopause, a woman's risk of death from heart disease does not rise very much, so she may want to consider starting hormone therapy later when her chances of dying of heart disease begin to equal those among men. A recent study showed that women who begin hormone replacement years after menopause can experience a benefit to their bones nearly as great as that associated with hormone use started at menopause.

[JEB, June 1997]

# A Tad of Testosterone Adds Zest to Menopause

**A** friend who remarried at 51 was feeling reborn, enjoying a renewed vitality and rejuvenated sex life with her new husband. But three years later, as she entered menopause and began hormone replacement therapy, her libido crashed. In great distress, she consulted her gynecologist, who suggested that she add a tiny dose of testosterone to her hormone regimen. Within weeks, she was back to feeling like her premenopausal self, once again enjoying sex.

For some women, the discomforting symptoms of menopause go beyond hot flashes, night sweats and vaginal dryness, symptoms that usually respond to estrogen replacement through medication or foods like soy and flaxseed. Some who undergo either natural or surgical menopause experience fatigue, lack of energy, depressed mood and loss of sexual desire that cannot be attributed to their external life circumstances. Rather, their symptoms are more likely the result of a decline in testosterone.

Although most people think of it as a male hormone, and indeed it is responsible for male characteristics like facial hair, muscles and a deep voice, women have testosterone too, though in much lower levels. In women, the hormone is mainly produced in the ovaries and adrenal glands.

If both ovaries are removed surgically from a premenopausal woman, her testosterone level will drop by a third or more. And when a woman's ovarian function declines in the years before and during natural menopause, so does the amount of testosterone she produces. Between a woman's 20s and 40s, the amount of testosterone circulating in her blood declines by about 50 percent, said Dr. Morrie Gelfand, an obstetrician-gynecologist at Sir Mortimer B. Davis Jewish General Hospital in Montreal. If, in addition, the woman starts estrogen replacement at menopause, her blood levels of testosterone drop even further as a result of a biochemical reaction.

As with the menopausal decline in estrogen, in different women the testosterone falloff causes symptoms of varying degrees, from negligible to highly distressing, and the ability of women to tolerate those symptoms varies widely as well. But for those who find their postmenopausal quality of life unaccountably deteriorating despite the use of estrogen, testosterone replacement may be worth trying. First, however, women and their doctors may have to shed some myths about this hormone, as well as consider its potential risks.

Both men and women produce testosterone throughout life in their sex organs, adrenal glands and in various tissues throughout the body. Testosterone is, as one author put it, "the hormone of desire," the substance that acts on the brain to stimulate sexual interest, sensitivity to sexual stimulation and orgasmic ability in both sexes.

Estrogen alone helps to maintain vaginal tissues and lubrication, making intercourse more pleasurable, but it has no direct effect on libido. While testosterone does affect libido and masculine characteristics, it also acts on the bones, brain, muscles, liver and blood vessels. It promotes bone formation and enhances cognitive functions. It has some negative effects as well, including inducing a susceptibility to baldness and increasing the risk of heart disease. But in men, the amount of testosterone emanating from the testes from puberty onward is vastly greater than what a woman produces in her ovaries.

The roles played by the small amount of testosterone circulating in a woman's blood are best deduced from the effects of its absence and replacement. The most common complaint associated with declining levels is an otherwise unexplainable loss of sexual enjoyment. Other symptoms may include depression, anxiety, anger, moodiness, insomnia, fatigue, lack of composure or vitality, memory problems and difficulty concentrating, Dr. Michael J. Rosenberg of the University of North Carolina at Chapel Hill notes.

Dr. Elizabeth Barrett-Connor, an expert on menopause at the University of California at San

Diego, pointed out that "one size doesn't fit all in hormone replacement." Rather, she said, "hormone therapy should be tailored to each individual according to symptoms, and combination estrogen-androgen therapy can be significantly better for some women than estrogen alone."

Dr. Gloria A. Bachmann, an obstetrician-gynecologist at the University of Medicine and Dentistry of New Jersey and Robert Wood Johnson Medical School, said testosterone therapy "may be underutilized because many women don't know that they could feel better." She and others believe that the decision to try testosterone replacement should be based on a woman's symptoms and her desire to eliminate them. Most experts say there is little point in trying to measure a menopausal woman's blood level of testosterone, since at the very low levels a woman produces the measurements are not very accurate or meaningful.

Dr. Susan Rako, a psychiatrist in Newtonville, Massachusetts, and author of *The Hormone of Desire*, listed the following as the most obvious signs of testosterone deficiency: overall decreased sexual desire, diminished vital energy and sense of well-being, decreased sensitivity of the clitoris and nipples to sexual stimulation, overall decreased arousability, diminished capacity for orgasm and thinning and loss of pubic hair. "The wipeout of sexual desire that results from a critical reduction in testosterone is different from the fluctuations we experience with the various ups and downs of life and relationships," she wrote.

Dr. Barbara Sherwin, a professor of psychology and obstetrics and gynecology at McGill University in Montreal, says many doctors harbor mistaken notions about testosterone therapy for women. They think, incorrectly, that it will turn women into men, make them grow a beard or make them overly aggressive or sexually demanding. "Of course," Dr. Sherwin said, "it doesn't do any of that in the doses used postmenopausally. The goal is to reinstate what the woman had before menopause, to bring her back to what she was and how she felt." Many of the myths stem from high-dose testosterone treatments for other, unrelated medical conditions, which can cause virilization—growth of facial hair, loss of scalp hair, deepening of the voice and weight gain. If even the hint of such changes occurs in a woman who is being treated with postmenopausal testosterone, the dose can be reduced and the symptoms reversed, except for voice changes.

The one major medical concern is a testosterone-induced decline in a woman's blood levels of protective HDL cholesterol. But the therapy also lowers harmful LDL cholesterol and triglycerides. And, unlike estrogen, which merely slows postmenopausal bone loss, testosterone therapy increases bone mass and is therefore more effective than estrogen in preventing osteoporosis.

[JEB, February 1998]

## Keeping Clinical Depression Out of the Aging Formula

Depression among older people is an often unrecognized and untreated problem that can tarnish the golden years for millions of people who might otherwise find joy, not anguish, in their old age. That includes older people in nursing homes as well as those living independently. Experts estimate that as many as 90 percent of depressed elderly Americans are not being treated.

More than five million Americans age 65 and older—nearly one in six—suffer from serious, persistent symptoms of depression, and another one million have major clinical depression, an immobilizing disorder that can lead to suicide. From 1980 to 1992, suicide rates rose by 9 percent among all Americans 65 and older and by 35 percent among those aged 80 to 84. Only a small percentage of those deaths are believed to represent a calculated escape from an incurable, incapacitating illness.

Most older people contemplating suicide see their primary care doctor within the month before killing themselves, and 40 percent make that visit in the week before committing suicide. Rarely do these doctors detect suicidal potential in older people before it is too late.

The failure to treat depression in the elderly, as in younger people, is a costly mistake. It can lead to a loss of self-reliance and the ability to live independently, which in turn increases the burden on other family members and the cost of daily care and medical care. Depression increases the likelihood that a serious physical illness will develop or get worse. Depressed older people make more medical visits, require more tests and stay longer in hospitals. Also lost is the contribution they can make to their families and society, including caring for children and elderly friends, meal preparation, tutoring and volunteer work for myriad social and cultural organizations.

Many mistaken beliefs and expectations about depression and aging impede effective treatment that would brighten the days of older people, improve their physical health and enhance their relationships with family members and friends.

**MYTH**—It is natural to become increasingly depressed with age.

**FACT**—Dr. Barry D. Liebowitz, an expert on the emotional disorders of aging at the National Institute of Mental Health, said, "Depression is not the outcome of natural processes of aging and should not be considered normal." Advancing age per se does not cause depression.

**MYTH**—Of course older people are depressed; their spouses and friends are dying all around them.

**FACT**—The death of spouses, companions and friends can cause profound sadness and sometimes even major depression, but at any age mentally healthy people bounce back from such losses and, within a year or so, find new sources of support and pleasure. Untreated depression, on the other hand,

often results in social isolation, which only exacerbates the depression.

**MYTH**—So many older people have serious health problems, why wouldn't they be depressed?

**FACT**—Mentally healthy people of any age who have chronic physical disabilities or diseases soon learn to adapt to their limitations and get the most out of life that they can. It is not so much that illness causes depression as that depression increases the risk of illness, functional decline and even symptoms of dementia.

Sometimes, however, the biological consequences of a health problem—not the person's reaction to it—or the medications used to treat another illness can cause depression. For example, as many as 40 percent of stroke victims experience changes in brain chemicals, and those changes result in chronic depression. Experts also suspect that there are many other older people who become depressed following hidden strokes, including transient ischemic attacks.

**MYTH**—Older people who are healthy and financially secure have no reason to be depressed; they should be happy about their good fortune.

**FACT**—With rare exception, depression is a medical illness. People who are ill with diabetes or arthritis, say, are not expected to cure themselves by changing their mental outlook. If people who are depressed could "look on the bright side," "pull themselves together " or "be grateful for all the good things"—as they are often told to do—they would. What they need is concern, compassion and effective treatment.

At any age, depression can be difficult to diagnose because it has many different causes and symptoms. In older people, the picture is often complicated by the coexistence of other serious physical problems that overshadow the depression. Too often, depression is overlooked because it is seen as "understandable" in light of the person's other problems. But whether depression is precipitated by death of a spouse or a heart attack or it seems to strike out of the blue, it warrants professional attention. In every case, relief of the depression can facilitate a person's return to normal functioning.

Among the elderly, the classic symptoms of depression—deep sadness and lack of pleasure in people and activities they once enjoyed—are often replaced by irritability and apathy, a pervasive disinterest in life and what it may have to offer. Other common hallmarks of depression in the elderly include difficulty concentrating, memory lapses, loss of appetite, diminished energy and a physical slowing down. These symptoms are easily mistaken for signs of age—and disregarded.

Dr. Liebowitz, writing in *The Decade of the Brain*, a publication of the National Alliance for the Mentally

## Help for Depression

The following organizations can provide helpful information about the detection and treatment of depression for people of all ages.

**NATIONAL RESOURCES INCLUDE:**

- **National Alliance for the Mentally Ill,** 200 North Glebe Road, Suite 1015, Arlington, VA 22203, 1-800-950-6264, www.nami.org.

- **National Depressive and Manic Depressive Association,** 730 North Franklin Street, Suite 501, Chicago, IL 60610, 1-800-826-3632, www.ndmda.org.

- **National Foundation for Depressive Illness,** P.O. Box 2257, New York, NY 10116, 1-800-248-4344.

- **National Institute of Mental Health,** 5600 Fishers Lane, Suite 7C-02, Rockville, MD 20857, 1-800-421-4211, www.nimh.nih.gov.

Ill, pointed out that "depression is chronic and recurring and requires long-term treatment accompanied by lifestyle changes and, commonly, environmental manipulations. Social support—particularly from family members—is critical." In other words, treating depression in the elderly is similar to treating it in younger people.

But there are some important differences. Dr. Herbert W. Harris, also of the National Institute of Mental Health, noted that adverse reactions to antidepressant drugs are more common in older people, who tend to develop unwanted side effects even at relatively low doses. Doctors must also look out for adverse interactions with other medicines the patients take. Sometimes the patient must try several different treatments in succession before the one with the most benefit and fewest side effects is found.

Older people who are depressed can also be their worst enemies. Compliance with treatment tends to be poor and short-lived, particularly in light of drug side effects, the number of drugs many of them have to take for other conditions and the lack of follow-up by the prescribing physician.

Another inhibiting factor in effective treatment is the belief of doctors and families that depression is the least of an older person's problems. Yet, Dr. George S. Alexopoulos, a psychiatrist at Cornell University Medical College, reports that treating depression in a patient with Alzheimer's disease, for example, improves both the depression and the symptoms of dementia. And among patients with heart disease and those living in nursing homes, treating depression improves physical functioning, decreases pain, improves the person's outlook and prolongs life.

[JEB, November 1998]

# Test at Onset of Menopause Can Avert Bone Loss

My friend Carole and I paid a long overdue visit to the Osteoporosis Prevention Center at the Hospital for Special Surgery in New York to have the density of our bones measured. Carole is 59 and I am approaching 57, and we both should have had this test done for the first time when we entered menopause around age 50, repeating it, if warranted by the initial results and our risk factors, a few years later.

But neither of us had any reason to believe our bones would be anything less than perfect. We do not smoke or drink much alcohol and never did. We are not skinny and have never been anorexic. We do weight-bearing exercise every day. We both began estrogen replacement at menopause. Neither of us has a family history of osteoporosis. I have consumed a quart of milk a day for most of my life, and Carole takes a calcium supplement and a multivitamin containing vitamin D and calcium in addition to getting some dietary calcium from yogurt and tofu on most days. Why wouldn't our bones be in great shape?

So we were confident as we lay on the examining table while the arm of a special X-ray machine passed over our lower spines and right hips. The test, called dual-energy X-ray absorptiometry, uses the amount of radiation one would get flying from New York to Los Angeles and is the most reliable way to measure the mineral content of one's bones. It involves no injections, dyes, sedation, special diets or any other advance preparation, just the ability to lie still for about one minute. You do not even have to get undressed. And most insurance plans cover the cost, which ranges from about $150 to $300.

As it turned out, the bone density of my spine and hips were good—nearly as good as that of a 35-year-old woman with healthy bones. In most women, bone density peaks between the ages of 30 and 35, making this the benchmark for maximum bone density. But Carole was shocked to discover that while the density of her hip bones was borderline normal, the density of her spine was well below normal, approaching the level that the World Health Organization defines as osteoporotic and that many doctors now treat with bone-enhancing drugs.

Had Carole known earlier that her bones were thinning at an accelerated rate, she could have made some dietary changes years ago to increase her calcium intake and thus slow the loss of bone. Judith Andariese, the nurse-practitioner at the osteoporosis center who evaluated Carole's test results, also gave Carole a urine test to see whether her bones were being broken down faster than they reformed, which fortunately they were not.

Ms. Andariese advised Carole to keep up her exercise regimen, handed her a comprehensive list of calcium-rich foods and told her to eat more of them and to double her calcium supplement to achieve a total calcium intake of 1,500 milligrams a day. Ms. Andariese also recommended that Carole repeat the bone density test in a year to check on her progress and determine whether more aggressive treatment with a bone-building drug was warranted.

Men get osteoporosis, too—one in five patients is male—and the National Osteoporosis Foundation recommends a bone density test for men as well as women with several risk factors for bone loss, including a family history of the disease and a personal history of smoking and drinking.

Concern about bone density should start decades before menopause. Theresa Galsworthy, director of the center, said that failure to build strong bones through a calcium-rich diet in childhood, adolescence and young adulthood leaves one with a slender bank account of bone mineral when the withdrawals start exceeding the deposits after age 35 and especially when those withdrawals accelerate greatly at menopause. Although hormone replacement and weight-bearing exercise can slow postmenopausal bone loss, they cannot do much for bones when calcium is in short supply. But consuming enough calcium through foods or supplements or both is not as simple as many women think.

The current recommended calcium intake for women over 50 who are on hormone replacement is 1,000 milligrams a day, rising to 1,500 milligrams for women not on hormones and for all women over 65. But if your diet is rich in animal protein—say, more than four ounces a day of meat, poultry or fish—your calcium needs rise even further, to about 1,500 to 1,800 milligrams even if you take estrogen. In addition, without an adequate supply of vitamin D, your body cannot properly absorb and utilize calcium.

There are three sources of vitamin D: foods like fortified milk and products made from fortified milk (yogurt is not among them), as well as some fish; supplements (either a multivitamin with vitamin D or calcium with D); and sun-exposed skin. Although it takes only 15 minutes a day of sun on the face to produce enough vitamin D, current advice to avoid the sun and always use sunscreen have greatly decreased the body's ability to manufacture vitamin D from sunlight. Also, in winter in northern latitudes, the oblique angle of the sun means fewer effective rays reach the skin.

Milk and milk products are still the best all-around sources of dietary calcium; nonfat and low-fat versions have more calcium than their fattier cousins. Eight ounces of skim or 1 percent milk provide nearly 300 milligrams, and a cup of nonfat yogurt has 400 milligrams. You can increase the calcium content of milk even further by adding some nonfat powdered milk to liquid milk or by preparing a more concentrated solution of powdered milk than the package calls for, say, by using one cup of powder to prepare 24 ounces of milk, which would give you about 502 milligrams of calcium per cup. If you are lactose-intolerant, you can buy lactose-reduced milk or add the enzyme lactase to regular or reconstituted powdered milk. Also, you should be able to digest yogurt with active cultures.

Hard cheeses (choose lower-fat varieties like Swiss and Jarlsberg) are better calcium sources than soft cheeses and cottage cheese; one-half cup creamed cottage cheese has 109 milligrams as against 260 in one ounce of Swiss.

Good nondairy sources of calcium include sardines and canned salmon eaten with the bones; calcium-fortified orange juice (200 milligrams in six ounces); tofu precipitated with calcium (check the package label or write to the manufacturer); dark-green leafy vegetables like arugula (the best, with 309 milligrams in half a cup), collards, bok choy, dandelion greens, kale, mustard and turnip greens, and figs.

But other calcium-rich vegetables like spinach, chard, sorrel, parsley and beet greens are not good sources because they contain oxalic acid, which inhibits calcium absorption. Also note that very high-fiber grains like wheat bran cereal reduce calcium absorption from milk by about one-third. However, neither coffee nor caffeine impedes calcium absorption.

If you must rely partly or entirely on calcium supplements, take them in divided doses (morning, noon and evening) with a meal to maximize absorption.

[JEB, March 1998]

## Guidelines Offer an Earlier Blueprint
## for the Battle Against Bone Loss

Osteoporosis is a silent disease. Just as a heart attack is often the first clue to the existence of atherosclerosis, a fracture is usually the first indication that a person's bones have become dangerously weakened. But it doesn't have to be that way. According to guidelines issued in 1998 by the National Osteoporosis Foundation, it is now possible to determine a person's propensity for fracture far in advance and offer preventive treatments for most people at risk of developing osteoporosis.

This is not a problem to be dismissed lightly. Osteoporosis is responsible for about 1.5 million fractures a year that incur medical costs of $38 million each day. An estimated 28 million Americans have already lost enough bone to be at great risk of suffering a fracture. Half of all women over 50 and one in eight men over 50 will suffer an osteoporosis-related fracture in their lifetimes. And when the fracture involves the hip, as it does in 300,000 people a year, it is fatal in 20 percent of cases.

Nor is osteoporosis a concern only for the elderly. Bone loss starts around ages 30 to 35, and in women who do not take hormone replacement, that loss accelerates rapidly in the first five or six years after menopause. By age 65, bones can be so weakened that even the best available remedies cannot prevent them from breaking. Yet, according to a survey last year of 30,000 Americans, 71 percent of women with osteoporosis do not know they have it, and 86 percent with the disease are not being treated. A bone density test is the only way to determine the health of your bones and how to preserve or improve it.

Ideally, all women aged 50 or older and men aged 65 or older should have their bone health checked. Given current limits to available medical resources and finances, the National Osteoporosis Foundation recommends a bone density test for the following individuals:

▶ All women 65 and older, regardless of other risk factors. Medicare now reimburses for bone density testing in eligible women.
▶ All women past menopause who have already had a fracture, including the vertebral fractures that cause a shortening and hunching of the spine.
▶ Women past menopause who have any risk factor for suffering an osteoporotic fracture.

Based on studies of many thousands of people, the foundation lists the leading risk factors as: a personal history of fracture as an adult, regardless of what caused it; a history of fracture in a first-degree relative (parent or sibling); current cigarette smoking; and having a small, thin frame, defined by a body weight of less than 127 pounds.

There is a much longer list of secondary risk factors, secondary only in that they may be less common or less well documented. But they are no less important. They include certain nonmodifiable factors: being of the Caucasian race, advanced in age, frail or in poor health or suffering from dementia. The more modifiable risk factors include having a diet low in calcium; having an eating disorder (anorexia or bulimia); and being estrogen deficient (including having undergone menopause before age 45 or having had more than a year without menstrual periods—other than during pregnancy—before menopause); and for men, having a low level of testosterone; consuming large amounts of alcohol and being sedentary or subject to repeated falls.

The new guidelines also suggest a bone density test for women considering treatment for osteoporosis if the test will help them reach a reasoned decision. They also recommend testing for women who have been on hormone replacement for many years, a suggestion that may seem strange, since estrogen after menopause protects the bones. However, Dr. Robert Lindsay, president of the foundation, explained that "many women are inconsistent in their use of hormones—they periodically stop taking them—and doctors should not assume that women on hormone replacement are not osteoporotic." Still other risks include the presence of any one of a long list of diseases, especially ones that interfere with the consumption or absorption of calcium or vitamin D, and long-term use of steroids and other drugs used to treat rheumatoid arthritis, epilepsy, thyroid deficiency, bipolar disorder (manic depression) and cancer.

Do not wait for your doctor to recommend a bone density test. If you fall into any of the high-risk categories, talk the matter over with your health care provider and, if necessary, ask to have your bones tested.

Regular X-rays are not able to detect bone loss until it is well-advanced. The foundation listed five tests that are considered "good predictors of future fracture risk." The Cadillac of tests is called dual-energy X-ray absorptiometry, better known as Dexa. It can accurately measure bone mineral density in the spine, hip or wrist, takes only a few minutes (the

---

## A Look at Those at Risk

The National Osteoporosis Foundation lists the following as risk factors.

### PRIMARY FACTORS

- A history of fracture as an adult, regardless of cause.
- A history of fracture in a parent or sibling.
- Cigarette smoking.
- Having a small, thin frame.

### SECONDARY FACTORS

**Nonmodifiable**

- Being Caucasian.
- Advanced in age.
- Frail or in poor health.
- Suffering from dementia.

**Modifiable**

- A diet low in calcium.
- An eating disorder.
- Estrogen deficient.
- Low testosterone, men.
- Drinking to excess.
- Physical inactivity.

---

patient stays clothed and no dyes are injected in any of the tests) and involves only a tiny amount of radiation—one-tenth of the amount in a standard chest X-ray.

However, Dexa is not available in all communities. The other four recommended tests are single-energy X-ray absorptiometry and peripheral dual-energy X-ray absorptiometry to measure the bones of the forearm, finger and sometimes the heel; radiographic absorptiometry to measure bones in the hand; quantitative computed tomography commonly used to measure spinal bone; and, the least precise, ultrasound densitometry to assess bones in the heel, calf, knee and other peripheral sites.

The status of the patient's bones is defined by comparing their density to that of a normal adult—usually a 35-year-old woman. The tests results are measured in standard deviations (S.D.s), and 1 S.D. below normal is equivalent to a 10 to 12 percent decrease in density. Thus, within 1 S.D. of normal, bones are considered healthy; between 1 and 2.5 S.D.s below normal, bone mass is low and at serious risk of becoming osteoporotic; and at 2.5 S.D.s or more below normal, the diagnosis is osteoporosis.

While it is never too late to slow bone loss and even improve bone density, the sooner preventive treatment is started, the better. New guidelines suggest that all men and women, regardless of bone density, consume adequate amounts of calcium and vitamin D (at least 1,200 milligrams of calcium and 400 to 800 International Units of vitamin D daily); get regular weight-bearing exercise like walking or dancing; avoid tobacco use and abuse of alcohol; and make sure vision is properly corrected to reduce the risk of falls.

The foundation also recommended drug treatment to improve bone density in women whose bones are below 2 S.D.s in the absence of other risks or below 1.5 S.D.s when other risk factors are present. Four drugs are approved to prevent or treat osteoporosis. They are hormone replacement therapy (associated with a 50 to 80 percent decrease in spinal fractures and a 25 percent decrease in other fractures with five years of use); alendronate, also known as Fosamax, which can reduce fractures of the spine, hip and wrist by 50 percent in patients with osteoporosis; calcitonin, delivered as an intranasal spray, which may reduce spinal fractures by about 40 percent; and the newest therapy, raloxifene (Evista), which prevents bone loss and may reduce the risk of spinal fracture 40 to 50 percent.

A final word: Parents now armed with the facts about bone density should make sure their children consume adequate amounts of calcium and vitamin D, stay physically active throughout childhood and into adulthood and avoid smoking and alcohol abuse. More than their bones is at stake.

[JEB, November 1998]

## New Drug Helps Delay Bone Loss

My friend Helen was certain that osteoporosis was one problem she would not have to worry about. She had been taking estrogen since menopause and calcium supplements for years. She quit smoking decades ago and remained unusually physically active throughout her adult life. Now in her 70s, she regularly walked for exercise, cycled to her tennis games and ice-skated daily all winter. Then one day last winter in the middle of a skating lesson, Helen found herself lying on the ice with a broken hip and arm. She had not tripped or slipped, suggesting that the fall may have resulted from her hip breaking rather than the other way around.

When I visited her in the hospital, Helen lamented: "My doctor wanted me to take Fosamax, and I didn't listen. He said every American woman over 65 has osteoporosis, but I was sure I was not among them."

Fosamax is one of several new drugs that can help people at risk of developing osteoporosis as well as those who have it. It is especially useful for the majority of postmenopausal women who cannot or will not take estrogen replacement, the treatment of choice for preserving bone density after the ovaries have stopped producing this bone-sparing hormone.

In Helen's case, instead of assuming that she was losing bone despite her daily regimen, the doctor should have sent her for a bone density test. Had Helen seen the extent of her risk of fracture from the results of such a test, she would almost certainly have taken this drug, which can increase bone density in the spine and hip and cut in half a woman's risk of spinal fractures.

Despite their solid appearance, bones are fluid structures. Bone is constantly being broken down (resorbed is the medical word) by cells called osteoclasts and rebuilt by cells called osteoblasts. Early in life, the action of osteoblasts outpaces that of osteoclasts and, as long as there is adequate calcium and vitamin D in one's diet, bone mass will increase. But even in the presence of estrogen, which helps to sustain the action of osteoblasts, in a woman's late 20s or early 30s bone rebuilding gradually begins to lose ground to bone resorption.

Then at menopause, the abrupt loss of estrogen greatly accelerates the process, and by age 65 or 70 a woman who has not taken estrogen could find herself with very fragile bones. An estimated 20 million American women have osteoporosis, and the fractures they suffer result in medical costs of $10 billion a year.

Many factors besides estrogen influence the risk of osteoporosis. Heredity is an important one, so if your mother had osteoporosis, you may be at greater than average risk of developing it as well. Women who are thin are more at risk than those who are heavier, and white women are more susceptible to osteoporosis than blacks. Cigarette smoking, excessive consumption of alcohol, inadequate calcium and vitamin D in the diet (especially during one's bone-forming years) and inadequate weight-bearing exercise increase the likelihood of reaching midlife with bones that are too thin.

The only way to determine the density of one's bones and an estimate of their likelihood of breaking is a bone density test. The best of these tests is called dual X-ray absorptiometry and it should be used to measure the density of the bones in the spine or hip or both, not just the wrist.

For someone who has already sustained significant bone loss or who has suffered one or more fractures related to osteoporosis (including people who have lost height when vertebral fractures compressed the spine), there are a few possible treatments. Estrogen replacement starting at menopause is the most widely used and best studied, but it is not suitable for every woman and cannot be taken by men. Of the new drugs, the best known is Fosamax, the brand-name for the drug alendronate sodium. It is absorbed into the latticework of bone, where it inhibits the cells that break down bone.

Fosamax, which is 100 to 500 times more potent

than a predecessor, Didronel, at inhibiting bone resorption, is suitable for men as well as women. In one study, a daily regimen of 5 or 10 milligrams of Fosamax increased bone mass in the spine and hip by 4 percent to 7 percent in just two years, comparable to the increase associated with estrogen replacement. Another three-year study showed that the drug significantly reduced vertebral fractures and prevented them in women with osteoporosis who had not yet suffered spinal shortening. And at a recent meeting of the American Society for Bone and Mineral Research in Cincinnati, Dr. Steven R. Cummings reported that Fosamax reduced the risk of spinal fracture by 44 percent among 2,214 healthy women with thin bones.

Dosing rules must be followed religiously to avoid serious erosion of the esophagus and digestive upset. It is taken daily upon awakening 30 to 60 minutes before eating, drinking or taking any medication. It should be swallowed with eight ounces of plain water (not mineral water, coffee, tea or juice), after which you must remain upright—standing or sitting—for at least 30 minutes. If you forget your morning dose, do not take it later in the day.

Fosamax should not be taken if you have an esophageal disorder, advanced kidney disease or low levels of calcium in your blood or if you are pregnant or nursing or cannot remain upright for half an hour.

A second option is a drug called calcitonin-salmon, administered as a nasal spray under the trade name Miacalcin. This drug was initially given by injection or rectal suppository, but is now available as a nasal spray administered daily in alternating nostrils. Miacalcin Nasal Spray is recommended for women five or more years past menopause who cannot or will not take estrogen. Calcitonin inhibits bone loss and can increase bone density when there are high levels of calcium in the blood. Those who use it should consume at least 1,000 milligrams of supplemental calcium and 400 International Units of vitamin D each day. Its main side effect is nasal irritation, which is usually mild and temporary.

Unlike Fosamax and Miacalcin, which slow bone breakdown, sodium fluoride, a treatment not yet approved for general use, stimulates the bone-forming osteoblasts. It is administered in a slow-release form, twice daily for 12 months, followed by a two-month hiatus before the drug is resumed. In a one-year study in postmenopausal women who had sustained vertebral fractures, sodium fluoride increased spinal bone density up to 5 percent and greatly reduced the fracture rate.

Another option is the custom-designed synthetic estrogen raloxifene, which has been shown to stimulate bone formation but not cell growth in the breast or uterus, and thus should be free of the cancer risks associated with postmenopausal estrogen therapy.

[JEB, September 1997]

# For Some Women, Losing Pounds Could Add Up to a Hip Fracture

It is taken as an article of faith that a leaner body is a healthier body. But for some people, losing weight appears to be a health hazard.

A study by the National Institute on Aging has found that women who lose a lot of weight beginning at the age of 50 significantly increase their risk of hip fractures. The increase is so pronounced that the researchers are recommending that doctors take the weight history of postmenopausal women into account when assessing their hip-fracture risks and prescribing preventive measures. The research is among the first to identify characteristics of healthy people that predispose them to debilitating hip fractures years later.

"A lot of what we know about hip fractures comes from studies of what happens to people when they get osteoporosis and from case studies of people with hip fractures," said Dr. Tamara Harris, one of the researchers, who is chief of the office of geriatric epidemiology at the institute. "We looked at what happens to people before they get sick."

Each year 250,000 Americans suffer hip fractures, studies show. In most cases, the immediate cause is a fall. But what makes the fall likely to cause the fracture is osteoporosis, an appreciable loss of bone mass that often comes with age. Seventeen percent of all 50-year-old white women will fracture a hip during their remaining years, as will 6 percent of men. White women are at especially high risk because they are among those most likely to develop osteoporosis.

Despite advances in hip replacement surgery, fewer than half the people with hip fractures fully recover. Ten percent to 20 percent of them die within a year of the injury, and half of those who survive remain disabled, living out their years in nursing homes or dependent on the care of relatives and friends, said Dr. Steven R. Cummings, chief of general internal medicine at the University of California at San Francisco.

The study, published in May 1996 in *The Archives of Internal Medicine*, followed 3,683 women who were 67 and older. Researchers asked them to recall how much they weighed at the age of 50, then charted their weight changes and incidence of hip fractures for eight years.

All the women in the study who lost 10 percent or more of their weight since age 50 increased their odds of fracturing a hip. The increase was greatest for the lean women—those who at 50 had the lowest body mass as measured by their weight in relation to their height. For example, Dr. Harris says, a woman standing 5'4" tall who weighed 110 pounds at 50 would fall into this category. The lean women in the study who lost as little as 5 percent or more of their weight increased their risk of hip fracture twofold, as compared with lean women whose weight remained stable.

The women of average body mass who lost 10 percent or more of their weight also had a twofold increase in risk. An example would be a woman who was 5'4" tall and weighed 140 pounds, Dr. Harris

said. Even the heavyset women in the study nearly doubled their risk of hip fracture if they lost 10 percent or more of their weight. An example would be a woman who was 5'4" tall and weighed 175 pounds, she said.

It has long been known that lean women have the greatest risk of hip fractures. The most obvious reason is that they have relatively low bone mass. They also have low levels of estrogen, a hormone that helps to maintain bone mass. And they have little fat to cushion their bones during falls. But the researchers believe that their study shows that weight loss after menopause is a risk factor apart from low body mass. "Our study suggests that weight loss increases the risk above just being skinny," Dr. Harris said.

Women often lose weight after menopause. Many postmenopausal women lose weight for the same reasons that younger people do—they go on diets or begin exercising. But many also lose weight because of illnesses like cancer, lung disease and rheumatoid arthritis.

The aging institute did not look at the reasons why the women in its study lost weight. But Dr. Kristine Ensrud, an internist and epidemiologist at the University of Minnesota in Minneapolis, has been studying whether certain kinds of weight loss are more dangerous than others. Researchers speculate that weight loss from a developing but perhaps undiagnosed illness accounts for most of the increased risk of hip fractures. They think that the illness causes general weakness, which predisposes people to falls, and that the weight loss causes bone loss, which increases the risk of fractures.

But experts believe that dieting after 50 can be risky, too. "If you lose weight by dieting, you lose bone density," Dr. Cummings said. It is not known whether losing weight by exercising is any safer. Weight-bearing exercise like walking is known to preserve bone, but Dr. Cummings said there might still be a net loss of bone in someone who had lost a lot of weight.

Dr. Harris and her colleagues hope that many hip fractures can be prevented if women become aware that significant weight loss after menopause is a risk factor. The researchers say that women who lose a lot of weight can do several things to help offset the damage to their bones, like taking supplements of calcium and vitamin D and talking with their doctors about the two medications that prevent hip fractures. Estrogen-replacement therapy and a new nonhormonal drug called alendronate each reduce the risk of hip fractures in people with osteoporosis by 51 percent, according to findings announced by the University of California at San Francisco.

For women who are unsure whether it is healthier to shed excess pounds or abandon all efforts to diet, Dr. Cummings had this advice: "Prevention of hip fractures is not a good reason to avoid losing weight if one is overweight." After all, obesity increases the risk of heart disease, and this kills more women than hip fractures. And so, he said, the best approach is to reach a normal weight and stay there.

[SG, June 1996]

# Women's Greatest Fear: Breast Cancer

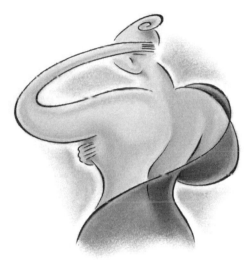

## DETECTION AND TREATMENT CONTINUE TO IMPROVE

For many women, no illness inspires as much dread as breast cancer. The disease is linked in women's minds to images of mutilating surgery, harsh drugs, suffering and death. And the numbers are chilling: 78,700 new cases in 1998, 43,500 deaths.

But researchers say that women overestimate their risk of getting breast cancer, and also overestimate the odds that the disease will be fatal. Few feel anywhere near the same dread of heart disease, even though it kills far more women, and few realize that lung cancer surpassed breast cancer 10 years ago as the leading cause of death from cancer in women. Much of the fear of breast cancer comes from the widely quoted statistic that over the course of a lifetime, one in eight women will develop breast cancer.

But contrary to what women have been led to believe, there is no decade in a woman's life in which her risk of developing breast cancer is one in eight. For women entering their 30s, it is 1 in 250, and for those in their 40s it is 1 in 77. It never exceeds 1 in 34, which occurs during a woman's 60s and 70s.

Survival rates are also better than many women realize. When the disease is treated early, before it can spread, 97 percent of patients are still alive five years later, according to the American Cancer Society. But if the cancer reaches lymph nodes, the five-year rate is 76 percent, and if it invades bones or other organs, the rate is only 21 percent.

Among all women with the disease, at all stages, 50 percent to 60 percent survive 15 years. But in women who are treated early, survival is higher.

The death rate actually declined 5.6 percent from 1990 to 1994, a drop that researchers attributed to better detection and treatment, and that some thought would turn out to be just the beginning of a major decrease in deaths.

# In Breast Cancer Data—Hope, Fear and Confusion

When they are asked to identify the greatest threat to their health, most American women name breast cancer. Most of them are wrong. Women overestimate their risk of getting breast cancer, researchers say, and they also overestimate the odds that the disease will be fatal. Few feel anywhere near the same dread of heart disease, even though it kills far more women, and few realize that lung cancer surpassed breast cancer 10 years ago as the leading cause of death from cancer in women.

Though some women have genes that greatly increase their risk of contracting the disease, the majority do not, and doctors worry that, over all, excessive fear of breast cancer may lead women to neglect the other conditions that are much more likely to kill them: to be cavalier about smoking or lack of exercise, for instance, or to refuse estrogen replacement therapy after menopause.

Even though estrogen is strongly recommended for women at risk for cardiovascular disease, some who would probably benefit from it turn it down, preferring to take their chances with a heart attack or stroke rather than accept what so far appears to be a small increased risk of breast cancer linked to the hormone.

Advanced heart failure "sounds like something you can live with, even though it's a fatal disease," said Dr. Barbara Weber, director of the Breast Cancer Program at the University of Pennsylvania Cancer Center in Philadelphia. "It sounds less painful than breast cancer. And taking blood pressure medicine and nitroglycerin doesn't sound so bad. But chemotherapy is frightening."

A study published in January 1999 reflected the lengths to which women would go in hope of avoiding the disease: The study included 639 women at high risk who chose to have both breasts removed while they were still healthy. The surgery, not commonly performed, did yield an 80 to 90 percent reduction in cases and deaths from breast cancer—but only 18 lives were saved, meaning that many of the women who had their breasts removed may have survived without the drastic procedure.

Of course, some fear of breast cancer is still not unreasonable. The numbers are daunting: 178,700 new cases in 1998, 43,500 deaths. Nearly every woman knows someone, or knows of someone, who died of breast cancer. In women's minds, the disease and the treatments for it are inextricably tied to disfigurement, suffering and death.

Women also associate breast cancer with dying young. Although more women die of heart disease every year—it accounts for 30 percent of all deaths among women, as opposed to 3 percent from breast cancer—it is also true that in some of their most vibrant years, their mid-30s to mid-50s, more women die of breast cancer than heart disease. Early deaths among family or friends loom large in many women's memories.

Some of the women who die young, particularly in families with many cases of breast cancer, may have carried a gene that predisposed them to the disease. Studies during the past decade have identified mutations in two genes, known as BRCA1 and BRCA2, that greatly increase a woman's risk of breast cancer, but inherited breast cancer is still thought to account for only 10 to 15 percent of cases.

Nevertheless, well-meaning public health campaigns may have made some of the fears even worse than they should be. The prediction that one in eight women in the United States will develop breast cancer is one of the most quoted and, to many women, most alarming statistics ever promoted by the National Cancer Institute and the American Cancer Society.

The number is technically correct. But it is also confusing and misleading, and it may serve to make a disease that is already bad enough sound even worse. When cancer specialists sit down with a woman to estimate her personal risk, one in eight is not the statistic they use.

"It's a double-edged sword," said Dr. Weber. "It has heightened women's awareness, and it's probably responsible for getting them to have mammograms and breast examinations. It may have helped get money for research. But the downside is that many people are overly frightened, and overestimate their risk."

Virtually every healthy woman she counsels about risk, Dr. Weber said, has an exaggerated notion, sometimes wildly so, of her own peril from the disease.

The one-in-eight statistic derives from research on large populations of women, studied from birth to death. When all the cases of breast cancer, including those in women who live past 85, are added up over the years, one in eight women, or 12.5 percent, get the disease.

But the one-in-eight figure does not mean that any individual woman, at any given time, has a one-in-eight risk of getting cancer that year—or even in the next 10 years. Rather, the figures apply to the population as a whole, and cannot predict individual variation in risk from one woman to another due to genetic and environmental differences, like obesity and alcohol intake.

In addition, the single lifetime statistic does not reflect the fact that a woman's risk actually changes with time.

Most important, doctors emphasize, is that the statistic does not mean that women have a one in eight chance of dying from breast cancer.

"Getting breast cancer is not the same as dying of breast cancer," said Dr. Kathy Helzlsouer, director of the Breast and Ovarian Surveillance Service at the Oncology Center at Johns Hopkins University. "We lose sight of that sometimes."

When the disease is treated early, before it can spread, 97 percent of patients are still alive five years later, according to the American Cancer Society. But if the cancer reaches lymph nodes, the five-year rate is 76 percent, and if it invades bones or other organs, the rate is only 21 percent.

Among all women with the disease, at all stages, 50 percent to 60 percent survive 15 years. But in women who are treated early, survival is higher.

The death rate actually declined 5.6 percent from 1990 to 1994, a drop that researchers attributed to better detection and treatment, and that some thought would turn out to be just the beginning of a major decrease in deaths.

When it comes to estimating individual risk, even some doctors have trouble understanding statistics and explaining them to patients. In a recent issue of *The New England Journal of Medicine*, researchers from Toronto recommended that doctors move beyond the one-in-eight lifetime statistic to a set of numbers that would make more sense to most women and that would be closer to the figures that cancer experts cite when they advise women about risk.

Instead of calculating lifetime risk, this approach figures the odds that a woman will develop cancer during the next five years, or the next decade. It does that by comparing her to a large group of women her age whose breast cancer rate during the time interval in question is known.

The method is based on actual rates of breast cancer in women of various ages in Ontario in 1995, which are comparable to those in the United States. The researchers used those rates to create a table showing how many new cases would be expected in 1,000 women at five-year intervals from birth through the age of 85 and beyond. The figures show that risk increases with age: It is very low in women in their 20s and 30s, and then begins rising.

The table can be used to calculate a woman's odds of developing breast cancer in a particular decade: That is done by dividing the number of women still alive by the number of cases of cancer during that decade.

The technique shows that, contrary to what many women have been led to believe, there is no decade in which a woman's risk is one in eight. For women entering their 30s, it is 1 in 250, and for those in their 40s it is 1 in 77. It never exceeds 1 in 34, which occurs during a woman's 60s and 70s.

Dr. Julia Knight, an author of the journal article and an epidemiologist at Cancer Care Ontario, a government agency, said many people were overwhelmed by the one-in-eight lifetime statistic. "Most people aren't used to dealing with numbers like that," she said. "I worry about the fear factor."

Dr. Knight said public health campaigns based on the one-in-eight statistic could have the unintended effect of making some women so frightened of breast cancer that they would go into denial about the disease and give up on tests aimed to detect it early. She said she and her colleagues had tried to develop a means of communicating risk that would be more realistic and also less threatening.

The table, she said, "is reasonable for a ball-park number."

Although the table reflects increased risk with age, Dr. Knight and her colleagues acknowledge that it represents the average woman and does not take into account individual differences, especially in women who have a higher than average chance of developing breast cancer.

Other researchers also agree that it makes more sense for women to look at their risk in 10-year intervals, rather than trying to make sense of their lifetime odds. For women with family histories or personal histories of breast problems that suggest a higher than average risk of the disease, some medical centers have created special clinics to provide risk assessment, counseling and extra examinations and mammograms when they are needed. In one such program, at the University of Pennsylvania, Dr. Weber said she and her colleagues started with population figures like those in the table created by Dr. Knight, and adjusted them for individual histories. "Our approach to a patient at 35 will be different than at 85, and we hope that what we know will be different by then, too," she said. "So, we take everything a step at a time."

[DG, January 1999]

## Coping with Fear: Keeping Breast Cancer in Perspective

**W**hat descriptions come to mind in connection with breast cancer? The ones I've heard often include tragic, terrifying, horrific, devastating, terrible, monstrous and "a woman's worst nightmare."

But how accurate are these words for the vast majority of women in whom breast cancer is diagnosed? And haven't we induced an unrealistic fear—indeed, a paralyzing terror—in many women in our efforts to stimulate research into this disease and raise awareness of the need to be vigilant and conscientious about checkups?

Elaine Ratner, a breast cancer survivor and author of the book, *The Feisty Woman's Breast Cancer Book*, maintains that all the publicity given in recent years to this disease has created the impression that it is far more common and more deadly than it really is, and the resulting fear has caused many women to avoid rather than seek the examinations that could save their lives.

Ms. Ratner wrote: "The fear of breast cancer among American women has reached epidemic proportions, not because the number of deaths is on the rise but rather because breast cancer has moved into the spotlight and is now a public issue. Negativity and morbidity prevail. In all the talk about breast cancer, you rarely hear the fact that most women who get it deal with it and go on to live out normal, healthy lives. You also rarely hear that fear itself, and a pessimistic attitude, can negatively affect a woman's ability to cope with the disease."

As a breast cancer survivor myself, I think it's time to replace fear with facts. Here are some important facts about this disease:

▶ The vast majority of women never get breast cancer. The "1-in-8 women" statistic is accurate, but only if you live to 85. And as you get older and remain free of cancer, the 1-in-8 figure starts dropping because you have already lived out many of the at-risk years. If, for example, you are now 70 and still cancer-free, your chances have dropped to 1 in 20.

▶ Seventy percent of women who get breast cancer do not die from it. And the death rate has been dropping steadily throughout this decade. Furthermore, if more women adhered to current detection guidelines and cancers were found while still in their earliest stages, upward of 95 percent could survive this disease.

▶ The probability that an American woman who lives to 90 will die of breast cancer is only 3.8 percent. Fifty percent will die of heart disease, yet this leading killer does not conjure up anything like the fear that breast cancer does.

▶ Lung cancer, not breast cancer, is the leading cause of cancer deaths in American women. This year, 68,000 women will die of lung cancer, 57 percent more than will succumb to breast cancer. Why are we not more terrified of lung cancer, which has a survival rate of only 12 percent?

▶ While it is true that breast cancer is the leading cause of death among American women in their 40s, it is also true that at age 40 only 1 woman in 250 and at age 50 only 1 woman in 50 gets breast cancer. Although cancer tends to be more aggressive in premenopausal women, with modern treatments, even these younger women will more than likely survive.

"It is time we turn some of our focus from the losers in the fight against breast cancer to the winners," Ms. Ratner said. "I do not belittle in any way the pain or tragedy of those who have succumbed. But it is only part of the story. Our preoccupation with those who die of breast cancer has kept us from being encouraged and inspired by the many more who live—long and well."

Among the many breast cancer survivors I know, for example, there is a champion amateur ballroom dancer and artist, an editor/literary agent and a community volunteer who spearheaded the redevelopment of downtown Cleveland. And there is me.

We are alive today because of improved methods of detection and treatment, combined with a willingness to participate in treatment decisions, a view that breast cancer was not the most terrible thing that could happen to us and a determination to beat the disease and get on with life.

Ms. Ratner, who chose mastectomy over lumpectomy followed by radiation, put it this way: "I consider myself fortunate that my cancer was in my breast. If I had to choose a body part to sacrifice, a breast would be my first choice. No other body part is as expendable."

In dealing with her disease, she wrote: "I decided that I would not let cancer take over my life. I decided to concentrate on continuing to feel fine. Maybe in the end cancer would get me and I would die, but for as long as I could, I would do everything possible to extend and enjoy my life." Worry, she insists, is a destructive force that can only make things worse.

I don't share Ms. Ratner's views on modern methods of treatment; her discussions of radiation therapy, chemotherapy and tamoxifen, a drug that can help to prevent recurrence and second cancers, fail to give enough weight to the lifesaving value of these procedures for many women. But I heartily endorse her emphasis on the importance of learning all you can about treatment options and not allowing doctors to make all the decisions for you.

I agree, too, with Ms. Ratner's plea to share one's breast cancer experience and concerns with good friends and others who can provide understanding and support through cancer treatment and recovery. "Human contact and emotional support have a great deal to do with anyone's ability to deal with illness," she wrote, noting that breast cancer strengthened her ties to her family and close friends.

Emotional support also aids survival. Dr. David Spiegel, a psychiatrist at Stanford University School of Medicine, demonstrated that even among women with advanced breast cancer, those who participated in support groups lived twice as long as other women with the same prognosis who were not in such groups.

With or without outside support, you can find much comfort as well as solid practical advice in another new book, *The Not-So-Scary Breast Cancer Book* by Carolyn Ingram and Leslie Ingram Gebhart, sisters who had breast cancer and who found many ways to ease the way through the experience. They discuss how to handle other people's reactions, keep the rest of your life going, and find the best ways to cope.

[JEB, October 1999]

## Software to Compute Women's Cancer Risk

t is an idea that women find either irresistible, or unbearable: a computer program that estimates a woman's personal risk of developing breast cancer. The software, called the "breast cancer risk tool," or "risk disk," was issued in fall 1998 by the National Cancer Institute, and can be obtained by calling (800) 4-CANCER or by requesting it from the institute's Web site at cancertrials.nci.nih.gov. The institute recommends that women go over their results with a doctor.

The software computes the risk of developing breast cancer, first within the next five years, and then over the course of a lifetime. The answers are compared with the numbers for someone who has no risk factors for the disease, and who is the same age as the woman using the software.

The software was originally developed to help determine whether a woman had a high enough risk to make it worth taking the drug tamoxifen, which can reduce the risk of breast cancer by about 50 percent in high-risk women.

The program bases its calculations on six questions: a woman's age, the age at which she began menstruating, the age when she first gave birth, the number of breast cancers in her mother and sisters, the number of breast biopsies she has had, the biopsy results and the woman's race.

The result is a reasonable estimate of risk, researchers say, though they said the program omits some essential questions, which might result in an underestimate of risk for some women in high-risk families. For instance, the program does not take into account the age of onset of breast cancer among relatives, or the history of breast cancer in the father's side of the family, which may be important in families carrying genes for breast cancer.

Dr. Kathy Helzlsouer of Johns Hopkins University described a case in which the disk indicated a relatively low risk for a woman whose mother had had breast cancer. But the woman's grandmother, and six of the grandmother's sisters, had also had the disease. The program was not designed to identify those cases, which Dr. Helzlsouer said indicated a much higher risk.

Other doctors also said that risk assessments carried out in person went into more detail. When women who are worried about developing breast cancer consult Dr. Patricia Ganz, who heads a program for high-risk women at the Jonsson Cancer Center at the University of California at Los Angeles, she discusses the factors on the software, but others as well, such as being overweight and drinking alcohol regularly.

Obesity, regular alcohol consumption, early menstruation and late or no childbearing all heighten risk by increasing lifetime exposure to estrogen, which can stimulate the growth of malignant cells in the breast. Some risk factors can be modified, Dr. Ganz said: women can exercise and try to stay lean, and cut back on alcohol.

For women who want to take replacement estrogen to quell hot flashes, insomnia and other symptoms of menopause, Dr. Ganz said studies had indicated that using the hormone for less than five years did not add substantially to the risk of breast cancer.

But many women may want to take it longer, because it is thought to protect against heart disease, the leading killer of women, and the bone-weakening disease osteoporosis. These women must weigh these benefits against the added breast cancer risk of long-term use.

Dr. Ganz said she recommended that women at

high risk for breast cancer take other drugs to lower cholesterol or prevent bone loss. But it is not known if the other drugs work as well as estrogen.

But some risk factors cannot be changed, and when a woman's risk is unusually high, doctors recommend more frequent breast examinations and mammograms, in hope of detecting tumors early enough to cure them. Extra monitoring is especially important for women with strong family histories of the disease, and those who have had a positive test for a mutation in the genes BRCA1 or BRCA2, which can produce a lifetime breast cancer risk as high as 50 percent to 80 percent. Those women are usually advised to begin having mammograms at an early age.

Some women from very high-risk families choose to have their breasts removed prophylactically, and while that is not something that most doctors encourage, Dr. Ganz said, many will support the decision if a woman has clearly given it careful consideration. But removal of the ovaries is often recommended for women who carry BRCA mutations, because the genes are also associated with ovarian cancer, which has a much higher death rate than breast cancer. Removing the ovaries, by reducing estrogen levels, can also help reduce the risk of breast cancer.

Extra monitoring may also be recommended for women with personal histories of breast lumps needing biopsies. Even negative biopsies may increase risk, researchers say, because the need for them may reflect an underlying problem linked to the tendency to develop cancer.

At the University of Pennsylvania, some women at high risk are being given both mammograms and magnetic resonance imaging scans, as part of a study to determine whether magnetic imaging can help doctors interpret suspicious spots that are hard to diagnose on mammograms.

Dr. Mitchell Schnall, a radiologist who is conducting the study, said that the magnetic scans might be able to detect cancers that a mammography missed. But that is not certain, he added.

Doctors in the special surveillance program at Memorial Sloan-Kettering Cancer Center in New York are also beginning to study magnetic imaging, said Dr. Alexandra Heerdt, a breast surgeon who directs the program. She said one of the greatest benefits for women who attended the clinic was peace of mind. Those with very high risk may be examined every three months, in addition to having yearly mammograms.

A mammogram looks for changes in the breast only once a year, Dr. Heerdt said. "But they could have minimal physical changes that I could pick up more quickly and readily," she said. "There's less stress because they don't feel that they have to take on the responsibility of doing all the breast exams in between. They feel that someone else is bearing the burden with them."

[DG, January 1999]

## Sorting Out Contradictory Findings About Fat and Health

Many health-conscious Americans are beginning to feel as if they are being tossed around like yo-yos by conflicting research findings. One day beta carotene is hailed as a life-saving antioxidant and the next it is stripped of health-promoting glory and even tainted by a brush of potential harm. Margarine, long hailed as a heart-saving alternative to butter, is suddenly found to contain a type of fat that could damage the heart.

Now, after women have heard countless suggestions that a low-fat diet may reduce their breast cancer risk, Harvard researchers who analyzed data pooled from seven studies in four countries report that this advice may be based more on wishful thinking than fact.

The researchers, whose review was published in *The New England Journal of Medicine*, found no evidence among a number of studies of more than

335,000 women that a diet with less than 20 percent of calories from fat reduced a woman's risk of developing breast cancer. Nor was risk related to the types of fats the women ate, the study reported.

Is this the final word on the subject, and does it mean that diet is not an important factor in breast cancer? Not at all. There are several possibilities still to be explored. One is the relationship between breast-cancer risk and fats consumed in childhood, adolescence and early adulthood. The current studies considered fat intake in mid-adult life. But evidence from other breast cancer studies, like those involving exercise and hormones, suggest that exposure to fats early in life plays a stronger role in determining risk.

Another factor to consider is the accuracy of women's dietary reports. People are notoriously poor at remembering what and how much they consume, especially if it involves foods that they think they should avoid, like fat-rich ice cream or cream cheese. A third factor is whether a diet share of less than 20 percent of calories from fat is low enough to be protective, and a fourth concerns the possibility that the kind of fat, not the amount, is the issue.

For example, in animal studies, monounsaturated fats like olive and canola oils do not promote tumor growth the way polyunsaturated fats do. And in Spain and Greece, women with breast cancer were shown to consume less olive oil than did healthy women. But until recently monounsaturated oils were not commonplace in American diets and may not have been well enough represented in the Harvard study to show up as protective.

Finally, and perhaps most important, there is the possibility that fat consumption may simply be an indicator of other dietary and life-style factors that play a more direct role in protecting against breast cancer.

The suggestion that dietary fat may influence the risk of breast cancer originally arose from international comparisons. Breast cancer is much less common in Asia and in poor countries that habitually consume a low-fat diet. Until recently, about 42 percent of the calories in the diets of American women came from fat (it is now at about 34 percent), whereas among Japanese women fat provided only about 10 to 15 percent of calories. But when Asian women move to the United States, their breast-cancer risk begins to climb, and in a generation or two it reaches the high level of American women, who face a one-in-eight lifetime risk of developing the disease.

Now the equivocal findings about the role of fats is prompting a closer look at other elements in the diets and lives of women that may account for international differences in breast cancer risk. In a review of breast cancer and diet in the January/February 1996 *Nutrition Action Health Letter*, the nutritionist Bonnie Liebman points out that when Asian women move to this country, they and their descendants gradually adopt Western eating habits.

For example, they start eating less soy and more meat. Soy foods like tofu, miso and soy milk contain substances called isoflavonoids, which act in the body like weak estrogens and may interfere with the action of estrogens the body produces. Since natural estrogens are known to promote the growth of breast tumors, anything that interferes with their activity should lower the risk of breast cancer. But this too may be a red herring; in two recent studies, Japanese women with breast cancer consumed no less soy than their healthy counterparts.

Another possibility is that in countries with low breast-cancer rates, women mainly subsist on plant-based foods: grains, vegetables, fruits and beans. Evidence is growing that plant foods, especially beans and vegetables, are rich in substances, including weak estrogens, that protect against cancers in general and specifically against cancers influenced by hormones. Supporting this possibility is the observation that in countries where women rarely get breast cancer, men rarely develop prostate cancer, which is also influenced by hormones.

Alcohol, too, may be an important factor. Although one drink a day helps to prevent heart disease, the leading killer of American women, it may raise the risk of breast cancer anywhere from 10 percent to 40 percent, and even more so among women who consume two drinks a day.

In every country that has a low rate of breast cancer, women traditionally get far more exercise than American women, most of whom have been rendered inactive by motor vehicles and labor-saving devices. Among Americans, Dr. Leslie Bernstein of the University of Southern California found that premenopausal women who exercised for one to three hours a week had a 30 percent lower risk of developing breast cancer than inactive women, and those who exercised for four or more hours a week had less than half the risk. An earlier study had linked exercise in adolescence and early adulthood to a reduced risk of breast cancer in mid-life.

Physical activity and a low-fat, plant-based diet are also related to yet another factor associated with breast cancer: body weight and especially distribution of body fat. Asian women are much leaner on average than American women. Among Americans, being overweight (by American standards) is associated with a slight increase in the risk of breast cancer, perhaps because body fat is a source of estrogen. But when fat gathers around the waist—the so-called apple shape, the relationship to breast cancer, as well as heart disease, is much stronger. Abdominal fat raises insulin levels in the blood and, at least in laboratory studies, insulin promotes the growth of breast cancer cells.

Height may also play a role. Tall women have a breast cancer risk that is 30 to 40 percent higher than that for short women. What makes women tall? In part, it is a childhood diet high in protein, which is common among Americans and, until recently at least, rare among the Japanese and other peoples with a low risk of breast cancer. Another possibly protective factor, at least for premenopausal women, is prolonged breast-feeding—for 4 to 12 months—which until recently has been rare among "modern" American women.

[JEB, February 1996]

## Studies Confirm Relationship of Alcohol to Breast Cancer

An analysis of six long-term studies conducted among a total of more than 300,000 women has confirmed that drinking alcohol can raise a woman's risk of developing breast cancer. But the increase in risk is very small for those who consume no more than one drink a day.

The findings, published in the *Journal of the American Medical Association*, showed that a woman's risk of breast cancer rose with the amount of alcohol she regularly consumed, strongly suggesting that by drinking moderately or not at all a woman could reduce her chances of getting breast cancer.

But breast cancer is not the only disease influenced by alcohol intake. Excessive alcohol consumption increases the risk of several digestive tract cancers. On the other hand, moderate drinking has been linked in numerous studies in several countries to a reduced risk of heart disease and increased longevity overall.

In the study, the researchers found that women who were relatively heavy drinkers, consuming two to five alcoholic drinks each day, were 41 percent more likely to develop breast cancer than nondrinkers. But for moderate drinkers who consumed three-fourths to one drink, or 10 grams of alcohol, a day, the risk was only 9 percent higher than among nondrinkers.

Put another way, a woman who lives to age 85 in the United States has a 12.5 percent chance of having breast cancer at some time in her life. If she consumes one drink a day, the analysis suggests, her chances of having breast cancer would increase to 13.6 percent.

By contrast, cigarette smoking can raise a woman's risk of developing lung cancer by as much as 1,000 percent. Lung cancer is the leading cancer killer of women, causing 67,000 deaths among women annually, 23,500 more deaths than are caused by breast cancer.

Among the women studied, the risk of developing breast cancer rose by an average of 9 percent for each additional 10 grams of alcohol consumed daily. No risk difference was found for various forms of alcoholic drinks; comparable amounts of beer, wine and hard liquor had similar effects. One shot of hard liquor contains 15 grams of alcohol, 12 ounces of beer contain 13 grams and 4 ounces of wine, 11 grams.

In speculating on reasons for the relationship between alcohol and breast cancer, the authors of the report noted that alcohol raised levels of estrogen, which is known to stimulate breast cancer growth. They said that drinking two to five drinks a day confers a breast cancer risk comparable to that associated with having a family history of breast cancer or starting to menstruate before age 12.

The authors also pointed out that alcohol consumption is one of the few factors linked to breast cancer within a woman's control. They suggested that in deciding whether to drink and how much, women should consider alcohol's benefits to the heart and their own risks of developing heart disease and breast cancer.

"Our study suggests that the link between alcohol and breast cancer risk applies to most women," said Dr. Stephanie Smith Warner, lead author of the study.

In an interview Dr. Smith-Warner added, "Women should consult with their personal physicians to evaluate their cardiac and breast cancer risk factors and determine if moderate alcohol consumption is advisable for them." Dr. Smith-Warner is a research fellow in nutrition at the Harvard School of Public Health.

If, for example, a woman was at high risk for heart disease but low risk for breast cancer, consuming one drink a day might be better for her health than no drinks. But drinking alcohol may be more hazard than help to a woman who is free of the known risk factors for heart disease.

Deaths from heart disease greatly exceed those caused by breast cancer. Each year more than 500,000 American women die of heart disease, compared with 43,500 who die from breast cancer. According to a large long-term study published by the American Cancer Society, having one drink a day raises a woman's risk of dying of breast cancer by 11 percent but diminishes overall mortality by 20 percent because of alcohol's protective effects on the heart.

Dr. Smith-Warner and her colleagues noted, however, that there are ways other than drinking alcohol to reduce a woman's cardiac risk, including regular exercise, maintaining a normal body weight, controlling blood pressure and cholesterol, taking aspirin and not smoking.

There are also some things a woman can do to reduce her breast cancer risk. Women who smoke, for example, have higher breast cancer rates, and those who get regular physical exercise before menopause face a breast cancer risk that is 30 to 50 percent lower than that among sedentary women. This study is the largest ever to examine the relationship between diet and breast cancer. Dr. Smith-Warner and her colleagues pooled data from six "prospective" studies in four countries—the United States, Canada, the Netherlands and Sweden.

In a prospective study, information is gathered at the outset about diet and other characteristics that might influence the risk of disease; the subjects are then followed for years to see what happens to their health. In the six studies, the women were followed for up to 11 years.

More than 50 percent of American women age 18 and older are current drinkers, according to data gathered by the National Center for Health Statistics. Of those who drink, during the two weeks before being surveyed, 29 percent consumed no alcohol and 46.4 percent drank "lightly," consuming no more than three drinks a week.

If the trend shown in the new analysis applies to this low consumption rate, these women would have about a 5 percent greater risk of developing breast cancer than women who never drink. An additional 21 percent of women who drink reported consuming 4 to 13 drinks a week, which would confer an added risk of about 7 percent to 18 percent. Only 3.4 percent reported drinking 14 or more drinks a week, which would be associated with a breast cancer risk up to 40 percent higher than among nondrinkers.

[JEB, February 1998]

# Do Breast Self-Exams Save Lives?
# Science Still Doesn't Have Answer

If examining her own breasts once a month is not actually the lifesaving tool it is cracked up to be, Estelle Bolofsky does not want to hear about it.

Ms. Bolofsky, 47, an office supervisor in Manhattan, is a devout acolyte of the protocol the American Cancer Society recommends for all women over the age of 20. Once a month, she doggedly inspects and massages each breast and armpit, all the while fighting off the fear that she will discover a lump like the one that sent her to the gynecologist in a panic two years ago. That lump turned out to be benign, but Ms. Bolofsky is not taking any chances. "You have to know your own body," she said. "If you don't take care of yourself, then who's going to take care of you?"

But despite the determination of Ms. Bolofsky and millions of women like her to believe in breast self-examination, medical research has not yet been able to prove that the complex monthly routine does save lives.

Instead, it remains one of the most disputed issues in preventive medicine, pitting experts and policy makers against one another, while doctors and patients dangle in the middle, and researchers try to figure out why a maneuver whose merits seem so intuitively obvious should be so remarkably resistant to scientific validation.

Before mammography became widely used in the 1980s, breast cancer was routinely diagnosed by touch: a doctor discovered a lump in the breast, or, more often, a woman found one herself. Even now, in the mammography era, "a significant proportion of breast cancers are found on self-exam, particularly among women less than 50," said Dr. Hiram S. Cody 3d, a breast surgeon at Memorial Sloan-Kettering Cancer Center in New York.

Simple logic would thus dictate that the more regularly and methodically a woman examines her breasts, the more likely cancer is to be found at the earliest possible moment and the less likely the woman is to die of the disease. But this logic is evidently so confounded both by the complex biology of breast cancer and by the complicated psyches of women at risk that studies from around the world have been unable to confirm it.

The evidence that the procedure is worthwhile remains lukewarm enough for the United States Preventative Services Task Force, one of the pre-eminent advisory bodies for disease screening policies in the country, to state recently, "There is insufficient evidence to recommend for or against the teaching of breast self-examination."

Yet many cancer experts feel so strongly about the importance of self-examination, in conjunction with regular mammograms and breast examinations by doctors, that they argue that if science cannot support self-examination, then the science must be wrong.

"I tell everybody to do it," Dr. Cody said. "If we tell women it's not important to examine themselves, we might be making a big mistake." And a New York oncologist, who spoke on the condition that he not be identified, said: "I don't care what the studies show. Self-examination clearly is a way of early detection. It's a wise thing to do."

But Dr. Susan Love, a California surgeon who has written extensively on breast cancer and other women's health issues, has dismissed breast self-examination for years as overrated, pointing out that although many women find breast lumps themselves, it is usually in the course of ordinary living, without an intensely fear-provoking monthly ritual.

Even proponents of breast self-examination acknowledge that especially in younger women, the ritual results mainly in periods of dreadful anxiety and unnecessary surgical procedures. Since breast cancer is more common in women over 50 than younger ones, the lumps younger women find in their breasts, like the one that sent Ms. Bolofsky into a tearful weekend panic two years ago, are far more likely to be false alarms than cancer.

Still, when breast cancer occurs in younger women, it is far deadlier than in older women, making a high rate of false alarms, at least in theory, a cost worth tolerating.

"But by the time a woman picks something up, it's really large," said Dr. Diane M. Harper, a family doctor at Dartmouth Medical School in Hanover, New Hampshire. Tumors found on self-examination average more than a half-inch in diameter, much larger than tumors found on mammography. Some experts believe that finding tumors this large a few months earlier may make very little difference in their response to treatment. If the tumors are aggressive enough to spread out of the breast, markedly reducing chances of survival, they are likely to have done so already, these authorities say.

In fact, early detection of these tumors may only increase the length of time a woman has to live with a diagnosis of cancer, without actually changing her prognosis. That may be one reason why no study has found that self-examination saves lives.

Another reason may be the difficulty of coaxing women to overcome the fear of what they may find when they examine their own breasts.

"Only about 25 percent of our patients do it right," said Dr. Kathryn Kash, director of Psychosocial Services at Strang Cancer Prevention Center in New York. Despite the intensive instruction in breast self-examination technique the center provides, Dr. Kash said: "The high-risk women that we see are terrified to do it. They're so worried they might find something."

And yet, doing it right may make all the difference. A handful of studies, among them one reported in November 1997 in *The Canadian Medical Association Journal*, suggest that breast self-examination may save lives, but only in women using good techniques.

Studying almost 90,000 Canadian women, researchers found no decrease in the number of fatal breast cancer cases among those taught to examine their own breasts. But the women who looked at the contour of the breasts carefully and used the pads of their three middle fingers to examine them were somewhat less likely to develop fatal disease two years later.

## How to Do a Breast Self-Exam

Breast self-examinations should be done each month at the same time, preferably a few days after the menstrual period ends. Most lumps detected are not cancerous, but any breast changes, like unusual lumps or discharges, should be reported to a doctor. What to look for:

### Changes in skin texture
Stand in front of a mirror and look at both breasts. Is there any puckered, dimpled or scaly skin or any discharge from the nipples?

### Changes in shape
Clasp your hands behind your head and press your hands forward. Continue looking as you firmly press your hands on your hips. Bend slightly toward the mirror as you hunch your shoulders and pull your elbows forward.

### Lumps or thicknesses
Use one of the following patterns to examine your breasts, as well as the underarms and upper chest, for lumps or thicknesses:

**METHOD 1:** Begin in the underarm area and move your fingers down until they are below the breast. Move your fingers in toward the center and go slowly back up. Cover the whole area, going up and down.

**METHOD 2:** Begin at the outer edge of the breast, moving your fingers slowly around it. Work toward the nipple in a spiral.

**METHOD 3:** Start at the outer edge of the breast and move your fingers toward the nipple and back. Do the whole breast, covering one wedge-shaped section at a time.

Raise one arm and put your hand behind your head. With the opposite hand, use the pads of your fingers, not the tips, to check the breast, the area between the breast and underarm, the underarm itself and the area above the breast, up to the collarbone and over to your shoulder. Some women prefer to do this step in the shower.

Repeat the breast examination while lying flat on your back with your right hand behind your head and a pillow or folded towel under your right shoulder. With your left hand, carefully examine the right breast and area around it. Then switch hands and repeat the procedure for the left breast.

*Source: New York State Department of Health*

"The overall message is that, yes, breast self-exam does seem to help, but you have to do it well," said one of the researchers, Dr. Cornelia J. Baines, an associate professor in the department of public health sciences at the University of Toronto.

Women who know they are at relatively lower risk of developing the disease may do the self-examination better than others, Dr. T. Gregory Hislop, an epidemiologist at the University of British Columbia in Vancouver, observed in a commentary on the study.

And what will probably become the definitive study on the value of self-examination, now under way in China, has yet to confirm the finding. In it, more than 100,000 Shanghai factory workers have been carefully instructed in self-examination techniques and are not only regularly supervised while examining themselves, but also receive periodic reminder visits from study workers.

A preliminary report published in *The Journal of the National Cancer Institute* in March 1997 showed that after five years, the breast cancer death rates among these highly trained self-examiners were no different from those in a similar group taught techniques for preventing lower-back pain instead.

But Dr. Baines said that even when the Shanghai study is finished, in 5 or 10 years, "it's unlikely the results will apply here." Breast cancer rates in China are lower than those in the United States and Canada, and because screening mammography is unavailable in China, self-examination may be more important for screening.

This means that the uncertainty about whether breast self-examination is worth the time and effort spent learning to do it correctly—and the money spent promoting it—is likely to persist here for years, forcing doctors to find a compromise they and their patients can live with.

"I don't push it," said Dr. Eileen Hoffman, associate director for education at the Mount Sinai Women's Health Program in New York. "I don't like to make women feel that they're responsible when they don't find their lumps 'soon enough.' I'm careful to tell them that the goal is not to find lumps but to get to know what normal is."

Dr. Soheyla D. Gharib, co-director of the Women's Health Center at Brigham and Women's Hospital in Boston, said: "If it pushes all someone's panic buttons, then I say, don't do it. Then I may see them in the office a little more frequently. But it's such an easy and cheap thing to do. It's good to get to know your own landscape."

Dr. Harper at Dartmouth said: "For new patients, I get a read on who the patient is, her body image, her sexuality and her self-esteem. Some really don't want to think of their breasts just as objects waiting to become diseased. But women who are doing it already, I don't discourage them. Usually they're doing it because they're good citizens."

But Dr. Harper said her patients often admitted that " 'I'm doing it because I'm supposed to, but I haven't the vaguest idea of what I'm doing.' "

[AZ, January 1998]

## Living Proof: Mammograms Are Not Always Enough

In 1988 I wrote a column that might have been called "the myth of the negative mammogram." In it I discussed the fact that 10 to 15 percent of breast cancers do not show up on a mammogram and cautioned women that any suspicious area in the breast should be biopsied even when the mammogram is negative.

In February 1999, I became living proof of the value of that advice. I'd been having annual mammograms for about 13 years with no evidence of anything wrong. Likewise at my exam this year, my radiologist for the last eight years, Dr. Doreen Liebeskind, delivered the news that my X-rays looked fine. However, this time I feared something was the matter.

The matter was an area of thickening in my left breast that we'd been watching for years. My mammograms were consistently negative and sonograms had shown nothing more than fibrous tissue, a normal aberration common in many women. But from time to time the area hurt and it had been especially painful two weeks earlier. I had begun to wonder how I would know if something went awry. Even if I suspected all was not well, would I fail to act after being reassured for seven years that there was nothing to worry about?

Then Dr. Liebeskind did a manual exam and said, "It feels a little different from last year, a little more nodular. Let's get another sonogram." Sonography, a way of viewing tissue using ultra-high-speed sound waves, is an excellent noninvasive tool for investigating suspicious areas in the breast that are picked up either by a mammogram or physical examination. It is also useful for screening women at high risk either because of family or personal histories of breast cancer, according to Dr. Peter I. Pressman, breast cancer surgeon at New York's Lenox Hill Hospital and Beth Israel Medical Center and co-author, with Dr. Yashar Hirshaut, of *Breast Cancer: The Complete Guide*.

When Dr. Liebeskind compared my sonogram to the one taken the year before, she said, "There's something new there now, and I think we should do a needle biopsy and see what it is." Guided by ultrasound, a thin hollow needle was inserted into the suspicious area and cells were sucked out for microscopic analysis.

It was all so swift and matter-of-fact that I wasn't even scared when Dr. Liebeskind said she saw something in the cells that wasn't quite normal. She handed over the slides of my breast cells to Dr. Grace Yang, cytopathologist at New York University Medical Center. Several years ago, Dr. Yang developed a rapid stain technique that enabled her to make a diagnosis within 10 minutes—no three days of agonized waiting for biopsy results. I don't know why her technique is not used everywhere by now.

Dr. Yang was also matter-of-fact. "This is cancer," she said, tempering her grim report with, "But you're very lucky. It's small, one centimeter, and very early and of low nuclear grade, meaning it's not an aggressive cancer." Surgery a week later and a complete microscopic analysis of the tumor and lymph nodes into which my breast drains confirmed her diagnosis.

I was very lucky, if someone with cancer could ever be considered lucky. My chances are better than 95 percent that the surgery, a lumpectomy and sentinel node biopsy, and subsequent five weeks of radiation (five days a week) will be a permanent cure. In a lumpectomy, the surgeon removes the tumor and a small amount of surrounding tissue, and the sentinel node biopsy removes only those underarm nodes into which the breast drains. And just to be sure, since my tumor cells, like those of most breast cancers, respond to estrogen, I'll be taking the antiestrogen drug tamoxifen for the next five years. Just last year, a major multicenter study showed that tamoxifen reduced the risk of breast cancer recurrence and the chances of developing cancer in the opposite breast by about 45 percent.

My experience should in no way discourage any woman from having regular mammograms. My advice is also the recommendation of the American Cancer Society and the National Cancer Institute: an annual mammogram starting at age 40. Mammography is an excellent surveillance tool that can detect 85 percent of breast cancers. It can pick up tumors when they are too tiny to be felt, before they have spread beyond the area where they arose, when the potential for cure is greatest.

Early detection through mammography is one of the main reasons for the declining death rate from breast cancer. The other factors are the widespread use of radiation therapy for five or six weeks following a lumpectomy and postoperative chemotherapy, which, depending on the cellular nature of the tumor, is now often given even when there is no evidence that cancer has spread beyond the breast if the tumor is larger than mine or there are indications that it is more aggressive.

Mammograms are lifesaving, and I will continue to have them annually. But as with the recently removed tumor, I will not rely on them 100 percent. If something feels wrong, I will make sure to have it examined by ultrasound and biopsied if there is a suspicious lesion.

I will repeat what Dr. Liebeskind told me in 1988: "Every lump should be biopsied unless it disappears on its own in a month or two or it is shown to be a benign fluid-filled cyst that collapses and does not recur when the fluid is removed." A mammogram alone cannot distinguish between an innocent cyst and a cancer. If ultrasound is available, it can show if the cyst is filled with fluid, and guided by ultrasound, a needle can be used to suck out the fluid.

Despite the value of mammography, a negative mammogram does not rule out cancer. Mammograms are most likely to miss cancers in women under 50 who have dense breast tissue. Breast size, however, is not a factor. Although annual mammography is not recommended before age 40 (except, perhaps, for women with a strong family history of early breast cancer or who carry genes that place them at high risk of cancer), many radiologists recommend that a baseline mammogram be done at age 30 or 35, when everything is likely to be normal. That way future deviations from normal will be easier to spot.

Too many women with worrisome lumps are falsely reassured by doctors when their mammograms are negative. Some are advised to return in three or six months for another look, but others are not examined again for another year. One of my friends who had a mammogram-negative lump was followed for a year with periodic mammograms before her doctor decided to do a biopsy, which revealed a cancer.

Money should not be a concern that deters women from having regular mammograms. Many states now have laws mandating insurance coverage, at least for women over 50, and Medicare now covers annual mammography for all Medicare-eligible women. For those not fully covered by insurance, there are low-cost mammography services almost everywhere. To find one, call the American Cancer Society at (800) 227-2345.

And don't forget breast self-examination. Even with the increased use of screening mammography, today most women with breast cancer come to the doctor with a tumor they have found themselves, usually by accident. This speaks to the value of doing regular breast self-examination because a woman who checks her own breasts every month is most likely to be sensitive to subtle changes that could mean trouble. And the earlier trouble is discovered, the less aggressive the therapy needs to be and the greater the likelihood of cure.

As Dr. Liebeskind put it, "A woman doesn't have to know what she is feeling, only that it feels different from before." She emphasizes that monthly examinations by a woman who is familiar with every nuance in her breasts are far more likely to pick up an early cancer than is an annual breast examination by a health professional.

[JEB, March 1999]

## Cancer Gene Tests Turn Out to Be Far From Simple

When scientists identified two genes, BRCA1 and BRCA2, as the culprits in most hereditary cases of breast cancer, the discovery prompted much excitement and hope. Women with family histories of breast cancer would at last be able to determine if they, too, were likely to get the disease. And so armed, they could take preventive action.

But as with most highly promising developments in cancer, the decade-long story of the breast cancer genes, while it has revealed important insights and greatly increased scientists' knowledge, has turned out to be far from simple, both from a scientific perspective and a personal one.

From studying the behavior of the breast cancer genes, for example, researchers now know that a woman can inherit a high risk of breast cancer from her father as well as from her mother, so it is not enough to consider only the mother's cancer history when estimating a woman's risk.

In addition, the three mutations in BRCA1 and BRCA2 initially identified as rendering a woman highly prone to breast cancer have since multiplied into hundreds of mutations, each of which may confer a different degree of risk. Moreover, the genes appear to play a role in other illnesses besides breast cancer, and to affect men as well as women.

Mutations in the genes, for example, greatly increase a woman's risk of developing ovarian cancer, which is both harder to detect and much harder to cure than breast cancer. And a recent report in the *Journal of the National Cancer Institute* linked mutations in BRCA2 to an increased risk of developing cancers of the prostate, pancreas, gallbladder, bile duct and stomach, as well as malignant melanoma. Other studies have suggested a modestly increased risk of colon cancer.

To complicate matters further, the same gene defect may not behave the same way in all families. In some families, in which few or no cases of cancer have yet occurred, the gene's "penetrance"—that is, its tendency to express itself—may be much lower than in other families, where several cases of breast or ovarian cancer have occurred in blood relatives.

Finally, many researchers strongly suspect that BRCA1 and BRCA2 are not the only genes that can go awry and raise the risk of breast cancer. As more is learned about the human genome, other breast cancer genes may show up.

One of the most common misconceptions about breast cancer is that some cases are genetically influenced and some are not. It is true that only a small percentage of all cancers, including breast cancer, is inherited, that is, the likelihood of getting them is transmitted at conception from parent to son or daughter, either through the egg or through the sperm that fertilized it. In such cases, the gene defect appears in every body cell, including blood cells.

But genetic defects are at work even in cancers that are not inherited: for a normal cell to become a cancer cell, a genetic mutation or deletion must first occur, destroying the mechanism that puts the brakes on the cell's ability to reproduce. As a result, cancer cells multiply endlessly, like the broom in the Disney version of *The Sorcerer's Apprentice*.

As Dr. Michael G. Muto, director of the Familial Ovarian Cancer Center at the Dana-Farber Cancer Institute in Boston, and Dr. Janet E. Shepherd, a gynecologist in Boulder, Colorado, pointed out in a journal article, "Cancer is always a genetic disease."

A mutation that allows uncontrolled cell growth can occur at any time during life, induced either directly or indirectly, by exposure to a toxic substance like tobacco smoke or to a chronic irritant like alcohol or stomach acid. Such mutations can also occur spontaneously, when a mistake is made during cell division that is not detected by the cell's built-in surveillance system.

A cancer-causing mutation in a breast or ovarian cell acquired during a woman's lifetime cannot be passed on to her children. But researchers studying the genetics of breast cancer say it is possible, even likely, that all breast cancers involve mutations in BRCA1 or BRCA2 but that in only a small percentage of these cases is the mutation inherited from a woman's mother or father. Dr. Mary-Claire King, geneticist at the University of Washington in Seattle, said, "There is increasingly good evidence for a close connection between inherited and noninherited forms of breast cancer, although what that connection is is not yet clear."

There are three main types of genes involved in cancer: oncogenes, tumor-suppressor genes and mismatch/repair genes. Oncogenes dictate the production of proteins that stimulate normal cell growth. If a mutation occurs in an oncogene, cells can proliferate at a greatly accelerated rate. Excessive cell proliferation—as, for example, might happen in an esophagus chronically exposed to stomach acid—greatly increases the chance that mutations will occur that could result in cancer.

Tumor-suppressor genes, as their name implies, place brakes on cell division. If a mutation inactivates a tumor-suppressor gene, cell multiplication can continue unchecked. BRCA1 and BRCA2 are tumor-suppressor genes that seem to be especially important in controlling cell multiplication in the breast and ovaries.

The mismatch/repair genes have the job of correcting mistakes made in the cell's DNA when it is copied, which happens every time a cell divides to form a new cell. Because DNA is the stuff that genes are made of, when mismatch/repair genes do not function properly, mutations can accumulate in other genes, including oncogenes and tumor-suppressor genes.

One hereditary form of colon cancer, the kind that does not involve the formation of polyps, has been linked to mutations in mismatch/repair genes. These same mutations have also been linked to a three to four-fold risk of developing ovarian cancer.

In 1971, Dr. Alfred Knudson of Fox Chase Cancer Center in Philadelphia, proposed a scheme by which an inherited mutation might result in a predisposition to cancer. The scheme, called the two-hit hypothesis, still stands for many cancer genes, including BRCA1 and BRCA2. Each cell contains two copies of every gene, and for cancer to result, both copies must be abnormal, the hypothesis holds. Thus, an alteration must occur in each of the two genes inherited from a person's mother and father.

Consider, for example, a woman who has inherited a mutated gene from her mother and a normal one from her father. According to the two-hit hypothesis, cancer would develop only if something happens to the normal gene in a single breast cell or ovarian cell during the woman's life.

For cancers that are not inherited, the two-hit hypothesis suggests that alterations must occur in both copies of a normal gene. Because two hits are less likely than one to occur during a person's lifetime, the risk of an inherited breast cancer is much greater than the risk of a cancer that develops without any hereditary predisposition.

The risk of developing a nonhereditary breast cancer is about 12 percent; that of nonhereditary ovarian cancer only 1 to 2 percent. But for women who start life with one copy of the BRCA1 gene already mutated, the risk of developing breast cancer by age 70 is as high as 85 percent, and the risk of developing ovarian cancer at any time in a woman's life is as high as 44 percent.

For a woman with an inherited BRCA1 mutation, the risk of developing either breast cancer or ovarian cancer by age 70 has been estimated to be as high as 95 percent, which has prompted some women with a BRCA1 mutation to have their breasts and ovaries removed while these organs are still healthy. The risk of breast cancer associated with BRCA2 mutations is similar, and, although lower for ovarian cancer, it is still very much higher than for women born without one mutated gene. Unlike BRCA1, BRCA2 mutations increase a man's risk of developing breast cancer.

As genes go, BRCA1 and BRCA2 are huge. BRCA1, on chromosome 17, has about 100,000 base pairs of DNA and codes for a protein made of 1,863 amino acids. BRCA2, on chromosome 13, is twice that size; its protein contains 3,418 amino acids.

The very size of these genes leaves lots of opportunity for things to go wrong in the DNA base pairs that could cause the gene to malfunction. Thus far, more than 340 mutations in BRCA1 have been identified, and most can disrupt the gene's tumor-sup-

## Looking at Cancer on the Genetic Level

Three different gene types are linked to the development of cancer cells.

ONCOGENES

Dictate the production of proteins that stimulate normal cell growth. When mutations occur, cells multiply at an accelerated rate.

TUMOR SUPPRESSORS

Inhibit cell division. When mutations deactivate the gene, cell mutiplication can continue unchecked.

MISMATCH/REPAIR

Correct mistakes in the cell's DNA when the cell replicates. When they function improperly, mutations of other genes are passed from one generation to the next.

pressor ability. For BRCA2, more than 100 mutations have been identified, and researchers expect that many others will be found that can impair the gene's function.

Only 1 in 400 Americans harbors an inherited mutation in BRCA1 or BRCA2. However, certain mutations in these genes have been identified as occurring with unusual frequency in Ashkenazi Jews, whose ancestors came from Eastern Europe. About 90 percent of Jews in the United States are of Ashkenazi origin. And more than 2 percent of Ashkenazi Jews have been found to carry one of three mutations in a DNA base: On the BRCA1 gene, the loss of two nucleic acids in position 185 or the insertion of an extra nucleic acid in position 5382; on the BRCA2 gene, the loss of one nucleic acid at position 6174. Just as dialing one wrong digit in a phone number connects the caller with the wrong person, these seemingly minor errors are enough to impair a gene's ability to function normally. Certain BRCA mutations also are found more often in people from some Scandinavian countries.

A number of laboratories can now test a blood sample for the presence of the three mutations common in Ashkenazi Jews, at a cost of about $400. Blood cells can also be analyzed for all the mutations thus far identified in BRCA1 and BRCA2, at a cost of $2,500. But the results, in terms of disease risk, are often much harder to interpret than for the mutations found in Ashkenazi Jews. And the results of such testing are most useful when a mutation found in a woman who has had cancer is also found in her still healthy blood relatives.

A woman with a family history of breast cancer is most likely to have a mutated BRCA gene if the cancers in her blood relatives occurred before menopause. In an analysis of 798 families, women who developed breast cancer before age 50 had a 25 percent chance of carrying a BRCA mutation if they had any blood relative who also developed the disease before age 50.

However, interpretive difficulties arise when a woman with a family history of breast or ovarian cancer tests negative for BRCA mutations. Dr. Kenneth Offit, director of clinical genetics at Memorial Sloan-Kettering Cancer Center in New York, explained that the cancers in the woman's family could have been the result of different genes than the ones that were tested for. Or the cancers may have been caused by some other nonhereditary factor.

Since by age 85 one in eight American women will get breast cancer and more than 90 percent of those cases are not hereditary, "by chance alone, more than one woman in a given family may have breast cancer," Dr. Offit said.

[JEB, August 1999]

# Breast Cancer Drug Dilemma: Who Should Take It, and When?

When Bernice Olson heard in 1992 that a nationwide study was under way to determine whether the drug tamoxifen could prevent breast cancer in high-risk women, she volunteered right away. One of her sisters, who is now healthy, had had the disease in 1980, at the age of 43. That, combined with Mrs. Olson's own age, 51, defined her as high risk.

In April 1998 she and others in the study received a letter marked "urgent," notifying her that the experiment had been halted a year early, because tamoxifen had shown such a powerful protective effect—45 percent fewer cases of breast cancer in the women taking it—that the scientists felt ethically bound to offer the drug to all the women in the study, some of whom had been assigned to a group that were taking placebos.

But the letter did not tell Mrs. Olson whether she

should start taking the drug, which can have dangerous side effects. Even the researchers were surprised by the need to cut the study short, and they have not yet analyzed enough data to develop recommendations. "We're working feverishly," said Dr. Leslie Ford of the National Cancer Institute said.

Twenty-nine million American women may be waiting for the answer. That is how many Federal health authorities say are "potentially eligible" for preventive treatment with tamoxifen. The group includes all women over 60, who are at increased risk simply because of their age, and also many younger women whose personal or family history indicates a high risk. Most of them are perfectly healthy, and are being asked to consider taking a powerful drug to prevent a disease that they may never get.

The study involved more than 13,000 women, assigned at random to take either tamoxifen or a placebo for five years. Tamoxifen had already been in use for 20 years to treat breast cancer, but it was not known whether it could also prevent the disease.

Each group had its drawbacks: tamoxifen can have side effects, including small increases in the risk of serious disorders like blood clots and uterine cancer. But if it did prevent breast cancer, women on placebos would have missed out on five years of protection.

Mrs. Olson, who lives in Coon Rapids, Minnesota, did not mind. "I thought somebody has to do it, and I'm willing to because I'm so grateful my sister is still alive," she said. Four of her six sisters also joined the study (the one who had had cancer was not eligible, and another lived too far from the study site).

The letter Mrs. Olson received revealed that she had been in the placebo group, and said she could now ask her doctor to prescribe tamoxifen, or she could enter another study in which patients would be given either tamoxifen or a similar drug, with no one getting placebos.

A few days after receiving the letter, Mrs. Olson had not decided what to do. "I've thought about it a lot," she said. "I do not want cancer. If my doctor said to go on tamoxifen, I'd do it today."

To help decide who really would benefit from tamoxifen, Dr. Ford said she and her colleagues were trying to provide information that women and doctors could use to assess an individual woman's risk of developing breast cancer, and of suffering serious side effects from tamoxifen. But Dr. Ford cautioned that the group would not be able to offer a simple set of guidelines that would apply to everyone; each woman's risk profile is different.

For women who should take tamoxifen, the next thing the scientists hope to determine is when they should take it, Dr. Ford said. For prevention, a single five-year course of treatment is recommended, but it is not clear when a woman should begin that course. "Is one five-year period better than another?" Dr. Ford asked. "If you come from a family where everyone with breast cancer had it young, that would probably enter into the decision."

Another question is whether tamoxifen helps women who carry the genes BRCA1 or BRCA2, which greatly increase a woman's risk of developing breast cancer. Blood samples from women in the study are being tested for the genes to answer that question, but the results will not be given to individual patients because the samples were stored anonymously.

Dr. Ford said that the researchers would also be looking for other side effects, including depression. One of Mrs. Olson's sisters, Jackie Kristenson, of Lake Elmo, Minnesota, dropped out of the study after less than a year because the depression she had suffered in the past became far worse. She encountered another woman who had the same experience, and when the study was stopped, Mrs. Kristenson learned that she had indeed been taking tamoxifen. She was offered four more years of treatment with the drug, she said, but hopes never to take it again.

It is already clear that not every woman can take tamoxifen. Because it can increase the risk of blood clots, it may not be safe for women with other conditions that add to that risk, like previous blood clots, hypertension, diabetes, obesity or cigarette smoking. Blood clots are serious: Two women on tamoxifen in the study died from clots in their lungs.

Dr. P. J. Flynn, a cancer specialist in Minneapolis who coordinated the study in Minnesota, said that clots sometimes form even in people who lack the known risk factors. "There is nothing you can do to test the general public to tell who is prone to clotting," he said.

Other women who should not take tamoxifen, the cancer institute says, include those who are pregnant, and those who do not wish to stop taking birth control pills or hormone replacement after menopause.

The other serious concern is that tamoxifen can increase the risk of uterine cancer. Dr. V. Craig Jordan of Northwestern University Medical Center in Chicago, made that discovery in 1988 and urged doctors to monitor women taking tamoxifen. The risk increases because the uterus, like the breast, has estrogen receptors. But in the uterus, instead of acting as an estrogen blocker, tamoxifen actually mimics estrogen and can stimulate tumor growth.

That seeming paradox occurs, Dr. Jordan said, because although the estrogen receptors themselves are probably the same in both places, other proteins in the breast and uterus differ, and may determine what happens next after tamoxifen binds to a receptor. In the breast, he said, proteins called co-repressors may stick to the complex formed by the drug and the receptor, and inhibit cell growth. But in the

uterus, co-activator proteins may team up with the complex to switch on genes that stimulate cell growth.

The risk of uterine cancer is small: in women ages 60 and over, two cases occur per 1,000 women who take tamoxifen, as opposed to one case per 1,000 women who do not use the drug. The risk is similar to that in postmenopausal women who take estrogen-replacement therapy. Uterine cancer is usually detected early enough to be cured. Nonetheless, few patients or doctors are comfortable with any increase in cancer risk.

In addition to studying other drugs to see if any might offer the same benefits as tamoxifen, without raising the threat of uterine cancer, Dr. Ford said that researchers were also trying to find out whether adding other drugs to tamoxifen might protect the uterus. "But we can't answer these kinds of questions unless people volunteer for studies," she said.

Mrs. Olson said that she and some of her sisters were ready to sign up for the next round. "Anything to help women in the future," she said. "I have three lovely daughters and a granddaughter."

[DG, April 1998]

## Round 3 in Cancer Battle: A 5-Year Drug Regimen

Having completed the first two phases of treatment for an early breast cancer—a lumpectomy and six weeks of radiation therapy—I have now begun the third and, in a way, the most exciting phase: five years of daily treatment with the drug tamoxifen.

Unlike traditional cancer chemotherapy, tamoxifen does not kill cells and does not cause nausea and hair loss. Tamoxifen is more like a growth regulator. It is an estrogen-like compound that acts in the breast as an antiestrogen, preventing the natural hormone from stimulating the growth of breast cancer cells.

Tamoxifen has been around for about 20 years. It was first used to treat advanced breast cancer, then to prevent recurrence of less advanced disease. Now it is

being used to prevent breast cancer from occurring in the first place in women at high risk of developing the disease.

Factors that contribute to a woman's risk of developing breast cancer include being over 60, having a family history of breast cancer, having had a noninvasive breast cancer or precancerous breast abnormalities, having begun to menstruate before the age of 12 and having had no children or a first child after age 30.

I admit to being confused and disappointed when my surgeon announced gleefully that my cancer was highly sensitive to hormone stimulation, as indicated by a test for estrogen and progesterone receptors on the cancer cells. To me that meant I would probably never again be able to take postmenopausal hormones, which could protect my heart, bones and brain from premature deterioration and which prevented hot flashes and vaginal dryness.

The surgeon was pleased because being estrogen-receptor-positive meant that my tumor was slower growing, and that I could reap the maximum protection from tamoxifen, which has been shown to cut in half the risk of recurrence of the original breast cancer as well as the development of a second cancer in the opposite breast.

Estrogen receptors are found in about 65 to 80 percent of breast cancers in postmenopausal women and 45 to 60 percent of cancers in premenopausal women.

The higher the level of estrogen receptors in a woman's tumor, the greater the survival benefit associated with taking the drug. Women whose cancers are estrogen-receptor-negative reap some benefit from tamoxifen as well, suggesting that the drug has other as-yet undiscovered actions.

Studies have indicated that five years of daily tamoxifen is more protective than one or two years and as good or better than taking the drug for 10 years. Its protective effects have been shown to persist for at least five years after the drug is stopped.

Most exciting, in 1998, tamoxifen was shown in a study of more than 13,000 women to reduce by 50 percent the development of a first cancer in women considered at high risk for the disease. This made tamoxifen the first drug found to prevent cancer, although it is still not known for sure whether the protection is permanent. But tamoxifen may not be helpful in women who carry cancer-promoting mutations of the genes BRCA1 and BRCA2.

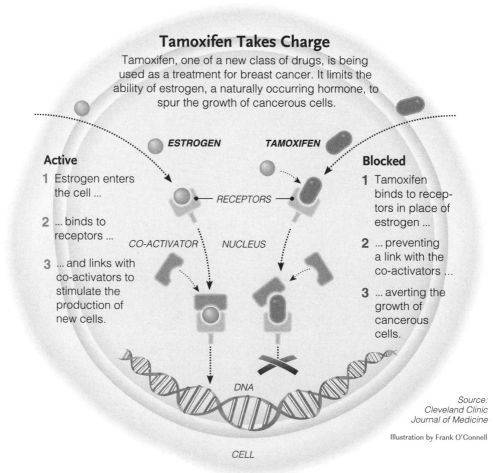

**Tamoxifen Takes Charge**

Tamoxifen, one of a new class of drugs, is being used as a treatment for breast cancer. It limits the ability of estrogen, a naturally occurring hormone, to spur the growth of cancerous cells.

*ESTROGEN*     *TAMOXIFEN*

**Active**

1 Estrogen enters the cell ...

2 ... binds to receptors ...

3 ... and links with co-activators to stimulate the production of new cells.

RECEPTORS

CO-ACTIVATOR    NUCLEUS

**Blocked**

1 Tamoxifen binds to receptors in place of estrogen ...

2 ... preventing a link with the co-activators ...

3 ... averting the growth of cancerous cells.

DNA

CELL

*Source:
Cleveland Clinic
Journal of Medicine*

Illustration by Frank O'Connell

Dr. D. Lawrence Wickerham, an oncologist at Allegheny University in Pittsburgh and a co-leader of national tamoxifen studies, said, "The cancers that developed in tamoxifen-treated women tended to be smaller and were found at an earlier stage," meaning they were more readily cured. Describing other benefits found in the studies, Dr. Wickerham said: "Women taking tamoxifen suffered fewer bone fractures of the wrist, hip and spine and their cholesterol level dropped by 12 to 20 percent. Furthermore, there is no evidence that tamoxifen is associated with weight gain, depression, nausea or cancers of the ovary, liver and gastrointestinal tract."

The effects of tamoxifen on the brain are unknown, though there is no evidence of any ill effect, like memory impairment.

But for all the good tamoxifen does, it has certain major and minor disadvantages. Like estrogen, it raises the risk of developing a relatively uncommon cancer of the uterus, endometrial cancer, a disease that can be detected early through routine monitoring and cured by surgery and, if needed, radiation therapy. Its other serious side effect—one that is shared by estrogen as well—is an increased risk of blood clots, which are occasionally fatal. Nonetheless, Dr. V. Craig Jordan of Northwestern University's cancer center, who did pioneering research on tamoxifen, said the survival benefit from the drug for a woman like me who has had breast cancer outweighs the risk of death from its effects on the uterus and blood by about 30 times.

Stimulation of the growth of the endometrium, or uterine lining, which could increase the risk of cancer, occurs in a small percentage of women who take tamoxifen. Nonetheless, women may be advised to have a baseline uterine examination before starting tamoxifen, followed by annual checkups to see if the drug is stimulating growth of the endometrium. This examination can be done in a doctor's office as an endometrial biopsy or painlessly by transvaginal ultrasound. A woman who experiences an unusual vaginal discharge or bleeding while on tamoxifen should report that to her gynecologist without delay.

On a less serious note, tamoxifen also causes hot flashes in a quarter to a third of users and an annoy-ing vaginal discharge in about 5 to 10 percent of women. The hot flashes may seriously disrupt a woman's life. But they usually diminish with time, and their intensity may be diminished by daily consumption of soy products like tofu and ground flaxseed.

Tamoxifen, sold as Nolvadex, is the first of a new class of drugs called SERMs, for selective estrogen receptor modulators. These compounds compete with natural estrogen for a docking site on cells throughout the body. When these sites, called receptors, are occupied by tamoxifen, estrogen cannot hook on properly and exert its usual effects.

A more recent addition to this class is raloxifene, sold as Evista, which seems to share most of the characteristics, good and bad, of tamoxifen, and several other such drugs are in various stages of development. The ultimate goal is to find a compound that does all the good that estrogen does, including reducing the risk of heart disease and osteoporosis, stimulating brain cells and preventing menopausal symptoms, but that has none of estrogen's bad effects, especially raising the risk of cancers of the breast and uterus and causing blood clots.

Raloxifene, which is approved for the prevention of bone loss, also appears to protect the breast and heart but without stimulating cell growth and cancer in the uterus. But like tamoxifen, it can increase clotting and induce hot flashes, and it is not yet known whether it is as good as or better than tamoxifen in preventing breast cancer.

A study to determine this, called STAR (for Study of Tamoxifen and Raloxifene), began in 1999. The study, sponsored by the National Cancer Institute, will involve 22,000 women and is expected to last 5 to 10 years.

"At the moment, it's too early to use raloxifene to prevent breast cancer outside of a clinical trial," Dr. Wickerham said during a teleconference sponsored by Cancer Care Inc. "We don't yet know raloxifene's long-term benefits or risks."

More information on tamoxifen can be found in the paperback book, *Tamoxifen* by Dr. John F. Kessler and Greg A. Annussek.

[JEB, May 1999]

# Drugs to Fight Breast Cancer Near Approval

An advisory committee of the Food and Drug Administration voted unanimously in September 1998 to recommend approval of the drug tamoxifen to reduce women's risk of developing breast cancer. Although the drug, which was already on the market, is intended only for women at high risk of breast cancer, and the advisory panel was cautious in its wording, tamoxifen's approval represents a milestone in efforts to prevent cancer.

"As far as I know, this is the first drug approved for the prevention of cancer," said Dr. Leslie Ford, the associate director for early detection and community oncology at the National Cancer Institute.

Also in September 1998, the advisory panel unanimously recommended approval for a new drug for women with advanced breast cancer. Officials say that the drug, Herceptin, made by Genentech, is intended for use by the estimated 30 percent of breast cancer patients who have too many copies of a gene called HER2/neu, making the cancer aggressively spread through the body.

Herceptin is not a cure, but has been shown in clinical trials, either alone or with chemotherapy, to delay the progression of the disease.

Tamoxifen had already been on the market as a treatment to prevent recurrences of breast cancer. Because doctors can prescribe drugs for other than their approved uses, they could give tamoxifen to healthy women even without the F.D.A.'s approval. But approval of tamoxifen as a drug to reduce cancer risk allowed the company to advertise and market it widely for this purpose and health insurance companies are more likely to pay for it for women who have never had cancer.

Supporters expressed delight that women would have a new avenue to prevent one of the diseases they dread the most. "We're very pleased," said Susan Braun, the president and chief executive of the Susan G. Komen Foundation, an advocacy group for women with breast cancer.

But tamoxifen is not a panacea, experts warn, and the 11-member advisory panel said it did not yet have enough information to determine which women were at high enough risk of breast cancer to make the drug's hazards, including potentially fatal blood clots as well as cancer of the uterine lining, worth its benefits.

Skeptics said they feared that the drug would be overpromoted and that more women might be harmed than helped. "The message we try to get across is that not everyone is at high enough risk to make this worthwhile," said Cindy Pearson, executive director of the National Women's Health Network. "It isn't like putting iodine in your salt or chlorine in your drinking water. Women have already died taking this drug." It is still not clear, she said, that in the long term it will save lives.

Alan Milbauer, who is vice president for external affairs at Zeneca Pharmaceuticals, the Wilmington, Delaware company that makes tamoxifen, said the company planned to advertise the drug directly to women in 1999, after first educating general practitioners about its use. Mr. Milbauer said that tamoxifen costs $80 to $100 a month.

Dr. Robert Justice, who is acting director of the division of oncology drug products at the F.D.A., said "potentially tens of millions of women" could be candidates for tamoxifen. He said Zeneca, a unit of Zeneca Group Plc, applied to market the drug for the prevention of breast cancer at the behest of the agency and the National Cancer Institute. He called the advisory committee's decision to recommend that the drug be approved for this purpose "courageous."

Already demand for tamoxifen is starting to build. Dr. Barbara Weber, who directs the breast cancer program at the University of Pennsylvania Medical Center, said that "more and more women are calling me," about the drug and that other doctors have had the same experience.

Cancer experts had long hoped that tamoxifen might prevent breast cancer. Its biochemistry was promising, because it prevented the hormone estrogen from stimulating breast tissue. "It's holding up across the board—in any setting where you get reduced exposure to estrogen, you get less breast cancer," Dr. Weber said.

For example, women who start menstruating late or who reach menopause early are less likely to develop breast cancer. But the notion of testing tamoxifen as a breast cancer preventative in healthy women was controversial because it would mean exposing women to the known risks of the drug to provide a possibly elusive benefit.

Nonetheless, the cancer institute went ahead in 1992 with a large study involving 13,388 women who had at least double the average risk of breast cancer. Half of the women took tamoxifen and the others took a dummy pill. The institute abruptly halted the trial in April 1998, 14 months before it was scheduled to end, announcing that it was unethical to continue because the data were clear that women who took the drug were less likely to develop breast cancer. Eighty-five women taking tamoxifen had developed breast cancer, compared with 154 women taking a placebo, a 45 percent reduction.

But 33 women taking tamoxifen developed cancer of the uterine lining, as opposed to 14 of women taking the placebo; 17 women using tamoxifen had blood clots in their lungs, as against 6 taking the placebo.

And the picture was soon further muddied. While the cancer institute's study was awaiting publication in September 1998, two European groups published results from their own studies in *The Lancet*, and the data were not so encouraging. A British study of 2,471 women and an Italian study of 5,408 women found no reduction in breast cancer risk in women who took tamoxifen.

Some at the cancer institute suggested that the European studies were too small to see tamoxifen's benefit. In addition, noted Dr. Ford, who directed the tamoxifen trial for the cancer institute, the women in the European trials were at lower risk of developing breast cancer. But, wrote Dr. Kathleen I. Pritchard of the University of Toronto in an accompanying editorial in *The Lancet*, "The failure of these trials to confirm the results of the U.S. study, however, casts

doubt on the wisdom of the rush, at least in some places, to prescribe tamoxifen widely for prevention."

By that time, momentum was already building for the approval of tamoxifen for healthy women at increased risk of breast cancer. In April 1998, shortly after the American tamoxifen study ended, officials from the F.D.A., the cancer institute, and the American tamoxifen study met and decided that the agency should consider allowing Zeneca to market tamoxifen as a breast cancer preventative, Dr. Justice of the F.D.A. said. "They were encouraged to submit an application to us as soon as possible," he added.

The advisory panel, headed by Dr. Janice Dutcher, a professor of medicine at Montefiore Medical Center in the Bronx, was unhappy with the wording of the agency's questions, which asked if tamoxifen should be approved as a way to "prevent" breast cancer. That had not been demonstrated, the group said, noting that it remained possible that the drug merely staved off cancers that would eventually occur. So it changed the words to "reduce the risk" of breast cancer and voted unanimously to recommend approval for that purpose.

Dr. Ford said that the cancer institute and its tamoxifen researchers had been preparing for this day, developing a computer disk for women and doctors that would calculate an individual's risk of developing breast cancer as well as compare her risk to that of the women in the large tamoxifen study. Those who want the disk can order it, Dr. Ford said, through the cancer institute's clinical trials Web site: http://cancertrials.nci.nih.gov/.

Herceptin is the first genetically engineered drug for the treatment of advanced breast cancer. Herceptin has not yet been tested in earlier-stage breast cancer, but some specialists said they believed it could also prevent or delay the spread of the disease.

Although Herceptin has the potential to delay tumor progression in less than one-third of patients whose breast cancer has spread, or metastasized, cancer specialists said it represented an important step toward a new method of treatment. Unlike chemotherapy, which kills fast-multiplying cells, healthy as well as cancerous, Herceptin targets a specific genetic alteration linked to the cancer. Thus, it has relatively few side effects.

Dr. Debu Trepathy, director of clinical trials at the breast care center of the University of California at San Francisco and a principal investigator of the drug, called the drug a breakthrough. "There is no doubt in my mind that this is the beginning of a whole new wave of biological drugs that modulate the causes of cancer," he said.

Herceptin was developed by Genentech Inc., based in South San Francisco, California, which is 67 percent owned by Roche Holdings Ltd., of Basel, Switzerland. Herceptin is a genetically engineered copy of an immune system protein known as a monoclonal antibody.

Herceptin was recommended for the treatment of patients with advanced metastatic breast cancer whose tumors produce excessive amounts of a gene known as HER2, for human epithelial growth factor receptor-2. When several copies of an HER2 gene exist in a cancer cell, excessive amounts of a protein are produced on the surface of cells.

About 25 to 30 percent of metastatic breast cancer patients produce too much HER2. In turn, an excess of HER2 often means the patient's cancer will spread faster and prove fatal sooner than in patients producing smaller amounts of HER2. Patients in clinical trials of Herceptin were screened using laboratory tests to determine if they produced large amounts of HER2.

"The ability to ask functional questions about cells, and about what causes a normal cell to become malignant, and then to intervene to fix what is broken, that has been the promise," of molecular biology in cancer, said Dr. Dennis Slamon, director of the Revlon U.C.L.A. Women's Cancer Research Program in Los Angeles. "HER2 and Herceptin, in that context, represent to my mind the first real-world real-

ization of that hope," he said. Dr. Slamon was a principal investigator of Herceptin.

In clinical trials of patients with metastatic disease who had not received chemotherapy, tumors progressed more slowly in those treated with Herceptin and chemotherapy than those treated with chemotherapy alone.

About 28 percent of women treated with Herceptin and chemotherapy did not show tumor progression at one year, compared with 14 percent who were treated with chemotherapy alone.

A second trial, of women who were not helped by chemotherapy showed that Herceptin alone delayed tumor progression to some extent in a fifth of the patients.

For most patients, the main side effect of Herceptin was a fever, treatable with Tylenol. In a minority, however, who received Herceptin along with a class of chemotherapy drugs called anthracyclines, the combination caused cardiac problems, such as congestive heart failure. These effects typically ceased when the drug was withdrawn.

"It's a very big advance," said Dr. Larry Norton, medical director of the breast center at New York's Memorial Sloan-Kettering. "All by itself, it's definitely going to help a lot of people and it dramatically augments the Taxol effect," he said, referring to a chemotherapy drug that has been particularly effective against breast cancer.

"The key issue is not the efficacy, although that's very exciting," Dr. Norton said. "The key issue is that this is the beginning of the whole new approach in the treatment of cancer."

The panel voted to approve the use of Herceptin alone, or with Taxol, but voted against its use with anthracyclines.

[GK and LMF, September 1998]

# Hope for Sale: Business Thrives on Unproven Care, Leaving Science Behind

For years, Dr. Larry Norton tried to conduct a medical study to determine, once and for all, whether bone marrow transplants could really save the lives of women desperately ill with breast cancer. His efforts—and those of dozens of other doctors—were largely futile. Year after year, few women were willing to participate in the clinical tests, which, to be scientifically valid, required patients to be randomly assigned to either the experimental treatment or standard chemotherapy.

Many believed the experimental treatment was their only hope, and were unwilling to leave anything to chance. So most chose to get transplants from a growing number of hospitals and cancer centers that are part of a multimillion-dollar industry that sells experimental treatments. There, for more than a decade, many women were told that the procedure was the only thing that could save their lives—when, in fact, no one knew for sure whether it was better or worse than the standard treatment.

"I got so angry," Dr. Norton said. "Fifty years from now, we will look at this period with horror and say 'How could this have happened?'" But Dr. Norton, head of the division of solid tumor oncology at Memorial Sloan-Kettering Cancer Center in New York, said he understood why the women refused to join the study: Few patients, faced with advanced and likely fatal disease, would risk passing up a supposedly cutting-edge treatment simply to advance scientific knowledge.

Experts say that tens of thousands of such personal decisions, made under enormous emotional strain, are significantly slowing the search for cures for dire diseases like cancer. The wide availability of unproven procedures sops up the vast majority of potential test subjects, they say, making it difficult, or impossible, to assess which treatments work and which do not.

To better understand the workings of this system, *The New York Times* examined one of the most widely offered procedures—bone marrow transplants for solid tumor cancers like breast cancer. The examination found that this procedure entered the medical marketplace in the 1980s before studies to test its effectiveness had even begun. By the time testing was under way, the business had taken on a life of its own. Patients were unavailable and tests were delayed for years or had to be abandoned.

The issue arises because medical procedures, like the bone marrow transplants or new surgical techniques, are not regulated, reflecting the Government's usual reluctance to interfere with doctors' practice of medicine. By contrast, Federal rules require that new drugs or devices like a heart valve be proven safe and effective before being sold to the public.

Doctors, of course, can voluntarily regulate themselves and those in one tiny specialty, pediatric cancer, have done so. These doctors have agreed to provide experimental procedures only to patients who participate in valid research. As a result, the advances in this field have been phenomenal, far outracing anything seen in adult medicine.

In breast cancer, testing of bone marrow transplants took twice as long as anyone expected. Throughout the 1990s, doctors and hospitals reported to a national registry that about 15,000 women had purchased bone marrow transplants for treatment of breast cancer. Medical experts said that the voluntary reporting system missed about half of the women who actually received the procedure. Yet, while as many as 30,000 women had bone marrow transplants for breast cancer, only 1,000 participated in the scientific studies.

In ovarian cancer, it proved impossible to even conduct a trial of bone marrow transplants. Doctors at more than 100 medical institutions nationwide spent two and a half years seeking 285 women who would participate. They enlisted just 25. In April 1999, researchers admitted defeat. The ovarian cancer trials collapsed. Many doctors, like Dr. Maurie Markman, director of the Taussig Cancer Center at the Cleveland Clinic, were unable to enroll a single patient despite monumental efforts. "It's a tragedy that we can't do a randomized trial in the United States to answer this," Dr. Markman said. "Unfortunately, if someone says they can cure you and I say I can't, it is very logical that people will drift to those who can give you hope."

Those who sell experimental procedures have a different view. They say they are helping patients who have run out of options and that researchers who are only focused on determining whether a treatment works are out of touch with the needs of patients suffering with a disease now. "These are not guinea pigs, this is not a fascist society," said Dr. William H. West, chairman of Response Oncology, a publicly traded, for-profit company that sells the procedure. "We are an open marketplace, and that's true in clinical trials."

But other experts point out that the same arguments could be made about drugs and medical devices. In those cases, the Government has decided that treatments must be proven safe and effective before they are offered on a large scale. Abandoning that standard for procedures, these experts said, is perilous.

"Physicians must demand the same high standards of science for new procedures as we do for new medicines,' said Dr. C. Warren Olanow, professor and chairman of the department of neurology at the Mount Sinai School of Medicine in New York. "The alternative is uncontrolled human experimentation."

Today, in bone marrow transplants, the uncertainty lives on, tearing at women as they face the decision of whether to undergo this difficult procedure. With so many years having passed since the idea of bone marrow transplants first emerged, they struggle to understand how a medical system so advanced could not yet answer a question so basic: Does the treatment work?

Catherine Porter, 44, who has breast cancer that has spread to other parts of her body, is among those wondering. Seven years ago, Mrs. Porter, of Imlay City, Michigan, had a breast removed to combat her cancer. She felt certain she had been cured. Then,

recently she learned the cancer was back, worse than ever. Figuring she would take a gamble, she elected to have a bone marrow transplant at the Barbara Ann Karmanos Cancer Institute in Detroit. Now, she waits, wondering if the experimental treatment she received will help her, and why medical science still cannot answer that question for so many thousands of women. "Something has got to be done," she said, "So we don't have to keep doing this."

In 1979, when the options for treating breast cancer were limited, Dr. Gabriel Hortobagyi was one of a handful who ventured into uncharted territory: treating the cancer with a bone marrow transplant. When the first patient appeared to do well, Dr. Hortobagyi offered the procedure to another woman, and another.

It was not an easy procedure. Known within the field as high-dose chemotherapy followed by bone marrow transplant or stem cell rescue, the experimental treatment is based on a simple concept: If a little chemotherapy killed some of the cancerous cells in a woman's body, a lot might kill them all.

So doctors remove some bone marrow or red blood cells from the patient, then load her with huge amounts of toxic drugs, quantities that destroy the bone marrow. The hope is that the high doses will eliminate the cancer and that the saved bone marrow, when returned to the body, will grow back quickly enough so that the patient does not die from infection. A version of the procedure, using donations of bone marrow, had long been established as effective for blood cancer, but solely because the cancer was in the marrow that was being replaced. The use of the treatment for breast cancer involved a completely different—and untested—reasoning.

Even though Dr. Hortobagyi and a handful of other pioneers at academic centers selected patients who were young and otherwise healthy, they could not save some from the terrible effects of the powerful anticancer drugs. Fifteen to 20 percent of the women in those early days died from the harsh drugs alone; others had permanent injuries, including hearing loss, nerve damage and heart damage.

The pioneers became heroes by the late 1980s, when they began announcing what looked like amazing outcomes. The data were not scientifically valid proof that the treatment worked—each medical center looked at less than a few dozen patients and had to infer how they would have fared without a transplant. But the data appeared to make a startling point. Women with advanced breast cancer who had had transplants experienced remission rates of 50 to 60 percent. The general population of women with advanced breast cancer who had received conventional chemotherapy had remission rates of just 10 to 15 percent.

"Those of us who were involved got very, very excited," Dr. Hortobagyi said. "We told our patients, 'Look at the results we're getting.'" The patients were not the only ones who looked. With the apparent success of the bone marrow transplants, a new business had been born. "It seemed so logical," Dr. Norton said. "It started getting accepted without clinical trials."

Data from a voluntary registry, the Autologous Blood and Bone Marrow Transplant Registry of North America, show the growth in the popularity of this procedure. The registry, which records about half of the bone marrow transplants in the United States, found that 271 women with breast cancer had transplants in 1989. Two years later the number had jumped to 749. By 1997 there were 2,853 bone marrow transplants for breast cancer reported. For-profit corporations offering bone marrow transplants emerged by the late 1980's. Response Oncology, one of the first, started offering the procedure in 1989 as part of what it called a "clinical trials program."

That program involved only trials that gave everybody the procedure and watched how they fared. These studies cannot be used to demonstrate whether the procedure is any better than the standard treatment, because there is no comparison group of similar patients. Therefore, there is no way of knowing how the patients would have fared with conventional treatment.

But the trials did help Response Oncology earn profits. Dr. West, the chairman of the company, said the profit margin from bone marrow transplants is 15 percent. All told, Response Oncology brought in $128 million in revenue in 1998, largely from its cancer centers providing bone marrow transplants.

Private hospitals also joined the fray. Institutions like a hospital in Zion, Illinois, owned by Cancer Treatment Centers of America, advertise heavily for patients and even pay for patients to travel there for the procedure. Hospitals associated with giant for-profit chains, including the Columbia/HCA Healthcare Corporation and Tenet Healthcare, opened bone marrow transplant programs that offered the treatment to women with breast cancer.

But the academic medical centers—even those trying to recruit patients for clinical trials—did not stand aside and let all the profits go elsewhere. By the early 1990s virtually every major medical center was offering bone marrow transplants for breast cancer patients and a growing number of community hospitals were offering them as well. At academic centers, bone marrow transplant programs quickly became "the cash cow for the cancer service," said Dr. William McGuire, an ovarian cancer specialist at Mercy Medical Center in Baltimore.

Every entity offering the experimental procedure tried a different sales pitch. Some promoted the prestige of their institutions, others the convenience of their locations, others their caring attitudes and patient support, and others, like Response Oncology, their lower prices.

Paying for the procedures turned out not to be a problem for many patients: Their insurance companies ended up footing the bill. The insurers at first refused, pointing out clauses in their policies saying they would not pay for experimental procedures. But under pressure from patients, doctors, lawyers and lawmakers, most insurance companies gave in.

Take the case of Rita Hartmann, a 60-year-old elementary school teacher from Wooster, Ohio. When her ovarian cancer recurred, Mrs. Hartmann and her husband agonized over what to do. Cancer Treatment Centers of America told her she had a 30 percent chance of a cure if she had a transplant, but her insurance company said it would not pay. Mrs. Hartmann's husband wanted to mortgage their house, sell all they owned to raise the money. But Mrs. Hartmann held back. "I said, 'That's too traumatic,'" she said.

Instead, she called a staff aide for her Senator,

Mike DeWine, a Republican. The aide in turn reached Mrs. Hartmann's insurance company. In addition, Mrs. Hartmann and 20 of her friends wrote pleading letters to her insurer. Three months later, on Valentine's Day 1998, the company agreed to pay. Mrs. Hartmann had her transplant. Her cancer returned within nine months.

Under pressure from doctors and patient groups, Congress even mandated in 1994 that insurers for Federal employees pay for bone marrow transplants for women with breast or ovarian cancer. Soon, lobbied by doctors, hospitals and patient groups, about a dozen states adopted their own mandates that the experimental procedure be covered. Lost in the rush to offer the treatment to more cancer patients with solid tumors was the fact that the procedure still had not been shown to work even for breast cancer, where it got its start.

"It evolved into a standard of care," said Dr. John Glick, director of the Cancer Center at the University of Pennsylvania. "It isn't."

After being assured that her insurance company would pick up the $150,000 bill for a bone-marrow transplant for ovarian cancer, Deborah Holmes traveled halfway across the country for the treatment, from her home in Hamden, Connecticut, to the hospital in Zion, Illinois, operated by Cancer Treatment Centers of America. To Ms. Holmes, it was worth the trip. "There was so much hope there, so much positive energy down to the nurses and the doctors," Ms. Holmes said.

At Brown University in Rhode Island, a 90-minute drive from Ms. Holmes's home, the mood was far less positive. Despite the happy assurances of 30 percent cure rates at places like Cancer Treatment Centers, researchers at the university knew the truth: No one could say whether this procedure worked for ovarian cancer patients like Ms. Holmes.

Ms. Holmes, unaware of the national clinical trial, believed what Cancer Treatment Centers of America had told her—that transplants could cure women like herself. When her cancer returned five months after her transplant, Ms. Holmes said she guessed she was just one of the unlucky ones. She died nine months later.

Breast cancer clinical trials had begun several years before, in 1990, but struggled to find patients. There were two national trials: one for women whose breast cancer had spread throughout their bodies and another for women whose cancer had spread to at least 10 of the lymph nodes under their arms. Researchers expected it would take about three years to enroll about 1,000 women in the two studies. Instead it took seven years. For every 10 women who could have been in a clinical trial, one actually enrolled, Dr. Norton said.

Medical centers had to make a choice: Offer only the randomized clinical trials—and watch patients leave in droves—or offer bone marrow transplants outside the randomized trials for those who would not participate in the research studies.

Dr. Andrew L. Pecora, chief of the adult blood and marrow stem cell transplant program at Hackensack University Medical Center in New Jersey, gave women an option of having a transplant outside a randomized trial. "I offered the clinical trial to every patient," he said. "But I did not force them to do it." Few entered the trial, he said. Dr. Norton refused to provide transplants outside the trial. His patients went elsewhere. "I was disheartened but I wasn't surprised," he said.

As the business was booming and the trials staggering, Dr. Hortobagyi, one of the pioneers who had helped get transplants started, was having second thoughts. Those initial stunning results he and others had reported were with carefully selected patients younger than 60 and otherwise healthy—no heart disease, no emphysema, nothing that might make the high doses of drugs even more risky.

The researchers had compared their outcomes with the outcomes of conventional chemotherapy for all women with advanced breast cancer, even though most breast cancer patients were older and sicker than those who had transplants. Dr. Hortobagyi decided to go back and compare the outcomes in the women who had transplants with those of women who were just as young and healthy but who had conventional chemotherapy.

The women, he discovered, did just as well when they had conventional chemotherapy. The women he had provided with transplants did not survive in greater numbers because of the procedure. They survived because they were healthier to begin with. It was a hard fact to face. In promoting transplants, "we deceived ourselves and we deceived our patients," Dr. Hortobagyi said. "We oversold it."

But that realization came too late. In May of 1999 a crowd of breast cancer specialists filled a conference room half the size of a football field at the Georgia World Congress Center in Atlanta. Those who came too late to get seats spilled into two smaller rooms nearby with closed circuit television screens. Few at the annual meeting of the American Society of Clinical Oncology wanted to miss this moment when the leaders in their field would present the long-awaited data from clinical trials of bone marrow transplants for women with advanced breast cancer.

The results were not the triumph that many had hoped for. In four of the five clinical trials, there was no difference in survival between women who had transplants and those who had conventional therapy. Only in the South African study did the women who received bone marrow transplants outlive the patients in the group who received standard therapy. But on closer inspection of the data, even that success seemed suspect: The women who had transplants lived about as long as the women in the other studies. But the women who had conventional chemotherapy in the South African study did far worse. The results did not indicate that transplants improved survival, but that the outcomes for the control group were poor.

No one on the podium that day claimed that the studies showed that transplants were a triumph. Indeed, the trials' failure to show the expected benefits of transplants gave rise to a troubling question: When the best available data provided no evidence that bone marrow transplants were any better than conventional chemotherapy, should transplants continue to be promoted and sold?

For the National Breast Cancer Coalition, which represents cancer patients, the data spoke for themselves: Bone marrow transplants had been tested and had failed. "How can anybody look at these data and think this is something we should continue doing or

that they are inconclusive?" asked Fran Visco, the coalition's president. The group put out a news release saying, "It is time to move beyond the infrastructure" created around transplants.

But cancer specialists were less definitive. Many said they still saw promise in transplants, arguing that it was too soon to say for sure that the procedure offered no benefits. They urged that nothing change for the time being while the women in the studies were followed for longer periods to see if those who had transplants eventually did better. They also said that chemotherapy had improved over the last decade and because the studies used older drugs, it remained possible that bone marrow transplants with new drugs might be better than conventional chemotherapy.

Reflecting these views, the American Society of Clinical Oncologists put out a news release saying that the papers presented at the meeting "report mixed early results" and that more years of study are needed. Dr. Allen S. Lichter, the departing president of the society and dean of the University of Michigan Medical School, urged that nothing change for the time being while new studies get under way and the women in the initial studies continue to be followed.

"As a nontransplanter and a keen observer of this research, I don't think there is enough information to say it should die," Dr. Lichter said. He also said that because not every woman is eligible for a clinical trial or has ready access to one, transplants should still be available outside trials. "I for one am not ready to say that this should only be done in a clinical trial," Dr. Lichter said.

Dr. West of Response Oncology said his company intended to keep selling transplants. Calls to stop offering them are "an oversimplification," he said, because the trials were not definitive. More trials and years of further study are needed, he said. At bottom, he said, critics are missing the point. What matters, he said, is not whether the treatment has been shown to work but whether studies are producing more knowledge.

So now oncologists and companies say they will press ahead, continuing to sell a painful, expensive procedure that the best available science says is no improvement over standard care, which is less traumatic. Some patient advocates and doctors find this a troubling abandonment of the rigors of science.

"I don't have a problem with oncologists who say, 'We really have to do something for these patients, they are facing a terribly short future,'" said Dr. Alan Garber, a professor of medicine at Stanford University. "The problem is when they start to do things that have been tested and have not proven effective. Then you are leaving the arena of science and going into blind faith."

[GK and KE, October 1999]

## Reactions of Women With Cancer

Until a few months ago, Donna Bowers's life mirrored a million other women's lives. She juggled family and career, rearing her two little girls and working as a lawyer and health information manager at Baylor University Medical Center in Dallas. The future stretched ahead to a far horizon, and like most people, she did not think about the prospect of her time running out.

That changed abruptly in February 1999, when Ms. Bowers, who is 38 years old, found out that she had breast cancer and that it had already spread to the lymph nodes under her arm. The more cancerous lymph nodes a woman has, the worse her outlook. Ten or more put her in a bleak zone with a high risk that the disease will recur, spread and kill her. Ms. Bowers learned she had 16 positive nodes.

"That was sort of devastating," she said. And the news plunged her into a terrible dilemma: should she take her chances with conventional breast cancer chemotherapy, or risk the rigors of high-dose chemotherapy followed by a bone-marrow transplant?

She knew that some doctors recommend the second choice, even though the treatment itself is so dangerous that some women die from it. She had several friends with breast cancer who had undergone the treatment, in which patients are given such high doses of chemotherapy that the immune system is practically destroyed. To restore it, doctors usually remove some of the patient's own bone marrow before treatment, and return it to her afterward.

But Ms. Bowers's doctor, Dr. Joyce O'Shaughnessy, a breast cancer specialist at Baylor, did not recommend a bone-marrow transplant. Dr. O'Shaughnessy recommended that Ms. Bowers go ahead with the less extreme chemotherapy program and wait for the results of several major bone-marrow transplant studies before deciding whether to have a transplant.

That made sense to Ms. Bowers. "If she tells me my chances of survival are enhanced, I would do it," she said. "If the statistics show a 10 percent increase or better, I'd probably do it. Eight or 9 percent, maybe."

In the meantime, she and her husband, a doctor, decided that she should have "the most aggressive treatment known," she said. "I told Dr. O'Shaughnessy to load me up with the most toxic stuff she had and I'd let her know if I could handle it. My goal is to survive."

After seeing the results, Dr. O'Shaughnessy said she still would not recommend a bone-marrow transplant for Ms. Bowers. But she said she wanted to see whether the findings would change over the next few years. And Ms. Bowers said that if her cancer should recur in the future, she would consider having the treatment.

Women who have already had the procedure have also been awaiting the studies, sometimes with anxiety over what the findings might predict about their own fates. One woman in her 30s, who spoke on condition of anonymity, said, "Part of me wants to know, but part of me doesn't."

She is the patient described (though not named) by Dr. Jerome Groopman, a cancer specialist at the Harvard Medical School, in a *New Yorker* magazine article in fall 1998. She had the treatment in January

1998, for breast cancer that had spread, or metastasized, to her liver and bones. She knew that only 20 percent of women with metastatic breast cancer lived five years, and it seemed to her that the high-dose treatment was her only chance of survival. Because of rumors and news reports that the studies would be negative, she said, friends and relatives had called her ahead of time to warn her to brace herself for bad news.

Kathy Rich, a 43-year-old writer in New York who had the high-chemo treatment in 1995, said she felt a bit skeptical about the negative report on metastatic cancer, because it was only one study. "Cancer is so complex and individual," she said. "Who knows if it's helping one kind of breast cancer and not another?"

Ms. Rich, who has written a book about her experience called *The Red Devil: To Hell With Cancer—and Back*, was first treated for breast cancer in 1989. She learned in 1993 that the disease had spread to her bones, including her spine. By 1994 the spinal tumors had nearly paralyzed her. Radiation shrunk them, but she knew they might grow back.

She had joined a support group of about a half dozen women who had metastatic breast cancer, but by early 1995 all the other members had died, including a woman whose disease had spread to her bones. Then a mutual acquaintance told Ms. Rich that this woman wished she had had a transplant, and she began thinking it was time for her to consider it.

But she knew better than to expect a cure. "One of the really heartbreaking things with this is that you'll find people whose cancer comes back after a month," she said. "I knew someone like that."

But so far Ms. Rich has fared better. After the treatment, she said, "I had no evidence of disease for three years. A year ago I had one positive node in the adrenal gland. It's just been sitting there and hasn't done anything for about a year. It could stay that way for years."

Asked if she thought the transplant had brought about her recovery, she said, "I have no idea if the transplant helped or not."

[DG, April 1999]

## Breast Surgeons Turn to a Gentler Biopsy

**B**reast surgeons at several hospitals are perfecting a new technique that can spare many women with newly diagnosed breast cancer the pain and complications of a major surgical procedure.

The new technique, sentinel node biopsy, is replacing a routine part of breast cancer surgery called axillary dissection, in which surgeons remove a cluster of lymph nodes in the armpit near the affected breast and examine each of them under a microscope. These lymph nodes are the first destination for cancer cells spreading from the breast. If any contain cancer, the chances of a woman's survival are sharply reduced, and she becomes a candidate for aggressive anticancer treatment.

Sentinel node biopsy is a simpler procedure than axillary dissection; it takes less than an hour and is often done on an outpatient basis. To do it, doctors identify the first lymph node that cancer cells would reach within the cluster of pea-sized nodes under the arm, and only that one, the sentinel node, is removed for microscopic examination. The sentinel node's status seems to predict accurately whether the other nodes under the arm will be free of cancer.

Dr. Hiram S. Cody 3d, a breast surgeon at Memorial Sloan-Kettering Cancer Center in New York City, said that among 60 women at his hospital with small breast tumors, a negative sentinel node test meant, with 99 percent accuracy, that the other nodes would also be free of cancer. Dr. Cody's group is offering women with small tumors the option of forgoing axillary dissection entirely in favor of the simpler procedure.

The procedure was developed several years ago by Dr. Armando E. Giuliano of the John Wayne Cancer Institute in Santa Monica, California. He reported in the June 1997 issue of *The Journal of Clinical Oncology* that among 100 women with small tumors, the sentinel node predicted the status of the other nodes under the arm 100 percent of the time.

Dr. Giuliano's group finds the sentinel node by injecting a blue dye into the breast tissue around the tumor, then making a small incision in the armpit several minutes later and looking for the blue node. Dr. Cody's group and others in Florida and Vermont also inject a radioactive isotope solution into the breast tissue before the procedure, then use a probe that can detect radioactivity to help steer them to the blue sentinel node.

Once the node is found, it is removed for immediate examination under the microscope. If the node contains tumor cells, the surgical incision is enlarged and the remaining 20-odd nodes in the area are removed in a standard axillary dissection procedure that rids the body of as much tumor tissue as possible. But if the sentinel node is free of cancer, as it is in roughly 80 percent of women with small tumors, the procedure is over, and the other nodes are left in place.

A sentinel node biopsy spares these women the frequent side effects of axillary dissection: swelling, numbness and tingling in the arm and pain and stiffness in the arm and shoulder. The sentinel node biopsy has none of these complications, Dr. Giuliano said.

Dr. Cody said the sentinel node biopsy seemed less accurate in women with larger breast tumors. In a minority of cases, the cancer cells are not found in the sentinel node until the laboratory analysis several days after the procedure, and women must return to the hospital for a second operation. So far, the biopsy has been tested only in women.

But for most women with early breast cancer, the new procedure offers a way to avoid aggressive surgery, much as removing a breast tumor alone (lumpectomy) has become an attractive alternative to removing the entire breast (mastectomy). Still, Dr. Giuliano cautioned, a sentinel node biopsy can be done accurately only by an experienced surgeon. "Before you abandon the old procedure," he said, "you have to know that you can do the new one."

[AZ, August 1997]

## Removal of Healthy Breasts Is Found to Cut Cancer Risk

For women with a high risk of breast cancer, a study published in January 1999 offered hope, but at a cruel price. Removing both breasts while they are still healthy reduces the risk of getting breast cancer by 90 percent. The findings, from a study of 639 women who had their breasts removed from 1960 to 1993, are widely regarded as the most reliable information to date on the long-term effectiveness of the operation.

Surgeons had been performing the procedure, bilateral prophylactic mastectomy, on such women, since the 1960s, assuming it would reduce a woman's cancer risk. But they did not know whether it really did, or by how much, since there is no guarantee that all the problem tissue has been removed.

One way high-risk women can try to protect themselves is by having regular mammograms and breast examinations in hopes of detecting the disease early enough to cure it with surgery, chemotherapy and radiation. The only other way such women can protect themselves against breast cancer is by taking the drug tamoxifen, which in a large study in 1998 was shown to reduce the risk of the disease by about 45 percent.

But women are supposed to take the drug for only five years because it is thought to be ineffective after that time. In addition, tamoxifen may cause blood clots or uterine cancer in some women, and although it reduces the risk of breast cancer, studies have not shown that it lowers the death rate from the disease, as mastectomy does.

The study of the surgery, by researchers at the Mayo Clinic in Rochester, Minnesota, was published in *The New England Journal of Medicine*. The women in the study were considered at high risk because of a strong family history of breast cancer or a personal history of breast lumps needing biopsies. Tests developed in the 1990s to detect genetic mutations also provide an indication of women who may be at risk.

"This is a very important paper," said Dr. Patrick Borgen, chief of breast surgery at Memorial Sloan-Kettering Cancer Center in New York, who was not involved in the study. "It's the first credible calculation."

But Dr. Borgen and other cancer experts, including the authors of the paper, said the findings should not be used to pressure women into having their breasts removed. "The study doesn't mean we should sell the surgery to more women," he said. "But women who are considering it now have a hard-core fact to use as they're making their calculation."

The data reflect rates of illness and death for the participants as a group. Individual women involved in the study and others who have undergone the procedure have no way of knowing whether it spared them from cancer that might have killed them, or cost them their breasts to protect them from a disease they would never have contracted.

Dr. Lynn Hartmann, a medical oncologist who directed the study of breast removal, said, "This report is not meant as a universal recommendation for this procedure. It's meant to provide data for a tough and controversial area. I think that to date only a minority of high-risk women are interested in this procedure."

Dr. Patricia Ganz, director of the division for cancer prevention and control research at the Jonsson Cancer Center at the University of California at Los Angeles, said that despite the warnings, "a lot of physicians and surgeons scare women, and there is fear in the medical community that they will say to

women, 'You ought to have your breasts removed.'"

Among the 639 women studied, the researchers concluded that at least 20 and as many as 40 women would have died if they had not had their breasts removed. But there were only 2 deaths. Dr. Barbara Weber, an expert on breast cancer genetics at the University of Pennsylvania, and co-author of an editorial that accompanied the study, pointed out that although the procedure theoretically saved 18 lives, 621 other women who had their breasts removed probably would have survived without the drastic operation. She also noted the paradox of finding evidence supporting breast removal in healthy women, when treatments for women who already have cancer are aimed at saving the breast whenever possible.

By contrast, she and other researchers said, many women with strong family histories of breast and ovarian cancer are urged to have their ovaries removed. But that surgery is not disfiguring, and ovarian cancer, unlike breast cancer, is difficult to detect early enough to save a woman's life.

Dr. Larry Norton, director of the Lauder Breast Center at Memorial Sloan-Kettering Cancer Center, said the study was convincing and important. But the surgery "is not for everybody," Dr. Norton said. "I would like very much to make this not an option, to have better ways of preventing breast cancer in ways that do not involve surgery," he continued.

The number of women in the United States who have had their breasts removed in hopes of preventing cancer is not known. There is no registry of cases. Dr. Hartmann and other researchers said that women who wanted it tended to be those who had seen mothers, aunts and sisters die young from breast cancer.

Dr. Borgen said there had been a recent increase in interest in the surgery, but he did not think the number of procedures had risen with the development during the 1990s of tests for mutations in the genes BRCA1 and BRCA2, which greatly increase a woman's risk of developing breast or ovarian cancer.

"Now that we had a way to identify women who had an 85 percent chance of developing breast cancer, women said, 'What can you tell me about prophylactic mastectomy?'" Dr. Borgen said. "All we could say was, 'Gee, we think it works. But no studies have been done.'"

Although it might seem reasonable to assume that a woman without breasts cannot get breast cancer, proof was needed. Mastectomy can remove only 90 to 95 percent of breast tissue, and many researchers feared that the tissue left behind might harbor rogue cells that could one day turn malignant.

Dr. Hartmann and her colleagues sought to fill the information gap by conducting a retrospective study, involving women who had had the surgery in the past, rather than women going through it now. They used the Mayo Clinic's records to identify 639 women who had prophylactic mastectomies there from 1960 to 1993. The women were 18 to 79 years old when they had the surgery, with a median age of 42 years. Half the women had had the surgery 14 or more years before, and all had had it at least five years previously.

The team classified 214 of the women as high risk because of their family histories, Dr. Hartmann said. Many had mothers or sisters, or both, with the disease, and in 150 of their families, there were three or more breast cancers among close relatives. The women were not tested for mutations in BRCA1 or BRCA2 genes, but Dr. Hartmann said the tests are under way.

High-risk families like those in the study account for 5 to 10 percent of the 180,000 new cases of breast cancer diagnosed each year, Dr. Hartmann estimated.

The other 425 study subjects, even though they had their breasts removed, were considered to have been at only moderate risk. They had fewer close relatives with the disease than the high-risk women did, but, Dr. Hartmann said, many had chosen the surgery because of their own histories of multiple breast lumps that required repeated biopsies.

"Each one is an exercise in anxiety control," Dr. Hartmann said. She said some women with that kind of history reach a point where they look ahead and see an endless series of painful, nerve-wracking biopsies, one of which they imagine will finally give the result they have been dreading all along. And they decide they might as well get it over with.

The researchers tried to determine how many breast cancers would have developed and how many women would have died if the surgery had not been performed. Then they compared the expected numbers to the real ones.

For the 214 at high risk, they compared the women with their own sisters, who had not undergone the preventive surgery. Since siblings are similar genetically and usually share the same environment growing up, they assumed the sisters' risk of breast cancer would be similar.

On the basis of the breast cancers that developed in the untreated sisters after the subjects had mastectomies, the researchers calculated that 38 would have been expected in the subjects. But only three

---

**BY THE NUMBERS**

## Relief From Fear, At a High Cost

For the first time, researchers have shown that removing the breasts can prevent cancer in women with higher than normal risk of the disease.

| Of **425** women who were at MODERATE RISK: | Of **214** women who were at HIGH RISK*: |
|---|---|
| Expected cancers **37.4** | Expected cancers **30-52.9** |
| Actual cases **4** | Actual cases **3** |
| Reduction **89.5%** | Reduction **90%-94.3%** |
| Expected deaths **10.4** | Expected deaths **10.5-30.6** |
| Actual deaths **0** | Actual deaths **2** |
| Reduction **100%** | Reduction **80.9%-93.5%** |

*Because of differences in the statistical methods used, results for high risk women are given as a range, rather than a single number.

*Source: Mayo Clinic*

occurred—a reduction in risk of more than 90 percent. Similarly, 10 deaths from breast cancer would have been expected, but only two occurred—an 80 percent risk reduction.

A computer model predicted 37.4 cases of breast cancer among women in the moderate group, and only four occurred, for a 90 percent reduction in risk. Ten deaths were expected and none occurred—a 100 percent risk reduction.

The Mayo Clinic did not disclose the names of women who participated in the study. But a woman who had the surgery elsewhere agreed to be interviewed. Staci Mishkin, 40, from Springfield, Virginia, was delighted to hear of the study, which, she said, "validates what I did."

In 1997, Ms. Mishkin had both breasts removed. She was perfectly healthy, but her mother, maternal grandmother and two of her mother's sisters had died of breast cancer before they reached 50. "I knew growing up, my whole life, that women in my family got breast cancer and died," said Ms. Mishkin, who tested positive for a mutation in BRCA1. "It was not a question of, will I get it?" she said. "It was a question of when."

Ms. Mishkin said she believes doctors have been overly hesitant about recommending the procedure to high-risk women. "They wouldn't recommend it or not recommend it," she said of her own operation. "But now, with this study, they can say this will reduce your risk 90 percent. They'll have to tell their patients it's an option."

Dr. Susan Love, a breast cancer expert and professor of surgery at the University of California at Los Angeles, said that, thanks to the study, "Women who want to do this know they will at least have some benefit. But it should drive us hard to find better prevention."

Dr. Love said she did a few prophylactic mastectomies, but only after several months of discussions with patients. "Sometimes your sister or mother gets diagnosed and you're so panicked you want a quick fix," she said. "I would suggest that women not choose to do this at that moment in time."

She also said it was important to remember that seven women in the study got breast cancer even though their breasts were removed. "Nobody should come away thinking it's a guarantee," she said.

[DG, January 1999]

## Study Says Few Women Rue Preventive Breast Operation

A recent survey of women who took a drastic measure to prevent breast cancer, having both healthy breasts removed, shows that nearly 70 percent are satisfied with their decision and would make the same choice if they had it to do over.

The operation, bilateral prophylactic mastectomy, is an uncommon procedure that has been performed since the 1960s in women with a personal or family history that puts them at high risk for breast cancer. There are no statistics on how many women have had the operation.

The surgery is a subject of debate, regarded by some as an indefensible mutilation of healthy women and by others as an option that women at high risk have a right to consider.

The study, in which 572 women were surveyed, is not the first to examine the question, but it is larger and more representative than earlier ones. A major study on the same women published in January 1999 showed reliably for the first time that the surgery reduced the risk of getting cancer by 90 percent—though some risk remained because it was impossible to remove all breast tissue.

The women in the recent survey had the operation at the Mayo Clinic between 1960 and 1993. Many had a mother, grandmother or aunt—or all three—with breast cancer, or a personal history of multiple breast lumps requiring biopsies. Now, 74 percent say that the operation helped diminish their emotional concerns about developing the disease.

But the relief from worry had a price: 25 percent also said they felt less feminine after the surgery, and 36 percent were less satisfied with the way their bodies looked. Eleven percent were dissatisfied with their decision; 9 percent very dissatisfied.

Dr. Marlene Frost, a nurse and research associate at the Mayo Clinic in Rochester, Minnesota, presented the findings at a cancer conference in Atlanta held by the American Society of Clinical Oncology. She pointed out that because "prophylactic mastectomy is irreversible," the survey provided "important information that women need in contemplating this decision."

"The decision is very complex and personal," Dr. Frost said, "and a woman herself must take the lead. Our role is to provide women with the best data, both positive and negative."

She and her colleagues sent questionnaires to the women asking how they had decided to have the surgery and how they felt about it later. They were also asked to explain why they were satisfied or dissatisfied.

In important areas of their lives, many women said the operation had not changed their feelings: self-esteem, sexual relationships and emotional stability. Factors that contributed to the women's overall satisfaction included positive feelings about their appearance, lower levels of stress and worry afterward, satisfaction with sexual relationships and absence of problems with breast implants. Although 95 percent of the women had their breasts reconstructed with implants, those who did not were among the most satisfied.

"Our thought is that women who went into this with the decision that they wouldn't have reconstruction were those who probably placed less emphasis on their breasts in measuring their self-esteem," Dr. Frost said.

She said she and her colleagues were concerned that 25 percent felt a loss of femininity after their mastectomies. "But a lot of people are making claims that this is mutilating, and in light of that, 25 percent isn't a phenomenal number," she said. A study in 1998 by other researchers had even more positive results, finding that only 5 percent of 370 women surveyed in 43 states regretted the operation.

Dr. Patrick Borgen, lead author of the January 1999 study and chief of breast surgery at Memorial Sloan-Kettering Cancer Center, cautioned that the study may have been unrealistically positive, because the women who took part were those who answered magazine advertisements inviting them to participate. Those in the Mayo Clinic study, by contrast, were sought by researchers who identified them from medical records.

Dr. Borgen said his team had found that the women most likely to have regrets were those who felt they had let themselves be pressured into the operation by their doctors. But Dr. Lynn Hartmann, an oncologist at the Mayo Clinic, said there were also women who regretted being talked out of the procedure. She described a patient whose mother, grandmother and aunts had had breast cancer. But when the woman asked her doctor about prophylactic surgery, he said, "Why would you want to do that to yourself?" When she went to the Mayo Clinic several years later, she had metastatic breast cancer, and only a 20 percent chance of surviving five years.

[DG, May 1999]

# Breast Reconstruction: All at Once or Not at All?

At a recent medical conference, a plastic surgeon proudly showed a slide of a woman with breast cancer who had undergone a mastectomy and then a reconstruction of her breast. The surgeon challenged the audience to detect which breast was natural and which he had created in the operating room. Few could tell.

The slide show demonstrated the tremendous strides that plastic surgeons have made in creating natural-looking breasts for women who have lost theirs to cancer. The new breasts can be made of tissue from another part of the body that has flesh to spare, like the buttocks, abdomen or back. Or the surgeon can use saline-filled implants.

Regardless of the type of reconstruction, though, doctors agree that the best-looking results occur when the cancer surgeon and the plastic surgeon plan the operation together, and the reconstruction is done at the same time as the mastectomy, with the two surgeons working in concert. It is an approach that is being recommended to more and more women; many say they are delighted with the results.

But jumping right into reconstruction is not for everyone. Women with advanced cancer who will need further treatment may be advised to postpone the procedure; those receiving radiation may not be able to have it at all, because some damage to the skin may have resulted. And if there is a mistake in the diagnosis, and the cancer is more advanced than initially thought, the reconstruction may interfere with treatment.

Even some women who are eligible for the procedure prefer to delay it so that they can recover from the mastectomy and make sure the cancer is taken care of first. And some wind up feeling that they don't need to bother with reconstruction, after all.

A recent survey of nearly 600 women from around the country who were at high risk for breast cancer and had healthy breasts removed in the hope of preventing the disease found that the vast majority had undergone reconstruction. But when all the women were asked how they felt about their decisions to have mastectomies, the most satisfied were those who had not had reconstructive surgery.

Dr. Marlene Frost, a researcher and nurse at the Mayo Clinic in Rochester, Minnesota, who presented the survey findings in May 1999, at a cancer conference in Atlanta, said that the women may have been more comfortable with their decisions because they avoided trouble with implants or because they were women whose self-esteem did not depend on having breasts.

Dr. Jeanne Petrek, a cancer surgeon and the director of the surgical program at the Evelyn H. Lauder Breast Center at Memorial Sloan-Kettering Cancer Center in New York, said that when women find out that they have breast cancer, many do not know what they want to do about reconstruction.

Delaying the procedure gives them time to decide. In addition, Dr. Petrek said, it means less surgery, less time under anesthesia and less stress on the body during the mastectomy. A mastectomy alone can take one and a half to three hours, Dr. Petrek said. Reconstruction can add one and a half hours, for implants, to as many as eight hours, if the woman's own tissue is used.

For a woman who is fighting cancer, a simpler and shorter operation may have its advantages. The drawback to waiting is that if a woman does decide to have reconstruction, she must undergo general anesthesia again.

Dr. Lynn Hartmann, an oncologist at the Mayo Clinic, called reconstruction a big procedure and agreed that some women find it hard to make decisions about cosmetic details while they are also dealing with life-and-death questions about treating their cancers.

"Occasionally, they will come back and say, 'If I had known how much this would require, I'm not sure I'd have made the same choice,'" Dr. Hartmann said. That reaction seems more likely to occur, she added, when the reconstruction uses implants and is done in several steps that require many visits to a surgeon. By contrast, reconstruction with the woman's own tissue is more difficult at first, Dr. Hartmann said, "but once done, it's done."

Reconstruction tends to be more important to younger women than to older ones, she said, though not in every case. If a woman is uncertain whether she wants the procedure, Dr. Hartmann said, "I would definitely urge her to wait and see how she feels following the mastectomy alone."

Judi Fibush, a 60-year-old retired executive from Cornelius, Oregon, had both breasts removed in 1998 because of cancer, and decided against reconstruction. She said she had no regrets, and in fact enjoyed going braless in a T-shirt, something she had never felt comfortable doing before, because her breasts were large.

"I don't think a woman should feel embarrassed if she doesn't have breasts again," Ms. Fibush said. "As long as you feel confident and comfortable with yourself, that's what counts. Who says we all have to look a certain way?"

But Ms. Fibush also said that if she had been in her 30s or 40s, or still going to the office every day, she might have felt differently.

From what she had read about reconstruction, though, she thought that it sounded like more trouble than it would be worth. "Even with the new saline implants, there is the problem that a mammogram cannot detect breast cancer because of them," she said.

Experts agree that implants can make a mammogram harder to read. "I don't want something that's going to keep me from being alive," Ms. Fibush said.

Occasionally, reconstruction can interfere with the cancer treatment. A 38-year-old woman, who asked that her name not be revealed, had a double mastectomy and simultaneously began the reconstruction process, which required that tissue expanders with metal parts be implanted in her chest. After the surgery, though, her doctors discovered that the cancer

was more advanced than they had realized, and that they needed an M.R.I. scan to help gauge how far it had spread. But the metal implants made an M.R.I. impossible. Removing them would have been arduous. And so she had a CAT scan instead, though the M.R.I. would have been more useful. "For sure, I wouldn't have had the reconstruction had I known," she said.

Ms. Fibush could not see the point of putting herself through the surgery for breasts that lacked normal sensation. A reconstructed breast very rarely retains the natural nipple, and so its sensations are gone. "The breast is an erotic zone, and if you have no feeling there, what's its purpose?" she said. "Who is it benefiting?" Her husband supported her decision. "I was very concerned about his reaction," she said. "He said it made no difference to him whatsoever."

Gayle Feldman, a 47-year-old writer in New York, also felt no need for reconstructive surgery after both her breasts were removed. "I didn't want to have more operations," she said. "I thought, I still feel that I'm a woman, an attractive woman. I think one always feels, and you'd be lying if you said otherwise, the regret of the loss of the breasts. But far more important to me was the feeling that I was alive and had come through the thing and would just carry on."

And if the cancer ever recurs, she said, it will be far easier to detect with no implants in the way. But she also said that she probably would have made a different decision had only one breast been removed. "You can't go around as a lopsided lady," she said.

Ms. Feldman recalled the first time she went to the beach after her breasts were removed. "I was concerned when I put a bathing suit on that people would notice and stare," she said. "That's when I felt the most fear over self-consciousness. But I found there were lots of ladies on the beach who were very small-breasted and didn't look much different from me. Nobody stared."

[DG, June 1999]

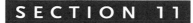

# Heart Disease

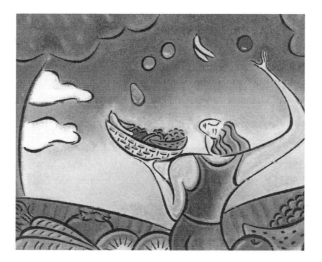

## MORE NEEDS TO BE DONE TO CURB THE NUMBER ONE KILLER OF WOMEN

**M**any people seem to think that heart disease is mainly a man's problem and that women have little to worry about. But that is not the case: Heart disease is the leading cause of death in American women. It is true that in people under age 50, heart attacks are far less common in women than in men. But after menopause, women's risk begins catching up to men's, and overall, women who suffer heart attacks fare worse than men. A 1999 study revealed that the sharpest and most alarming difference in survival occurs in people under 50. When women in that age group do have heart attacks, they are twice as likely to die as men with the same diagnosis. The reasons are not clear, but researchers say that women are more likely than men to form large clots in the coronary arteries, and to have artery spasms that squeeze the vessels shut. Those conditions may produce especially damaging heart attacks.

Women can take measures to lower their risk. The most important is to stop smoking, which, in just a year, can reduce the risk of heart attack by 50 percent. Even exposure to secondhand smoke can almost double the risk of heart attack, and researchers estimate that 50,000 heart attack deaths a year may be caused by secondhand smoke.

Exercising and controlling weight can help to lower high cholesterol and blood pressure, and to ward off Type-2 diabetes, a major contributor to heart disease. Unfortunately, women tend to exercise less and less as they grow older, compounding the increase in heart attack risk that occurs anyway as a consequence of aging.

Diet can also help to lower risk. A diet that can protect the heart and perhaps also help prevent cancer includes plenty of fruits, vegetables, soy products, fiber from whole grains, beans, olive oil and oily fish like mackerel and salmon. Meat is also included, but in small amounts. Such a diet is low in saturated fat, trans fats and refined flour, and high in antioxidants like vitamin C and vitamin E, and the B vitamins folate and B6. Alcohol, the equivalent of one glass of wine a day, can also help to protect the heart, by making clots less likely and raising the blood level of HDL, or high-density lipoprotein, the "good cholesterol." Tea also appears to be protective. All of this may seem too good to be true, but the good news seems to be that the most healthful eating regimen is one that many people find delicious.

# Paradox or Not, Cholesterol in France Is on the Rise

Americans, famous for wanting their cake and eating it too, were delighted to learn that even though French foods seem to be rich in fat, much of it artery-clogging saturated animal fat, the French are not nearly as likely to be cut down in midlife by heart attacks. This intriguing phenomenon is called the French Paradox, and it has drawn comment, criticism and speculation during much of the 1990s.

But a recent treatise on the subject, published in *The British Medical Journal*, suggests the paradox may not be so paradoxical after all. Rather, the authors maintain, it is only a matter of time before the fatty French diet exacts its coronary toll. These scientists, Dr. Malcolm Law and Dr. Nicholas Wald, specialists in preventive medicine at St. Bartholomew's and the Royal London School of Medicine and Dentistry, point out that for decades until 1970, the French ate much less animal fat and had significantly lower blood cholesterol levels than did Britons, who were in no better shape than Americans.

But as the French diet grew richer, French cholesterol levels did too. "Only between 1970 and 1980 did French values increase to those in Britain," the authors noted, adding that since only about 1 percent of men die of heart disease before age 50, it takes decades of exposure to a high-fat diet to exact this toll.

Though the new British report is the most thorough analysis of this "time-lag hypothesis," it has been put forward before as an explanation for French diet and health. Dr. Marion Nestle, chairwoman of the department of nutrition at New York University, noted several years ago that it was not until 1985 that French consumption of fat caught up to that of Americans.

In an interview, Dr. Nestle said, "There's been a steady increase in fat consumption in France over the last 20 years as the French diet has become more Americanized." She noted that the French were now eating more meat and fast foods, snacking more, eating fewer regular relaxed meals, exercising less and drinking less wine than in the past. And, predictably, they are getting fatter. Wait a few more decades, Dr. Nestle predicted, and the French will no longer enjoy a coronary death rate that is less than half that of Americans.

Still, even if the French did not reach American levels of fat consumption until recently, something still seems to have been protecting their hearts. How else could they have gotten away with their apparent penchant for eggs, butter and cream, not to mention pâtés and rich cheeses full of saturated fat and cholesterol?

Several health experts, commenting on the report by Dr. Law and Dr. Wald, have offered possible explanations that could prove helpful to Americans seeking to lower their risk of heart disease without forgoing all the pleasures of dietary fat.

Dr. Meir Stampfer and Dr. Eric B. Rimm of the Harvard School of Public Health stress in their commentary that coronary disease is not due to any single factor and that preventing it cannot result from only one adjustment in living habits, like eating less saturated fat. Although they do not dismiss the idea that time will take its toll on the French heart, they cite several other differences in dietary habits between the French and Britons (and, by extension, Americans) that studies strongly suggest play an important role in heart disease. For example:

**Alcohol.** "Law and Wald may be too quick to dismiss the role of alcohol as a partial explanation," the Boston researchers wrote. Many studies have shown a strong relationship between an increased intake of alcohol and a lower level of cardiac deaths. Alcohol raises blood levels of protective HDL cholesterol, which helps rid arteries of fatty deposits. Red wine in particular, the favored beverage in France, contains chemicals that lower the risk of blood clots that could touch off a heart attack. Also important may be the pattern of alcohol consumption. In France wine is drunk slowly with meals.

"The evidence of benefit from moderate consumption of alcohol is very, very strong, and it seems to be strongest when alcohol is taken with meals on a moderate, regular basis as opposed to weekend binge-ing or alcohol consumed alone," Dr. Stampfer said in an interview. Moderate consumption means a daily limit of two glasses of wine for men and one glass for women.

**Fiber.** The French consume two to three times more fiber from whole grains and grain products than do Britons and Americans. These cereal fibers have been linked in at least three major studies to a decreased risk of heart disease. One of the studies, examining nearly 69,000 middle-aged nurses, was published in the *Journal of the American Medical Association.* Each increase of five grams a day of cereal fiber (the amount in a half-cup of bran-flake cereal) was associated with a 37 percent decrease in coronary risk among these women. Similar associations were found in the Iowa Women's Study and in men in the Health Professionals Follow-Up Study.

**Nuts.** The French eat about twice as many nuts as Americans do. Several studies that followed tens of thousands of men and women in this country showed that "even modest amounts of nuts were associated with a markedly lower risk of coronary heart disease, a benefit greater than would be predicted from their effects on serum cholesterol," Dr. Stampfer said. The fat in nuts is the unsaturated kind that lowers the level of harmful LDL cholesterol. "Ironically, many health-conscious Americans have been avoiding nuts because they are high in fat," he

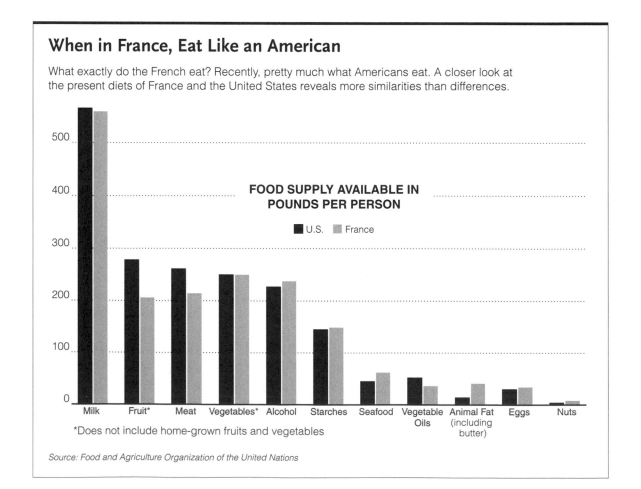

## When in France, Eat Like an American

What exactly do the French eat? Recently, pretty much what Americans eat. A closer look at the present diets of France and the United States reveals more similarities than differences.

FOOD SUPPLY AVAILABLE IN POUNDS PER PERSON

■ U.S.  ■ France

*Does not include home-grown fruits and vegetables

*Source: Food and Agriculture Organization of the United Nations*

noted. Over all, for the last 30 years, the French intake of heart-sparing polyunsaturated fat has been nearly twice that in Britain, Dr. Stampfer and Dr. Rimm noted.

**Folate.** When Americans visit France or dine in fancy French restaurants in this country, they tend to eat rich, fancy foods. "But the French people don't eat fancy foods day to day," Dr. Stampfer said. "They eat many more fruits and vegetables," including those that are rich in a B-vitamin called folate (or folic acid), which has been associated with a decreased risk of heart disease. Good sources of folate include dark-green leafy vegetables and orange juice.

**Glycemic Load.** Frequent consumption of foods that quickly raise the level of sugar in the blood has been linked to an increased risk of developing heart disease and diabetes. When blood sugar rises, insulin is released to process it, which stimulates the production of a harmful form of triglycerides, a known coronary risk factor. In general, whole foods and minimally processed grains (including pasta, which is made from crushed as opposed to finely ground semolina wheat) produce a low glycemic load, while sweets, pastries, white bread and potatoes produce a high glycemic load. Americans who snack on sweets and refined carbohydrates raise their glycemic load and, in turn, their risk of heart disease.

**Cheese and Foie Gras.** Dr. Serge Renaud, research director at France's National Institute of Health and Medical Research, maintains that there is something different about the fats in duck and goose liver and in cheese that makes them less damaging and possibly even protective of the heart. His evidence in part comes from the heart of foie gras country, the Gascony region of southwest France, where the coronary death rate among middle-aged men is about half that of the rest of France. He has said that "goose and duck fat is closer in chemical composition to olive oil than it is to butter and lard." What, if anything, may be special about the fats in cheese is now under study.

**Portion Size.** Rich foods or not, the French simply eat less than Americans do. French portion sizes tend to be a third to a half of American portions, and until recently, the French sat down to eat leisurely meals three times a day and rarely ate between meals, Dr. Nestle said. French visitors to America are typically aghast at the amount of food piled on plates in American restaurants and homes. The French are more gourmets than gluttons, as evidenced by the difference in obesity rates: 30 percent here versus 8 percent there.

Despite their dietary advantages, the French still get heart disease. Dr. Dean Ornish, cardiac specialist at the University of California at San Francisco, has pointed out that while "heart attacks are less frequent in France, they are still the leading cause of death there."

And as Dr. Nestle noted, French habits are changing, and not for the better. Children are now given soft drinks, not wine, to drink; wine consumption overall has dropped to about half of former levels; snacking is now commonplace, more and more family meals are coming from pizza parlors and McDonald's and more people are driving to big markets to shop instead of walking to local groceries.

As she and others have said, it is only a matter of time.

[JEB, June 1999]

# What Women Can Do to Escape Heart Disease

**B**y now most women surely are aware that heart disease is an equal opportunity killer, especially in those past the age of 50. Slightly more than half the deaths from heart disease in the United States now occur among women, and this share is likely to increase as the population ages.

But what are women doing to stem this rise, particularly those in their 50s and 60s, the decades when their coronary death rate begins its steep climb? Not nearly enough, according to recently published reports. Women with two or more major controllable coronary risk factors—cigarette smoking, lack of physical activity, high blood cholesterol, high blood pressure, diabetes and overweight—are more the norm than the exception. Three factors—smoking, sedentary habits and overweight—were featured in recent reports.

The United States Public Health Service estimated that in 1990, 61,000 American women over 35 died from cardiovascular diseases caused by smoking. The chances of suffering a heart attack can be cut in half within just one year of quitting smoking, but only 2.5 percent of women who smoke successfully quit each year. As of 1993, the most recent year for which national data are available, 22 million women—more than one in five—were regular smokers.

According to a February 1995 report from the Centers for Disease Control and Prevention in Atlanta, while 73 percent of female smokers 12 and over told Government interviewers that they wanted to quit, their efforts were notoriously unsuccessful. A major hindrance to becoming and staying former smokers, the national survey of 7,137 women revealed, is addiction to nicotine and the subsequent unpleasant symptoms that accompany efforts at withdrawal.

Four out of five female smokers aged 12 and older reported one or more indicators of nicotine addiction: feeling dependent on cigarettes, needing more cigarettes to get the same effect, being unable to cut down and feeling sick when trying to cut down or quit.

Over all, 75 percent reported feeling dependent on cigarettes, and the more cigarettes they smoked each day, the greater the dependency. In those 12 through 24, 80.6 percent who smoked 6 to 15 cigarettes a day felt dependent; the comparable number for women over 25 was 76.1 percent.

Among those who had tried to cut smoking in the preceding year, 81.5 percent of the younger women and 77.8 percent of those over 25 were unsuccessful. Among those who smoked only 6 to 15 cigarettes a day, an overwhelming majority had been unable to cut back, let alone quit.

Even among those who smoked fewer than six cigarettes a day, more than half reported one or more symptoms of addiction. More than a third of all smokers questioned reported feeling "sick" when they tried to reduce their smoking.

Withdrawal symptoms seem to be a far greater deterrent to quitting than the weight women tend to gain when they stop smoking. And the women were not even asked about other symptoms of withdrawal, including anxiety, irritability, anger, difficulty concentrating, hunger or intense cravings for cigarettes.

An estimated 87 percent of girls and women who smoke every day began smoking by the age of 18, often with the strong belief that they could quit any time they wanted to. This turns out to be a misconception that ends up robbing women of many healthy years of life. The easiest way to quit is never to start.

Even moderately intense activity, like housework, gardening and walking, has significant health benefits for women, including a reduced risk of coronary heart disease, some cancers and osteoporosis. The bad news is that in a newly released national survey conducted in 1992 as part of the Federal Behavioral Risk Factor Surveillance System, only 27.1 percent of 55,506 women 18 and older said they got 20 or more minutes a day of vigorous leisure-time activity on three or more days a week or 30 or more minutes a day of moderate activity on five or more days a week.

Physical inactivity accounts for about 25 percent of

all deaths from chronic disease in this country, mostly diseases of the heart and blood vessels, experts say. Yet more than 70 percent of American women are sedentary or irregularly active. And, the survey revealed, as women get older, they become increasingly sedentary just when they most need the cardiovacular benefits of exercise. While a quarter of women from 18 to 34 were inactive, 42.1 percent of those 65 and older did not have the recommended level of activity.

Increasing the level of activity among American women requires more than education and encouragement by doctors. Public health experts suggest that employers schedule exercise breaks or provide incentives for participation in exercise programs. Impediments to participation must also be addressed, including safety and child care questions and availability of walking and cycling trails, recreation sites and something as simple as sidewalks.

A continuing study of nearly 116,000 female nurses has revealed an unsettling fact: Women who gain weight as adults increase their risk of suffering and dying of a heart attack at any age and particularly after 50. A gain of just 11 to 18 pounds after the age of 18 increased the heart attack risk by 25 percent, and a gain of 18 to 25 pounds increased it by 60 percent. For those who gained more than 25 pounds as adults, the risk rose as much as 200 to 300 percent when compared with the rates among women who gained less than 11 pounds as adults. The risk was lowest among women who gained nothing or perhaps lost some.

How can such gains be prevented? By eating fewer calories and/or expending more as women age. Women still have a long way to go in cutting calorically dense dietary fat, now at about 34 percent of calories. By replacing most fatty foods with vegetables and fruits and moderate amounts of low-fat starches, they will further improve their chances of escaping both heart disease and cancer. Regular exercise will not only help to keep off heart-damaging pounds, it can also keep blood pressure down and coronary arteries open.

[JEB, March 1995]

## For More Help

- The American Heart Association has published a very helpful 27-page pamphlet, *Silent Epidemic: The Truth About Women and Heart Disease*. Single copies are available free from chapters of the heart association. Call 800-242-8721 for locations.

- *The Healthy Heart Handbook for Women*, a 90-page guide developed by the National Heart, Lung and Blood Institute, is available from New Orders, Superintendent of Documents, P.O. Box 37154, Pittsburgh, PA 15250-7954. Refer to booklet S/N 017-043-001222-2.

- For more detailed explanations, consult *The Woman's Heart Book: The Complete Guide to Keeping Your Heart Healthy and What to Do if Things Go Wrong*, by Dr. Fredric J. Pashkow and Charlotte Libov, or *The Women's Guide to Fighting Heart Disease* by Dr. Richard H. Helfant.

## Protein May Be Heart Risk Factor

Just when it may have seemed that all the important risk factors for heart disease had been identified, researchers are puzzling over what appears to be another one: a blood protein that, in some people at least, may indicate that their chances of suffering a heart attack are two or three times the normal rate. The protein appears to mark a particular risk for white men and women under 65.

The substance, lipoprotein(a), or Lp(a), is a form of low-density lipoprotein, the so-called bad cholesterol, which can be deposited on artery walls and eventually cause heart disease. But the exact role of

Lp(a) in the development of heart disease is still unclear, and it is not certain for which people it might be a risk factor. It is also not known what can or should be done to reduce elevated blood levels of Lp(a). However, the association between Lp(a) and heart disease may help to explain why heart attacks occur in some people who have otherwise low cholesterol levels and who have no other major coronary risk factors.

In the newest study, conducted among nearly 600 women 65 or younger in Sweden, those with the highest levels of Lp(a) were nearly three times as likely to experience a heart attack or the chest pains of angina as those with the lowest levels. The study, published in January 1997 in *Circulation*, a journal of the American Heart Association, found an increased coronary risk associated with high blood levels of Lp(a) in women both before and after menopause.

Among the 292 women who had heart attacks or angina, blood levels of Lp(a) averaged 38 percent higher than among 292 healthy women who were otherwise comparable in age and other coronary risk factors, Dr. Kristina Orth-Gomer of the Karolinska Institute and her collaborators reported.

Lp(a) levels typically rise after menopause, but not among women who take estrogen replacement therapy, suggesting that estrogen plays an important role in determining Lp(a) levels in women.

In a study published in August 1996 in the *Journal of the American Medical Association*, Dr. Andrew G. Bostom of Tufts-New England Medical Center in Boston and his colleagues linked elevated Lp(a) levels to an increased risk of heart disease in men under age 55. In that study, more than 2,000 men participating in the Framingham Heart Study whose Lp(a) levels had been measured in the early 1970s were followed for an average of 15 years. But experts are puzzled because that research found that black men tended to have much higher Lp(a) levels than white men without incurring the increased coronary risk seen in white men.

In a previous study, Dr. Bostom and his colleagues had linked raised Lp(a) levels to the development of premature heart disease in more than 3,000 women participating in Framingham who were followed for an average of 12 years. However, both studies used indirect measurements of Lp(a), which some experts say can lead to spurious results.

Unlike well-established coronary risk factors like blood pressure, cigarette smoking and cholesterol, Lp(a) is not simple to measure. It comes in various shapes and sizes, with a highly variable number of repeating chemical sequences that can skew test results, said Dr. Helen Hobbs, an Lp(a) expert at the University of Texas Southwestern Medical Center in Dallas.

Lp(a) levels are nearly entirely determined by a person's genes. Diet, exercise and other habits appear to have no influence on Lp(a) levels in blood. About the only way known to reduce Lp(a) levels is with niacin, or nicotinic acid, an established cholesterol-lowering agent that can have unpleasant side effects, but even that does not work in all people.

Researchers are still unsure about how Lp(a) may act in the body to contribute to coronary risk. In laboratory studies, the protein interferes with the activity of plasminogen, a substance in blood that helps break down clots, Dr. Hobbs said. And it may increase the fatty deposits that accumulate on artery walls. Dr. Hobbs said that Lp(a) was found in such fatty deposits, or atherosclerotic lesions, in proportion to the amount of Lp(a) present in blood plasma.

How important might Lp(a) be in the grand scheme of things? Dr. Bostom has pointed out that smoking is a far greater risk factor, accounting for 55 percent of the cases of premature heart disease among the men in the Framingham study. At this time, the primary value of finding that someone has high levels of Lp(a) would be in deciding who should be treated most aggressively to reduce the other coronary risk factors, he suggested.

[JEB, January 1997]

# Study Finds Secondhand Smoke
## Doubles Risk of Heart Disease

Secondhand cigarette smoke is more dangerous than previously thought, Harvard researchers reported in a study with broad implications for public health policy and probable direct impact on at least one major lawsuit. The 10-year study, which tracked more than 32,000 healthy women who never smoked, has found that regular exposure to other peoples' smoking at home or work almost doubled the risk of heart disease. Many earlier studies have linked secondhand smoke to heart disease, but the new findings show the biggest increase in risk ever reported, and the researchers say that it applies equally to men and women.

The women in the study, who ranged in age from 36 to 61 when the study began, suffered 152 heart attacks, 25 of them fatal. The results mean that "there may be up to 50,000 Americans dying of heart attacks from passive smoking each year," said Dr. Ichiro Kawachi, an assistant professor of health and social behavior at the Harvard School of Public Health and the lead author of the study, which was published in the journal *Circulation*.

By contrast, lung cancer deaths from passive smoking are estimated to be far fewer, at 3,000 to 4,000 a year. Because heart disease is much more common than lung cancer, even a small increase in risk can cause many deaths. Before this study, it was known that passive smoking caused increased risk for several ailments, including asthma and bronchitis, as well as middle-ear infections in young children. But the increased risk for heart disease had been estimated at about 30 percent.

"This is a very important study," said Dr. Stanton A. Glantz, a professor of medicine at the University of California at San Francisco, who has done extensive research on passive smoking but who was not involved in the Harvard study. "It's exceptionally strong and from a very solid group." Dr. Glantz also praised the Harvard team for what he called its careful analysis of workplace exposure to smoke, which had rarely been done before.

"That's important because of the effort to create laws controlling smoking in the workplace," he said.

"This study will be of enormous help to legislative bodies, statewide and locally, who are trying to get limits on smoking, especially in controversial areas like restaurants and bars, where the tobacco industry has worked closely with restaurant associations to block legislation to make these places go smoke free," said Edward L. Sweda, a senior lawyer with the Tobacco Control Resource Center at Northeastern University in Boston.

The study was particularly pertinent for one lawsuit. "From our standpoint, that's a wonderful study," said Stanley Rosenblatt, a Miami lawyer who represented flight attendants in a class-action suit against tobacco companies that went to trial in 1997. That suit was the first class-action suit based on the effects of secondhand smoke. It involved 60,000 former and current flight attendants, who contended that they were harmed by smoke in airplane cabins when smoking was legal on most flights. Most of the plaintiffs had had lung cancer or respiratory ailments. In 1998, tobacco producers settled the case for $300 million.

The Philip Morris Companies, which is named in the flight attendants' suit, declined to comment on the study. The Tobacco Institute, an industry group, said it could not comment on the study because it had not seen a copy of it.

The data being reported are from the Nurses' Health Study, a project that began in 1976 with 121,700 female nurses filling out detailed surveys every two years about their health and habits. To measure the effects of passive smoking, the researchers asked the women in 1982 about their exposure, and then monitored new cases of heart disease for the next decade. The analysis did not include all the study participants, but only the 32,046 who had never smoked and who at the outset did not have heart disease or cancer.

The women who reported being exposed regularly to cigarette smoke at home or work had a 91 percent higher risk of heart attack than those with no exposure. Even though the women worked in hospitals, some were exposed to smoke on the job because at the time of the study many hospitals allowed smoking in certain areas. The study was set up to make sure that other risk factors like diabetes and high blood pressure did not account for the difference between the two groups.

Laboratory studies of the effects of passive smoke on the body support the survey findings, Dr. Glantz said. In studies of both people and animals, Dr. Glantz and other researchers have identified several ways in which the chemicals in secondhand smoke can contribute to heart disease. Besides reducing a person's oxygen supply, the substances damage arteries, lower levels of the beneficial form of cholesterol known as HDL and increase the tendency of blood platelets to stick to one another and form clots that can trigger a heart attack. A study last year of healthy teenagers and adults exposed to passive smoking for an hour or more a day detected artery damage. The higher the exposure was, the greater the damage.

But once the exposure ceases, the damage may quickly heal. "In active smokers, the risk of heart disease drops immediately," half of the way to that of a nonsmoker within a year, Dr. Glantz said. "It never gets quite back to the nonsmoker's level, but it comes close," he said. "One would expect the same to be true for passive smoking."

The Harvard study may supply ammunition for more lawsuits against the tobacco industry. "I think it could have very profound implications legally," said John Banzhaf, a law professor at George Washington University and executive director of Action on Smoking and Health, an antismoking group. "We now have proof which will meet the legal threshold requirement. In an ordinary civil suit, you have to prove something by what we call a preponderance of evidence, which means it's more probable than not."

The doubling of risk shown in today's study satisfied that requirement, Mr. Banzhaf said, adding, "You're right in that striking range with regard to the quantum of proof which we need." Because passive smoke can cause heart problems more quickly than it causes lung cancer, Mr. Banzhaf said, it will be easier to prove the connection to juries.

[DG, May 1997]

## Study Cites Risks for Women Under 50 With Heart Attacks

In people under 50, heart attacks are far less common in women than in men, but when they do occur, women are more than twice as likely to die.

Researchers had long known that overall, women with heart attacks fare worse than men, but the large difference in the younger age groups was not known before a recent study. The difference between women and men who have heart attacks diminishes with age, as men's risk goes up, but women's risk of death stays higher than men's until the age of 75.

The reasons for the difference are not fully understood, and scientists say that the recent findings, based on a study of the hospital records of 155,565 women and 229,313 men who had heart attacks and were treated at 1,658 hospitals, mean that younger women who suffer heart attacks are a high risk group needing special study and attention. The research was published in July 1999 in *The New England Journal of Medicine.*

A second study in the same issue of the journal, involving 3,662 women and 8,480 men with heart problems, also found that overall, women with heart attacks were more likely than men to die. They were more likely to have weakened heart muscle, dangerously low blood pressure and electrocardiograms that initially made it difficult to tell whether they were having a heart attack. Women also had more complications from treatment, particularly bleeding from blood-thinning drugs routinely given to heart attack patients.

In addition, women's heart attacks tended to have different causes than men's: In men, blocked arteries were more likely to bring on heart attacks, whereas women had clearer arteries. But the women still had heart attacks, which researchers said were probably caused by large blood clots and spasms in arteries.

"These studies are eye-opening to both physicians and their female patients," said Dr. Nieca Goldberg, a cardiologist and chief of the women's heart program at Lenox Hill Hospital in New York who was not involved in either study.

Heart disease is the leading cause of death in the United States. According to the American Heart Association, 9,000 women age 29 to 44 had heart attacks in 1997, compared with 32,000 men. The association did not have death rates, but in the larger study, 6.1 percent of women under 50 died from their heart attacks, compared with 2.9 percent of the men.

Dr. Viola Vaccarino, an assistant professor of epidemiology at the Yale University School of Medicine and lead author of the larger study, said, "Heart disease is less common in these young women, but those who get it prematurely appear to have more severe disease in some ways, and they have more severe heart attacks."

Dr. Vaccarino said younger women needed to realize that they could develop heart disease. "Women need to work on what we know to be risk factors, such as high blood pressure, high cholesterol, smoking, obesity and diabetes," she said.

Dr. Goldberg said that women from families in which heart disease occurs at an early age needed to be especially vigilant about risk factors.

Dr. Judith Hochman, lead author of the second study and director of the cardiac care unit and cardiac research at St. Luke's-Roosevelt Medical Center in

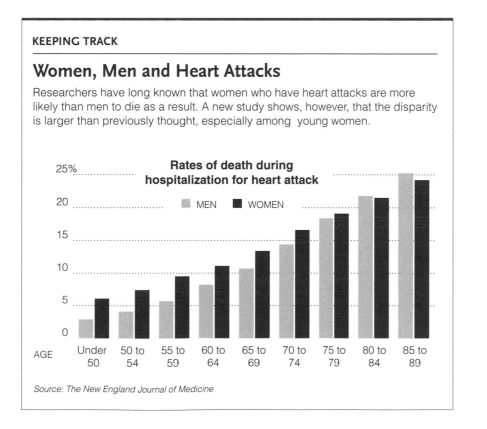

**KEEPING TRACK**

## Women, Men and Heart Attacks

Researchers have long known that women who have heart attacks are more likely than men to die as a result. A new study shows, however, that the disparity is larger than previously thought, especially among young women.

**Rates of death during hospitalization for heart attack**

◻ MEN   ◼ WOMEN

AGE — Under 50 · 50 to 54 · 55 to 59 · 60 to 64 · 65 to 69 · 70 to 74 · 75 to 79 · 80 to 84 · 85 to 89

*Source: The New England Journal of Medicine*

New York, said that an encouraging finding from her study was that women actually did better than men when they were treated for a condition called unstable angina, a type of chest pain that often precedes a heart attack.

"The message is, don't ignore symptoms," Dr. Hochman said. "Don't delay seeking care."

Women with heart attacks do not always have typical symptoms like chest pain, Dr. Hochman said. Some just become short of breath or feel discomfort in the upper part of the stomach, throat or neck.

Dr. Vaccarino said that three factors accounted for part of the difference in survival between men and women. Women with heart attacks were more likely than men to have other conditions that worsened their outlook, including diabetes and stroke. In addition, they tended to delay going to the hospital, and when they got there were less likely than men to be given prompt treatment for a heart attack, which includes aspirin, other blood-thinning drugs and beta blocker drugs. Even so, those three factors combined accounted for only about a third of the difference in death rates.

The researchers had several theories about the rest of the difference. Dr. Hochman said that because of their higher estrogen levels, most younger women were less likely than men to develop atherosclerosis, the build up of fatty plaques that can trigger heart attacks by blocking the arteries that supply blood to the heart muscle.

But the destructive process of forming plaques can have a good side, Dr. Hochman said. Often, as plaques develop and blood flow through the arteries is gradually diminished, the body compensates by sprouting new blood vessels. But women are less likely than men to sprout those new vessels.

Total blockage of the arteries can develop in women even if they do not have severe atherosclerosis, though. Some studies have shown that women tend to form large blood clots that can shut down an artery. The clots form because women's platelets, blood cells involved in clotting, tend to clump together more, initiating clot formation.

Dr. Hochman also said some women may be more likely than men to have artery spasms, which can trigger a heart attack. Women are more prone to other conditions related to artery spasm, including migraine headaches and Reynaud's syndrome, which causes the hands and feet to become cold and numb.

Dr. Vaccarino said that more research was needed to explain women's higher risk, but also to find better ways to detect heart problems in younger women. "The symptoms and signs we have now are based on what we know about men and older women," she said. "What we are doing may not be good enough."

[DG, July 1999]

## Yet Another Reason to Fight the Fat

Do you know your triglyceride level? New evidence strongly suggests that it is time to add triglycerides to the substances in the blood that influence your chances of developing heart disease. Triglycerides are basic particles of fat carried through the bloodstream by various molecules. They are derived from fats eaten in food or made in the body from other energy sources like carbohydrates.

The new evidence indicates that blood levels of triglycerides that have long been considered "normal"—200 milligrams in 100 milliliters of blood serum—are actually too high and should be monitored and controlled along with other coronary risk factors. Researchers at the University of Maryland Medical Center in Baltimore have found significant cardiac risks above 100 milligrams. They say longstanding uncertainties about the importance of triglycerides arose in part from mistaken assumptions about where to draw the line between safe and hazardous levels.

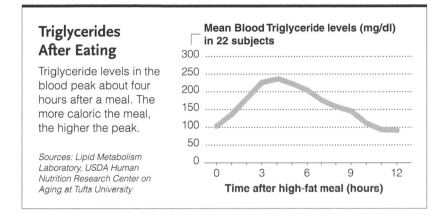

**Triglycerides After Eating**

Triglyceride levels in the blood peak about four hours after a meal. The more caloric the meal, the higher the peak.

*Sources: Lipid Metabolism Laboratory, USDA Human Nutrition Research Center on Aging at Tufts University*

**Mean Blood Triglyceride levels (mg/dl) in 22 subjects**

**Time after high-fat meal (hours)**

The recent studies also call into question the way triglyceride levels are measured, after a 12-hour fast. Dr. Michael Miller, who directed the Baltimore study, said the level achieved after a fatty meal might tell more about a person's chances of developing clogged arteries.

The National Cholesterol Education Program lists 200 milligrams as a normal blood level of triglycerides. Levels of 200 milligrams to 400 milligrams are considered borderline, warranting changes in diet to bring them down. Drug therapy to lower triglycerides, according to the national guidelines, should be reserved for those with levels higher than 400 milligrams as well as those with levels of 200 to 400 who have other coronary risk factors like smoking, diabetes and high cholesterol.

However, the Baltimore study found that those with triglyceride levels at or above 100 milligrams (as measured after a 12-hour fast) were 50 percent more likely than those with levels below 100 to suffer heart attacks, need bypass surgery or angioplasty or die from heart disease. This study, which followed 350 men and women for 18 years, was published in the May 1998 *Journal of the American College of Cardiology.*

Dr. Miller, director of preventive cardiology at the University of Maryland, said his was just one of several recent studies "suggesting that we may have been missing the big picture" regarding triglycerides, because clinicians and medical researchers had failed to look low enough when they assessed the contribution of triglycerides to coronary risk.

Furthermore, researchers had assumed that if high triglyceride levels were hazardous, the higher the level the greater the risk would be. But this is not always the case. In fact, some people with very high triglyceride levels—1,000 milligrams or more—are no worse off than those with levels of 200.

Further complicating the picture, when triglyceride levels go up, blood levels of protective HDL-cholesterol go down, suggesting that low HDLs, not high triglycerides, are really responsible for any increased coronary risk found in people with high triglycerides. "We showed that a fasting triglyceride level above 100 milligrams is an important risk factor independent of the level of HDLs," Dr. Miller said.

An earlier finding from the decades-long Framingham Heart Study had also shown that in women and in people over 65, rising triglyceride levels increased coronary risk independent of any cholesterol measurements.

And a Danish study of 3,000 initially healthy middle-aged and elderly men found that the risk of suffering a first heart attack rose substantially when triglyceride levels were above 140, regardless of HDL levels. In a report in March 1998 in the journal *Circulation,* the team from Copenhagen University Hospital reported that the Danish men with the highest triglyceride levels were more than twice as likely to suffer a heart attack as those with the lowest levels.

Finally, in an analysis published in 1997 in the *Journal of Cardiovascular Risk* that combined the results of 17 triglyceride studies among a total of

46,413 men and 10,864 women who had been followed for years, Dr. John E. Hokanson and Dr. Melissa A. Austin of the University of Washington in Seattle reported, "Triglyceride is a risk factor for cardiovascular disease for both men and women in the general population, independent of HDL."

Missing from this impressive set of data is a large long-term study showing that reducing triglyceride levels that are above 100 or even 200 milligrams can prevent serious heart problems. It took studies like this to convince physicians and the public that it was worth the money and effort to lower cholesterol levels. Small studies indicate that lowering high triglycerides may be as effective in preventing coronary artery disease as lowering the level of heart-damaging cholesterol.

Some people with extremely high triglyceride levels do not get heart disease because their triglyceride complexes are too large to damage arterial cells, whereas others with much lower levels are in danger because their triglyceride complexes are small.

Triglyceride levels in the blood reach their peak about four hours after a meal; the more caloric the meal, the higher the peak and the longer it takes the body to clear excess triglycerides from the blood. And, since triglycerides raise the risk of clotting, having too much in the blood for too long could precipitate a heart attack.

Diets high in saturated fats (from meats and dairy foods), sugars (including natural sugars in fruit), alcohol and refined carbohydrates (white bread, white rice, etc.) can raise blood levels of triglycerides. If people on a very low-fat diet replace fats with sugars and refined starches, triglyceride levels may rise and protective HDLs fall.

Some experts say that if weight is not a problem, it may be better to replace artery-clogging saturated fats with heart-healthy olive and canola oils and to eat more fish rich in omega-3 fatty acids like mackerel, sardines, herring, bluefish and salmon.

Being overweight (particularly fat around the middle) and sedentary also contribute to high levels of triglycerides. The treatment here is obvious: Eat fewer calories and burn more through exercise. It is also better both for reducing triglyceride levels and weight to consume many small nutritious meals a day instead of a few large ones. Triglyceride levels may also rise somewhat in postmenopausal women who take estrogen by mouth and in people who take bile acid sequestrants, a common medication for lowering cholesterol.

If changes in diet, weight loss and exercise fail to bring elevated triglycerides down to a safe level, effective drug treatment is available.

[JEB, July 1998]

## Savory Diet That's Good for the Heart? Let's Eat

A generation ago, Dr. Ancel Keys and colleagues at the University of Minnesota published findings that, if heeded then, would have extended millions of American lives during the last 30 years and millions more in the years to come.

The researchers examined the relationship between diet and heart disease rates in seven countries and found that people who lived along the Mediterranean Sea suffered only a tiny fraction of the heart attacks and coronary deaths experienced by Americans and people in other Western industrial-

ized countries. Among people along the Mediterranean, dietary fat consumed was mostly of vegetable origin; among the others, diets were rich in highly saturated animal fats from meat and dairy products.

In the years since the seven-countries study other researchers have helped to tease out the various influential features of what has come to be called the Mediterranean diet, and a number of cookbooks have been published promoting delicious foods that just happen to protect hearts and blood vessels and, as a bonus, may also help prevent several common cancers.

Various studies have substantiated Dr. Keys's initial observations and shown that deaths from coronary heart disease are far less common in countries along the Mediterranean than in northern Europe. In addition, some researchers have tested the benefits of a Mediterranean-style diet in people who face a high risk of dying of heart disease.

A recent study, published in February 1999 in *Circulation*, the journal of the American Heart Association, is a four-year follow-up of more than 400 men and women in France, all of whom had already suffered one heart attack and therefore were at risk of another. About half the participants were told to switch to a Mediterranean-type diet rich in fruits, vegetables, cereals, fish and beans, and the other half were advised to eat a more traditional Western diet that was relatively low in fat, saturated fat and cholesterol.

Those following the Mediterranean diet were 50 to 70 percent less likely than the comparison group to develop recurrent heart disease, including fatal and nonfatal heart attacks.

Perhaps the most surprising, and gastronomically pleasing, feature of the dietary scheme that has emerged from this research is that the diet may not have to be low in fat to protect the heart. Rather than insisting, as does Dr. Dean Ornish, that no fat be added to food and that all fat-containing animal foods be avoided, advocates of the Mediterranean diet include a fair amount of fat, nearly all in the form of oils: olive oil, nut and seed oils and fish oil.

However, meat in the traditional Mediterranean diet is only a sometime thing, used more as a condiment than as the main ingredient in meals. Instead, the diet features lots of fruits and vegetables, legumes and nuts and all manner of grains (bread, pasta, rice, bulgur and the like), often cooked and/or seasoned with olive oil.

The predominant animal foods are fish, yogurt and cheese (usually low-fat feta). Wine is typically consumed in moderation with meals. A featured item of Greek meals, for example, is a large salad of tomatoes, cucumbers, olives, onions and feta cheese, dressed with vinegar and olive oil and eaten with bread.

In the recent study, conducted by Dr. Michel de Lorgeril and colleagues in Lyon, France, 30 percent of calories in the experimental Mediterranean diet came from fat and 8 percent from saturated fat, compared with 34 percent fat calories and nearly 12 percent saturated fat calories in the other group's diet. Cholesterol intake averaged 212 milligrams a day on the Mediterranean diet; on the control diet, 312.

The levels of fats and cholesterol reached in the Mediterranean diet approached those recommended by the American Heart Association for people who have heart disease or high levels of cholesterol in their blood, whereas the comparison group's diet closely resembled that of typical Americans, half of whom die of heart disease.

The Mediterranean diet group also consumed more dietary fiber, antioxidants and B vitamins found in fruits and vegetables, all of which may slow the arterial damage that precedes heart disease.

What is so special about olive oil or, for that matter, the oils in nuts and seeds, like walnut oil, canola oil and flaxseed oil? They are, first of all, unsaturated oils that do not raise blood levels of cholesterol. And they are rich in a kind of fatty acid called alpha-linolenic acid, an omega-3 fatty acid that is found only in plants and is an essential nutrient in the human diet.

Along with fish oils, which are also rich in omega-3 unsaturated fatty acids (eicosapentaenoic acid, or EPA, and docosahexaenoic acid, or DHA), these oils have several effects in the body that would be expected to prevent or reduce coronary heart disease. Studies in animals and people have pointed to such effects as a reduced risk of blood clots, prevention of abnormal heart rhythms, less inflammation and clogging of blood vessels by deposits of fat and cholesterol and prevention of sudden cardiac death (this last effect is linked mainly to fish oils).

As might be expected, in the Lyon study, those participants who had higher blood levels of omega-3 fatty acids had a lower risk of developing a recurrent heart attack or other cardiac problems. This finding should not be interpreted to mean that blood levels of cholesterol are unimportant; countless studies have clearly demonstrated that they are. The higher the cholesterol level, the greater the risk of heart disease.

In fact, Dr. de Lorgeril and colleagues suggested that the protection afforded by the Mediterranean diet might be enhanced by drugs that lowered blood levels of cholesterol. But, according to Dr. Alexander Leaf, professor emeritus of clinical medicine at Harvard University Medical School, the Lyon study indicates that "there are other powerful risk factors within the realm of diet that must be considered if we are to achieve maximal dietary benefits in reducing this Number One cause of mortality in the world today."

One interesting finding of the Lyon study was that although the project was officially terminated after 27 months (the benefits of the Mediterranean-type diet were so drastic that the researchers concluded it would be unethical not to give the comparison group a chance to go on it), most of the participants who had been in the experimental group continued to follow the diet. In other words, the diet was well-tolerated and probably enjoyed.

If you are serious about wanting to avoid a heart attack, or a worsening of heart disease, numerous

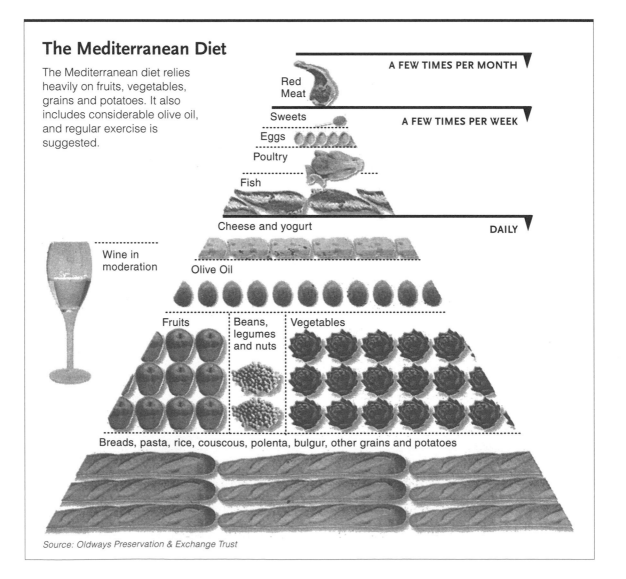

## The Mediterranean Diet

The Mediterranean diet relies heavily on fruits, vegetables, grains and potatoes. It also includes considerable olive oil, and regular exercise is suggested.

Red Meat — A FEW TIMES PER MONTH

Sweets — A FEW TIMES PER WEEK
Eggs
Poultry
Fish

Cheese and yogurt — DAILY

Wine in moderation

Olive Oil

Fruits | Beans, legumes and nuts | Vegetables

Breads, pasta, rice, couscous, polenta, bulgur, other grains and potatoes

*Source: Oldways Preservation & Exchange Trust*

studies have strongly indicated that you'd be wise to eat fish at least once or twice a week. Here is a quick summary of some of the most telling findings:

▶ In a study, in Seattle and surrounding suburbs, of 334 people who suffered a cardiac arrest compared with 493 people who had not, eating one fatty fish meal a week was associated with a 50 to 70 percent lower risk of a fatal heart attack, according to a report by Dr. David S. Siscovick and colleagues at the University of Washington. This finding strongly suggests that eating fish can prevent potentially fatal disruptions of heart rhythms, an effect that has been demonstrated in laboratory animals given fish oils.

▶ A British study found that people who regularly ate fish, especially fatty fish, were less likely to suffer heart attacks. The researchers, writing in the *British Medical Journal*, suggested that fish oils reduced the thickness and stickiness of the blood, which in turn meant less chance that a blood clot would form and precipitate a heart attack.

▶ A 30-year study of 1,800 men in Illinois showed that men who consumed one or two servings of fish a week (about 7 ounces) had a significantly lower risk of suffering a fatal heart attack. The lead researcher, Dr. Martha Daviglus of Northwestern University Medical School, concluded, "The good news is that small amounts of fish, amounts all of us can easily fit into our diets, may make a difference."

[JEB, March 1999]

## There's Plenty of Choice in a Diet for a Healthier Heart

Is your cholesterol level a little too high? Have you been told to de-fat your diet or take costly medicines to bring it down? Eating à la Dr. Dean Ornish (about 10 percent of calories from fat) is too much of a challenge for most people, and many currently healthy people would rather not take cholesterol-lowering medications (all have some side effects) if there are safe, effective and more pleasant options to achieving a desirable cholesterol level and a reduced risk of heart disease.

Recent studies have highlighted a wide variety of foods and beverages that offer the promise of a healthier heart, often with other protective benefits as well. In fact, if weight is not a problem, you may not have to eat low-fat at all, as long as the fats you eat are the right kinds of fats.

Don't assume that any of the choices below is the Holy Grail that will allow you to subsist on a cheeseburger-and-fries diet. Saturated fats must still be kept to a minimum. They are found in significant amounts in chicken fat (30 percent saturated), vegetable shortening (31 percent), lard (40 percent), beef fat (50 percent) and butter (62 percent).

However, in a special report published in November 1998 by the journal *Postgraduate Medicine*, Dr. Lisa A. Hark, director of the nutrition education and prevention program at the University of Pennsylvania School of Medicine in Philadelphia, said that reducing total dietary fat appeared to be less effective in lowering coronary risk than simply replacing saturated fat with unsaturated fat and consuming less trans fats, which act in the body like saturated fat and are formed when unsaturated vegetable oils are partially hydrogenated.

Data from the continuing Nurses' Health Study showed that every 5 percent increase in saturated fat in the diet resulted in a 17 percent increase in the risk of cardiovascular disease.

Heart-healthy fats include those found in fish, olives, avocados, seeds and nuts. For cooking and salad dressings, you can choose among olive, canola, sesame seed, peanut and walnut oils. But be sure to use them with discretion. Even heart-healthy oils are high in calories, about 120 calories a tablespoon, and if you gain weight, your cholesterol level and coronary risk will rise. For a table spread, choose a margarine that is trans-fat free.

You've no doubt heard about any number of foods and drinks purported to be good for the heart: fish, soy, whole grains, various fruits and vegetables, garlic, alcohol and particularly red wine. Here's the current scoop:

**Fish.** Just one fish meal a week may cut in half a man's risk of sudden cardiac death. The Physicians' Health Study found that men who ate fish—for example, shellfish, canned tuna, salmon, sardines, mackerel, herring, bluefish or swordfish—at least once a week reduced their risk of sudden death by 52 percent when compared with men who ate fish less than once a month. Eating fish more often than once a week did not further reduce the risk, but those who benefited most consumed fish as part of an overall low-fat diet. Eating fish appears to protect against fatal abnormal heart rhythms and the oils in fish reduce the risk of arterial clogging.

**Soy Foods.** Eating soy protein daily can lower the blood level of heart-damaging LDL cholesterol and raise protective HDL cholesterol. However, a lot of soy protein is needed to achieve a significant improvement—between 25 and 50 grams a day. One ounce of powdered soy protein contains 23 grams, 4 ounces of tempeh has 17 grams, 4 ounces of tofu has 6 to 13 grams and 1 cup of soy milk has 4 to 10 grams. The beneficial substances in soy appear to be plant estrogens called isoflavones, antioxidants which may have an added benefit of reducing the risk of breast cancer.

**Whole Grains.** A continuing study of more than 34,000 postmenopausal women in Iowa has shown that eating one or more servings of whole-grain foods (in place of refined grains) can reduce the risk of death from heart disease by a third. Such foods include cereals like Wheaties, Cheerios and Shredded Wheat, brown rice, oatmeal, corn, bran,

wheat germ and breads in which the first ingredient listed is whole wheat. Check the nutrition information label and look for cereals with 3 to 6 grams of fiber and breads with 2 grams of fiber per serving.

**Soluble Fiber.** Foods rich in soluble fiber reduce cholesterol by increasing its excretion. Last month the Kellogg Company introduced grain products, under the trade name Ensemble, that are enriched with psyllium, the soluble fiber in the stool softener Metamucil. If you try psyllium-rich foods, introduce them gradually, be sure to consume plenty of liquid with your meal and don't be surprised if they increase intestinal gas and bowel frequency. Other foods rich in heart-protective soluble fiber include dried beans and peas, oats and oat bran, barley, apples, citrus fruits, corn and flaxseed. Flaxseed, which should be ground to derive its full benefits, also contains the kind of heart-protective oil found in fish and substances called lignans that may act as cancer blockers. Ground flaxseed can be added to cereal, yogurt and the batter for pancakes, breads and other baked goods.

**Supplements.** The study of Iowa women also highlighted dietary calcium, either from foods or supplements, as heart-protective, probably because it helps lower blood pressure. Most helpful was a diet that contained more than 1,400 milligrams of calcium a day, about the amount in a quart of skim milk or yogurt or calcium-fortified orange juice.

A dietary supplement, Chinese red-yeast-rice, sold as Cholestin, contains the same cholesterol-lowering compounds found in the cholesterol-lowering statin drugs like pravastatin and simvastatin. It is highly effective and much cheaper than the statins, but it may have the same potential side effects of liver and muscle damage, and the Food and Drug Administration is trying to reclassify it as a drug.

Two B vitamins—folate and B-6—may reduce the risk of fatal heart attacks by lowering blood levels of a substance called homocysteine, which, like high cholesterol, damages coronary arteries. Good sources of folate include dark green leafy vegetables, dried beans and peas, orange juice, fortified whole-grain cereals and breads and multivitamin supplements. B-6 is found in whole-grain cereals, bananas, beef, chicken and vitamin supplements.

A clove of garlic a day can be beneficial as well. But if a dried deodorized garlic supplement is chosen, be sure it is enteric-coated, which will protect it from stomach acid and allow the formation of the odoriferous active ingredient that lowers cholesterol and another blood fat, triglycerides.

**Tea and Alcohol.** Tea, with or without caffeine, is beneficial to the heart. Regular black tea is a rich source of flavonoids, the protective antioxidants in soybeans that are believed to retard the development of atherosclerosis. In a study of nearly 700 men and women in Boston, those who drank one or more cups of regular (not herbal) tea a day had nearly half the risk of suffering a heart attack as those who drank no tea.

Moderate consumption of alcohol, one drink a day, has been linked in numerous studies to a reduced risk of heart disease, a benefit that apparently results from an alcohol-induced rise in protective HDL cholesterol. Studies have singled out red wine as especially beneficial because of antioxidant and anticlotting substances in the skins of red grapes. These substances are also present in purple grape juice, which may also reduce the risk of atherosclerosis by keeping LDL cholesterol from attaching to coronary arteries.

[JEB, April 1999]

## Drink a Day Can Lower Death Rate By 20 Percent

One drink a day can be good for health, scientists are reporting, confirming earlier research in a new study that is the largest to date of the effects of alcohol consumption in the United States. The study, which examined mortality in nearly 500,000 people between the ages of 35 and 69, found that those who took one drink a day of wine, beer or hard liquor had a death rate 20 percent lower than nondrinkers during a nine-year period.

"That's a whopping big effect," said Dr. Meir Stampfer, an epidemiologist at the Harvard School of Public Health who has conducted similar studies but was not involved in this one. Although the same effect has previously been reported, Dr. Stampfer said, confirmation by the new findings is important because such a large study leaves little room for doubt.

Dr. Eric B. Rimm, another Harvard epidemiologist, said: "This is one of the best studies you could do on alcohol and mortality. We're not going to get much better answers than what we have in this paper." He also noted that it was one of the first large studies to include data on the health effects of alcohol in people who already have heart disease.

The study, published in December 1997 in *The New England Journal of Medicine*, was conducted by scientists from the American Cancer Society, the World Health Organization and Oxford University. Subjects included 490,000 people between the ages of 30 and 104, who described their drinking habits in 1982 and whose death rates were then recorded for nine years. Most subjects were white, middle-class and married, and more likely than the rest of the United States population to be college-educated.

The researchers said the finding of a benefit from one drink a day applied equally to married and single people. Dr. Michael Thun, the lead author of the study and the director of analytic epidemiology for the American Cancer Society, added a note of caution to the results of the study, saying: "The study does not represent the major hazards of alcohol abuse. It does not include people who drink themselves out of a home or a job, and does not include anyone under age 30, but it does reflect the experience of large numbers of people with fairly stable drinking patterns in middle age and beyond."

One drink was defined as 5 ounces of wine, 12 ounces of beer or one cocktail.

Researchers found that nearly all the benefit from moderate drinking was because of a reduction in the risk of cardiovascular disease. People with the most to gain were men and women at high risk for heart attack or stroke because of hypertension, high blood cholesterol or who already had heart disease.

Alcohol can help the heart in two ways: by reducing the likelihood of blood clots, which can trigger heart attacks, and by raising the blood levels of HDL cholesterol, which is protective. The anti-clotting effect takes place quickly, within hours of drinking, but HDL takes several weeks to rise with daily drinking and may take a year or so to reduce a person's risk, Dr. Stampfer said.

Despite the clear advantage of moderate drinking, the researchers presented their findings with strong caveats, emphasizing that too much alcohol is dangerous, and that 100,000 deaths a year in the United States are related to alcohol abuse. Study subjects who took four or more drinks a day were three to seven times as likely as nondrinkers to die from cirrhosis, alcoholism and cancers of the mouth, throat and liver. And in people under 30, alcohol is linked to an increased risk of death from accidents, violence and suicide in young people, Dr. Thun said.

In another discouraging finding, the study confirmed that the same one-drink-a-day ration that lowered the overall risk of death also increased by 30 percent a woman's chance of dying from breast cancer. "Breast cancer is the one disease in which the basically cardiovascular benefits of a drink a day are directly in conflict with cancer," Dr. Thun said.

But women are still far more likely to die of heart disease than breast cancer. In the study, many more women died from cardiovascular disease than from breast cancer, so more would stand to benefit from reducing the heart disease risk. "But women may not be equally concerned about the two diseases," Dr. Thun said, acknowledging that many seemed to fear breast cancer more than heart disease. Ultimately, he said, deciding whether or not to drink will be an individual decision.

All the researchers agreed that the findings did not mean that teetotalers concerned about their hearts should take up drinking. "We can lower the risk of heart disease in other ways if we try, through diet, physical activity and watching weight," Dr. Stampfer said.

[DG, December 1997]

## High Intake of 2 Vitamins May Lower Coronary Risk

A high intake of two B vitamins found in fruits, vegetables and other common foods appears to reduce by nearly half a woman's risk of suffering a heart attack, a study has shown. The study also confirmed that drinking moderate amounts of alcohol had a protective effect on women's hearts.

The study, conducted among more than 80,000 women who are nurses, is the first to show a direct link between these B vitamins, folate and B-6, and protection against coronary disease. It suggests that eating more fruits, vegetables and whole grains or getting these B vitamins from supplements is as important as quitting smoking, lowering high cholesterol and controlling blood pressure in preventing premature death from the nation's leading killer.

The new finding, published in the *Journal of the American Medical Association*, also suggests that the current Recommended Dietary Allowance, or R.D.A., of folate and B-6 for adults other than pregnant women is inadequate to provide maximum protection against heart disease. The Food and Nutrition Board of the National Academy of Sciences currently suggests that to prevent nutrient deficiencies, adults should consume 180 micrograms of folate and 1.6 milligrams of B-6 each day. But the most cardiac protection in the new study was achieved with daily intakes of more than 400 micrograms of folate and more than 3 milligrams of B-6. B vitamins from either foods or supplements were found to be protective.

"Everyone should be at two to three times the current R.D.A. for folate and B-6 to achieve the maximum reduction in risk," said Dr. Eric B. Rimm of the Harvard School of Public Health, who directed the study. "The exciting news is that a substantial reduction in risk can be achieved easily, without a dramatic change in diet," he said. "You don't have to give up everything you eat. You just have to eat more foods like fortified cold cereals, orange juice, spinach and other leafy greens, whole grains, bananas, potatoes, chicken and fish."

The Food and Drug Administration recently authorized the fortification of flour with folic acid, which is the form of folate used by the body and the form found in multivitamin supplements. Although the agency's primary goal was to prevent the birth of children with spinal deformities, fortification is also likely to increase significantly the folic acid intake among children and adults and thus should help protect against heart disease.

"The findings of the current study encourage the view that with intervention through supplementation, fortification, improved dietary intakes of folate and vitamin B-6 and better food processing and distribution methods, the decline in U.S. cardiovascular mortality and morbidity will continue," Dr. Kilmer S. McCully wrote in an editorial accompanying the new report. The researchers said they expected that the findings would also apply to men. Previous studies in men and women showed that folate and B-6 consumed through foods or through foods and supplements reduced blood levels of the amino acid homocysteine and protected against narrowing of the arteries that feed the brain. Other studies had linked high levels of homocysteine in the blood to a greatly raised risk of suffering a heart attack. Homocysteine is believed to increase coronary risk by one or more of several mechanisms: damaging cells that line arteries, fostering blood clots and narrowing blood vessels by promoting growth of smooth muscle cells.

In his editorial, Dr. McCully noted that several clinical and population studies have concluded that moderately high blood levels of homocysteine are "a powerful independent risk factor for arteriosclerosis, comparable with hypercholesterolemia," or elevated cholesterol, "smoking and hypertension."

The new study also supported previous research that has linked a moderate intake of alcohol to protection against heart disease. In the study, the women who consumed the most folate and who also had at least one alcoholic drink a day had the lowest risk of suffering a heart attack—78 percent lower than those who consumed the least amount of the B vitamin and who drank no alcohol.

The study, by researchers at the Harvard School of Public Health, Brigham and Women's Hospital and Harvard Medical School in Boston, involved 80,082 nurses whose diets and health status were first evaluated in 1980 and then periodically reevaluated for the next 14 years. During that time, 658 of the women had nonfatal heart attacks and 281 died of heart attacks. The women were classified into one of five groups, depending on how much of each vitamin they routinely consumed through foods and supple-

## Asparagus to Spinach

A daily intake of more than 400 micrograms of folate and more than 3 milligrams of B-6 may cut a woman's risk of a heart attack nearly in half, a new study indicates. Many cereals and grains are fortified with added B vitamins. Below are some other foods rich in those vitamins.

| FOLATE in micrograms per cup: | B-6 in milligrams: |
|---|---|
| Orange juice: 45 | Plantain, 1 medium: .54 |
| Black-eyed peas: 210 | Banana, 1 medium: .68 |
| Cooked asparagus: 262 | Chicken, 1 cup: .66 |
| Cooked spinach: 262 | Beef liver, 3 oz.: .77 |
| Cooked lentils: 358 | |
| Chicken liver: 1,078 | |

*Source: United States Department of Agriculture*

ments in 1980. Dr. Rimm said there was relatively little change in the women's diets during the follow-up period. The researchers took all major and many minor risk factors for heart disease into account in analyzing their data.

During the next 14 years the women consuming the most folate were 31 percent less likely to suffer a heart attack than those who consumed the least folate. Likewise, those who consumed the most B-6 were 33 percent less likely to have a heart attack than were those who consumed the least. However, among those at the highest level of consumption of both vitamins, coronary risk was reduced by 45 percent, suggesting that each nutrient benefited the heart somewhat independently.

The American Heart Association cautioned that additional research, in which people are randomly assigned to take vitamins or not take them, would be needed to confirm the role of these vitamins in reducing risk of heart disease. In the new study, an even greater reduction in risk was noted among women at the highest intake of both folate and B-6 who also drank at least one alcoholic drink a day. Their risk was reduced by 75 percent, a benefit that was "much stronger than we anticipated and needs to be confirmed by others," Dr. Rimm said. Among the nurses who drank the most alcohol, he added, about 90 percent consumed no more than one or two drinks a day.

Alcohol, which raises the level of protective high-density lipoprotein (HDL) cholesterol in the blood, has been linked in numerous studies to a decreased risk of heart attack in men and women. However, alcohol consumption has a negative effect on folate. Even in moderate amounts, alcohol inactivates folate and decreases its availability to the body. "If you drink alcohol and consume low levels of folate, you're not going to get much benefit from folate," Dr. Rimm said. "A woman who drinks may need to consume more folate to lower homocysteine levels."

[JEB, February 1998]

# Image and Self-Image

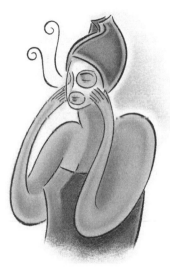

## THE SURGICAL PATH TO APPEARANCE CHANGES

I f there is a body part that women have not despised and yearned to alter, it has yet to be discovered. Breasts too small or too big, flabby thighs, a crepey neck, yellow teeth, frown lines, unwanted eyeglasses: you name it, and there's an operation to fix it. It is a matter of opinion as to whether the drive to remake oneself reflects a healthy interest in looking one's best, or an unhealthy, insecure fixation on appearance.

What are women looking for? The obvious answer is beauty, which in American culture usually means youth—or at least the appearance of youth. Plastic surgeons can often restore some semblance of it, but occasionally there is an extra price to pay in terms of risks or disappointing results.

Breast implants, which fell out of favor in 1992 amid concerns over possible health risks from silicone, are making a comeback. Implants today are filled with salt water rather than silicone. But plastic surgeons and many women say that silicone-filled implants have a more natural feel than saline, and some surgeons think that silicone implants may one day make a comeback as well, especially since an expert panel declared during the summer of 1999 that silicone implants could not be linked to any systemic illnesses.

That does not mean that implants, silicone or saline, are harmless: the same panel that found a lack of systemic disease also said some women had localized problems, including scarring and hardening of breast tissue from their implants.

Nose jobs, unlike breast implants, have declined in popularity in some parts of the country, as more and more young women and girls decide to keep their natural looks as a matter of ethnic pride.

Doctors have raised questions about the safety of an enormously popular procedure, liposuction, in which fat is sucked out the body to reduce bulges in the hips, thighs, arms, belly, back or just about anywhere they occur. A handful of deaths have been linked to the procedure, and although it seems minuscule compared to the number of procedures done, doctors say it is of great concern because liposuction is not medically necessary, and is done on healthy people.

The key to safety in cosmetic surgery is the same as with any other type of operation: finding a skilled surgeon who does the procedure in question frequently, as often as several times a week.

# A Question of Beauty: Is It Good for You?

have an image of perfect health. It's a photograph of a young woman smiling, her teeth white, her hair shining, her skin glowing, her body thin and muscular—the sort of picture that appears on the cover of magazines like *American Health*. It's the true me, of course, the me if I did everything right and took an anti-aging pill.

Of course, it's ridiculous. Yet somehow, that loosely defined word "health" and that loaded word "beauty" are so intricately entwined that many of us confuse them, consciously or subconsciously, in our incessant dream of perfect health—or is it perfect beauty?

The icons of health and beauty assault me relentlessly. I can't forget my favorite advertisement for breakfast cereal, which showed a bicyclist in the golden light of dawn, or the advertisements for bottled water that featured slim and sweaty athletes downing a drink. Then there are the clothing catalogues that show up, unbidden, in my mailbox, with young models cavorting in sparkling blue surf. The health-and-beauty industry suffuses our society and our economy, luring us to buy food, clothing, cosmetics, exercise equipment, even cars—the Chevrolet Web site features a young father mounting bikes on top of his minivan; my local BMW dealer displays a folding BMW bicycle as prominently as its autos.

If there is anything to the notion of subliminal messages linking health and beauty, I've clearly been seduced by them. I find it hard to think of health without envisioning someone young and beautiful. Even the words we use are a sort of double-speak. "Health" clubs? At the health club I frequent, few of us are sweating away on the elliptical cross-trainers for our health. Yes, we feel good after a tough workout. But we love the machines because they burn so many calories. I lift weights for muscle definition, not explicitly to make myself healthier.

Most "health foods" have more to do with beauty than health; they tend to be ones that are low in calories, allowing us to eat more. I somehow doubt that most of us who buy them do so because we think that we'll prevent an illness. Disease prevention seems so distant and beauty so immediate. If I take care of myself, I might slightly diminish my risk for heart disease in the future. But I might look better next week.

Yes, of course, there is probably a health benefit to all that dieting and exercising. But there is also an implicit self-righteousness. When the slothful person gets sick, colleagues whisper: "Of course. What can you expect if you don't take care of yourself?"

The idea that health and beauty are linked goes back to Alfred Russell Wallace, who, with Charles Darwin, developed the theory of evolution. Like Darwin, Wallace was puzzled by the observation that male birds tend to be brightly colored, even though their fiery plumage can make it hard to hide from predators. Darwin's idea was that male birds evolved to have brilliant colors because females wanted them that way. Wallace concluded that females chose the more brightly colored males because they were healthier.

Thus an academic endeavor was born. Since the puzzle of the birds was described in the mid-to-late 19th century, it has become almost a sine qua non that what people think is beautiful is in some way correlated with good health.

But is it? Researchers have asked whether animals that are sexually attractive are also healthy, getting mixed results. It appears to be true for some species, not for others. When it comes to humans, the evolutionary biology hypothesis was harder to test. Yet it certainly has a ring of truth.

"If you look at any sign of ill health, it's the opposite of what we consider beautiful," said Dr. Nancy Etcoff, a psychologist at the Harvard Medical School and the author of the new book *Survival of the Prettiest: The Science of Beauty*. "There is no culture in which yellow, cracked teeth or thinning hair or broken bones are not considered unattractive or ugly." On the other hand, she added, "Youth and strength, clear skin, shining eyes, thick hair and good teeth are associated with the things we consider beautiful."

Some doctors, who are focusing on health, not beauty, say they nonetheless use a patient's appearance as an indicator of illness. Dr. Suzanne Fletcher, a professor of ambulatory care and prevention at the Harvard Medical School, said that when she sees a new patient, she guesses the person's age before asking. One sure sign of ill health, Dr. Fletcher said, is looking much older than you are.

"I'm picking up on wrinkled skin and the color of the hair," Dr. Fletcher said. "But it's really a brightness of movement as much as anything else. It's an expression of a face and the eyes, it's their alertness and understanding of what's going on around them. Almost any illness can affect these things, and they also are signals of what we call aging."

But the hypothesis goes only so far. On an individual basis, there is no relationship between the prettiest person and the healthiest, according to S. Michael Kalick, a psychologist at the University of Massachusetts at Boston, who has searched for an association to no avail.

Professor Kalick used data from a study that began in the 1930s in Berkeley and Oakland, California. Hundreds of residents agreed to be photographed and to have their health assessed on an annual basis from the ages of 11 to 18. They each had an additional health assessment when they were in their 30s and again between the ages of 58 and 66. In Professor Kalick's study, volunteers looked at photographs of the subjects' faces when they were 17, 17½ and 18 and rated them on how attractive they were. Dr. Kalick and his colleagues knew from the study records how healthy these people were as teenagers and how healthy they would be later. They could thus determine whether the healthiest people were rated as the most attractive.

It turned out that they were not. Those with the fewest and least severe illnesses were no more attractive than those who always seemed to be sick. And those who had the fewest medical problems when they grew older were not better looking than those plagued with ill health.

"We did not find a relationship," Professor Kalick said. "That was kind of surprising." But when he asked another group of volunteers to look at the photographs and guess how healthy the study subjects were, the raters assumed that the most attractive people were the healthiest. "People really think that attractiveness indicates health," Professor Kalick said. "It's just that they're mistaken about it."

Elizabeth Haiken, a history professor at the University of British Columbia in Vancouver, and author of the recent book *Venus Envy: A History of Cosmetic Surgery*, said her research indicated that the perceived relationship between health and beauty became entrenched early in the 20th century with a popular-psychology movement that said if you felt better about yourself, you would be healthier, stronger, more able to act—a sort of health-through-self-esteem movement. And what better way to feel good about yourself, or so advertisers proclaimed, than to make yourself as beautiful as you could be?

"These things are all sort of intertwined together," Professor Haiken said.

The ultimate example, of course, is plastic surgery, which began in earnest after World War I, according to Professor Haiken's book, and has now reached a point where new words are being used to describe ordinary body variations. "Bat-wing deformity" is "redundant skin and tissue hanging from the upper arms." "Aging neck deformity" is wrinkled skin on the neck. Others, like "spare-tire deformity" and "violin deformity," also called "saddlebags," are just what you think they are.

"It brings you face to face with your own boundaries," Professor Haiken said. "I mean, what is a deformity and what is unattractive? Where is the line? I was driving through Kentucky and I heard an ad on the radio: 'Are you not satisfied with your life? Do you think things are missing? Do you need a change that is more than skin deep?'" she recalled. "I thought it would be an ad for personal growth." But as she continued to listen, she discovered what it really was: an advertisement for plastic surgery. "Isn't it funny that in the 20th century, self-improvement has become this sort of physical thing?" she mused.

Cosmetics and skin care came of age along with plastic surgery, and they, too, catered to our desires to improve ourselves, seizing on devices like the ubiquitous makeover promoted by women's magazines.

In her book *Hope in a Jar: The Making of America's Beauty Culture*, Kathy Peiss, a history professor at the University of Massachusetts at Amherst, told how the industry emerged. Companies noticed early on that women took advertising slogans for cosmetics and soaps to heart. A study commissioned by Woodbury Facial Soap in the early 1920s, for example, found that college students "quoted advertising slogans verbatim, 'a skin you love to touch,' a 'schoolgirl complexion' when describing and evaluating their own faces," Professor Peiss writes.

Now companies are exploiting the health and beauty image for all it's worth. On Clinique's Web site, you can click on "What's New" and learn about "Superfit Makeup." Lancome suggests on its Web site, "Take a destressing moment with Hydra Zen, Lancome's newest moisturizer." Revlon features "Age-Defying Makeup," crowing: "Don't lie about your age. Defy it." Nexxus tells Web page readers to "Feed your head" with its hair products. Jergens advertises a "daily nourishing cream" with "alpha and beta hydroxy complex."

"You have to come up with new ways of selling stuff," Professor Haiken said. " 'Feed your skin.' That sort of stuff. For a generation that is pretty much obsessed with health, that is what sells." It's an illusion, of course. And, in particular, the vitamins, minerals and herbs that are suffusing beauty products these days do nothing for the health of the skin, said Dr. Albert M. Kligman, a professor of dermatology at the University of Pennsylvania School of Medicine in Philadelphia.

"Let's say you have a good cream, so you add a little vitamin A," Dr. Kligman said. "Then you add vitamin B, then you add C and D and E. Now suppose you want to add a little selenium and a little copper, and suppose you want to add an antioxidant. Now we have a cocktail. I know a product that has 67 active ingredients." He worries about the long-term effects of using an untested mix of chemicals on the skin and the lack of regulation of the cosmetics industry.

But most of the added chemicals are useless, Dr. Kligman said. The doses are tiny—"homeopathic," in many cases—and the chemicals, when they are used in a cosmetic formulation, are often unstable. Vitamin A, for example, breaks down almost instantly in a cream.

"You make it up, and two days later you have half of what you put in. Two months later, you ain't got nothing," Dr. Kligman said.

Nonetheless, many cosmetics, regardless of vitamins, minerals and herbs, can give that glow of youth. Hair color can make gray disappear. Cosmetic dentistry promises shiny white teeth. Plastic surgery claims to wipe years from your face. And now, with even bifocal contact lenses, maybe we do have a chance to look healthier. (Read "more beautiful.")

Yet, if the evolutionary biology hypothesis has but a germ of truth, and if we have radar for signs of health, are we purposely flying below the radar screen when we take advantage of the plethora of products to make us look youthful and beautiful? "We've totally confused the radar," Prof. Etcoff said. "We're looking younger and younger and healthier and healthier. We're master cheats, I think."

And master dreamers. I know I'm being conned by the advertisements and the images. I refuse on general principle to buy beauty products with added vitamins, minerals or herbs. I laugh at the word "health," mocking it for pretending to be some nirvana of perfect harmony that is always just out of reach. But with health (read "beauty") beckoning, it is hard to escape the illusion that, someday, if I just put in a bit more time and a bit more effort, I might get there.

[GK, June 1999]

# Life's Wrinkles, Some of Them Ugly, Afflict the Beautiful, Too

Ask anyone: It is better to be beautiful. To be a "dish," a "knockout," a "babe." To be an object of desire. To be the kind of woman who can silence a chattering room with a toss of her hair. It is better, if possible, to have high cheekbones, large eyes, a diminutive chin, long, shapely legs, full, moist lips, a waist that a man can close his hands around.

These attributes, American culture dictates and researchers have found, buy a woman attention and give her an edge from the cradle onward. And every woman who possesses them is grateful. Or is she? Certainly, beautiful women are grateful that they are not unattractive. And they enjoy, to an extent, the power attractiveness bestows.

But with all its advantages, beauty has its perils. A beautiful woman is not just admired, she is idealized, lusted after and envied. She is often viewed as a mountain to be conquered or a competitor to be vanquished. And in the lives of most beautiful women there are stories that will never make the pages of the fashion magazines, difficulties rarely discussed in company.

Consider a 22-year-old woman in Texas who cut her waist-length blond mane short, dyed it black and gained 30 pounds in an attempt to discourage the unrelenting stares, come-ons and buttocks-pinching that seemed her lot every time she displayed her fortunate set of genes in public.

Then there's the 36-year-old massage therapist in Woodstock, New York, who quit the modeling business because she was tired of men who "think that you could just jump into bed with them." The attention, she said, "was not necessarily the kind you want." She marvels, for example, at the stranger who grabbed her crotch in public.

For many beautiful women, a solitary evening stroll may mean running a gauntlet of sexual threat, and entering any personal relationship often involves negotiating a mine field: If she is with men, she worries that her friendliness is perceived as flirtation or that his friendship masks a desire to become her lover. With women, she is under a microscope, dodging resentful comments and perpetually watching her back.

Such laments typically elicit little sympathy. "I don't take those kinds of complaints very seriously," said Ellen Berscheid, Regents' Professor of Psychology at the University of Minnesota. "Were attractive women to walk in the shoes of someone who was physically unattractive, and to encounter the reactions these people encounter—the penalties in educational opportunities and occupational opportunities! I would say those complaints are rather minuscule."

Yet researchers, who have spent years documenting the benefits of attractiveness, which are substantial, are finally beginning to explore the costs that may attend good looks, especially for women. If, as studies have found, attractive women are seen by other people as healthier and happier, they are also stereotyped as selfish, as less likely to be faithful and as less likely to be good mothers. Their achievements may be discounted by others, who assume they got ahead because of their looks, and they may be passed over by employers looking for authoritative managers. "Attractiveness is a commodity that, like wealth, brings with it a host of problems," said Michael Cunningham, the acting chairman of psychology at the University of Louisville, in Kentucky.

Of more concern, said Dr. Nancy Etcoff, an instructor at Harvard Medical School and author of *Survival of the Prettiest: The Science of Beauty*, men are likely to make assumptions about beautiful women, increasing the likelihood that they will approach such women in a sexual way. Men assume that attractive women have a higher sex drive, are more sexually permissive and more sexually confident. Studies have shown that in interacting with any woman, attractive or not, a man is more likely to interpret social cues— a friendly smile, for example—as an invitation to sex.

A result is that many attractive women feel bombarded by male sexual attention, not all of it benign. "The male gaze can be appreciative, but on the other hand it can be aggressive," Dr. Etcoff said.

Though there are no studies of any links between rape and the victim's attractiveness, researchers find that young women are more likely to become rape victims—their age, perhaps, a signal of the period when attractiveness is at its peak. And in very preliminary work in his laboratory, Dr. Cunningham and his colleagues are finding that male stalkers are likely to prey not on the most attractive women, but on women who are very attractive but also friendly.

Similarly, one attractive woman put forward "the B-plus theory." She has found that it is not women at the apex of beauty—the Naomi Campbells and Cindy Crawfords—who encounter an onslaught of sexual attention from men; most men assume that such women are out of reach. Men may sense that they have a shot with women who are beautiful, but at a less exalted level, she said; these women consequently draw more sexual attention.

When a woman marries, her attractiveness may cause aggressive behavior in her mate. In a study of 107 married couples, David Buss, an evolutionary psychologist at the University of Texas at Austin, found that men married to attractive women were more likely to engage in mate-guarding behaviors, like following their wives around, snooping through their mail and making them feel guilty about talking to other men. But the men were also more likely to display signs of treasuring their wives, giving them more resources and offering more expressions of love and commitment.

For some women, having a boyfriend or a husband is a way to deflect unwanted male attention. "It's like I always need that there, and I end up in this relationship I don't want to be in," one woman said. "But I'm scared to get out," because it affords her protection. Other women wear wedding rings even if unmarried or don baggy clothes to lessen the impact of their looks.

For women whose physical attractiveness falls in the normal range, the antidote for many pressures in life is a good heart-to-heart with a female friend. But attractive women say they often have difficulty forging friendships with other women, who are likely to envy their looks and subject them to an even harsher scrutiny than men. "If you're attractive or reasonably attractive and then on top of that have some ambition, that's a deadly combination," said a 29-year-old graduate student who, like many of the women interviewed, asked not to be identified because it seemed too risky to admit that she knew she was attractive.

Ruth Berenzy, the former model, said wives of male friends often do not like her. One male friend of 15 years has still not introduced her to his wife. In response, some attractive women say they seek female friendship only with women as good-looking as they are, women who share the same set of experiences and are less likely to harbor resentment. "I have a bunch of beautiful friends, who've been in the same boat," said the Texas 22-year-old.

Studies support the notion that attractiveness stimulates competition and jealousy in other women. Attractive women, researchers find, may be rated as more popular by other women, but they are also more disliked. In part, social scientists say, women's antipathy toward the most attractive of their sex may have its roots in biology: nobody likes to be outshone. Lee Dugatkin, a biologist at the University of Louisville, has found that male guppies, for example, prefer to swim near other males whose poor success rate with females makes them look, by comparison, like the Tom Cruises of the guppy world. And Dr. Etcoff cites studies showing that men are less eager to date women with average looks after gazing at photographs of beautiful faces.

Given such complications, it's no wonder that for some attractive women, aging, though difficult in many respects, offers a not unwelcome respite. Not that looks fade without regret: when a woman is used to commanding men's attention, the loss of that ability takes some adjustment.

An ophthalmic surgeon in the Baltimore area who is 46 said that even six years ago, she knew "if I went to a meeting, I could have a group of men standing around me just because of the way I looked." At a recent conference, she sat down at the lunch table and realized that things had changed. "I was very much aware that if someone was going to talk to me, I was going to have to put my personality out there," she said.

Yet, in the dulling of her attractiveness, there was a positive side as well. When she moved into her neighborhood, she said, she quickly became friends with a woman down the street. "Looks didn't enter into it," she said, "and that was kind of a relief."

[EG, June 1999]

## Cosmetic Breast Enlargements Are Making a Comeback

Boarding a flight from LaGuardia to Minneapolis, passengers could not help noticing Ana Voog. Strikingly attractive, with huge brown eyes, flawless skin and cropped platinum hair, Ms. Voog, who is 5'2" tall and weighs 90 pounds, also has remarkably large breasts for such a petite woman. Her clingy white pullover bore a startling inscription: YES, THEY'RE FAKE.

Two years ago, when she was 30, Ms. Voog, a rock musician in Minneapolis, gave in to her longtime craving for a bust line, and had saline breast implants—pouches full of salt water—surgically inserted into her chest. She went into the operating room, she said, "totally flat, like not even enough for a training bra," and came out a D-cup.

"It was the most surreal thing I've ever experienced," Ms. Voog said.

Surreal or not, the experience is one that more and more American women are seeking. Cosmetic surgery to enlarge the breasts (which does not include reconstruction after mastectomy) is regaining popularity after falling out of favor in 1992. That year, the Food and Drug Administration banned silicone-gel-filled implants amid worries about potential health problems from silicone leaking out of the pouches. The number of operations plunged to 32,607, from a high of an estimated 120,000 to 150,000 in 1990.

But the count has been climbing back up and exceeded 122,000 last year, according to the American Society of Plastic and Reconstructive Surgeons. The states with the most operations are Florida, Texas and California, and plastic surgeons report that women in

Texas request bigger implants than those in any other state. Silicone gel is still banned from most cosmetic implants, but it has been replaced by saline implants like Ms. Voog's.

Why the resurgence? Plastic surgeons say the interest never died. There have always been women who wanted bigger breasts, but many were scared away by reports that silicone might be unsafe. Saline implants then gained acceptance as a safer alternative. Even though the covering is made of a rubbery form of solid silicone, it has not been linked to health problems.

Lawsuits have tried to link the silicone implants to autoimmune illnesses like lupus and scleroderma, but those links are still being debated because of an absence of conclusive evidence. Some women take that as reassurance that implants are safe. The recent $3.2 billion settlement between the Dow Corning Corporation, a joint venture of the Dow Chemical Company and Corning Inc., and 170,000 women who claim to have been injured by implants did not resolve the question of whether silicone can cause systemic illness.

"I think people are feeling more sanguine about implants not being poison," said Dr. Bruce Cunningham, chief of plastic surgery at the University of Minnesota.

But saline implants are not without risk: Infection and complications of anesthesia can occur, as with any surgery. Painful scar tissue can harden the breasts, and the implants can rupture, go flat and need replacing. They can also interfere with mammography.

But women are undeterred. Breast operations are just part of a larger picture: All types of plastic surgery are on the upswing, partly because a surge in the economy means that people can afford the operations, even though insurance does not cover them, said Dr. Scott Spear, professor and chief of plastic surgery at Georgetown University in Washington. Breast enlargement surgery usually costs between $5,000 and $6,000.

Dr. Roxanne Guy, a plastic surgeon in Melbourne, Florida, said that for some, breast implants have become a statement, like a tattoo or pierced eyebrow. "Women are more empowered, bold, more unabashed and free about their bodies," said Dr. Guy.

Dr. Diana Zuckerman, a psychologist and board member of the National Women's Health Network, does not see implants as a sign of empowerment. In many cases, she said, they reflect an urge to conform to an image of sexiness defined by magazines and lingerie catalogues full of models with implants.

Dr. Cunningham said he expected to see more implant operations as baby boomers work to defy aging. "'I'm going to emphasize how young I look,'" he said, describing the attitude. "'Large breasts show I'm young and vital and full and happy.' I think you will see more of that, like you'll see more men on Harleys."

Not only are more women getting implants, but they want them bigger than ever, said Dr. Joel Studin, a New York City plastic surgeon who performs two or three breast enlargements per week. "Women are understandably concerned about appearing that they have breast implants, so they tend to be conservative," he said. "But all too frequently these same women return a year later saying that while they're happy with their implants, they wish they had gone a little bit bigger. And many do decide to make the change."

Few women are neutral on the subject of breast enlargement. Some shudder at the thought of having surgery just to fill a bigger bra, and assume that women who submit to it must lack self-esteem or intelligence. But others see implants as one more means of looking better, albeit a bit more extreme than hair dye, mascara and pierced ears.

Plastic surgery appeals to some people, said Dr.

Spear, whereas "another segment would never do it and can't see why anybody else would. The key thing is not to let one group tell the other what they can do." His patients have included doctors, lawyers and judges, he said.

Many women want implants because their breasts shrank and sagged after childbirth. One, a 31-year-old mother of two young children from Wayne, New Jersey, who spoke on the condition of anonymity, said she had always been "small-chested," but developed "big, beautiful breasts" during pregnancy and nursing. Once she stopped breastfeeding, though, they became smaller than ever. She wanted the big ones back.

"I felt really depressed," she said. "I felt inadequate when I was intimate with my husband. It was nothing he did. I just didn't feel feminine." Trying on clothes, especially bathing suits, she thought she looked downright masculine. Once, hoping to look good in a strapless gown, she resorted to using masking tape to try to create cleavage.

Implants took her from an A cup to a C. The operation was more painful than she had expected, and recovery took longer, but she thinks it was worth it. "Our sex life is so much better because I feel so much better about myself," she said. "I feel sexy and I guess my husband picks up on that. I buy sexy lingerie all the time where before I never did."

Ms. Voog debated with herself about implants for 10 years before she finally got them. She said that before the surgery, her chest was so flat she had almost no breasts at all. "Clothes sort of just hung on me," she said. Now her clothes look smashing, she said, but her D-cup anatomy is a bit more than she expected. "I think my surgeon went a little hog wild," she said. "I think I wanted to be a C."

There were other surprises. For a week after the surgery, she was in such severe pain that moving her arms became difficult, and her boyfriend had to take care of her. Her nipples have normal sensation, but scattered spots on other parts of her breasts are a bit numb. And her breasts do not feel the way she had expected they would. "I thought they would feel natural, and they don't," she said. "That was a shock. I'm self-conscious when I hug anybody."

Ms. Voog's breasts are round, high and firm looking. But her nipples are not centered; the implants have left them high and outside.

People respond differently to her appearance. Intellectual men, she said, seem less inclined than before the surgery to take her seriously. Feminists act disdainfully. Men she thinks of as "jocks" have suddenly become more interested in her. Some stare at her chest instead of looking her in the eyes while talking to her. "It's beyond their control," she said. "They become totally dumb, like deer in the headlights."

She printed YES, THEY'RE FAKE on her shirt with a marker to attend a party in Manhattan, just to head off questions, smirks and smug remarks. "People are always wondering," Ms. Voog said. "I just wanted to put it out of their minds."

[DG, July 1998]

## Panel Confirms No Major Illness Tied to Implants . . .

An independent panel of 13 scientists convened by the Institute of Medicine at the request of Congress has concluded that silicone breast implants do not cause any major diseases.

"Some women with breast implants are indeed very ill and the I.O.M. committee is very sympathetic to their distress," the group wrote in its report. "However, it can find no evidence that these women are ill because of their implants."

The report, more than 400 pages long, says the "primary safety issue" with implants is their tendency to rupture or deflate and to lead to infections or hardening or scarring of the breast tissue. There is little argument about these localized problems, which can be painful and disfiguring and which often lead women to have additional surgery.

But the report asserts in forceful terms that there is no reason to believe that the implants cause rheumatoid arthritis, lupus, or any other systemic disease. Women who say their implants have caused them to suffer these or related problems have turned breast implants into a leading source of liability litigation.

The report is the latest in a series of evaluations that have concluded that there is no scientific evidence to support the lawsuits. Because it comes from the Institute of Medicine, the medical arm of the National Academy of Sciences, the nation's most prestigious scientific organization, it is expected to be influential in setting scientific agendas and encouraging women to accept settlements from implant makers rather than take their cases to court.

In preparing the report, panel members held public hearings, met in private and evaluated more than a thousand research reports. The Institute panel did not conduct any original research. Rather, the panel relied primarily on research and other materials reported by scientists and submitted by companies and advocates for women with implants. But the report said that since lawsuits were first filed in the late 1980s and early 1990s, there have been many scientific studies upon which to make an evaluation.

Scientists appointed by the judge overseeing implant liability litigation, Sam C. Pointer Jr., of Federal District Court in Alabama, came to a similar conclusion as the Institute panel and as a report issued by scientists in Britain who had been charged by the British minister of health with reviewing implant safety. Scientists appointed by Judge Robert E. Jones of Federal District Court in Oregon, reached a comparable conclusion.

Meanwhile, Dow Corning, a subsidiary of the Dow Chemical Company, which filed for bankruptcy citing the burden of its breast implant litigation, has agreed to pay women $3.2 billion to settle their claims. Other implant manufacturers, Baxter International, Bristol-Myers Squibb, and 3M, have agreed to a total settlement estimated to be nearly $4 billion. In addition, thousands of women have settled their cases in private agreements with implant makers or gone to trial and won awards that reached millions of dollars.

The Institute of Medicine committee estimated that about 1.5 million to 1.8 million American women have had silicone breast implants, about 70 percent for breast enlargement and the rest as reconstruction after mastectomy.

Members of the committee, headed by Dr. Stuart Bondurant, a professor of medicine at the University of North Carolina at Chapel Hill, and Dr. Virginia Ernster, a professor of epidemiology at the University of California at San Francisco, were prohibited from discussing the report until it was officially made public.

Sybil Goldrich, founder of Command Trust Network, an information clearinghouse for women with silicone problems, said, "I find it extremely difficult to accept what the Institute of Medicine says because those studies are paid for by the manufacturers. They have not convinced me that their review is correct. It is as simple as that."

Tommy Jacks, a lawyer in Austin, Texas, whose firm has represented 425 women with implants, said he doubts that the report will be the last word on the matter. "This report is simply a review of the literature by a committee that's reached some conclusion," he said. "It is premature to conclude that reports like this are the last word that scientists and physicians will have about the safety of breast implants," he said.

But medical experts informed of the committee's conclusions, applauded them. Dr. Shaun Ruddy, chairman of the rheumatology, allergy, and immunology division at Virginia Commonwealth University's Medical College of Virginia in Richmond, said the conclusions were "very forthright and outspoken" and he was glad the group was attempting to put the disease hypotheses to rest. Dr. Ruddy, a past president of the American College of Rheumatology, said he had had no part in any of the litigation.

The Institute of Medicine committee was set up at the behest of Congress. Its work began with a scientific workshop, a day of deliberations and then a public hearing on July 24, 1997, when almost 700 people filled an auditorium at the National Academy of Sciences in Washington. Representatives of medical professional associations made statements, scientists spoke about their research, and women with implants spoke of how their lives had been ruined. Some said they were so ill that they needed canes or wheelchairs to get around, conditions they blamed on the implants. Others testified that after they breastfed their babies, their children developed the same debilitating symptoms.

Examining more than 1,200 references, the group addressed the major questions about implants: Do they cause established connective tissue diseases, like arthritis or lupus? Do they cause breast cancer, nerve diseases, like multiple sclerosis, or new diseases with symptoms like aches and pains and overwhelming fatigue? Are children of women with breast implants at risk for disease because of silicone transmitted across the placenta or in breast milk? Do breast implants produce immunological reactions that could cause disease?

In every case, the committee concluded, there was no convincing evidence that implants were at fault. When lawsuits were filed in the late 1980s and early 1990s there was a lack of research on the topic. Since then, according to the report, "a number of strong, well-designed epidemiological studies involving large numbers of women and clear results have been published."

For example, the group wrote, the evidence is "insufficient or flawed" that implants cause "atypical disease," a term covering signs and symptoms like weakness, fatigue and diffuse muscle pain. But the group said that evidence on the other side is strong. "Controlled epidemiologic studies cited" led the committee to conclude that there was "no novel syndrome."

On the question of established connective tissue diseases, like lupus and rheumatoid arthritis, the group reviewed 17 epidemiological studies, concluding that they were "remarkable for the consistency of finding no elevated risk or odds for an association of implants with disease."

After hearing a description of the report, David Bernstein, a law professor and adviser for the American Tort Reform Foundation, a business-sponsored group, said that, coming as it does in the wake of similar reports, the report "might have a dramatic effect in hastening the end of the litigation."

"It is a very strong statement," Mr. Bernstein said. But he added that it was a shame that the legal system had gone ahead with the litigation in the absence of science, with companies paying billions to compensate women with implants. "It would have been nice to have had this $7 billion ago," he said.

[GK, June 1999]

## . . . But Panel Calls for Study of Some Implant Risks

Members of an expert committee of scientists that assessed the safety of silicone breast implants formally issued their report, calling for more research on risks of rupture and other local complications that can arise from the devices.

Although there is no scientific evidence pointing to silicone implants as the cause of major diseases, the scientists said, women who have breast implants, whether they are filled with silicone or salt water, have the right to know what the chances are that the devices will slip or deflate or lead to infections or scarring.

The committee was established by the Institute of Medicine, part of the National Academy of Sciences in response to a request by Congress in 1997. Its members had no connection to companies that manufacture implants or to lawyers representing women suing the companies and had taken no prior positions on the safety of silicone breast implants, said Dr. Kenneth Shine, the president of the Institute of Medicine.

After reviewing thousands of papers and documents submitted by scientists, implant makers and groups representing women who had implants, the group reached a unanimous consensus: The primary safety concern with implants is their tendency to cause local complications like infections, pain and scarring and the possibility that women might have to have second or even more subsequent operations as a consequence.

The committee chairman, Dr. Stuart Bondurant, a professor of medicine at the University of North Carolina in Chapel Hill, said the group heard women tell them in testimony and letters that they had not known that their implants could cause local problems. "One of the notable things they told us is that they were told the implants would last a lifetime," Dr. Bondurant said. While emphasizing that that is the women's recollection, he noted that there were never any data to support such an assertion.

Dr. Virginia Ernster, a professor of epidemiology at the University of California at San Francisco, said that the best she could do in assessing the published data on the complications of implants was to come up with a range of risks. Women who had implants to augment their breasts had about a 24 percent chance of needing to go back to the operating room in three to five years to repair problems or complications with implants, Dr. Ernster said. Those who had implants after a mastectomy had a 23 to 40 percent chance of needing a second operation in three to five years.

In recent years, most women who had implants have received devices filled with saline—salt water—rather than silicone, Dr. Bondurant said. Preliminary studies suggest that these devices have fewer complications, with just a 1 to 3 percent chance of deflation per year, he said, but more research is needed.

Sybil Goldrich, founder of Command Trust Network, an information clearinghouse for women with silicone problems, said in a telephone interview that rupture was "not a trivial problem." Women whose implants rupture, she said, can "end up with a lifetime of medical bills that can be staggering."

The committee urged that women who have implants be tracked so investigators can get reliable data on the incidence of medical complications like rupture, scarring and infection. Such information "is an essential part of the informed consent process," the group said.

But the committee was insistent about what it described as its "very firm conclusions" on the diseases that some women and doctors have said were caused by implants—a list that includes cancer, connective tissue diseases like arthritis and lupus, neurological problems, a new disease characterized by symptoms like fatigue, muscle aches and pains and diseases in the children of women with implants. These were the diseases at the heart of the multibillion-dollar product liability litigation over breast implants.

Dr. Bondurant said that the group concluded that "women with implants are no more likely than other women to develop these systemic illnesses." More than 60 women with implants testified before the committee in a public hearing and hundreds more wrote letters telling of the severe medical problems they had suffered since having their implants.

"We were very moved by the testimony we heard," Dr. Ernster said. "But it does not appear that the implants were the cause of the systemic illnesses." Asked if another group of equally qualified and objective scientists could look at the same data and come to a different conclusion, Dr. Bondurant said, "No, I can't imagine that."

[GK, June 1999]

## Via Microtechnology, an Alternative to Glasses and Contacts

I'm lying on my back, clutching a stuffed toy elephant and a wad of wet tissues. My jaw is clenched, my limbs are tense, my shoulder blades are hot-wired to my chair. I am not having a breakthrough in therapy, though I am about to change my life. I am one moment away from having elective surgery on my eyes—both of them—and am well into white-knuckle territory.

"Bonnie, are you ready?" says a gentle voice directly behind my head.

Dr. John Seedor, the director of cornea and refractive surgery at New York Eye and Ear Infirmary, prepares to work. He will be performing a popular, reportedly painless, bloodless procedure, called Lasik (laser in situ keratomileusis, which means carving the cornea with a laser) and known affectionately by doctors as "flap and zap." Dr. Seedor has assured me that Lasik will correct my 20/400 vision—a nearsightedness (myopia) so severe that my hand looks fuzzy when held at arm's length. I sure hope he's telling the truth.

My eyeballs have been numbed with anesthetic

drops. The eyelashes of my right eye have been taped to my face. A device that looks like a giant's eyelash curler is holding my eye open. I stare into a small, innocuous-looking machine hovering overhead and see a blinking vermilion light. Desperate to suck oxygen into lungs too scared to fill, I squeak, "I'm ready."

Available in the United States for about three years, Lasik corrects vision by altering the shape of the cornea. It is the latest mousetrap in a decades-long line of vision-correction procedures based on this theory. Lasik depends on two high-technology devices, both approved by the Food and Drug Administration, but not for use together. The first, a microkeratome, slices a one- to two-millimeter-thick flap in the top of the cornea. The surgeon lifts the flap off the eye as if opening a flip telephone.

Then, a broad-beam excimer laser burns away some cells from the cornea's midsection, the corneal stroma. In myopes, like me, the cornea has too much curvature, and the laser will flatten it. For the farsighted, the laser will steepen the cornea. For an astigmatic cornea, which is bumpy, the laser will treat the areas that are very steep, making the curvature less severe. The zapping usually takes less than a minute. The surgeon closes the flap, floods the eye with saline solution, presses out the air bubbles with a tiny surgical sponge, drips in some antibiotics and, voila! Vision.

Lasik doesn't hurt. There are no stitches, no bandages, and the flap heals on its own. Most people can drive and work the next day. Within 7 to 10 days, vision is stabilized. Ninety percent of the time, the patient is left with 20/40 vision or better. The procedure has never caused blindness.

Still, it holds no guarantees. Patients need to sign extensive release forms warning that vision can be worse after surgery. During my pre-surgery consultation, Dr. Seedor made me repeat after him that I would be happy if my vision corrected to 20/30, which would mean that I might need glasses for driving, maybe for the movies. But I've worn glasses since age 6 and contacts since I was 12; 20/30 sounded like perfection to me—especially since I had developed allergies to most contact lens solutions, and I had a case of the "dowdies" every time I wore glasses in public.

After developing allergies, I asked my ophthalmologist, Dr. Maria Arnett, for an opinion. Her advice: If you don't need it, don't do it. This is, after all, elective surgery on fairly healthy eyes. I figured my allergies let me fit into one of her squishy categories. Besides, my glasses were making permanent indentations on the sides of my nose.

Six months later, I'm ready. Usually, in surgery, patients put themselves in the hands of a capable doctor and hope for the best. With Lasik, dutiful patients need to stay focused on that red light. "What happens if my eye wanders?" I ask, imagining my eyeball blowing up like a set piece in an action film. Quite simply, the doctor will stop zapping until I can refocus.

I'm twisting the elephant's trunk. "You're going to go gray or completely dark for a second—just keep looking into the light," Dr. Seedor says. There's tremendous pressure on my eyeball. Even though my eye is open, for a split second, I'm blind. Gears whine centimeters from my ear. It's the flap-maker. The

grinding stops, the pressure abates. I can see the red light again, only it's a tiny red blur.

The flap is lifted; it feels like a contact lens being removed. My vision is now smudged. I keep as steady as Philippe Petit on the high wire as the laser blinks for about a minute. Dr. Seedor closes the flap. The saline flooding my eyes is cool and uncomfortable, but it's a tolerable discomfort. "Ready for the other eye?" he asks.

Honestly, I wasn't sure. My body was still shuddering from the blindness, the gears, the acute smell of smoke that I imagined was from my burned corneal cells, but was actually from the laser. In 20 minutes, total, it was over. I released my grip on the elephant, and sat up.

"Your vision will improve every hour," Dr. Seedor says. He is standing about six feet from me. I peer at him as if through a windshield smeared with Vaseline. He is smiling. I can see his nostrils! I put on sunglasses and greet my husband. I hand him the two vials of eye drops, antibiotics and steroids that I will need to apply to my eyes four times a day for the next five days, along with a pair of plastic eye shields to wear to bed to protect the flap.

At home, I pass out from nervous exhaustion. I wake and look. Through haze, I see the cockeyed veil in my wedding photograph across the room. As the anesthesia wears off, my eyes ache and tear. I feel irritation rather than pain.

The next morning, my husband asks me to calculate the improvement. I squint at the bare branches on the tree in the neighbor's yard. Sixty percent improvement? An hour later, I'm at my one-day checkup. A hazy 20/30 in each eye, the doctor says. That afternoon, I go to the movies.

Later, I try to write, but the computer screen is fuzzy, and so are my notes. Working remains difficult for the better part of my post-operative week. That 20/30 vision comes and goes. I'm healing more slowly than I had expected.

At my one-week checkup, I complain of blurry, changeable vision. No one is prancing about, calling out fantastic numbers. My corneas are still slightly swollen, and Dr. Seedor assures me that my eyesight is right where it is supposed to be. He asks if I'm under stress, which, he explains, can actually affect my vision. I feel as if a bubble has burst; everything becomes much clearer. Including my vision.

"Stress? Me?" We laugh. I get in my car. Fourteenth Street is crystal clear.

Who can undergo Lasik? Dr. Seedor, the director of cornea and refractive surgery at New York Eye and Ear Infirmary, said 98 percent of the people who wear glasses. Prospective patients with health conditions, like diabetes, that affect eye health, must be carefully evaluated before choosing the procedure, Dr. Seedor said. Federal regulations require that the patient be over age 18. Some elderly patients can benefit, but progressive glaucoma, extremely dry eyes and unhealthy corneas can prevent healing.

The surgery will not correct presbyopia, the need for reading glasses, prevalent in people who are over 40, because the condition is not linked to misshapen corneas. Indeed, high myopes over 40 who undergo Lasik, but had not needed reading glasses before surgery, frequently need them afterward. That is because severe nearsightedness compensates for the aging crystalline lens in many myopes in their early 40s, creating perfect near vision. Once myopia is corrected, the crystalline lens acts its age, with nothing to compensate for it. About 15 percent of patients need "touch up," or "enhancement" surgery, after their vision stabilizes in three months. This entails lifting the flap and zapping more of the cornea.

Who performs Lasik? Dr. Seedor recommends seeking an ophthalmologist who has performed at least several hundred Lasik procedures. "You need someone who has a tremendous amount of experience," said Dr. Arnett, an eye surgeon affiliated with Beth Israel Hospital in New York, among others.

To perform Lasik, a surgeon must be certified by the laser company (in compliance with Food and Drug Administration guidelines), and the microkeratome manufacturer. Prospective patients should ask to speak with other Lasik patients, and should check the doctor's medical degrees, internship, residency and fellowship programs.

Cost? About $2,750 per eye, $5,500 total. The initial consultation should be free, even if you decide against surgery. The fee generally includes the surgery, follow-up visits for a year and any "enhancement" surgery, should it be required. Insurance generally does not cover the procedure.

To find a doctor, ask your ophthalmologist for a recommendation or check with the nearest teaching hospital or medical school.

[BRM, June 1999]

## Promise and Risks of Laser Eye Surgery

Dr. Mark Shulman, first fitted for glasses at age 5, was never happy about his dependence on them. They would fog up in winter or get clouded with sweat in summer when he pursued the outdoor activities he loved. To see clearly when he did his daily swim, he needed prescription goggles. Contact lenses didn't work for him. So at age 61 he invested about $5,000 in laser surgery to correct his myopia and astigmatisms by reshaping his corneas and to enable him to do everything but read without glasses.

Dr. Shulman, a retired professor of meteorology living in Woodstock, New York, couldn't be more delighted. His distance vision is now better than 20/20. He sees well at night and can drive without glasses despite a slight loss of depth perception.

Reports in the medical literature say that as many as 98 percent of patients have results as good or nearly as good as Dr. Shulman's. Dr. David Wallace, of Santa Monica, California, said: "People's response to the procedure is an overjoyed, almost child-like rediscovery of their capacity to participate fully in life's activities without the restrictions of optical devices. It doesn't just change eyesight; it literally changes lives."

But growing numbers of patients are warning others to weigh the risks very carefully before proceeding. Many say they were not sufficiently warned about what could go wrong and that mishaps, when they occur, may not be correctable by wearing glasses or contacts.

Some complain of seeing halos around lights, or of starbursts, clouding, dry eyes or impairment of night vision, though these conditions may be temporary. A common complaint among those less than pleased with the results of surgery is the feeling that they were pressured to undergo the procedure by professionals and receptionists who did not take their concerns seriously and whose opinions were clouded by the profit motive.

To counter these shortcomings and stimulate research to correct visual problems that surgery can sometimes cause, a grass-roots group in New York called Surgical Eyes has been formed and a Web site established (www.surgicaleyes.org) where people with unsuccessful surgery can post their problems.

For example, Mitch Ferro, 31, of Virginia wrote that he was never told that having large pupils or a high degree of astigmatism put him at high risk for complications. He ended up with a significant overcorrection of his nearsightedness and vision that is distorted by halos and starbursts in dim light and at night, an irregular astigmatism and floaters in one eye and dryness in both. His work and quality of life have suffered, he said, and, "I would pay any amount of money to get my pre-surgical corneas back."

Laser vision correction is a major growth industry, with the number of patients nearly doubling annually. Close to a million people in this country had the surgery in 1999. It can now be used to correct nearsightedness (myopia), astigmatism and farsightedness (hyperopia).

Laser surgery is considered a significant improvement over the original technique that involved making eight surgical slits in the cornea to change its shape. The laser method starts by either abrading the outer layer of the cornea (a technique called PRK, for photorefractive keratectomy) or slitting the cornea at one edge and lifting up a flap (a technique called Lasik, for laser insitu keratomileusis), then using a computer-guided cool beam of an excimer laser to precisely sculpt the surface of the cornea according to the correction needed to produce 20/40 visual acuity or better. After the surgery the outer layer of the cornea grows back in about a week (in PRK) or the flap reattaches itself in a few minutes (in Lasik).

The entire operation, usually done on one eye at a time (the second eye is usually done a week or two later as a precaution against infection), is performed on an outpatient basis with local anesthetic. It takes about 15 minutes. There are no sutures or patches, but PRK patients must wear a bandage lens until the corneal surface reforms. Lasik, the latest twist on corneal reshaping, is said to be painless, with only mild stinging and scratchiness for a few hours after the anesthetic wears off. However, patients are cautioned to protect the operated eye and to use antibiotic and anti-inflammatory drops for about a week. Full vision improvement and stabilization takes several weeks to months. In some cases, a second operation is needed to improve the correction.

Laser surgery is clearly not for everyone. The greater the degree of correction needed (in other words, the more severe the myopia or hyperopia), the more likely there will be complications. People with large pupils and extreme astigmatisms, like Mr. Ferro, are also more likely to have postsurgical problems. Also, ophthalmological surgeons will not operate on eyes that are not healthy to start with or on people with certain health problems, including autoimmune diseases, unstable diabetes, uncontrolled vascular disease, chronic herpes infections, connective tissue disorders or a tendency to scar excessively. Patients should be at least 21 years old, have stable vision and a strong desire to be free of glasses or contact lenses.

There is also the money factor. Because nearly all insurers consider the surgery a cosmetic procedure, most patients must pay for it entirely on their own—to the tune of about $2,200 an eye. Numerous follow-up exams are required at specific intervals, most of them performed by the referring eye specialist. Sometimes they are included in the cost of surgery, but otherwise they can add significantly to the cost.

Patients must realize that the surgery, even when it results in 20/20 distance vision, does not mean they will be free of corrective lenses forever. Laser surgery cannot correct presbyopia, the loss of clear close-up vision that occurs in everyone after age 40. Presbyopia results from an inflexibility of the lens of the eye, not a misshapen cornea. In fact, most people who are myopic and undergo laser surgery will eventually have to use reading glasses that they might have avoided had they stayed myopic.

Careful preoperative homework and consultation is important for everyone considering laser eye surgery to correct visual acuity. Dr. Shulman said he attended a seminar where he was well briefed on what was involved and the risks, including statistics on how often complications occurred. No pressure was put on patients to go ahead with the procedure if they were fearful or did not feel they were good candidates, he said. He also had confidence in the surgeon, who had done nearly 1,000 eyes before operating on his. If you are considering the surgery, be sure you will not be a guinea pig for a surgeon who has done only a few procedures before yours.

Also, if the surgeon you consult doubts your eligibility for the procedure, don't push to have it done anyway or go shopping for another doctor. The effects of laser surgery are permanent, and if things go wrong, you could end up with uncorrectable vision problems far worse than those you started with.

[JEB, September 1999]

## As Ethnic Pride Rises, Rhinoplasty Takes a Nose Dive

There was a time not so long ago when the Manhattan Eye, Ear and Throat Hospital on East 64th Street was as chic a destination for Christmas vacation as St. Barts or Telluride. That is where many teenaged girls would disappear during school holidays to get the ethnic bumps on their noses smoothed out. So crowded were the operating rooms at this time of year, recalled Dr. Gerald H. Pitman, a plastic surgeon, that he would set out 20 sets of rhinoplasty instruments in the morning and run out before the day was done.

But the crowd is thinning. In the midst of an explosion in cosmetic surgery, the number of nose jobs has dropped significantly. While the total number of cosmetic procedures increased 76 percent, to 697,000 from 395,000, between 1992 and 1996, the numbers of rhinoplasties, as they are known, fell 8 percent, to 46,000 from 50,000. And the decline was probably steeper between the 1990s and the 1970s, experts say, although no statistics are available before this decade.

The reasons are partly cultural and partly economic, according to plastic surgeons who have watched the evolution of a procedure that was once a benchmark in a young girl's life, especially among Jewish teenagers. "It was the thing to do," said Dr. H. George Brennan, who practices in Southern California. "You had your bat mitzvah and you got your nose done."

The heyday for nose jobs, experts agree, was in the 60s and early 70s, when the post-war baby boomers were teenagers. Parents of Jewish ancestry who knew first-hand of the Nazi atrocities were ever on the alert for stirrings of anti-semitism.

They wanted their own children spared discrimination. And to them, that meant fitting inconspicuously into the Protestant mainstream. "Jewish parents at that time didn't want their children to look Jewish," said Dr. James L. Baker Jr., who practices outside Orlando, Florida. "They feared a stigma left from the war."

The physical characteristic that most set Jews apart was their noses, and so legions of teenagers, usually girls, had them fixed. The technology was primitive compared to today's and so the results, through the 1970s, had a cookie-cutter similarity—little ski-jump noses with the bony bridge scooped away. But that was okay with the patients. "Everybody wanted to look like a shiksa," said Dr. Thomas D. Rees, a retired plastic surgeon who trained many of the high-priced doctors at work today along Park Avenue.

The leading practitioner back then was Dr. Howard Diamond of Manhattan, renowned for standardizing what had been a hit-or-miss operation. "Every girl on Long Island had a Diamond nose," said Dr. George J. Beraka, who said he can still pick them out on women now deep into middle-age.

But fashion was changing. Ethnic looks were coming into style. In the mid-70s, black models appeared for the first time on the covers of *Glamour* and *Vogue*. Blondes were not the only ones having fun. Lana Turner and Betty Grable were replaced by Barbra Streisand (who was afraid to have a nose job for fear it would change her voice) and Cher (who eventually had her nose fixed, along with many other body parts.)

Now, doctors say, their patients want to maintain their ethnic individuality, perhaps with slight refinement. Where once the button nose was the rage, women these days beg for a "natural" look. "They're not trying to erase their ethnic background anymore," said Dr. Darrick E. Antell, a Park Avenue surgeon.

Dr. Christopher Nanni of Brooklyn agreed: "There's a much broader definition of beauty. Not everyone needs to look like Barbie." Dr. Nanni noted that the preoccupation has shifted to flat stomachs and wrinkle-free faces. "It's youth they're looking for, not certain facial features."

Another factor in the decline of nose jobs, doctors say, is the new health care economics. In the old days, insurance plans covered the procedure if a patient complained of breathing difficulties. Now, insurers do not docilely accept that a cosmetic operation costing between $3,000 and $8,000 is necessary for a deviated septum. "They fight and fight," Dr. Pitman said, and many middle-class families are "reluctant to spend the college money."

The statistics available on rhinoplasty do not distinguish between primary and secondary surgeries, the return trips to the operating room to fix what was done before. Dr. Antell said he sees older women who have tired of their cute little ski-slope noses and "want to turn the clock back" and look like real people. He complies, transplanting cartilage from the septum to give them back the bump they once hated.

[JG, January 1999]

## In the Golden Age of Teeth, a Smile Can Be Perfected

Dentists call them Hollywood Chiclets—oversize, pearly white teeth that gleam so beautifully on the silver screen. Fifteen years ago, those celluloid teeth were most likely caps made of porcelain and gold, concealing filed-down tooth stumps, installed at a cost of thousands of dollars and many painful hours.

They still make for an expensive mouthful, but everything else about pearly whites has become easier. And not a moment too soon—at least for dentists, whose workload might otherwise be declining. For, by most accounts, America is in the golden age of teeth. Fifty years ago, 1 out of 3 Americans had no

teeth. Now that is 1 in 10 and falling. The rate of tooth decay has dropped by 50 percent, because of fluoridated water and better dental technology.

Visits to the dentist, once uniformly feared, are much less terrifying and painful. But how will dentists flourish if teeth are so much healthier? The answer: a supersmile in every mouth. By some estimates, 9 out of 10 dentists do at least basic cosmetic work, and a growing number of specialists are casting themselves as the tooth equivalents of plastic surgeons. No firm figures exist, but Dr. Jeff Morley, a San Francisco dentist and a co-founder of the American Academy of Cosmetic Dentistry, said that from his talks with practitioners around the country, he would estimate that the number has nearly doubled every year for the last few years.

The change began with a technological breakthrough in the mid-1980s, the porcelain veneer. Before, the only way to manufacture square, white teeth was to file away the tooth and cover the stump with a cap of porcelain and metal. The time, pain and expense were usually endured only by movie stars and the rich and vain.

Porcelain veneers are much simpler, if not a lot cheaper, especially considering that, in general, neither they nor caps are covered by insurance. The tooth is roughened with a laser so that the veneer can bond to it; then porcelain is molded and attached to the tooth. Metal is rarely used. Each tooth runs about $2,000, but the procedure, depending on how many teeth are done, lasts only a few hours. Dr. Larry Rosenthal, of the Rosenthal Group for Aesthetic Dentistry in Manhattan, described the procedure as "like bonding a baby's fingernail to each tooth." The perfect smile can cost from $750, for bleaching, to $20,000 for the works, including porcelain veneers and straightening.

Joan Spain, 55, a retired bookkeeper in Philadelphia, conceded that her reasons for redoing her smile "were purely frivolous."

"I had porcelain veneers put on 10 top teeth and 6 on the bottom," Ms. Spain said. "It took two visits, six hours. I had no pain and walked out happy."

Dr. Rosenthal, her dentist, is convinced that better teeth lead to a better smile. Veneers on the front top teeth can push the lips out, making them appear fuller, much as a collagen injection does, he said. Ms. Spain said that although her lips are naturally full, one side of her upper lip was thinning faster than the other because of age, and the veneers compensated. Ms. Spain has a checkup once a year, and this year is bringing a friend. "She has thin lips, and I'm betting she'll get work done," Ms. Spain said.

Dr. Wynn Okuda of Honolulu, a prominent cosmetic dentist, sees himself as an artist who works through the medium of teeth. "I used to be a general practitioner dentist, a long time ago," Dr. Okuda said. "What really triggered me to change my practice is

that I have a real love of art, and cosmetic dentistry connects art and dentistry." Before she saw Dr. Okuda, Carol Duarte, 55, a retired store manager living in Kauai, Hawaii, thought she was ready for false teeth. "I was living on aspirin, I couldn't chew my food, and I thought there was no hope for me," she said.

Her sister persuaded her to see Dr. Okuda, and every few weeks for two years Ms. Duarte commuted by plane to the big island of Hawaii, where she spent eight hours in the dental chair, having extensive work done, including tooth implants, bridgework and a root canal, as well as veneers.

"Now all my front teeth have porcelain veneers," she said. Ms. Duarte added that more than her mouth changed as a result: She made improvements in her diet and exercise habits as well, at Dr. Okuda's suggestion. "I felt that he had spent two years on my teeth," she said, "and I had to commit to maintenance, so I quit eating so much sugar and now I walk eight miles a day."

Cosmetic dentistry is not a regulated specialty. To perform cosmetic work, dentists need only order materials and read a few journals. But two professional groups, the American Academy of Cosmetic Dentists in Madison, Wisconsin, and the American Academy of Esthetic Dentistry in Naperville, Illinois, require certification and training to join; both provide referrals.

Specialists in the field, of course, are quick to describe problems caused by under-qualified practitioners—most commonly, unrealistically white teeth. A more serious drawback is that improperly applied veneers that are not adjusted to the patient's natural bite can chip and crack after a few years.

And it is important, Dr. Morley said, that the dentist, however specialized, "not overlook basic health principles" or less visible factors, like engineering the bite.

But the biggest hazard, cosmetic dentists assert, is that the patient does not get what he or she considers the most artistic result. Dr. Morley contends that a good cosmetic dentist can make a smile look more feminine or masculine. "For a more aggressive smile," he said, "the canines are the key." They have the most personality of all the teeth, he said. Making them longer and more pointed gives a smile an animalistic leer, perfect, perhaps, for a hungry executive on the rise.

The lateral incisors, which are on each side of the two front teeth, are the key to femininity. Making them slightly smaller and rounder softens a smile. Making the two front teeth more square gives a masculine cast. Eliminating cracks, chips and dinginess in front makes a mouth look younger.

To convince patients that the "after" will be a dramatic change from the "before," a growing number of dentists use computer simulations. Dr. Rosenthal, who has redone the smiles of Kathie Lee Gifford and the model Bridget Hall, likes to show a patient a split-screen display. While he describes the possibility, a technician sitting beside the patient manipulates the computer version of the patient's teeth to make the contrast clear, he said.

Of course, some people come in with a picture in mind. Dr. Hans Malmstrom, the director of general dentistry for the Eastman Dental Center at the University of Rochester, credits cultural influences, like the universally perfect teeth of movie stars and models. "You have people coming in now and asking about things like bleaching and veneers in a way you didn't see five years ago," Dr. Malmstrom said.

But not all patients want to be told that their smiles, though healthy, could be perfect for a price. One woman, who asked not to be named, was shocked when her dentist brought up cosmetic procedures. "I have very good teeth, very even, and he started talking about how the teeth had uneven transparencies, and he could put a veneer on them," she said. "I was offended and insulted, and I switched dentists."

That reaction is all too common, said Suzanne Boswell of Dallas, a consultant for doctors and dentists. Ms. Boswell visits their offices incognito, and reports back to them on how she was treated. "Dentists live in a tiny, tiny world," she said. "They work in a little room, on little mouths, on little teeth."

And people who go to a cosmetic surgeon know why they're going there; most visits to a dentist are for more mundane reasons. "Many people, especially baby boomers, have accepted how they look," Ms. Boswell said. "They don't want to sit in a dentist's chair and hear, 'we can take care of that space,' if they didn't bring it up. And most of the time an insulted patient won't confront their dentist, but will simply find another."

[WM, June 1999]

# The Joy of a New Neck

A friend of mine gave a party for her neck. Through the years it had grown worn and thick with the burdens of rubbernecking, bottlenecking and holding her head high. Recently it had developed a crepey wattle, which my friend took as a conspicuous sign that she would either be served up for Thanksgiving dinner or that the A.A.R.P. would soon be leaving its calling card. In the latter case, arthritis, Social Security and early-bird specials would surely follow.

And so, to hold back the spotted hands of time she bought herself a new neck. For three weeks she interviewed surgeons. Dr. Slash wanted to tighten her eyelids too. Dr. Paste suggested adding a chin. (She thumbed her nose at that.) Dr. Pull told her she looks like Ava Gardner (sure!) and offered to wipe away the jowls, smooth out the folds and vacuum her jaw line with a new technique that would lop 10 years off her age. She replied, "How soon?"

Now, four weeks later, her neck was ready to make its debut. I chose a turtleneck for the occasion. Two other women swathed themselves in Isadora-length scarves. Together we neckless wonders rang her bell. "Is your mother home?" one of them joked as our rejuvenated friend came to the door. "My God, you've lost so much weight," exclaimed another, her voice pure puce.

The truth was that a swan would have killed for that neck. It had been lifted, lipo'd, pulled and made girlishly taut: In fact, it seemed, so had her whole face. Between bites of gravlax, my friend shuttled us into the kitchen one by one to show us the inch-long incision under her chin (for the lipo) and the longer ones around her ears (for redraping the jowls). Proudly revealing her stitches, she let us feel the bumps of still-swollen tissue and basked in our dutiful ooohs and aaaahs.

Call it a neck job, but a demi-face lift is more like it. The two-and-a-half-hour procedure performed in the doctor's office cost $6,900 and required an overnight stay. It was less painful than root canal and worth every penny, glowed my friend as her husband beamed, "I feel like I'm with a younger woman."

Well, of course, he does, remarked one guest as we left. Did you see his eyes? When she went in for the tuck, he had his lids done. Today, if she turns her neck quickly and he squints, they find themselves in the throes of puppy love.

[MR, May 1998]

## Doctors' Review of 5 Deaths Raises Concern About the Safety of Liposuction

A team of doctors in New York is questioning the safety of liposuction, the immensely popular cosmetic surgery in which body fat is suctioned out through a tube to get rid of "thunder thighs," "love handles," pot bellies and other hated bulges. The warning, appearing in the May 13, 1999 issue of *The New England Journal of Medicine*, is based on the doctors' review of five deaths that occurred after liposuction from 1993 to 1998. Four of the deaths were in New York City, and the fifth was referred to the office of the city's chief medical examiner.

Although the number of deaths was small, and all surgery carries some risk, the researchers said the cases were cause for serious concern because liposuction is not medically necessary and is performed on healthy people. Nationwide, the number of complications and deaths from liposuction is not known, the authors of the paper said, because doctors do not have to report bad results to any central registry.

The researchers recommended that the procedure be studied further to assess its safety and that death records in other regions be examined. "Should there be any deaths from a cosmetic procedure?" asked Dr.

Rama B. Rao of New York University Medical Center and Bellevue Hospital, an author of the paper with a colleague, Dr. Robert S. Hoffman, and Dr. Susan F. Ely, a forensic pathologist in the office of the chief medical examiner in New York City.

Liposuction has become the most common cosmetic surgery in the United States, with more than 400,000 operations done in 1998. The patients who died, four women and one man, ranged in age from 33 to 54, and each was treated by a different doctor. Three died because their heart rate and blood pressure suddenly plummeted in surgery for unknown reasons. The fourth had a fatal blood clot in the lung, and the fifth died because doctors infused so much fluid into her body as part of the procedure that it seeped into her lungs and caused pulmonary edema, in effect drowning her.

Doctors who perform liposuction had mixed reactions to the new report, saying on one hand that it was unfair and sensationalistic to focus on a handful of deaths when most liposuctions were done safely. But they also said that like any surgery, liposuction could be dangerous if done incorrectly. They found it worrisome that the procedure had been taken up by many doctors, some with minimal training in the technique, who were eager to cash in on people's desperate desire to look sleek in shorts or a swimsuit.

"If you do the procedure correctly, it's very safe," said Dr. Alan Kling, a dermatologist who performs liposuction in his office in New York. "The problem is that so many people are trying to get in and make a fast buck, and they're not taking adequate precautions or getting adequate training."

Dr. Paul Schnur, associate professor and chairman of the department of plastic surgery at the Mayo Clinic in Scottsdale, Arizona, said, "If you just finished your internship yesterday and you want to do liposuction, you can, according to state law." Many doctors perform liposuction in their offices, and in most states they can do so without being tested or certified by any professional group, Dr. Schnur said, adding that doctors who wish to operate in hospitals require approval from the hospital's professional board.

Dr. Schnur, who is also president of the American Society of Plastic and Reconstructive Surgeons, said a handful of other widely publicized deaths from liposuction had led the group to create a panel that is studying the procedure and will recommend ways to make it safer. Dr. Ely, the forensic pathologist, said that in 1997 she investigated two deaths related to liposuction and became concerned about the procedure. A search of 48,527 autopsy reports in New York City for 1993 to 1998 turned up three more cases.

All five patients had had the most common form of liposuction, tumescent, in which doctors pump several quarts of fluid into the area of the body that is to be suctioned. The fluid is a salt solution containing a local anesthetic, lidocaine, to numb the patient, as well as a stimulant, adrenaline, to help prevent bleeding. The fat is sucked out through a tube attached to a vacuum pump. Some doctors use a general anesthetic as well as the local. Noting that high doses of lidocaine are used, compared with the amounts given for other procedures, the researchers suggested that the three unexplained deaths from low blood pressure and heart rate might have been a result of an overdose of lidocaine, or its interaction with other drugs.

Lidocaine is known to lower the heart rate and in fact is used as an emergency treatment for dangerously rapid heartbeats. Dr. Schnur says the plastic surgeons' society is concerned about the possibility of lidocaine overdose and has advised members to stay within a conservative limit. He said that in addition to potential problems from too much fluid and lidocaine, patients could be endangered if the surgeon tried to remove too much fat at one time. "The more fat you take out, the more trauma to the body," he said. "This is like an internal burn." The journal report did not say how much fat the doctors had been trying to remove from the five patients who died, but Dr. Schnur said lipsuction that removed 12 pounds of fat or more should be done in the hospital so that the patient could be carefully monitored.

Dr. Kling, the New York dermatologist, said that he never removed more than five or six pounds in one session and that he did not use general anesthesia. He said the cases described in the medical journal broke "every single rule of safety." The death from pulmonary edema was that of a 210-pound woman who had been given more than 13 quarts of fluid, 7 intravenously and 6 infused into surgical sites, in a procedure lasting four and a half hours. That was considerably more fluid than the other patients received. She also underwent more extensive surgery in one session, including breast enlargement and liposuction of her chest, arms, back, abdomen, thighs, buttocks and knees. She also had general anesthesia and at the time of surgery was being treated with seven psychiatric drugs.

[DG, May 1999]

# Herbs, Supplements and Alternative Medicine

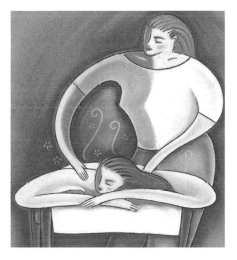

## CAUTION IS NEEDED
## AS OFFERINGS MULTIPLY

Americans are spending ever-increasing amounts of money on alternative, or complementary medicine, including herbs, vitamins and other dietary supplements, homeopathic remedies, chiropractors, massage therapy, aroma therapy and acupuncture. Supplements alone earned $8 billion in 1997, up from just $2 billion in 1994. Women spend $600 million a year on "natural" remedies for menopause.

What is driving the boom is not entirely clear. Some of it, surely, is the success of certain treatments. Acupuncture, for instance, has been found effective in treating some types of pain, and chiropractors and massage can help with back pain. Prayer and spirituality seem to improve the health of many people who have faith.

But some of the attraction of alternative medicine lies in so-called natural products, which many people assume to be pure and harmless and less likely to cause side effects than the chemicals synthesized by drug companies. Asian herbs have a special appeal for many people, who assume that any remedy that has been around for hundreds or thousands of years must have something going for it. Some people like to take charge and treat themselves, free from the control of doctors and managed care. And some find that practitioners of alternative medicine spend more time with them, listen better, and show more respect and compassion than members of the medical establishment.

Is there any harm in it? Maybe. People with serious ailments that could be cured or controlled by mainstream medicine may lose out if they spend too much time dabbling with supplements and unproved treatments. In 1999, doctors in Canada reported that several families rejected chemotherapy and radiation for children with cancer, in favor of supplements and herbal remedies.

In addition, supplements can be powerful, by themselves or in combination with other drugs. But in the U.S., supplements are loosely regulated and not subject to the rigorous tests of safety and efficacy that the Food and Drug Administration requires for drugs. Surveys have found that herbal products do not always contain the ingredients listed on the label, or the amounts stated. Impurities or dangerous ingredients are sometimes present: A study of Asian medicines sold in California in 1999 discovered many products that contained arsenic, mercury or lead. One, which contained a drug that had been banned in the U.S., caused a severe blood disorder in a young woman. A product imported from Germany was contaminated with digitalis, a heart medicine that can be fatal in overdose. It made patients sick. Another product, sold as a muscle builder, was actually an ingredient in paint thinner that put people into a stupor.

"Standardized" products, which provide a consistent amount of a given herb or supplement, are safer and more reliable than others, say advocates of herbal therapy. But it may not be clear what the proper dose of a product is. Manuals can help, and so can specialists in alternative medicine. But still, the buyer must beware.

# Alternative Medicine Makes Inroads, but Watch Out for Curves

Alternative medicine is clearly the largest growth industry in health care today. In 1997, 42 percent of American adults used some type of alternative care—herbal therapy, chiropractic, acupuncture, massage therapy or any of a number of other methods not taught in medical school, according to a nationwide telephone survey conducted for Landmark Healthcare Inc., a managed alternative care company in Sacramento, California.

Of the 1,500 adults interviewed in November 1997, 44 percent said they would use an alternative method if traditional medical care was not producing the desired results, and 71 percent predicted that consumer demand for alternative, or complementary, care would be moderate to strong in the future.

While most doctors shun such care and question its merits and reliability, Americans are voting with their feet and pocketbooks. Studies have shown that patients make more visits each year to alternative care practitioners than to primary care physicians, and most of them pay out of their own pockets for the care they receive.

Now, however, in response to the growing demand and in hopes of reducing health care costs, more and more health plans are including options for alternative methods, and a number of hospitals across the country have complementary care clinics.

At a meeting on complementary medicine sponsored by the Northern California Cancer Center and held at Stanford University, Dr. David Spiegel, a professor of psychiatry and behavioral science at Stanford, said patients who availed themselves of alternative care were seeking "caring attention, something they are getting less and less of from physicians under managed care."

Alternative care practitioners, including acupuncturists, chiropractors, herbalists and massage therapists, spend more time with patients—30 minutes on average, or 4 times more than physicians now devote to each patient, Dr. Spiegel said. "Patients want to be treated as a whole person, not just a disease," he said. "They want to be active participants in treatment, they want better communication with the practitioner and they want treatments that are not worse than their disease."

According to a 1993 study by the Kaiser-Permanente health care system, 56 percent of those who seek alternative care suffer chronic pain and 22 percent cite stress or a mental health problem as their chief complaint. Among the most common problems are back pain, anxiety, allergies, arthritis, depression and insomnia. Evidence is mounting that alternative techniques like acupuncture, hypnosis and some herbal remedies can help relieve such conditions.

Decades ago, physicians made an arbitrary separation between mind and body, and modern medicine is only now beginning to reintegrate them and more fully appreciate how they affect one another. Alternative care practitioners never forgot that people can get sick and can heal as much through their heads as through their bodies. Perhaps the most powerful testament to the healing power of the mind is the placebo, a look-alike but inactive remedy that, on average, benefits about one-third of those who receive it when active treatments are tested in clinical trials. Dr. Spiegel asked, "Even if an alternative remedy is just a placebo, if patients get better and there are no side effects, what's the harm in trying it?" (In some cases, of course, people will recover from an illness whether they take a drug, a placebo or nothing.)

Disastrous consequences, however, can come from an uneducated and careless foray into alternative medicine. Here are some important issues to keep in mind:

▶ Be sure you have received a correct diagnosis from a conventional doctor before seeking alternative care. Medical literature is filled with stories of patients receiving months of useless alternative remedies as an undiagnosed cancer grew unimpeded.

▶ Tell your medical doctor about any alternative methods, including dietary supplements, you are using or thinking of using. Discuss the risks and benefits and possible interactions with other treatments you are receiving.

▶ No matter what you may be told by a friend, neighbor or alternative care practitioner, never

stop an existing treatment without first consulting the doctor who prescribed it.

▶ Don't be fooled by the word "natural." Natural is not synonymous with safe. Arsenic, pennyroyal, botulinum toxin and urushiol (the rash-inducing substance in poison ivy) are perfectly natural—and highly poisonous.

▶ Beware of phony practitioners. Everyone who hangs out a shingle is not necessarily schooled or licensed. Anyone, including you and me, can take on the title "nutritionist" or "herbologist," and anyone can impress the uninitiated with phony credentials and certificates.

▶ Don't assume that products labeled "dietary supplement"—herbs, vitamins and minerals and other potions—are safe and contain what they say they do. Some are hormones, others are stimulants or sedatives that can have serious adverse effects.

These products are virtually unregulated. No one outside the company that produces them monitors them for quality control: the types and amounts of active ingredients, presence of contaminants or honest labeling. Independent studies have shown that some of these products contain little or none of the ingredient they are supposed to have, especially if that ingredient is a costly one.

Furthermore, because companies are not allowed to make health claims for their products, they are also not required to warn consumers of possible side effects or interactions. There are no guidelines for who should and should not use the product. To make matters worse, the Food and Drug Administration, which cannot require premarket clearance based on tests of safety and effectiveness for any dietary supplement, can act against a product only after a disaster.

[JEB, April 1998]

## Public Perceptions of Alternative Care

Many Americans are turning to alternative health care, from massage therapy to acupuncture to hypnosis. But many others remain cautious and skeptical of various techniques. Shown are findings of a nationwide random survey of 1,500 people, conducted by a marketing-research firm for Landmark Healthcare Inc. The margin of error is 2.5 percent. Findings were released in 1998.

### WHERE AMERICANS TURN

Shown are the therapies that respondents have used in 1997:

- Herbal therapy: 17%
- Chiropractic: 16%
- Massage Therapy: 14%
- Vitamin Therapy: 13%
- Homeopathy: 5%
- Yoga—5%
- Acupressure: 5%
- Acupuncture: 2%
- Biofeedback: 2%
- Hypnotherapy: 1%
- Naturopathy: 1%

### WHO USES IT

Households that have used alternative care in 1997:

- 42% said yes
- 58% said no

Source: "The Landmark Report on Public Perceptions of Alternative Care," 1998; survey conducted by InterActive Solutions of Grand Rapids, Michigan

# Taking Stock of Mysteries of Medicine

Many doctors continue to label alternative medicine "quackery" because proof of its effectiveness is lacking and the way the techniques work is often a mystery. Doctors are understandably turned off by seemingly irrational methods like reflexology (which treats the entire body through the foot) and by the mystical explanations offered for various techniques ("increases energy flow" is a common one) that cannot be observed or measured.

Still, millions of people attest to the benefits of the more than 200 alternative therapies that are said to be in use in this country. What critics often ignore is that many mainstream techniques, including most forms of surgery, also were never subjected to the acid test of science: the double-blind controlled clinical trial. Also forgotten is that many mainstream remedies, including aspirin and penicillin, became widely used long before experts knew how they worked.

So before dismissing the various therapies, it may pay to look more closely at some that are considered safe and effective and are even being prescribed by doctors as complements to conventional medicine. As Michael Castleman, author of *Nature's Cures* puts it, these techniques "don't replace what's taught in medical schools, but rather complete it." He notes, "They fill in what's been missing—an appreciation for the body's innate self-healing abilities."

Responsible practitioners of alternative medicine do not claim, for example, that they can cure cancer or multiple sclerosis. Rather, they believe their methods can marshal forces in the body that may help to combat illness in concert with conventional medicine. The biggest dangers of alternative medicine involve missing the diagnosis of an illness that requires medical treatment and the temptation to abandon conventional medicine. So before wandering into the likes of bioenergetics or herbal medicine, be sure to see a doctor to determine what may be causing your symptoms.

Stress and its sidekick muscular tension are common causes of pain and so-called functional complaints (that is, ailments for which no physical cause can be found). Or muscular tension may result from pain and increase its intensity. This is why relaxation-inducers like massage, yoga, meditation, deep breathing, therapeutic touch, tai chi and posture and movement techniques have won so many converts.

These methods, used either alone or with conventional medicine, are harmless and often helpful, for example, in relieving backaches and headaches, lowering blood pressure, speeding recovery from various ailments and enhancing quality of life.

Hypnosis produces a deep state of relaxation and heightened concentration in which people become highly suggestible. Hypnosis does not put people in a "trance" during which they can be made to do something they would not otherwise want to do. But as participants visualize a desired goal—for example, numbing pain or stopping a habit like smoking or thumb-sucking—remarkable effects can sometimes be achieved. According to a 1984 report in *The Lancet*, a medical journal published in Britain, hypnosis decreased abdominal pain and bowel symptoms and increased well-being in patients with irritable bowel syndrome to a degree greater than any drug has ever achieved.

Visualization, or guided imagery, a form of self-hypnosis, is also popular among athletes who use it to enhance their performance. The techniques are harmless and can be very helpful.

Acupuncture and acupressure rely on twirling needles (acupuncture) or point pressure (acupressure) applied to various parts of the body to relieve symptoms in other parts. They work in part by triggering the release of endorphins, the body's natural pain relievers. They are increasingly used or recommended by doctors to treat various health problems, especially pain resulting from both physical and functional ailments and addiction to drugs and tobacco. Many people have found acupressure applied to a point on the wrist to be very helpful in preventing motion sickness. Acupuncture also works in animals.

Like relaxation techniques, these alternative approaches are harmless as long as the practitioner knows what ailment is involved and the patient does not abandon the therapies of conventional medicine. For example, one acupuncture practitioner discovered that the man he was treating for fatigue really had leukemia and referred him to a cancer specialist.

It is challenging for a scientifically-trained doctor to imagine how homeopathy could possibly have a therapeutic effect beyond being a placebo. It starts with substances that cause symptoms like the ones being treated, then dilutes them hundreds or thousands of times until the solution contains only a memory of the original ingredient. Yet homeopathy is booming and enthusiasts swear by the effectiveness of its remedies. At least there is no dispute about its safety, since its potions contain too little of any active ingredient to cause harm.

Herbal remedies, on the other hand, can sometimes be dangerous. Keep in mind that a large percentage of conventional medications—from aspirin to toxic cancer drugs—derive their active ingredients from plants. All drugs, whether from a pharmacy or health food store, can have adverse effects, and sometimes very serious ones. They may be toxic or add to or counter the effects of traditional medicines. Large doses of garlic, for example, could interact dangerously with anticoagulants.

The form in which the herb is used can make the difference between benefit and harm. Mr. Castleman cites pennyroyal, used in flea collars as an insect repellent and in infusions to settle the stomach and relieve coughs and congestion. Yet, he warns: "As little as two tablespoons of pennyroyal oil can be fatal. Never ingest any kind of herbal oil."

Another problem with herbal remedies involves the purity of various products, which are not subject to premarket government regulation and may be adulterated by unscrupulous producers, especially if the active ingredient is very expensive or difficult to obtain. Furthermore, there are no regulations governing recommended dosages or warnings about interactions with other remedies or foods. Ephedra, a plant-derived stimulant used as a decongestant in conventional and herbal remedies, can produce dangerous increases in heart rate and blood pressure and has proved fatal when taken in excess.

Still, studies have pointed to real benefits with minimal risk from some herbal remedies used in moderate amounts, including St. John's wort to treat mild depression, echinacea to combat the common cold and saw palmetto to reduce prostate enlargement.

After a century of opposition, some conventional medical organizations have begun to embrace chiropractic, the manipulation of the spine. The technique can speed recovery from acute back pain, although long-term results are no better than are achieved through more traditional orthopedic methods. There is no proof of the chiropractic claim that since most nerves in the body run through the spinal cord, spinal "adjustments" can relieve all manner of ills.

[JEB, May 1998]

## Articles Question Safety of Dietary Supplements

People trying to treat their own ailments with remedies from health-food stores have become severely ill from pills and powders sold as "dietary supplements," according to six reports published in September 1998 in *The New England Journal of Medicine.*

Lead poisoning, impotence, lethargy, nausea, vomiting, diarrhea and abnormal heart rhythms were among the disorders described, resulting from powerful herbs, toxic contaminants or the presence of potent drugs or hormones in products that were supposed to be "all natural" and free of drugs. In addition, several children with cancer worsened when their parents rejected conventional therapy in favor of alternative methods.

The six reports—three articles and three letters to the editor—involved only about a dozen patients, but Dr. Marcia Angell, executive editor of the journal, said, "I think this is the tip of the iceberg." The six reports reached the journal over several months, Dr. Angell said, and were not solicited by the editors.

In a sharply worded editorial accompanying the reports, she and Dr. Jerome P. Kassirer, the editor in chief of the journal, criticized supplement makers and practitioners of alternative medicine for advocating unproven and potentially harmful treatments. "Alternative treatments should be subjected to scientific testing no less rigorous than that required for conventional treatments," they wrote.

Taken together, the editorial and multiple cases from the medical establishment amount to throwing down the gauntlet before the booming supplement industry. The cases demonstrate that consumers can be harmed by seemingly innocuous herbs and nutritional supplements, authors of the reports say, and lend weight to the argument that the loosely regulated industry should be held more accountable.

Unlike drugs, dietary supplements do not have to be proved safe and effective before they are put on the market. Dr. Angell said that if supplements were held to the same standard as drugs "the onus would be on the manufacturers to prove safety and efficacy, and I think most of them would shut down." She was especially critical of the Dietary Supplement Health and Education Act of 1994, which weakened the authority of the Food and Drug Administration to regulate vitamins, herbal remedies and other products classified as dietary supplements. The supplement industry boomed after the law was passed, to nearly $12 billion a year in 1997 from $8 billion in 1994.

Dr. Annette Dickinson, a spokeswoman for the Council on Responsible Nutrition, a trade association in Washington representing supplement makers, called the editorial an "unjustified broadside." Dr. Dickinson said that the law was adequate to safeguard the public, and that the industry had no more errors or mishaps than food or pharmaceutical producers.

Dr. William B. Schultz, Deputy Commissioner for Policy at the F.D.A., said that before 1994, if the agency had concerns about a supplement it could order the substance off the market until the manufacturer proved it safe. "The biggest impact," Dr. Schultz said, "was that a lot of products probably never got to market." In 1994, he said, "Congress changed the rules." The law stipulated that to take a product off the market, the F.D.A. would have to prove it unsafe. In practice, that means hazardous products may go undetected until someone is harmed by them, as in the cases reported in the journal.

In an especially impassioned letter, Dr. Max J. Coppes and his colleagues, pediatric cancer specialists at Alberta Children's Hospital in Calgary, described two cases in which parents of children with cancer decided to forego chemotherapy and radiation in favor of alternative treatments.

One patient was a 15-year-old boy with Hodgkin's disease, a cancer of the lymphatic system that can be cured in more than 80 percent of patients if standard treatment is begun promptly. But the family rejected conventional therapy and instead used an herbal product. Within a few months, the boy had become sicker, and the family wanted to switch to conventional therapy. By then, the disease had progressed, requiring higher doses of chemotherapy that would pose more risk from side effects than the treatment that had been planned originally.

"Until now, neither I nor my three colleagues had encountered families choosing alternative treatments as the only therapy for children with cancer," Dr. Coppes said, adding that during the past year they have had four such cases.

Doctors also sounded a warning about herbal products from Asia. One of the journal letters reported that 83 of 260 samples tested by the California Department of Health Services contained poisonous heavy metals like lead, arsenic or mercury, or drugs not listed on the label.

The products have harmed people, said Dr. Richard Ko, a food and drug scientist with the health services department. In a telephone interview, Dr. Ko told of one patient who had taken an herbal preparation she got from an acupuncturist and developed a condition in which she essentially had no white blood cells.

The woman's doctor thought she had leukemia. But the acupuncturist alerted the health department about the herbal preparation, zhong gan ling. It turned out to contain a drug, dipyrone, not listed on the label, that has been kept off the market in the United States because it is known to wipe out white blood cells. The woman recovered, though she suffered a severe infection as a result of the lowered white cell count.

---

A CLOSER LOOK

## Unexpected Ingredients

Supposedly natural supplements meant to cure all sorts of ills are flying off the shelves into consumers' hands. The concern is that some of these may contain surprising ingredients with decidedly adverse effects.

### ASIAN HERBAL REMEDIES

**Intended purpose:** One third of the American population has tried these for a variety of maladies.

**Possible problems:** May contain lead, other heavy metals or drugs not listed on the label.

### PC-SPES

**Intended purpose:** Taken as an alternative to estrogen to boost the immune systems of men with prostate cancer.

**Possible problems:** Actually promotes estrogenic activity causing swollen breasts and loss of libido.

### RENEWTRIENT

**Intended purpose:** Designed to stimulate muscle growth.

**Possible problems:** Causes intense drowsiness and unarousable sleep.

### PLANTAIN (herb, not fruit)

**Intended purpose:** Used to assist in cleansing of the body.

**Possible problems:** Contaminated batch caused nausea, vomiting and irregular heartbeat.

*Source: The New England Journal of Medicine*

---

In another case reported in the journal, two women were hospitalized last year in the United States because of severe nausea and vomiting, and irregular heartbeats. Both had taken herbal mixtures that were marketed as a "program" to clean out the intestinal tract. Tests showed that one ingredient in the mixture, plantain (an herb, not the fruit of the same name), had been contaminated with digitalis, a powerful heart drug that can be deadly in overdose. In tracing the source of the contaminated plantain, F.D.A. investigators led by Dr. Lori A. Love found it had been imported from Germany and shipped to more than 150 manufacturers, distributors and retailers. It was recalled, and later tests of other plantain supplies were negative for digitalis.

Dr. Dickinson, the spokeswoman for the supplement industry, said that the digitalis case actually showed that the law worked, because the F.D.A. and the industry worked together and quickly traced the contaminant and got products recalled.

Another letter to the journal describes an incident in which Scottsdale, Arizona, police officers stopped a driver who appeared drunk. He was lethargic, vomiting and sweating profusely, and was taken to an emergency room. But he had not been drinking. Rather, a half hour before being arrested he had taken two ounces of a liquid supplement called RenewTrient, marketed as a stimulator of growth hormone and an aid to body building.

Dr. Frank LoVecchio, an emergency-room doctor and toxicologist, and co-author of the letter about the case, said the supplement contained a chemical, gamma-butyrolactone, that is also used in paint remover. "There's no way it promotes muscle growth," Dr. LoVecchio said. The chemical depresses the central nervous system by acting on the same parts of the brain as alcohol and the drug Valium, he said.

The label on RenewTrient warns that one ounce will induce deep sleep for three to six hours, from which a person may be "unarousable." It also says that excessive doses will cause sweating, muscle spasms, vomiting, bed-wetting and diarrhea, and that the best treatment is to "sleep it off." A spokesman for RenewTrient's manufacturer responded to Dr. LoVecchio's report by saying that the patient had ignored the label and taken an overdose but recovered on his own within a few hours, and that the product is safe.

In another article, a team of doctors reported on a mixture of herbs called PC-SPES that many men are taking for prostate cancer. Dr. Robert DiPaola, an oncologist at the Cancer Institute of New Jersey in New Brunswick, said that some patients took the herbs on the assumption that they were a nonhormonal alternative to the female hormone estrogen, which has been used to slow the growth of prostate cancer.

But the researchers found that PC-SPES had "incredible estrogenic activity," Dr. DiPaola said. Like estrogen, the supplement did slow the progression of prostate tumors. But, also like estrogen, it caused marked adverse effects: sore, swollen breasts, loss of libido and, in one case, a blood clot in the foot. Dr. DiPaola said standard treatments like the drug Lupron were as powerful and less toxic than PC-SPES. Even so, he said, some patients chose to continue taking PC-SPES even after they learned the outcome of the study.

"This is an example of how patients can be taking herbal combinations and be unaware, and even the companies selling them can be unaware, of how they work and how potent and toxic they can potentially be," he said. "There is no such thing as a safe agent just because the word 'natural' is attached to it."

[DG, September 1998]

## Americans Gamble on Herbs as Medicine

Herbal medicine, the mainstay of therapeutics for centuries before modern purified drugs relegated it to the status of near-quackery, has in the last five years emerged from the fringes of health care with an astonishing flourish and now shows clear signs of joining the medical mainstream.

Despite many cautionary tales about adulterated and even dangerous products, herbs formulated as capsules, tinctures, extracts and teas—and increasingly as additions to common foods like potato chips and fruit drinks—are now routinely used by a third of American adults seeking to enhance their health or alleviate their illnesses. Each day the herbal realm wins new converts, particularly among those who have become disillusioned with the cost and consequences of traditional drugs, distrustful of conventional physicians and convinced that "natural" equals "good."

Yet, because herbal products are classified as dietary supplements, not drugs, and face none of the premarket hurdles drugs must clear, consumers have no assurance of safety or effectiveness. Indeed, scores of products sold in the United States are listed by European and American authorities as ineffective, unsafe or both, and manufacturing standards to assure high quality have been proposed but are not yet in force.

Thus, countless consumers are wasting their money on useless products or jeopardizing their health on hazardous ones. Among the serious side effects that have been linked to herbal remedies are high blood pressure, life-threatening allergic reactions, heart rhythm abnormalities, mania, kidney failure and liver damage. A few widely available products, including sassafras and comfrey, contain known carcinogens.

At the same time, according to a 1998 report in the journal *Psychosomatics*, unsuspecting consumers "have used herbal remedies with good results only to discover that the benefit was actually derived from the presence of undisclosed medicines," including steroids, anti-inflammatory agents, sedatives and hormones.

"The lack of quality standards is the Number One problem in the whole industry," said Dr. Varro E.

Tyler, emeritus professor of pharmacognosy (the study of active ingredients in plants) at Purdue University and a consultant and lecturer paid by a number of herbal companies.

Dr. Tyler, who has no equity connection to herbal products and is perhaps the nation's leading independent expert on herbal medicine, said: "I feel sorry for the typical consumer. How is he or she to know what is best, what products are reliable and safe? Even when a label says the product has been standardized, the consumer has no way to know if it actually meets that standard." Even if an herbal product has been reliably made in some standard dose, it does not mean that scientific studies have shown it to be effective.

The industry itself is promoting a "good manufacturing practices" doctrine. Annette Dickinson, director of scientific and regulatory affairs for the Council for Responsible Nutrition, a trade organization for producers of dietary supplements, said a consortium of associations submitted a document of manufacturing standards to the Food and Drug Administration in 1997. Although such a standard would say nothing about an herb's safety or effectiveness, it would result in reliable methods that the industry would have to use to insure the identity and quality of its products. The agency has issued a notice of proposed rules but no final ruling as yet.

Nonetheless, botanicals, as herbal products are more accurately known, are enjoying an annual retail market approaching $4 billion, up from $839 million in 1991 and growing about 18 percent a year. Hundreds of products made with virtually no Government oversight are crowding shelves of health-food stores, food markets and pharmacies nationwide. Supplements are also widely sold by marketers like Amway, through catalogues and on the Internet.

Now, even major pharmaceutical companies like Warner Lambert, American Home Products, Bayer and SmithKline Beecham are introducing herbal products, adding respectability to this marginalized market.

Some herbs—like echinacea, goldenseal, American ginseng and wild yam—have become so popular that their continued supply from natural sources is in danger. As the plants become scarcer and more expensive, products containing them are increasingly likely to be adulterated and may even contain none of the herb listed on the label. Peggy Brevoort, president of East Earth Herb Inc., a company in Eugene, Oregon, that produces botanicals, said that the demand for St. John's wort, used for mild depression, and kava, a calmative said to reduce anxiety, now exceeds their supply, introducing the "danger of adulteration" by "unscrupulous dealers."

At the same time, two major new publications—a 1,244-page *Physicians' Desk Reference for Herbal Medicines*, produced by the same company that publishes the *Physicians' Desk Reference*, and an English-language edition of Germany's therapeutic guide to herbal medicines, *The Complete German Commission E Monographs*—have been issued to help educate physicians, pharmacists and interested consumers about the known uses, proper dosages and safety concerns of more than 600 botanicals now sold in this country. The evaluations in both books are based on studies, most done in Germany and reviewed by teams of experts.

The National Institutes of Health lists on the Internet international bibliographic information on dietary supplements, including herbal products. In addition, a few medical and pharmacology schools have recently introduced courses in phytomedicine, the study of botanicals. Still, most doctors remain wary of botanicals, especially when patients choose self-medication with plant extracts over established medical remedies.

The very act of Congress that has fostered this growth—the 1994 Dietary Supplement Health and Education Act—has also permitted chaos to reign in the botanical marketplace, with no mechanism to assure that products are safe or effective. Pushed heavily by Senator Orrin G. Hatch of Utah, the home base of many supplement makers, and passed over the objections of the F.D.A., the law created a new product class, the dietary supplement, that was not subject to regulations applied to drugs. Now any substance that can be found in foods, regardless of amount or action and including substances that act as hormones or toxins, can be produced and sold without any premarket testing or agency approval.

Marketed as neither a food nor a drug, herbal products are not obliged to meet any established standards of effectiveness or safety for medicinal products, which require extensive laboratory and clinical trials before approval. As with other substances classified as dietary supplements, the F.D.A. can restrict the sale of an herbal product only if it receives well-documented reports of health problems associated with it. The agency took four years, and more than 100 reports of life-threatening symptoms and 38 deaths, to act against ephedra, often sold as the Chinese herb ma huang, a stimulant that can prove disastrous to people with heart problems.

With F.D.A. authority limited by the 1994 law, the Federal Trade Commission, which monitors advertising, has taken a more active role in monitoring supplement makers. In 1998, the F.T.C. took legal action against seven manufacturers that had broken rules requiring advertising be truthful and verifiable. The companies were selling remedies or purported cure-alls for ailments like impotence, cancer and obesity.

The commission also sent e-mail warnings to 1,200 Internet sites that it said had made "incredible claims" for drugs, devices and supplements, including herbal remedies that would supposedly ward off AIDS. Also in late 1998, the commission issued its first set of advertising guidelines aimed specifically at the supplement industry.

Still, the current regulations have created a quagmire of consumer confusion and set up potential health crises that even industry officials say could ultimately hurt producers as well as users of herbal products. Under the 1994 law, consumers have no assurance that an herbal product contains what the label says it does or that it is free from harmful contaminants. Independent analyses of some products, particularly those containing costly or scarce herbs, revealed that some have little or none of the purported active ingredient listed on the label.

Adding to the confusion is that botanical makers are allowed to describe products only in terms of their effects on the structure or function of the body, not their potential health benefits. Thus, a product label might say "promotes cardiac function" but it cannot say "lowers cholesterol." Likewise, although the law does allow health warnings on the label, most manufacturers have yet to include them.

Consumers are warned, however, that Federal drug safety officials are not watching the store. All botanicals must display a disclaimer on the label following the description of the product's structural or functional role: "This statement has not been evaluated by the Food and Drug Administration. This product is not intended to diagnose, treat, cure or prevent any disease." To which Dr. Tyler commented, "If that is true, why on earth would anyone use it?"

The seeds of the modern herbal market were sown in the 60s when "green, organic and natural became buzzwords," Dr. Tyler said. But they did not mature until the 90s with the growing consumer interest in "self-care and controlling one's destiny," he said. Many turned to herbs as a gentler way to treat health problems and a potential tool for preserving mental and physical health. The interest has spawned scores of Internet sites and hundreds of books on various herbs. But much of the literature is replete with poorly documented health claims and, with few exceptions (among them, Dr. Tyler's books), advocacy prevails over objectivity.

Because plants contain a mixture of relatively dilute chemicals, they naturally tend to have milder actions, both in their therapeutic benefits and side effects, than the concentrated, single chemicals in most drugs. Thus, botanicals generally take longer to act than regular pharmaceuticals and few have the potency of a prescription, the one possible exception being saw palmetto, which a well-designed study indicated may be as helpful for an enlarged prostate as the more expensive and riskier drug, Proscar.

The combination of chemicals in botanicals is potentially both a plus and a minus. When two or more chemicals enhance one another's activity, the therapeutic benefit could theoretically exceed that from an isolated substance formulated as a drug. Mark Blumenthal, who heads the American Botanical Council, noted that the herb St. John's wort, widely used in Germany and increasingly in the United States to counter mild depression, is standardized for

# Common Cures

With herbal remedies flying off the shelves, here is a look at what people are using them for. *Source: Preventive Magazine*

## Herbs Thought to Be Effective...

| HERB | Why It Is Used | How It Works | Cautions |
|---|---|---|---|
| **Black Cohosh** | Reduces symptoms of premenstrual syndrome, painful menstruation and the hot flashes and mood disorders associated with menopause. | It appears to function as an estrogen substitute and a suppressor of luteinizing hormone. | Occasional stomach pain or intestinal discomfort. Since no long-term studies have been done, use of black cohosh should be limited to six months. |
| **Capsicum** | Best known as the hot red peppers cayenne and chili. Applied topically for chronic pain from conditions like shingles and trigeminal neuralgia. It may also be helpful for cluster headache, muscle spasms and arthritis. | The active ingredient, capsaicin, works as a counterirritant and decreases sensitivity to pain by depleting substance P, a neurotransmitter that facilitates the transmission of pain impulses to the spinal cord. | Overuse can result in a prolonged insensitivity to pain. More concentrated products can cause a burning sensation. Users must avoid contact with eyes, genitals and other mucous membranes. |
| **Echinacea** | These species of purple coneflower appear to shorten the intensity and duration of colds and flus, help to control urinary tract infections and, when applied topically, speed the healing of wounds. | Though echinacea lacks direct antibiotic activity, it helps the body muster up its own defenses against invading microorganisms. | Experts warn against using echinacea for more than eight weeks at a time, and against its use by people with autoimmune diseases like multiple sclerosis and rheumatoid arthritis or by those who are infected with H.I.V. |
| **Feverfew** | The dried leaves of this plant have been shown to reduce the frequency and severity of migraine as well as its frequently associated symptoms of nausea and vomiting. | The active ingredient, parthenolide, appears to act on the blood vessels of the brain making them less reactive to certain compounds. It may also act as a serotonin antagonist. | Most commercial preparations recommend doses that are much too high. 250 micrograms a day of parthenolide—or 125 milligrams of the herb—is an adequate dose. |
| **Garlic** | Active against viruses, fungi and parasites. It also lowers cholesterol and inhibits the formation of blood clots, actions that can help to prevent heart attacks. | When fresh garlic is crushed, enzymes convert alliin to allicin, a potent antibiotic. Garlic tablets and capsules containing alliin and the enzyme can be absorbed when dissolved in the intestines and not the stomach. | More than five cloves of garlic a day can result in heartburn, flatulence and other gastrointestinal problems. People taking anticoagulants should be cautious about taking garlic. |
| **Ginger** | A time-honored remedy for settling an upset stomach, ginger has been shown in clinical studies to prevent motion sickness and nausea following surgery. | Components in the aromatic oil and resin of ginger have been found to strengthen the heart and to promote secretion of saliva and gastric juices. | May prolong postoperative bleeding, aggravate gallstones and cause heartburn. There is also debate about its safety when used to treat morning sickness. |
| **Ginkgo** | Used medicinally in China for hundreds of years, Ginkgo biloba was recently reported to improve short-term memory and concentration in people with early Alzheimer's disease. | It appears to work by increasing the brain's tolerance for low levels of oxygen and by enhancing blood flow to the brain and extremities. | Possible side effects include indigestion, headache and allergic skin reactions. |
| **Kava** | This South Pacific herb, also known as kava-kava, has a growing coterie of enthusiasts who use it to reduce anxiety, stress and restlessness and to facilitate sleep without developing problems of tolerance, dependence and withdrawal. | The active ingredients in the root and stem act as muscle relaxants and anticonvulsants. | Should not be used with alcohol or other depressants, by people who are clinically depressed or by women who are pregnant or nursing. Kava should also not be taken for longer than three months without medical supervision. |

| Herb | | | |
|---|---|---|---|
| **Milk Thistle** | One of the few herbs that has been demonstrated to protect the liver against toxins. Also encourages regeneration of new liver cells. | The seeds contain a compound called silymarin, which helps liver cells keep out poisons and promotes formation of new liver cells. | When used as capsules containing 200 milligrams of concentrated extract (140 milligrams of silymarin), no harmful effects have been reported. |
| **Psyllium** | A laxative that doesn't undermine the natural action of the gut. It may reduce the risk of colorectal cancer and produce a significant reduction in blood levels of cholesterol. | The seeds of this herb have coatings and husks that are filled with mucilage, a soluble fiber that swells with water in the intestines to add bulk and lubrication to the stool. | Increase in flatulence in some people, especially if a lot is consumed. |
| **Saw Palmetto** | German studies on patients with an enlarged prostate have shown that extracts of the fruits of this palm tree can reduce urinary symptoms even though the gland may not shrink. | Nonhormonal chemicals in saw palmetto appear to work through their antiandrogen and anti-inflammatory activity. | Large doses can cause diarrhea. Some experts are concerned that those taking the herb may have inaccurate P.S.A. readings, used as an early warning sign of prostate cancer. |
| **St John's Wort** | Numerous reports attest to this herb's ability to relieve mild depression. It may also have sedating and anti-anxiety activity. | Though products are commonly standardized for hypericin, the chemicals responsible for the herb's anti-depressant activity have not yet been certainly identified. | Based on the sun-induced toxicity of hypericin in animals, fair-skinned and photosensitive people who take St. John's Wort are advised to avoid exposure to bright sunlight. |
| **Valerian** | Perhaps best characterized as a mild tranquilizer. | The dried underground parts of this plant have anti-anxiety and mild hypnotic effects making it useful in treating nervousness and insomnia. | Long-term use can sometimes cause headache, restlessness, sleeplessness and heart function disorders. |

## ...And Herbs to Avoid

| HERB | Why It Is Used | Cautions |
|---|---|---|
| **Aconite, e.g. Bushi** | Pain, rheumatism, headaches. | Numerous poisonings in China. |
| **Belladonna** | Spasms, gastrointestinal pain. | Contains three toxic alkaloids, including atropine. |
| **Blue Cohosh** | Menstrual ailments, worms. | Can induce labor. |
| **Borage** | Coughs, diuretic, mood booster. | May contain liver toxins and carcinogens. |
| **Broom** | Intoxicant, diuretic, heart problems. | May slow heart rhythm; contains toxic alkaloids. |
| **Chaparral** | Arthritis, cancer, pain, colds. | Can cause severe hepatitis, liver failure. |
| **Comfrey** | Cuts, bruises, ulcers. | Contains toxins linked to liver disease and death. |
| **Ephedra** | Stimulant, decongestant. | Contains cardiac toxins resulting in dozens of deaths. |
| **Germander** | Digestion, fever. | Contains stimulant that can cause heart problems. |
| **Kombucha Tea** | Insomnia, acne. | Can cause liver damage, intestinal problems and death. |
| **Lobelia** | Mood-booster. | Large doses can cause rapid heartbeat, coma and death. |
| **Pennyroyal** | Stimulant, gastric distress. | Liver damage, convulsions, abortions, coma and deaths have been reported. |
| **Poke root** | Emetic, rheumatism. | Extremely toxic; low blood pressure, respiratory depression and death. |
| **Sassafras** | Stimulant, sweat producer, syphilis. | Contains the carcinogen safrole. Banned from use in food. |
| **Scullcap** | Tranquilizer. | Can cause liver damage. |
| **Wormwood** | Tonic, digestion. | Can cause convulsions, loss of consciousness and hallucinations. |

*Sources: The Physicians' Desk Reference for Herbal Medicines; Tyler's Honest Herbal by Dr. Varro E. Tyler with Steven Foster; Tyler's Herbs of Choice by Dr. Tyler with James Robbers; Journal of the American Dietetic Association, October 1997;The Mayo Clinic Health Letter, June 1997.*

a substance called hypericin. But, he explained, "hypericin is not directly linked to its antidepressant activity." Rather, other substances in the herb seem to have diverse actions on brain chemicals, all of which work together to counter depression.

But, equally possible when using an herb with two or more active chemicals is that one will cancel the benefits of another or introduce a hazard. Without careful chemical tests and large, well-controlled clinical trials such actions are often hard to detect.

Consumer confidence in herbal medicine is bolstered by the common but erroneous assumption that "natural" equals "safe" and the public's failure to realize that many plants contain chemicals that are potent drugs or outright poisons. Natural laxatives like the herb Cascara sagrada are just as habit-forming and harmful to the colon as laxatives sold as drugs.

Indeed, one quarter of prescription drugs and hundreds of over-the-counter products were originally isolated from plants. Ephedra, for example, contains a natural stimulant that is approved for use as a decongestant and bronchial dilator in some pharmaceutical products. However, when used in uncontrolled dosages or by people with certain underlying health problems, it can cause a dangerous rise in blood pressure and, in its herbal form, has been responsible for serious adverse reactions and dozens of deaths, mainly among people who inappropriately used it as a stimulant or diet aid.

Complicating the safety issue is the fact, shown in several recent surveys, that most patients fail to tell their physicians they use herbal supplements and thus sometimes risk dangerous drug interactions or endure costly tests or treatments when an herb causes an unrecognized side effect. Experts say many patients withhold information about herbal drug use because they fear being ridiculed by their doctors. Although all German physicians must take courses on herbal remedies, only a handful of American medical and pharmacology schools offer courses in this field.

In 1998, the President's Commission on Dietary Supplement Labels recommended that the F.D.A. appoint a committee to evaluate the safety and effectiveness of herbal products. "This could be the most important step in the United States toward legitimizing herbal medicine," Dr. Tyler said. However, the agency responded that it lacked the budget to support such an effort. American physicians have completed and published only a few well-designed studies of some popular botanicals. Among them were studies showing that saw palmetto can shrink an enlarged prostate and ginkgo biloba can improve memory in patients with early Alzheimer's disease.

The Office of Dietary Supplements at the National Institutes of Health is helping to finance a three-year multicenter study of St. John's wort as a treatment for clinical depression and a study of plant-based estrogens as a preventive for postmenopausal health problems.

However, thousands of studies of botanicals have been completed abroad—mainly in Germany—that strongly suggest a health-promoting role for more than 200 plant products. Germany's Commission E evaluated 380 botanicals, approving 254 as safe and reasonably effective and disapproving 126 as ineffective, unsafe or both.

The Germans use a different criterion to assess an herb's benefits—a doctrine of "reasonable certainty" that the herb has the desired effect and is safe, Mr. Blumenthal said. Whereas standard testing of a drug for approval by the United States F.D.A. can cost as much as $500 million per product—a prohibitive amount for companies to spend on botanicals that cannot be patented—tests to establish "reasonable certainty" would cost only $1 million to $2 million, Dr. Tyler estimated.

In June 1996, Dr. Robert Temple, director of medical policy for the F.D.A.'s Center for Drug Evaluation, suggested that, rather than subjecting botanicals to the extensive tests required for drugs, the agency might consider applying less stringent criteria to assess an herb's effects, at least when a product is to be used only for a short time. He said, "A long history of safe use might provide sufficient safety information for products that are intended for short-term use."

More than four dozen botanicals or botanical formulations have been submitted to the agency as investigational new drugs. If any meet the agency's criteria for safety and effectiveness and are eventually approved as drugs, they would be allowed to make direct health claims—instead of just structure and function statements—on labels and in advertising.

Meanwhile, Dr. Joerg Gruenwald, medical director of a German phytomedicine company and primary editor of the new *Physicians' Desk Reference for Herbal Medicines*, said professionals can rely on that volume for current, documented information about botanicals. The volume, to be issued annually, updates the Commission E reports and adds several hundred other products sold in the United States, listing effects, side effects and conditions in which their use is inadvisable.

[JEB, February 1999]

## Seeking Help for the Body in the Well-Being of the Soul

Early Sunday mornings in a chapel at Riverside Church in New York, a service begins with meditation enhanced by aromatherapy and music. The communion includes laying on of hands, an ancient rite for the sick. Finally, congregants gather in the church's new Wellness Center, where they discuss topics like nutrition and cancer.

Most of the congregants are women. Whether for social or biological reasons or both, said the Rev. Diane Lacey Winley, the center's coordinator and a board member of New York City's Health and Hospitals Corporation, "women find it easier to use prayer and meditation to find energy, strength and healing."

But women aren't alone in exploring the connection between spirituality and health, nor are clergy members the only professionals who talk of healing and religion in one breath. Just as more and more churches and synagogues offer liturgies to promote well-being, some 60 American medical schools now offer courses on health, religion and "spirituality." Both the religious and medical establishments are aware of polls showing that most Americans think that faith and prayer benefit health and that doctors should discuss the connection.

This hybridization of science and spirituality combines two of the baby boomers' greatest enthusiasms. As their huge generation ages, their increasing health concerns, from menopause to breast cancer, seem almost as likely to elicit a spiritual quest as a search for the best specialist. There is no denying that religion can "heal," in that it can greatly comfort the sick. But despite the testimony provided by polls and best-selling books, tapes, courses and other healing industry products, spirituality's effect on health remains a more hotly debated issue in science than in the rest of society.

The simplest and best-documented evidence of religion's salubrious effects concerns longevity. California's Alameda County Study and the National Health Interview Survey, which was financed by the Centers for Disease Control and Prevention, have tracked the health of thousands of randomly selected people, the first for decades and the second for eight years. These well-respected studies show that, even when allowing for individual differences, like medical problems or smoking, subjects who attend services weekly—the most common gauge of religiousness—live longer than those who do not. In the national health survey, frequent "attenders" died, on average, at age 83; those who never went to services died at age 75. In the Alameda study, the relative risk of mortality for male attenders was 10 percent lower than for other men; for female attenders, however, the risk was 34 percent lower than for other women.

By many measures—frequency of prayer, attendance at services, value placed on spirituality— women are more religious than men. Whether their greater fervor confers extra health benefits remains in question. The National Health Interview Survey, for example, did not reveal a significant gender gap. But in the Alameda study, according to William Strawbridge, an epidemiologist and the Alameda project's director, religion was found to be nearly as good for women's health as not smoking.

That religious men and women tend to live longer does not require supernatural explanations. Not surprisingly, people who frequent churches and synagogues are likelier to avoid risky behavior like drug abuse and promiscuity. But, Dr. Strawbridge said, compared with people who do not go to services, even less straitlaced attenders are likelier to "clean up their acts" by quitting smoking, say, or by drinking less alcohol. Explaining the connection between longevity and religion, Dr. Strawbridge pointed to "the difference between hanging out with the church choir or the Grateful Dead."

Drawing a parallel to marriage's well-established contribution to well-being, Robert Hummer, a sociologist at the University of Texas at Austin, who has analyzed the National Health Interview Survey, said religious involvement could influence not only health habits, but also relationships and the ability to cope with stress. "The general idea isn't that religion works instant cures or insures that anyone who walks into a church will live to be 85," he said, "but that it's linked with many factors that benefit health over a lifetime."

One Wednesday evening, about 80 people, some clearly frail, gathered for a healing service at Ansche Chesed, a synagogue on Manhattan's Upper West Side. Like the prayers and reflections, some simple songs gently acknowledged that, as Debbie Friedman, a composer and singer of Jewish spiritual music, said, "We all have to live with pain as well as joy." By the service's end, urban professionals had shed their reserve to sway together and sing.

Religion's potential health benefits are not limited to those who attend churches or synagogues. Herbert Benson, the director of the Mind-Body Medical Institute at Beth Israel Deaconess Medical Center in Boston, which is affiliated with the Harvard Medical School, said spirituality promoted health in two straightforward ways. Research has shown that belief in the effectiveness of a placebo, or sugar pill, can relieve illness. Therefore, Dr. Benson reasons, "so can

faith in the healing power of God—or nature, relationships or whatever resource the individual chooses."

And some spiritual practices, he said, have measurable metabolic effects. Whether produced by Zen breathing, Jewish davening (prayer) or reciting the Roman Catholic rosary, the quiet state that Dr. Benson calls the "relaxation response" can lower heart and respiration rates and slow brain waves. When performed daily, he said, this response acts as an antidote to the "fight or flight" response implicated in the stress-related ailments that motivate most visits to doctors and are resistant to drugs and surgery. The patient who combines standard medical treatment with this self-care, he said, "has all the bases covered."

Studies conducted by Duke University's Center for the Study of Religion, Spirituality and Health in Durham, North Carolina, indicate that deeply religious people are less likely to suffer from diastolic hypertension (high blood pressure when the heart muscle is relaxed) and depression, and tend to have lower levels of a protein called interleuken 6, which implies a strong immune system. "Religion offers powerful ways to cope with major life stresses, particularly health problems and experiences of loss," said Dr. Harold Koenig, a psychiatrist who is the center's director.

The idea that religion benefits health has its critics. In 1999, the prestigious British medical journal *The Lancet* published a report co-written by Dr. Richard Sloan, the director of the Behavioral Medicine Program at Columbia-Presbyterian Medical Center in New York. After reviewing hundreds of studies, he concluded, "There's no compelling evidence that religion affects physical health." It's not that religion could not do so, said Dr. Sloan, a psychologist. But with the exception of a few studies, like the Alameda survey, he said, "the vast majority" are flawed. Among his objections are poor matches between religious and control groups, as when nuns are compared with members of the general population.

Including spirituality in medical practice also raises ethical concerns. First, Dr. Sloan said, there is the problem of "blaming the victim," or the patient who fares poorly. Then, too, "prescribing religion isn't the same as prescribing a low-fat diet," he said, adding: "There's lots of evidence that marriage is good for health, but doctors don't tell their single patients to wed. That area of life is too personal and private."

Even researchers who are convinced that religion promotes health often express reservations about studies that try to ascertain whether sick people who are unaware that others are praying for them do better than those who are not being prayed for at all. As a scientist, Dr. Koenig said, "I steer clear of that area." As a Christian, he finds the idea of a God who favors those who have others praying for them hard to reconcile with the image of a "Good Shepherd who will look for that one lost sheep."

Sometimes religion aggravates health problems. Dr. Alice Domar, a psychologist and the director of the Center for Women's Health at the Mind-Body Medical Institute in Boston, has found that very devout patients, particularly Catholics, Jews and women raised with a punitive image of God, find it harder to cope with infertility. "They're likelier to regard it as their own fault—even as punishment," she said.

In a process called "cognitive restructuring," staff members help patients substitute destructive thoughts about infertility with constructive attitudes. When a woman who had suffered recurrent miscarriages said God was punishing her, Dr. Domar replied, "So, God kills babies?" The shocked patient said, "Oh, no, God would never do that!" Only after logic replaced her fear could the woman see infertility as a physiological problem.

A few good surveys now indicate that religion fosters health. But as illustrated by the efforts to establish the effects of smoking or aspirin, Dr. Strawbridge said, "Numerous studies must replicate an effect before medicine regards it as proved." Meanwhile, many compassionate religious and medical professionals continue to draw from both spirituality and science in their efforts to heal.

The Rev. Barbara H. Nielsen, an Episcopalian minister and fellow at the Mind-Body Medical Institute, has found that some patients who believe their prayers go unanswered appreciate learning what she calls "a new way to pray": One asks for what one wants, accepts what will be and, finally, meditates. Then, Ms. Nielsen said, "one can listen for the real answer to prayers." She recalled how a Catholic infertility patient who used this method began to see that the identity of Mary wasn't limited to maternity, but, like her own, included work, marriage and good character. "This woman got the message, that she's a fine person, from Mary," Ms. Nielsen said, "once she listened."

[WG, June 1999]

## Puzzle in a Bottle: In Vitamin Mania, Millions Take a Gamble on Health

Whatever health-conscious consumers might be looking for, there is a vitamin or mineral pill that promises it. Products for sale purport to offer cancer protection, a hardier heart, extra energy, enhanced immunity, less stress, a longer life, an antidote to pollution, stronger bones, less body fat, relief from premenstrual syndrome, athletic prowess and heightened sexual powers. "Vitamania," as some critics call it, is sweeping the country, with sales of vitamins and minerals soaring to record highs.

An estimated 100 million Americans spent $6.5 billion in 1996 on vitamin and mineral pills and potions, up from $3 billion in 1990, according to the Council for Responsible Nutrition in Washington, a trade group for the vitamin supplement industry. Consumers are, in effect, volunteering for a vast largely unregulated experiment with substances that may be helpful, harmful or simply ineffective.

The labels on the bewildering array of vitamin bottles in a drugstore or health-food store give few clues that the products can be harmful as well as helpful. And they do not mention that because the Food and Drug Administration considers vitamins and minerals "dietary supplements," no testing for safety or usefulness—or even for whether the supplements contain what they say they do—is required before they are marketed.

Clear and consistent information about vitamins and minerals is hard to get, even from experts in nutrition, because of a lack of good long-term studies, or from the Government, which has a bewildering array of standards and is in the process of revising them. "No rational person can understand this stuff," said Dr. Marion Nestle, chairman of the department of nutrition and food studies at New York University. "All the different numbers are almost guaranteed to make the situation more confusing rather than less."

The answers about how much of any vitamin a person needs often depend on the person's age, sex and stage of life. Nor is there a consensus about whether taking vitamins and minerals in addition to food is valuable for a person who is eating a relatively healthy diet.

Some facts are not in dispute. Vitamin and mineral pills can reverse or prevent deficiencies that can result in diseases like scurvy and rickets. But the questions that most Americans want answered are whether vitamin and mineral pills will fend off cancer, heart disease and osteoporosis and lead to overall well being and longer life.

There are no easy answers. Nutrition studies are filled with hints but few conclusions. Current evidence indicates some serious shortfalls in the consumption of essential vitamins and minerals, especially by young women and the elderly. And there are tantalizing indications that there could be significant health advantages from taking supplements of some vitamins and minerals in doses larger than those needed to prevent outright deficiencies.

At the same time, however, there are risks when nutrients are taken separately from the foods that contain them and in doses far larger than the body was designed to process. For the average healthy person who consumes a variety of foods, there is scant evidence that vitamin and mineral supplements are beneficial. Even for segments of the population who may need more vitamins—smokers, people who are ill or poorly nourished, the elderly and pregnant women—the long-term benefits are unclear at best.

And national surveys by Government and university scientists have shown that most of the people who take vitamins are those who are least likely to need extra nutrients: nonsmokers who do not drink heavily. They also consume more nutrients from foods, eat more fruits and vegetables, are better educated and have higher personal incomes than people who do not take vitamin and mineral pills.

Despite all those advantages, vitamin takers do not live longer or suffer fewer cancer deaths than those who do not take vitamins, according to a 13-year study of 10,758 Americans. A research team from the Federal Centers for Disease Control and Prevention in Atlanta reported in 1993 that the study "found no evidence of increased longevity among vitamin and mineral supplement users in the United States."

The team also failed to find any mortality benefits from supplements among people with special nutritional needs, like smokers, heavy drinkers and people with chronic diseases. And there is little, if any, evidence that taking vitamin and mineral supplements can compensate for dietary deficiencies that result from careless eating habits.

Furthermore, there are known dangers of vitamin use. High doses of vitamin E can interfere with the action of vitamin K, which promotes blood clotting. Large amounts of calcium can limit the absorption of iron and perhaps other trace elements. Zinc can reduce the level of copper in the body, impair immune responses and decrease the level of protective high-density lipoproteins in the blood, often called the "good" cholesterol. Folic acid can react badly with anticonvulsant medications and mask signs of a B12 deficiency. Iron supplements can be deadly to small children. In fact, the most common cause of poisoning deaths among children is not caustic cleaning agents or aspirin, but iron supplements intended for adult use.

There is unfortunately only one simple path through the vitamin and mineral maze. And it is to follow the same boring but tried-and-true advice that parents and health classes have been giving out for ages. Eat a balanced and varied diet that is low in fat and high in fruits and vegetables and complex carbohydrates.

The current boom in the vitamin and mineral business got a lift in October 1994, when Congress passed the Dietary Supplement Health and Education Act, which for the most part keeps the F.D.A.'s hands off vitamin and mineral supplements unless something goes wrong. Matthew Patsky, an analyst with the investment firm of Adams, Harkness & Hill in Boston, follows the broad field of dietary supplements, which includes vitamins, minerals and herbs, hormones like melatonin and hard-to-classify substances like shark cartilage. All are somehow considered "dietary," even those that would not normally be part of anyone's diet.

Mr. Patsky said in an interview that the stocks of the manufacturers of dietary supplements that he follows, which dropped in 1994, surged 70 percent in 1995, 57 percent in 1996 and 42 percent in the first half of 1997. The business "wildly outperformed the overall market and continues to do so in 1997," he said.

The dietary supplement law was passed after a struggle between the F.D.A. and the manufacturers. The agency, in re-evaluating its labeling rules, had been planning to apply existing regulations for items like drugs to vitamins, minerals, herbal preparations and other supplements. Those rules would have prevented manufacturers from making health claims of any sort for any supplements without agency approval. The industry responded with intensive lobbying, aided by a letter-writing campaign by consumers who feared that Government rules would limit their access to supplements of all kinds.

An end result, the 1994 law, was something of a compromise. Labels on vitamin and mineral products cannot make claims that a product cures a disease or has a specific beneficial health effect without special F.D.A. approval. The law does, however, allow general statements on the label about a vitamin or mineral's function in the body. At this time, the agency has agreed to allow companies to list direct

health benefits for only two supplements: calcium, to prevent bone loss, and the B vitamin folic acid for pregnant women, to prevent certain birth defects involving the brain and nervous system, including spina bifida.

In contrast, the label on a bottle of vitamin A capsules may say "essential for the normal function of vision," but it cannot claim that the product will prevent or treat vision problems. Vitamin B1 might be described as playing "a vital role in nerve function," but it cannot be called a neurological treatment.

Not that the lack of specific claims on labels has stopped people from assuming that the products offer therapeutic benefits, based on meager evidence, anecdotes and, sometimes, their doctors' recommendations, or based on extrapolations of the nutrients' normal roles in the body. Claims that products have direct benefits are made in many health magazines and newsletters, over the radio, by other media "experts" and by some employees of health-food stores.

Faced with a growing need for more research, the prestigious National Institutes of Health, at the behest of Congress, established an Office of Dietary Supplements in November 1995 to promote scientific study of dietary supplements. Although there are 40 known essential nutrients, almost all vitamins and minerals, "there are close to 1,000 dietary supplements," said the new office's director, Dr. Bernadette Marriott. "Where do we begin?" Dr. Marriott, a specialist in nutrition and behavior who had been deputy director of the Food and Nutrition Board of the National Academy of Sciences, sees her role as helping to stimulate research on the role of supplements in fostering optimal health. She said that although Congress had authorized an annual budget of $5 million for her office, that money had yet to be allocated. The office has been operating on $1 million a year in discretionary money from the director of the National Institutes of Health.

Meanwhile, the consumer who delves deeply into the guidelines for taking vitamins and minerals finds that different amounts of nutrients are suggested for people of different ages, weights and sexes, that the Government is in the process of changing its standards and that experts disagree about the amounts of vitamins needed and the amounts in various foods. The Food and Nutrition Board, which sets recommended intakes of vitamins and minerals, has just revised the Recommended Dietary Allowances, which vary for different people, and created guidelines called Dietary Reference Intakes to reflect, in part, the new interest in vitamins and minerals and their role in preventing disease.

In addition to the quantities needed to head off nutrient deficiencies, the board is creating a separate listing of higher amounts for some nutrients that appear to have important roles in preventing serious diseases and promoting optimal health. The board's Committee on the Scientific Evaluation of Dietary Reference Intakes has said it will "consider how the risk of chronic disease can be related quantitatively to nutrient intakes and dietary patterns."

New calcium recommendations have been set at higher levels that might help prevent osteoporosis rather than merely avoiding a calcium deficiency. In addition, the committee issued new recommended intakes in summer of 1997 for phosphorus, magnesium, vitamin D and fluoride. It expects to develop the same guidelines for all nutrients and for food components like fiber and phytoestrogens, plant-derived hormones, by 2000. But the D.R.I.'s are not the numbers that most people see. The F.D.A. requires the makers of vitamins and minerals to print the agency's Reference Daily Intakes. That list is derived from the numbers of the Food and Nutrition Board and is loosely meant to be an amount that would stave off deficiency in a healthy adult. But these are not true recommendations, and some are, in fact, higher than the board's recommendations.

Details on any given vitamins aside, experts agree that many, and perhaps most, Americans are short-changing themselves on one or more essential nutrients and that in the process, they may compromise their chances for living long healthy lives.

"The style of eating in this country has changed dramatically in the last decade," Dr. Marriott observed. "There's a lot more eating out, which is bound to affect nutrient intake. Americans are fatter than ever, but that doesn't necessarily mean they are well nourished."

Most people who are interested in supplements do not focus on avoiding deficiencies but rather hope to achieve more subtle and often long-term health effects, like improved stamina, protection against heart disease and cancer, and treatment of a whole host of conditions, like carpal tunnel syndrome and premenstrual tension. Some of the goals are reasonable; some are not.

The National Cancer Institute maintains that if Americans consumed at least five servings of fruits and vegetables a day, they would be most likely to take in the amounts of nutrients linked, in laboratory and population studies, to protection against several major cancers and that they would not have to worry about pills. But with the national clamoring for hamburgers, french fries and pizza, only 15 percent of Americans eat that many daily servings of nutrient-packed foods. Such nutrients can also lower coronary risk. About a third of middle-age and elderly people have high blood levels of an amino acid, homocysteine, which studies suggest may be as important as smoking and even more important than cholesterol as a risk factor for heart disease and stroke.

Homocysteine levels rise when a diet is relatively deficient in certain B vitamins, particularly folic acid, which is primarily found in dried beans and peas and dark green leafy vegetables, as well as B6 and B12. This is one case where there is strong support for taking supplements, said Dr. Jeffrey Blumberg, a professor of nutrition at Tufts University. "These people should be doing two things," he said, "eating more foods containing B vitamins and taking a B-complex supplement. Even though we don't yet have placebo-controlled clinical trials to prove it, the data are compelling enough now to justify people doing something about it."

Dr. Blumberg is a strong advocate for bringing nutrition into the medical mainstream, and he said he hoped that researchers determined what levels of vitamins would improve overall health. "We're seeing a paradigm shift in thinking beyond the minimum nutrient intakes to prevent deficiencies to levels that can promote health and prevent chronic diseases," he said.

The Nationwide Food Consumption Survey, conducted in 1987 and 1988 among 5,884 adults by the

Department of Agriculture and analyzed by Dr. Suzanne P. Murphy, a research nutritionist at the University of California at Berkeley, revealed that 22 percent of those surveyed were eating diets that provided at least two-thirds of the recommended daily amounts of 15 essential vitamins and minerals. There were deficiencies of nutrients like calcium, zinc, folic acid, magnesium and vitamins A, B6, C and E. The most poorly nourished were young women 19 to 24. For women 20 and older, average intakes were below the recommended amounts for six nutrients: vitamins B6 and E, calcium, magnesium, iron and zinc. For men, there were deficiencies in zinc and magnesium.

Fewer than one-fourth of the women and fewer than half of the men consumed the recommended amounts of calcium, magnesium and zinc. Although the data from the 1994 Food Consumption Survey have not been fully analyzed, a preliminary review shows little or no improvement over the earlier findings, Dr. Murphy said.

Can vitamins and minerals in pills compensate for dietary deficiencies that result from careless eating habits? Most experts, even those who believe in supplementing a seemingly balanced diet, say no. They emphasize that there are many health-promoting substances in foods other than vitamins and minerals and that haphazard diets are likely to be unhealthy, even if people use vitamin and mineral supplements to bring their consumption of essential nutrients up to the recommended levels.

Though doctors, who are largely unschooled in matters of nutrition, often shy away from all megadoses, some studies by nationally recognized researchers have indicated that extra doses of some vitamins and minerals can help prevent several devastating health problems, including serious birth defects, heart disease, sight-robbing eye disorders, osteoporosis and even some cancers.

In 1970, Dr. Linus Pauling announced that megadoses of vitamin C could prevent the common cold. Although its ability to prevent colds has yet to be proved in a well-designed scientific study, vitamin C in large doses has been shown to attenuate the symptoms of many colds. But its more important role may be as an antioxidant, a substance capable of defusing highly reactive agents that can injure cell membranes or genes or transform innocuous chemicals into damaging ones. Nutrients known to be antioxidants include vitamin E, beta carotene and selenium.

In studies at the Southwestern University Medical Center in Dallas, researchers showed that megadoses of vitamin E—amounts way beyond those to prevent a deficiency—could block the change in low-density lipoprotein cholesterol that allows it to be deposited on artery walls. Other laboratory studies have documented the anticlotting action of vitamin E. And a number of large long-term studies in men and women have correlated high intakes of vitamin E with protection against heart disease and strokes caused by blood clots.

As for selenium, a study of 600 men found that taking a daily supplement of 200 micrograms for 10 years dramatically reduced the incidence of prostate, esophagus, colon-rectum and lung cancers and cut total cancer deaths in half. Earlier studies had linked a low intake of selenium to an increased risk of developing heart attacks, strokes and other diseases related to high blood pressure.

Thus far, however, virtually all the evidence for health benefits derived from supplements of individual nutrients or groups of nutrients is considered suggestive but not conclusive. Until, and unless, long-term studies are performed on large numbers of healthy people who are randomly assigned to take supplements or placebos, the evidence remains indefinite. Given the enormous cost of studies that are years long, the definitive studies may never be conducted.

Attempts to counter illness with vitamin supplements can also backfire. Dr. Larry Norton, medical director of the Lauder Breast Cancer Center at the Memorial Sloan-Kettering Cancer Center in Manhattan, said research at his institution showed that large doses of vitamin C could blunt the beneficial effects of chemotherapy for breast cancer. The research showed that breast cancer cells had large numbers of receptors, or docking places, for vitamin C, suggesting that the vitamin acted like a growth tonic for the cancer cells. And a recent experiment showed that free radicals, chemicals that damage cells in ways that may lead to cancer, are also necessary for some of the mechanisms that stop cancer once it gets going. So a substance like vitamin C, in large doses, could have unpredictable effects. It is also known that folic acid can negate the effects of methotrexate, a drug used to treat cancer.

"I'm not antivitamin," Dr. Norton said. "But the safest thing to do is to have a healthy life style and consume vitamins in foods."

An excess of a vitamin or mineral can sometimes be just as harmful as a deficiency, whether or not a person is already ill. Nutrients known to be harmful when excess amounts are consumed include vitamins A, D and B6; the minerals zinc and selenium, and perhaps even vitamins C and E. For example, too much vitamin A can cause headaches from increased brain pressure, liver and bone damage, hair loss, skin disorders, psychiatric symptoms and, when taken in early pregnancy, birth defects. Too much B6 can damage nerves. Too much vitamin C can interfere with tests for blood in the stool. And in men and post-menopausal women, who tend to accumulate iron in their bodies, supplements containing iron could result in heart disease, cancer and serious infections.

For the majority of vitamins and minerals in tablets and capsules that are sold in pharmacies and health-food stores, the numerous hints of benefits far exceed the facts. In a recent position statement on supplements, issued in January 1996, the American Dietetic Association, the nation's largest organization of nutrition professionals, advised, "The best nutritional strategy for promoting optimal health and reducing the risk of chronic disease is to obtain adequate nutrients from a wide variety of foods."

The reason is that there are many unknown compounds in foods that can have powerful biological effects, like preventing cancer. Many dietary experts now question the wisdom of isolating single nutrients from the usual company they keep in foods. That concern was fueled by two large long-term studies that have seriously tempered enthusiasm for a very popular supplement, beta carotene, a nutrient in fruits and vegetables that the body converts to vitamin A.

Beta carotene is a potent antioxidant that has long been heralded as a possible preventive of common lethal cancers. Though there were undeniable shortcomings in both studies, their findings showed no benefits, instead indicating that supplements of beta carotene might increase, rather than quell, the chances of developing cancer. One possible explanation for the findings emerged from two studies at the University of Arizona Cancer Center. Both laboratory animals and people who were given beta carotene supplements had low blood levels of vitamin E, which may be more important than beta carotene in protecting health.

Furthermore, growing evidence suggests that—at least for beta carotene and the 40 other carotenoids in common foods—it is the combination of food-borne nutrients and other substances in plant foods, like fiber and various plant chemicals, that may provide specific benefits. Thus, taking supplements of one or two of those substances is unlikely to have the desired effects on health.

Also worrisome, the dietetic association says, is the risk of chemical excesses or nutrient imbalances that may result from taking pills rather than eating the foods themselves. For beta carotene and other essential nutrients, particularly the "trace" minerals needed in minute amounts, taking too much of one nutrient may increase the need for another, creating a deficiency. Or supplements may interact adversely with other drugs or worsen disorders.

"If you're taking large amounts of single nutrients," Dr. Marriott said, "that's cause for concern. Patients should be sure to tell their health-care practitioners what supplements they're taking."

Most toxic reactions to vitamins and minerals come from taking something out of a bottle, not from food. In the case of selenium, for example, the toxic dose for adults is only five times the amount recommended for daily intake. Dr. Marriott cautioned: "Buyers need to beware. They must be very careful about choosing supplements. They should look critically at the information. Maybe the study had only six participants, all young men. How does this apply to me, a woman over 50? People are so enthusiastic about nutrition, they tend to jump on every study that's published."

[JEB, October 1997]

# Vitamins and Minerals: What You Don't Know Can Hurt You

When vitamins and minerals are consumed in food, they are just about always good for you. In pill form, however, particularly in high doses, they should be approached with caution.

The trouble in calculating how much is enough, or too much, is that there is no single level of any vitamin or mineral that can be considered the optimum intake for everyone. Needs vary, often widely, with age, sex and stage of life, the scientific evidence is often unclear, and the maze of government numbers for reasonable intakes is confusing, even to the experts. The numbers below are not the ones consumers see on the bottles of supplements; those are so-called labeling standards, good mainly for making comparisons between brands. The numbers here, the best available in an uncertain science, are drawn from the Recommended Dietary Allowances developed by the National Academy of Sciences. The amount for women is right for a healthy premenopausal 40-year-old woman who is neither pregnant nor lactating. For men, the amount given is for a healthy 40-year-old. For vitamin D and calcium the academy did not make a definite recommendation, since it did not have enough evidence, and created another category: Adequate Intake.

The chart also lists good food sources of many commonly supplemented nutrients, their functions and the risks of high doses, even though in many cases, experts are not certain how much is dangerous. In a few cases the Government has established upper limits, levels that are considered unlikely to cause problems for healthy people.

JANE E. BRODY

| VITAMIN | Food sources | Daily Intake | | Function | Risks of high doses |
|---|---|---|---|---|---|
| **A (retinol)** | Liver, egg yolks, fortified milk and dairy products, margarine, fish oil | **Women** 800 micrograms (retinol equivalents) or 2,667 international units | **Men** 1,000 micrograms (retinol equivalents) or 3,333 international units | Needed for normal vision; helps keep bones, skin and red blood cells healthy; essential for the immune system. | Numerous temporary effects, including dry skin, headache, irritability, vomiting, bone pain and vision problems, which disappear after pills are stopped. In children, bone and skin symptoms can persist. Pregnant women should be wary: at 5 to 10 times the recommended levels, there is a link to birth defects |
| **Beta carotene** | Carrots, sweet potatoes, spinach and other dark green leafy vegetables; cantaloupes, apricots | (none established; included in vitamin A recommendation) | | An antioxidant, protects cells against oxidation damage that can lead to cancer; converted as needed into vitamin A. | Excess, while not poisonous, can cause yellowing of skin; suspected but unconfirmed link to increased risk of cancer adds to evidence for consuming foods, not supplements. |
| **C (ascorbic acid)** | Citrus fruits, melons, berries, peppers, potatoes, cabbage, broccoli, tomatoes, fortified cereals | **Women** 60 milligrams | **Men** 60 milligrams | Helps in healing cuts and bruises and in the body's absorption of iron; strengthens bones, cartilage and skin; protects against cancer-causing cell damage. | High doses interfere with tests for hidden blood in stool, which are used in screening for colon cancer; high doses are also inappropriate for people with genetic conditions that cause iron overload, like thalassemia and hemochromatosis, and can interfere with some cancer treatments. |

| VITAMIN | Food sources | Daily Intake | | Function | Risks of high doses |
|---|---|---|---|---|---|
| | | Women | Men | | |
| D | Vitamin D-fortified milk, egg yolks, eel, herring, salmon, liver | 5 micrograms (200 i.u.) (Adequate Intake) Upper limit 50 micrograms (2,000 i.u.) | 5 micrograms (200 i.u.) | Promotes calcium absorption and makes it available to bones; also obtained from action of sunlight on skin. | From supplements (not from skin synthesis or normal food intake), nausea, weakness, irritability. Birth defects in experimental animals suggest pregnant women should avoid supplements. |
| E | Vegetable oil, nuts, wheat germ, whole grains, green leafy vegetables | 8 milligrams alpha-tocopherol equivalents (8 i.u.) | 10 milligrams alpha-tocopherol equivalents (10 i.u.) | Needed for healthy blood cells and tissues; antioxidant, protects cells against cancer-causing damage. | Appears safe at doses up to 50 times the standard level, but high doses increase the action of anticoagulant drugs and interfere with absorption of some other fat-soluble vitamins, especially vitamin K, which promotes blood clotting; supplements should not be taken before surgery. |
| Niacin (nicotinic acid) | Meats, fish, liver, dried beans and peas, fortified grain products, nuts, potatoes | 15 milligrams niacin equivalents | 19 milligrams niacin equivalents | Needed for healthy skin, nervous system and digestive tract; vital for metabolism of carbohydrates, fats and proteins. | Causes itching, skin flushing, gastrointestinal distress. |
| B6 (pyridoxine) | Poultry, fish, pork, whole grains, dried beans and peas, bananas, avocados | 1.6 milligrams | 2 milligrams | Essential for protein metabolism, nervous system and immune function; involved in synthesis of hormones and red blood cells. | Long-term use of doses 500 times the recommended level may damage the sensory nervous system. |
| B12 | Meats, dairy products, eggs, liver, fish | 2 micrograms | 2 micrograms | Needed for synthesis of RNA and DNA, building red blood cells and maintaining nerve cells. | No direct toxicity reported. |
| Folic acid (folate) | Leafy green vegetables, oranges, bananas, liver, dried beans and peas | 180 micrograms | 200 micrograms | Protects against birth defects like spina bifida and other neural tube defects. Helps form DNA, RNA and protein; may reduce risk of heart disease by metabolizing the amino acid homocysteine. | No direct toxicity reported; can mask B12 deficiency at high doses; interferes with certain seizure and cancer drugs |

| Mineral | Food sources | Recommended amounts | Function | Warnings |
|---|---|---|---|---|
| Calcium | Dairy foods, some green leafy vegetables like broccoli and collards, tofu, calcium-fortified foods | **Women** 1 gram  **Men** 1 gram  (Adequate Intake) Upper limit 2.5 grams | Needed for healthy bones, normal muscle contraction and blood clotting. | High intakes may cause constipation and impair kidney function and iron absorption. |
| Magnesium | All unprocessed foods; highest concentrations in nuts, legumes and unmilled grains | **Women** 320 milligrams  **Men** 420 milligrams  Upper limit 350 milligrams (as supplements, in addition to that from food and water) | As with many minerals, is involved in many physiological processes, including nerve signaling, bone building and muscle contraction. | People with impaired kidney function can accumulate magnesium, which can be fatal. |
| Iron | Meat, poultry, fish, eggs, vegetables, tofu and cereals, especially ones fortified with iron | **Women** 15 milligrams  **Men** 10 milligrams | Key component of hemoglobin; involved in oxygen transport. | Iron overload can increase risk of heart disease or even cause multiple organ failure in people with hereditary conditions that cause abnormal iron absorption. Children can be poisoned, sometimes fatally, by taking supplements meant for adults. |
| Zinc | Meat, liver, eggs, seafoods and cereals | **Women** 12 milligrams  **Men** 10 milligrams | A constituent of many enzymes involved in body chemistry; a component of insulin; involved in sense of taste. | Excessive intake can cause gastrointestinal irritation, impaired immune function and copper deficiency. |
| Selenium | Seafoods, kidney, liver, other meats, some grains and seeds | **Women** 55 micrograms  **Men** 70 micrograms | Deficiency linked to heart disease; an essential component of a key antioxidant enzyme. | Heavy exposure may cause reversible changes in hair and nails, gastrointestinal distress and neurological problems, like weakness and slower mental function. |

**International units are defined differently for different vitamins, and calculated differently for different nutrient sources.

Sources: Federal Register (Reference Daily Intakes); United States Department of Agriculture publications (food sources); "Recommended Dietary Allowances, 1989," National Research Council (National Academy Press); "Handbook of Vitamins," L. J. Machlin, editor (Marcel Dekker); "Vitamin and Mineral Safety," Council for Responsible Nutrition (maximum safe levels); Food and Nutrition Board; Dr. Marion Nestle and Lisa Young/department of nutrition and food studies, New York University; "Modern Nutrition in Health and Disease," M. E. Shils, et al. (Lea & Febiger) (functions and risks of unsafe doses).

# U.S. Panel on Acupuncture Calls for Wider Acceptance

An independent panel of experts concluded that the ancient practice of acupuncture was an effective therapy for certain medical conditions, especially those involving nausea and pain, and should be integrated into standard medical practice for these problems. The panel emphasized that acupuncture was remarkably safe, with fewer side effects than many well-established therapies. Currently, more than one million Americans are believed to be relying on acupuncture to treat a wide range of ailments, from headache and bowel disorders to arthritis and stroke.

The panel's findings, summarized in a 16-page consensus report of the National Institutes of Health, are expected to encourage more patients and physicians to consider acupuncture as an alternative or complementary treatment for some common health problems, including nausea associated with pregnancy and cancer chemotherapy, and pain following dental surgery. The report may also foster the use of acupuncture to treat chronic problems, like low back pain and asthma, for which standard medical treatments are inadequate or costly or may entail serious side effects.

The panel said its report should prompt medical insurers, including Medicare and Medicaid, to consider covering the costs of acupuncture, at least for conditions where there is clear evidence of its benefits.

Acupuncture, which originated in China more than 2,500 years ago, involves stimulation of certain points on or under the skin, mostly with ultrafine needles that are manipulated manually or electrically. Other acupuncture methods, used less often or still considered by acupuncturists to be experimental, involve the use of herbs and heat, or low-frequency laser beams, at the various acupuncture points. Although acupuncture originally involved only 361 such points, there are now upward of 2,000 recognized by licensed acupuncturists.

Acupuncture has been slow to gain acceptance by the Western medical establishment, largely because traditional Chinese explanations for its observed effects were based on theoretical concepts of opposing forces called Yin and Yang, which, when out of balance, disrupt the natural flow of Qi (pronounced chee) in the body. But the panel cited growing evidence of acupuncture-induced biological effects that could at least partly explain the benefits observed in scores of studies and in clinical practice. For example, the report said, there is considerable evidence that acupuncture causes a release of natural pain-relieving substances like endorphins, as well as messenger chemicals and hormones in the nervous system. Further, it said, acupuncture appears able to alter immune functions.

"There is sufficient evidence of acupuncture's value to expand its use into conventional medicine and to encourage further studies of its physiology and clinical value," the panel concluded after spending a day and a half hearing and reviewing presentations on acupuncture research. The panel evaluated 17 scientific presentations summarizing hundreds of studies conducted in recent years, primarily in Western countries.

But critics of acupuncture, some of whom call it "quackupuncture," said the presentations could not have resulted in a reasoned consensus, because no naysayers had been invited to give their views. "I fail to see how they can arrive at a consensus when only one view is presented," said Dr. Wallace Sampson, a member of the National Council Against Health Fraud who prepared the council's position paper on acupuncture, published in 1991. Dr. Sampson pointed out that for the most part, the best-designed studies of acupuncture showed the poorest results for it, a fact also mentioned by several experts who made presentations to the panel.

The 12-member panel, headed by Dr. David J. Ramsay, a physiologist who is president of the University of Maryland at Baltimore, represented a wide range of scientific disciplines and included some physicians who perform acupuncture or have been treated by it. The members were charged with determining the quality of evidence for the benefits of acupuncture, the conditions for which it might be effective and what studies were needed to further define its value. The panel, which based its conclusions almost entirely on studies that meet criteria for well-designed research, was convened by various agencies of the National Institutes of Health, including the Office of Alternative Medicine.

The panel did not issue a ringing endorsement of acupuncture. But it did find the procedure to be especially useful for treating painful disorders of the muscle and skeletal systems, like fibromyalgia and tennis elbow, and possibly safer than currently accepted remedies for those disorders. As for other pain problems, including postoperative pain and low back pain, the panel said, available data suggest that acupuncture may be a reasonable option. Among further areas cited as possibly amenable to treatment by acupuncture, usually together with standard remedies, were drug addiction, stroke rehabilitation, carpal tunnel syndrome, osteoarthritis, headache and asthma.

Although the panel lamented the paucity of well-designed clinical studies of acupuncture, it found that in many cases "the data supporting acupuncture

are as strong as those for many accepted Western medical therapies." Nonetheless, it said, larger, better and longer studies are needed to establish properly acupuncture's therapeutic benefits and limitations.

A major barrier to mounting such studies is lack of financial support from commercial sources, which have no vested interest in a technique that cannot be patented. Most presenters here focused only on the relatively few studies that met the "gold standard" for modern clinical research: those entailing random assignment of patients to treatment and control groups, and independent, well-documented assessments of the results. Even some of these studies were considered limited, a number of them because they involved too few or too infrequent acupuncture treatments, or even incorrect acupuncture points.

Further, a major problem in designing acupuncture studies is selection of a control treatment that does not prejudice the results. For example, most studies have used other, nearby points on the skin for comparison with the effects of manipulating real acupuncture points. But this "sham acupuncture" has some biological effects as well, and they make it harder to determine the true benefit of real acupuncture.

[JEB, November 1997]

## The Arthritis Is at Bay, Thank You

The two questions I was asked most often in 1997 were "Is that dietary supplement still helping your arthritic knees?" and "Are there results yet from the studies being done on this side of the Atlantic?"

In late 1996, following my arthritic spaniel's dramatic improvement upon taking a supplement containing two substances that play a role in the formation of cartilage, glucosamine and chondroitin sulfate, I decided to try the stuff myself. Two months later, ignoring bemused queries like "Are you barking yet?" I reported about a 30 percent improvement—

not an absence of pain and stiffness, but less of them and little or no swelling after activities like tennis and ice skating that gave my knees a workout.

In early 1998 my dog and I were still taking the supplement, though at lower daily doses. My dog, who turned 13 that June, is free of pain and stiffness. He walks two hours a day, goes up and down stairs easily and regularly climbs a mountain road with me. I continue to play singles tennis two to four times a week and skate four or five times a week, and I have added a daily three-and-a-half-mile brisk walk to my activities.

Despite recent X-rays showing advanced arthritis in one knee and moderately advanced arthritis in the other, my knees do not swell anymore and are no longer stiff after prolonged sitting. I do not have pain-free knees, but I no longer have disabling discomfort, a chronic limp or difficulty going down stairs, and I have greatly reduced my use of ibuprofen, which while relieving pain and swelling may contribute to joint deterioration.

My dog and I are not alone. My mailbox has been stuffed with testimonials from others who have ventured into this form of alternative medicine to cope with their arthritis. One elderly Brooklyn man said that after three years of crippling pain, he has thrown away his cane and now walks a mile a day. An Arizona woman in her 70s who could hardly walk now walks a mile and a half every morning with her once equally crippled 13-year-old dog. A 67-year-old man in North Carolina reports that after being sidelined by arthritis, he has resumed square dancing.

An orthopedic surgeon in Rochester, New York, told of one patient who canceled knee replacement surgery after improving with the supplements. And the Arizona doctor who in January 1997 turned glucosamine and chondroitin into a national craze, Dr. Jason Theodosakis, author with Brenda Adderly and Barry Fox of *The Arthritis Cure*, said he was among thousands of patients helped by one or both substances, neither of which is covered by medical insurance because they are sold as dietary supplements, not drugs.

In a follow-up work, *Maximizing the Arthritis Cure*, Dr. Theodosakis includes additional testimonials, among them ones from a 70-year-old man who said he was able to dance for the first time in 10 years and a priest who was no longer stiff getting off his knees in church.

No dietary supplement alone can be expected to cure osteoarthritis, the wear-and-tear degeneration of the cartilage that cushions the ends of bones in each body joint. Dr. Theodosakis devotes the bulk of the second book to exercises that foster aerobic conditioning, muscular strength and flexibility and a diet that counters overweight. I can testify to the value of both. My knees hurt when I carry just 10 extra pounds in my arms for any distance. If those pounds were on my frame, they would be carried by my knees as well. Furthermore, not everyone improves on the supplements. If cartilage has completely worn away, it cannot be rebuilt. On average, about half those who try the supplements report reduced pain and stiffness.

But anecdotes do not establish facts. Well-designed studies are needed to prove, or disprove, the value of a remedy. Patients must be randomly assigned to take either the substance in question or a look-alike inactive or comparison remedy, and neither patients nor evaluating physicians can know who is on what until the study is completed. And, while positive results from good studies continue to be published in Europe, there are still no published results of such studies in people on this side of the Atlantic. Two unpublished American studies, good but less than perfect, have been completed using the combination treatment and a third more exacting study, in Canada, is nearly finished. It enlisted 100 patients in a 16-week trial of glucosamine alone.

The Canadian physician, Dr. Joseph B. Houpt, a rheumatologist at the University of Toronto, maintains that there is little point in testing the combination regimen before defining the benefits of the individual components. Other researchers, pointing to extensive studies in Europe of glucosamine alone and a few studies of chondroitin, believe the combination is synergistic, that is, the two together produce greater benefits than would be expected simply from adding together their individual effects.

Dr. Houpt also explained that "these are difficult studies to do." Each patient must be thoroughly evaluated to document the extent of arthritic changes within the joints, pain, stiffness, swelling and functional disabilities like trouble climbing up and down stairs, walking or getting up after prolonged sitting.

Dr. Amal K. Das Jr., an orthopedic surgeon in Hendersonville, North Carolina, has completed a study of nearly 100 patients treated for six months with both glucosamine and chondroitin sulfate. He said, "We found the combination of 1,500 milligrams glucosamine and 1,200 milligrams of chondroitin daily to be effective for treating the pain of mild to moderate arthritis confirmed by X-ray." Patients were evaluated using numerous measures of pain, including their discomfort when walking and climbing stairs. Dr. Das said, as have others, that the supplements had caused no adverse reactions.

Another study, of 34 Navy Seals and divers by Dr. Alan Philippi and Dr. Christopher Leffler at the Portsmouth Naval Medical Center in Virginia, is said by other researchers to have found significant relief of knee pain but no improvement in function after eight weeks on the supplements.

Several university-based studies of arthritic horses and dogs as well as basic laboratory studies continue to point to functional benefits and healthy changes in joint cartilage associated with the supplements. For example, Dr. Louis Lippiello, a biochemist at Medical Professional Associates of Arizona, found in cell cultures and in dogs that each substance independently increased synthesis of cartilage components and that the two together did even better.

[JEB, January 1998]

## Kava May Soothe Jagged Nerves, but Is It Safe?

A pill that calms you down without making you dull, sleepy or addicted? It may seem too good to be true, but the prospect of inner peace with no strings attached is tempting more and more Americans to try kava, an herbal product derived from the roots of a pepper plant grown in Fiji, Vanuatu and other Pacific islands.

To many people who suffer from anxiety and insomnia, kava might seem an ideal "natural" alternative to Valium and the other potentially addicting drugs prescribed to soothe ragged nerves. Kava is said to have been used for thousands of years in the Pacific to help people relax and socialize. Unlike alcohol, which can make people boisterous or belligerent, kava users report that the herb calms them without dulling the mind or causing hangovers.

There have been no scientific studies of kava in human beings in the United States. Nonetheless, Americans spent $15 million on kava in 1996, and twice that much in 1997, according to the *Nutrition Business Journal*, which projects sales of almost $50 million this year. Ed Smith, president of Herb Pharm, in Williams, Oregon, one of about 40 American companies that sell kava, said, "Kava was virtually unknown three years ago, and now our sales are going through the roof."

The wholesale price, $14 to $20 for a kilogram of dried root (2.2 pounds), nearly doubled in the last few years, Mr. Smith said. Kava has become the subject of several popular books, and numerous Web sites sell it.

Scientific trials of kava have been conducted overseas, especially in Germany, and have found it helpful in alleviating anxiety and easing symptoms of menopause, like hot flashes, sleep disturbances and emotional problems. The active ingredients are chemicals called kavalactones, which have a mildly depressing effect on the nervous system. The German researchers found no side effects or withdrawal symptoms when people stopped taking kava.

But important questions about kava have yet to be answered. It is not known whether the products sold in the United States have the same properties as the ones tested in Germany or the traditional kava-based drinks prepared fresh in the Pacific. Researchers also do not know whether kava can be used safely for a long time or whether it can be combined with other drugs or natural products. Because it depresses the nervous system, some doctors warn patients not to take it with alcohol or drugs like Valium that have the same effect.

Kava is not totally benign. Road signs on some Pacific islands warn people not to drink kava and drive. In addition, there have been rare instances of kava abuse among Pacific islanders, resulting in problems with the skin and liver. All apparently clear up when the person gives up kava.

The original kava is a far cry from the hermetically sealed bottles now stocked in American health-food stores. An 18th-century traveler to Polynesia wrote that kava was prepared in a "most disgustful manner." The freshly dug roots were cut up and chewed (preferably by virgins), spat into a communal bowl and mixed with coconut milk or water. The resulting fluid was then strained and passed around. People had such a good time drinking kava that Christian missionaries tried to ban it.

On some islands, kava was pounded rather than chewed. Traditionally, only men drank it. Westerners who have tried kava say it is bitter and tastes like dirt. It also numbs the mouth. In his book, *Kava: Medicine Hunting in Paradise*, Chris Kilham wrote that he was glad he had worn shoes to a kava bar on Vanuatu, because the patrons did so much spitting to get the taste of kava out of their mouths that there wasn't a dry spot on the floor.

Needless to say, the kava sold in the United States is not prepared in the traditional manner. The roots are dried and ground by machines into a powder that can be sold as is, for blending into drinks; put into pills or capsules, or made into an alcohol-based extract.

Dr. Michael J. Balick, curator of the Institute of Economic Botany at the New York Botanical Garden, said the demand for kava was leading growers in Micronesia to begin cultivating upland forests that should be preserved as watersheds. The Nature Conservancy, he said, is trying to encourage the growers to use low-lying tracts that are not so critical to the region.

Kava is sold not as a drug but as a dietary supplement and, as a result, is largely exempt from the control of the Food and Drug Administration. Supplements, unlike drugs, do not have to be proved safe and effective and are not tested or inspected by any regulatory agency. The F.D.A. does not usually investigate a supplement unless people report problems. The agency has no evidence of health problems caused by kava, a spokeswoman said.

Under F.D.A. rules, manufacturers may not claim that their supplements can treat or prevent disease. They can, however, make so-called structure-function claims, saying, for instance, that a product promotes strong bones or supports the immune system.

For kava, Mr. Smith of Herb Pharm said: "We can make somewhat nebulous claims. We can say it enhances well-being, but we can't say it relieves anxiety." Nonetheless, he said, people are buying it in the hope that it will ease anxiety. If he could say anything he wanted, Mr. Smith said: "I would love to put on the label that it could be used for relieving anxiety. I know it does."

An Internet site devoted to inquiries about kava listed 660 messages in early October 1998. The writers ranged from people seeking help with anxiety to those looking for a new way to get high. Some described the results as pleasant, but others called kava useless. One wrote: "Got nothing from the first few small hits, then I downed the remaining two-thirds of the bottle and got a very mild, slightly relaxing effect for a couple hours."

Dr. Roberta Lee, an internist in Tucson, Arizona, who became familiar with kava while practicing medicine in the Pacific, was not surprised by that story.

## Remedy for Anxiety Has Long History

Although kava is emerging now in American stores as a natural remedy for stress and anxiety, it has had a long and important role in societies of the South Pacific Islands.

### THE HISTORY

**Early uses.** The kava root has been used in the South Pacific Islands for more than 3,000 years in ritual ceremonies for spiritual, medicinal and recreational purposes. It is deeply integrated into the culture of these societies.

**The Captain Cook travels.** Kava was first described by a Swedish botanist who accompanied Capt. James Cook in his maiden voyage to the South Pacific from 1768-1771.

**The kava bowl ceremony.** Traditionally served in a coconut half shell, kava is handed out to the ceremonial participants in order of rank.

There is no way of knowing how much active ingredient was in the product, she said, or how high the person's anxiety level might have been.

Still, Dr. Lee recommends kava to some of her patients. She said its effects were subtle, and that she urged her patients to use brands from large European manufacturers, which she declined to name. Because kava is considered a drug in Europe, she said, it is more carefully regulated than in the United States.

"I worry about patients having access to these herbal medications without a prescription or any regulation or even general advice," she said. "People in health-food stores are giving advice, and they're not pharmacists or medical people."

Dr. Lee would like to see the European studies of kava repeated in the United States. "I want to know what works on a sort of moderate anxiety level," she said. "My hunch is that it probably wouldn't be appropriate for someone with very major anxiety." Ultimately, she said, if kava does prove useful, it will be "just one tool" in treating anxiety, along with diet, exercise, counseling and other forms of therapy.

[DG, October 1998]

## Study on Using Magnets to Treat Pain Surprises Skeptics

No one was more skeptical about using magnets for pain relief than Dr. Carlos Vallbona, former chairman of the department of community medicine at Baylor College of Medicine in Houston. So Dr. Vallbona was amazed when a study he did found that small, low intensity magnets worked, at least for patients experiencing symptoms that can develop years after polio.

Dr. Vallbona had long been fascinated by testimonials about magnets from his patients, and even from medical leaders. But his interest in magnet therapy became more serious in 1994 when he and a colleague, Carlton F. Hazlewood, tried them for their own knee pain. The pain was gone in minutes. "That was too good to be true," Dr. Vallbona said.

Dr. Vallbona knew that the power of suggestion can fool both patient and doctor. But he also wondered: Could strapping small, low intensity magnets to the most sensitive areas of the body for several minutes relieve chronic muscular and joint pains among patients in his post-polio clinic at Baylor's Institute for Rehabilitation Research? Valid studies could allow consumers to make informed choices. And if magnet therapy were found to be safe and effective, it could relieve pain with fewer drugs—and their unwanted side effects.

Endorsements from professional athletes are one reason Americans spend large sums on magnets to seek pain relief. But most doctors take a "buyer beware" attitude because many claims lack scientific proof or explanation of how they might work. The Food and Drug Administration has warned doctors and manufacturers about health claims for magnets.

Aware of the medical profession's skepticism about magnet therapy, Dr. Vallbona sought to conduct science's most rigorous type of study. Participants would agree to allow the investigators to randomly assign them to groups getting treatment with active magnets or sham devices. But neither the patients nor the doctors treating them would know what therapy was used on which patient.

First, Dr. Vallbona informally tested magnets on a few patients. One was a priest with post-polio syndrome who celebrated mass with difficulty due to marked back pain that prevented him from raising his left hand. After applying a magnet for a few minutes the pain was gone, Dr. Vallbona recalled, and, "the priest said this was a miracle." Then a human experimentation committee allowed Dr. Vallbona to test 50 volunteers with magnets that at 300 to 500 gauss, were slightly stronger than refrigerator magnets. They were made in different sizes so they could fit over the anatomic area identified as setting off their pain.

It was difficult to design a system to prevent participants from learning whether they were being treated with a magnet or a sham. So Dr. Vallbona asked Magnaflex Inc., a magnet distributor in Corpus Christi, Texas, to prepare active magnets and inactive devices that could not be told apart. The devices were labeled in code. As a further precaution, a staff member observed the patients throughout the 45-minute period of therapy to make sure they would not try to find out—by testing with a paper clip, say—what treatment they were receiving.

After the investigators identified the source of the pain and then pressed on it, the 39 women and 11 men in the study graded the pain on a scale of 0 (none) to 10 (worst). Then after the experimental treatment, the participants rated their pain in a standard questionnaire. The volunteers were tested only one time. The 29 who received an active magnet reported a reduction in pain to 4.4 from 9.6, compared with a smaller decline to 8.4 from 9.5 among the 21 treated with a sham magnet.

The Baylor scientists emphasized that their study applied only to pain from the post-polio condition. Nevertheless, their report in the November 1997 issue of *Archives of Physical and Rehabilitation Medicine*, a leading specialty journal, has shocked many doctors who have scoffed at claims for magnets' medical benefits. In an article about magnet therapy for chronic pain published, Dr. William Jarvis, a professor of public health and preventive medicine at Loma Linda University in California and president of the National Council Against Health Fraud, dismissed magnet therapy as "essentially quackery."

Now, Dr. Jarvis said in an interview, the Baylor study changed his mind. "But like any other pilot study, it needs to be replicated," he said. Dr. Vallbona's findings have led him to try to carry out a larger study in several medical centers, and they are expected to lead other investigators to conduct their own studies.

Dr. Lauro S. Halstead of the National Rehabilitation Hospital in Washington, a pioneer in studying the post-polio syndrome, was among experts who said

that further studies were needed to answer questions like: Will various strength magnets produce different degrees of benefit? How long does the pain relief last? Will the effect wear off after multiple applications? For what other conditions might magnets work?

Dr. Vallbona said he did not know why magnets worked for many post-polio patients but not for others, or why some said they felt improvement in areas of the body far distant from where the magnet was applied.

Magnets' medical benefits have been proclaimed for centuries. So why has it taken so long to do studies to begin to answer the questions? The reasons involve economic, political, professional and human factors. Many doctors criticize the lucrative magnet industry for not investing in studies the way drug companies often do. "They don't do simple research," Dr. Jarvis said, and "it is hard to imagine an easier study to conduct than a magnet one for pain."

Yet doctors share the responsibility to do such research, and only rarely have they reported undertaking the scientifically controlled studies needed to settle major disputes about reported therapies. In many such debates, doctors demand a biological explanation for a therapy's benefits. Without documentation that satisfies them, doctors may summarily reject the claims. Yet in their everyday practices, the same doctors may use other therapies that lack scientific proof for why they work.

Scientists working in nonprofit medical schools and university hospitals are strongly influenced by economics because they need Government grants to pay for their overhead. Since scientific success is measured in part by the dollar amount of their grants, doctors tend not to pay for their studies, even if they are relatively inexpensive. The Baylor study was exceptional. It was done without a grant. Had it been done with Government aid, Dr. Vallbona said, it would have cost about $50,000. Magnaflex provided the active and inactive magnets free, the doctors donated their time and insurance companies were not charged for magnet therapy.

Until recently Government agencies and the scientists who judge applications to them have tended not to support studies on magnets and other therapies on the fringe. The reluctance is well-founded. Over history, so many claims for popular remedies have failed to hold up that many doctors are reluctant to put aside a promising project of their own to study something that may well turn out to be a fad.

Scientists are heavily influenced by peer pressure. Senior scientists often discourage younger investigators from replicating another group's studies because doing so is less likely to advance their careers than making novel findings. But in an age of medical consumerism, patient demand is changing some research agendas. For instance, the National Institutes of Health has created the Office of Alternative Medicine, which is paying for the magnet studies at the University of Virginia.

In tackling fringe areas, scientists usually know that they are stepping in deep water, risking scorn from colleagues who believe that what they are studying is theoretically unsound at best and quackery at worst. Even so, many with the courage may not know how deep the waters are.

[LKA, December 1997]

## Words of Caution About a Hot Potato

At health food stores, tiny tubs of wild yam cream sell well, despite their price ($20 or more). The lure is wild yam's reputation as a source of natural progesterone, a hormone that proponents of alternative medicine consider a palliative for menopausal discomforts. Natural progesterone creams have also become a hot commodity. In recent years, sales of wild yam salves, pure progesterone creams and hybrids containing both have accounted for a large chunk of the mushrooming $600-million market in natural remedies for menopause.

Many women believe these products replenish their dwindling progesterone. Satisfied users say they have fewer hot flashes and more supple skin, and that they are also protecting themselves from osteoporosis and uterine cancer. Natural progesterone is widely perceived as safer than progestin, its synthetic cousin and a common ingredient in hormone replacement therapy. This conviction was bolstered by the debut in December 1998 of the first prescription natural progesterone for menopausal women.

But do these products live up to the glowing testimony? And is the new oral prescription drug superior? Yam balms cannot supply the body with natural progesterone, said Gail Mahady, an authority on plant medicine at the University of Illinois in Chicago. "Only a pharmaceutical laboratory can convert the compounds in yams into progesterone," Professor Mahady explained.

Natural progesterone creams are not always what they seem to be, either. Aeron Life Cycles, a diagnostic testing company in San Leandro, California, screened 27 products and found that 15 of them contained no or little progesterone. The rest contained dosages that might be useful, but only if they were adequately absorbed—a big "if" for many doctors.

In fact, a report published in 1998 in *The Lancet*, the British medical journal, concluded that Progest, a relatively high-dose cream that is a top seller in the United States, does not raise blood progesterone levels sufficiently to protect the uterus from the cancer-inducing effects of taking estrogen alone; currently, that is the only use for which progesterone has been clinically approved. Many doctors find this result disturbing, because some women are substituting creams like Progest for the progestin normally prescribed in hormone replacement therapy. There is also little or no evidence to support the use of progesterone cream by itself to fortify bones or douse hot flashes, menopause experts said.

By contrast, the new prescription progesterone, a capsule sold under the brand name Prometrium, may offer genuine benefits to users of hormone replacement. While comparable to progestin in preventing estrogen's cancerous effects on the uterus, Prometrium is believed to offer better protection against heart disease. In clinical trials, it was better than progestin at preserving estrogen's positive effect on cholesterol levels.

Some women may also tolerate Prometrium better than Provera and other synthetic progesterones. But even though Prometrium is identical to the body's own hormone, it causes dizziness, headaches, sore breasts and other adverse reactions in 9 percent to 16 percent of women.

The drug is not cheap, either. A bottle of 100 capsules (roughly a seven-week supply) sells for $54, though most insurers will cover some or all of the cost.

[KM, June 1999]

# Behind the Hoopla Over a Hormone

In a culture that worships youth, many baby boomers and older people alike are ever in search of a fountain of youth. And if you believe the claims being widely disseminated in books, magazines and newsletters and on radio, television and the Internet, that Holy Grail is now available in dihydroepiandrosterone, or DHEA, a hormone that is selling briskly as a dietary supplement.

The claims for DHEA make it sound like a miracle drug that can stop and even reverse the aging process and the debilitating diseases that often accompany it. Some enthusiasts say that a daily dose of the substance has taken 20 years off their chronological ages.

Commercial proponents, true believers and a few less-than-cautious researchers say it can strengthen immunity; recharge a flagging libido; melt body fat and build new muscle; prevent cancer, heart disease, diabetes and osteoporosis; enhance energy; improve mood; relieve symptoms of lupus; treat Alzheimer's disease; and increase longevity. If even half these claims were established facts, DHEA might truly be a wonder drug. But before you rush out to buy a bottle, consider what is and is not known about its real and potential benefits and risks.

DHEA is a hormone, a weak androgen produced by the adrenal glands that can be converted in the body to testosterone and estrogen in both men and women. Its release into the blood peaks at various times: just before birth (slackening in childhood) and before puberty (slackening after age 25 or 30). Blood levels of the hormone in a 70-year-old are only about 25 percent of those in a 30-year-old, prompting some to suggest that aging may be a DHEA deficiency disease. But it could also mean that the hormone is not needed in large amounts by older people.

DHEA is a nonpatentable steroid that can be synthesized from pharmaceutical ingredients or extracted from wild yams. Although DHEA had been available over the counter for decades, the Food and Drug Administration deemed it in 1985 to be a drug for which unsubstantiated claims were being made and banned its sale. Then in 1994, the hormone, along with many other potent "natural" chemicals, re-emerged as a nonprescription supplement under the Dietary Supplement and Education Act, which blocks F.D.A. regulatory action unless a label makes unapproved claims or the product is proved dangerous.

**Warning No. 1:** The DHEA you can buy in health food stores and elsewhere has not been scrutinized by any official organization for quality or content. You may or may not be getting what you pay for.

**Warning No. 2:** There are no long-term studies of either the benefits or risks of the hormone. Nearly all of the relatively few studies completed in people have been small and short-term. Most of the claims made for it are based on studies in mice and rats, which, unlike people, do not produce significant quantities of the hormone at any time in their lives. Therefore, its effects in these animals may be quite different from those in people.

Furthermore, careful researchers say promoters have drawn unwarranted conclusions about the benefits of DHEA from their studies and have made claims based on small studies that have not been confirmed by others.

**Warning No. 3:** The overwhelming majority of researchers who are conducting well-designed studies of the hormone caution consumers against taking it without medical supervision. Given the many unknowns about how the hormone can be administered safely and what benefits it may bestow, the researchers say it should be used only by participants in an approved research study, in which they receive pharmaceutical-grade DHEA and are closely monitored for ill effects. The researchers also caution against doses higher than 50 milligrams a day.

For, despite its over-the-counter availability, the hormone may indeed have risks. As indicated by studies in animals and people, the possible hazards include stimulating the growth of prostate and breast cancer, damaging the liver, masculinizing women and increasing women's cardiac risk. Rather than administering the hormone as a pill that must pass through the digestive tract and be processed by the liver, some investigators believe that a safer route might be through the skin or under the tongue.

That said, once researchers have sorted things out, DHEA or a metabolite (a breakdown product) may indeed have a bright future as a hormone supplement in mid-life to late-life. At the University of California at San Francisco, Dr. Owen M. Wolkowitz and Dr. Louann Brizendine are evaluating the hormone's ability to improve memory and quality of life in patients with mild Alzheimer's disease, based on animal studies in which aged mice given DHEA performed as well on memory tests as young mice and on the finding that elderly people with lower blood levels of the hormone did not function as well as those with higher levels.

In another study of men and women with major depression, Dr. Wolkowitz said, the hormone produced significant improvement when compared with a placebo, or dummy pill.

The hormone's ability to enhance normal immune responses has been suggested in studies of older men and women, who produced higher levels of infection-fighting natural killer cells and less of a damaging immune substance, interleukin-6, while on the substance. Elderly patients on the hormone showed an improved response to influenza vaccine. And in patients with the autoimmune disease lupus, DHEA reduced the severity of symptoms and the amount of medication they required.

As for other claims, however, at best a modest decrease in cardiac risk for men and none for women was linked to higher blood levels of the hormone in a 10-year study of nearly 2,000 people in Rancho Bernardo, California, conducted by Dr. Elizabeth Barrett-Connor of the University of California at San Diego. Nor did she find an association between DHEA levels and bone density. Initial claims that the hormone might lower breast cancer risk have not been borne out by three studies. And two studies found higher levels of the hormone in women who developed cancers of the breast or ovary.

Anecdotal reports of a revival of sexual desire and prowess stimulated by DHEA remain just that: anecdotes. *Nutrition Action* newsletter reported in March 1997 that volunteers in one study experienced no change in sexual desire while taking 50 milligrams of the substance daily for three months, and no study has yet examined the hormone's effects on sexual activity.

Likewise with studies of the hormone's effects on energy and mood. A small three-month study described "improved physical and psychological well-being" in people given 50 milligrams of DHEA a day, but a second study of a 100-milligram dose taken for six months did not produce such reports.

And Dr. Arthur Schwartz of the Temple University School of Medicine in Philadelphia said that contrary to claims on the Internet, his studies had not shown that the hormone aids in weight loss. Six other studies found no benefit from the hormone on levels of body fat in men and women.

[JEB, February 1998]

# INDEX

## A

abdominal exercises, 26, 35–37, 41–42
abortion, 157–58
  emotional impact of, 82–84
abusive relationships:
  aggressive behavior of women, 113–14
  battered women, 105–14
  emotional abuse, 109
  planning to escape from, 110–11
  sexual abuse, 196
  stalking, 106, 117–21
  within stepfamilies, 106, 114–16
*ACE FitnessMatters*, 42
aconite, 335
acupuncture and acupressure, 323, 325,
  327–28, 348–49
Adderly, Brenda, 350
Adelman, Dr. Ronald, 87
adopted children, 151–52
Aeron Life Cycles, 355
African-Americans:
  birth rate for unmarried, 206
  fibroids among, 185
  hypertension among, 7
aggression, female, 113–14
aging, *see* elderly; menopause and aging
AIDS, 144, 145, 179, 206, 333
Alameda County Study of religion and
  longevity, 337, 338
Alan Guttmacher Institute, 206, 207
alcohol, 2, 15, 159, 160, 235
  abuse of, 100, 209–10, 234
  breast cancer and, 247, 248–49, 298
  heart disease and, 280, 281–82, 297–98, 300
  teenagers and, 188, 195, 196, 209–10
alendronate (Fosamax), 234, 235–36, 238
Alexopoulos, Dr. George S., 230
allergies, 325
  reactions to herbal remedies, 331
Allison, Dr. David, 21–22
alpha-linolenic acid, 70, 293
alternative medicine, 323–57
  cautionary advice, 325–26, 328–31
  as complementary to conventional medicine, 327
  diagnosis by convention doctor prior to
   using, 325–26, 327
  growth in popularity of, 325, 326
  harm of rejecting mainstream medicine,
   324, 329

"natural" remedies, cautions about,
  323–24, 326, 328, 336
  phony practitioners of, 326
  practitioners, appeal of, 324, 325
  *see also specific forms of alternative medicine,
   e.g. acupuncture and acupressure;
   herbal remedies*
Alzheimer's disease, 102, 103, 104, 213–14,
  221, 222, 230, 336
Amador, Dr. Xavier Francisco, 91, 92
*Ambiguous Loss: Learning to Live with
  Unresolved Grief* (Boss), 102
American Academy of Cosmetic Dentistry,
  318, 319
American Academy of Esthetic Dentistry,
  319
American Academy of Family Physicians,
  165
American Academy of Pediatrics, 179, 209
American Association of Retired Persons,
  88, 101–102
American Association of University
  Women, 195
American Cancer Society, 12, 15, 21, 240,
  241, 242, 249, 254, 297
American College of Obstetrics and
  Gynecology, 27, 165, 182, 185–86
American College of Sports Medicine, 40
American Council on Exercise, 42
American Diabetes Association, 12
American Dietetic Association, 14, 344
American Heart Association, 7, 21, 40, 285,
  286, 293, 300
American Home Products, 332
American Institute for Cancer Research, 16
*American Journal of Clinical Nutrition*, 4
*American Journal of Obstetrics and
  Gynecology*, 5
American Podiatric Medical Association, 30,
  32
American Psychiatric Association, 201
American Psychological Association, 112
American Society of Clinical Oncologists,
  269
American Society of Plastic and
  Reconstructive Surgeons, 308
*Am I Thin Enough Yet?* (Hesse-Biber), 196,
  198
Anderson, Dr. Ross E., 40
Andrews, Lori, 149

androgens, 132–35
  testosterone, 43, 123, 131, 132–34, 219,
  227–28
Angell, Dr. Marcia, 329
angina, unstable, 290
Annussek, Greg A., 261
anorexia nervosa, 188, 193–94
Antell, Dr. Darrick E., 318
antibiotics, 159
antioxidants, 280, 297, 343, 344
anxiety, 80, 117, 199–200, 325
  kava for, 332, 351–53
Archer, Dr. John, 113
*Archives of Internal Medicine*, 237
*Archives of Pediatrics and Adolescent
  Medicine*, 211
Arnett, Dr. Maria, 314
Arnot, Bob, 15
aroma therapy, 323, 337
arsenic, 326, 329
arthritis, 54, 233, 325, 349–51
*Arthritis Cure, The* (Theodosakis et al.), 350
artificial sweeteners, xiv
Ashkenazi Jews, 257
Asian herbs, 324, 329–30
asthma, 348, 349
astigmatism, laser surgery to correct,
  313–17
atherosclerosis, 290, 297
Atkins, Dr. Robert C., 64–67, 68
Atkinson, Dr. Richard, 71, 72
attractiveness, *see* beauty
Austad, Dr. Steven N., 217
Austin, Dr. Melissa A., 292
Autologous Blood and Bone Marrow
  Transplant Registry of North America,
  267
avocados, 295
axillary dissection, 271–72
Aydin, Dr. Vulent, 157

## B

Bachmann, Dr. Gloria A., 228
back pain:
  acupuncture for, 348, 349
  alternative medicine for, 325, 327
  chiropractors for, 323, 328
Baines, Dr. Cornelia J., 252
Baker, Dr. James L., 203, 204, 317
Balanchine, George, 192

Balick, Dr. Michael J., 352
ballerinas, eating disorders among, 191–94
Bancroft, Dr. John, 125
Banting, William, 65
Banzhaf, John, 288
Barnes, Dr. Lawrence C., 170
Barnett, Dr. Rosalind C., 86, 87
Barrett-Connor, Dr. Elizabeth, 227–28, 357
Bartsich, Dr. Ernst, 182–83, 184
Batman, Dr. Phillip, 177
battered women, 105–14
    profiles of batterers, 107–109
    sources of help for, 110–11
Baxter International, 310–11
Bayer, 332
Baylis-Ungaro, Alycea, 44, 45
Baylor Institute for Rehabilitation Research, 353–54
beans, 8, 223, 280, 296, 342
beauty:
    cosmetic surgery to enhance, *see* cosmetic surgery
    disadvantages of, 306–308
    health and, association between, 303–305
    sexual selection among animals, 303
    stereotyping of attractive women, 306–307
Becker, Dr. Anne E., 201
Becker, Paul, 48, 50
Beebe, Christine, 11–12
*Behavioral Research and Therapy*, 56
Bell, Dr. Alan, 135, 136
belladonna, 335
Bellino, Dr. Frank, 220
belly dancing, 35–37
Benson, Herbert, 338
Beraka, Dr. George, 204, 318
Berenzy, Ruth, 307
Berger, Vivian, 122
Bernstein, David, 311–12
Bernstein, Dr. Leslie, 248
Berscheid, Ellen, 306
beta carotene, 343, 344, 345
Betancourt, Marian, 110, 111
Bielenson, Dr. Peter, 146
bilateral prophylactic mastectomy, 241, 246, 272–76
bile duct, cancer of the, 255
biopsy:
    needle, 253
    sentinel node, 271–72
bipolar disorder, 233
Birnbach, Dr. David, 172

birth control pills, 124, 127–29, 134, 182
Black, Dr. Susan, 155
black cohosh, 334
bladder cancer, 16
Blair, Dr. Steven, 39–40
Bliske, Anne, 122
blood clots, 129, 293
    alcohol and, 280, 281
    heart attacks in women and, 279, 289
    secondhand smoke and, 288
    tamoxifen and, 247, 258–59, 261, 262
    triglycerides and, 292
blood clotting, vitamins and, 340
blood pressure, 40, 54
    alternative medicine for lowering, 327
    calcium and, 1, 4, 6–7, 296
    ephedra's effect on, 52, 75–76, 328, 336
    high, *see* hypertension
blood sugar, 54, 283
    diabetes and, *see* diabetes
    fiber and, 1
blue cohosh, 335
Blum, Michael, 46
Blumberg, Dr. Jeffrey, 342
Blumenthal, Mark, 333–36, 336
body mass index (B.M.I.), 53–54, 55, 56
*Body Project: An Intimate History of American Girls, The* (Brumberg), 190, 196
Bolaji, Dr. Ibrahim I., 174
Bondurant, Dr. Stuart, 311, 312, 313
bone density test, 219, 231, 233–34
    dual-energy X-ray absorptiometry (Dexa), 233–34, 235
bone marrow transplants, 265–70
bones, 357
    age at peak bone mass, 7
    calcium for, *see* calcium, for bones and teeth
    fractures, 233–34, 236–38
    menopause and bone loss, 214, 218, 226, 231–38
    osteoporosis, *see* osteoporosis
    vitamin D and, *see* vitamin D
borage, 335
Borgen, Dr. Patrick, 273–74, 276
Boss, Dr. Pauline, 102–104
Boswell, Suzanne, 320
botanicals, *see* herbal remedies
botulinum toxin, 326
Boykin, Dr. Alan, 183
brain, the, 70, 170
Braun, Susan, 262
Braverman, Dr. Andrea, 150, 151
breakfast, 3–4
breast cancer, 71, 239–78, 240, 357

abortion and, 157–58
alcohol and, 247, 248–49, 298
axillary dissection, 271–72
bilateral prophylactic mastectomy, 241, 246, 272–76
birth control pill and, 129
bone marrow transplants for, 265–70
BRCA1 and BRCA2 genes, 222, 241, 246, 254–57, 258, 273, 274
breast reconstruction, 277–78
chemotherapy for, 268, 269, 270
clinical trials for bone marrow transplants, difficulty of running, 265–70
death rate from, xiii, 240
diet and, 15, 16, 17, 21, 70, 246–48
exercise and, 247–48
fear of, coping with, 243–45
as genetic disease, 255
hormone replacement therapy and, 214, 221–24, 241, 245
inherited risk of cancer-causing mutations, 254–57
lumpectomy, 253, 272
mammography to detect, 252–54, 308
needle biopsy, 253
radiation therapy for, 253
radical mastectomy, xiii, 272, 277
self-examination to detect, 250–52, 254
sentinel node biopsy, 271–72
smoking and, 249
software to compute risk of, 244–48
statistical risk of, 239–44
support groups, 244
survival rates, 240, 242, 244
tamoxifen and, 246–47, 253, 257–63
testosterone and, 134
*Breast Cancer: The Complete Guide* (Hirshaut), 253
*Breast Cancer Prevention Diet, The* (Arnot), 15
breast-feeding, 178–80, 181, 248
breast implants, 301–302, 308–13
    safety of, 310–13
    saline, 301, 302, 308, 312
    silicone, 301–302, 308, 310–13
breast reconstruction, 277–78
breast self-examination, 250–52, 254
Brennan, Dr. H. George, 204, 317
Brevoort, Peggy, 332
Brind, Dr. Joel, 158
Brinton, Dr. Louise A., 225
Bristol-Myers Squibb, 310–11
*British Medical Journal*, 4, 174, 207, 281, 295
Brizendine, Dr. Louann, 357

Brodman, Dr. Michael, 175
broom (herb), 335
Brown, Sarah, 190–91
Brownell, Dr. Kelly D., 57–58, 59
Brumberg, Dr. Joan Jacobs, 190, 196
Buel, Sarah, 110
bulimia, 188, 193–94, 196, 201
Burkitt, Dr. Denis P., 12–13, 14
Busch, Dr. Trudy, 224
Buss, David, 307
butter, 21, 69, 246
Byers, Dr. Tim, 62

**C**

Caesarean births, 173–75
caffeine, 8, 159, 160, 232
calcitonin (Miacalcin), 234, 236
calcium, xiv, 4–9, 66, 233, 234, 343, 347
    blood pressure and, 1, 4, 6–7, 296
    for bones and teeth, xiv, 1, 4, 5,
        231–32, 235
    colon cancer and, 1, 4, 6
    food sources of, 7–8, 17, 219, 231–32
    iron absorption and, 340
    PMS and, 1, 4, 5
    recommendations, 6, 223, 232, 342
    supplements, xiv, 8–9, 19, 231, 238,
        296
    vitamin D and absorption of, 4, 5, 8,
        9, 10, 223, 232
California Department of Health, 329
calories, 3, 62–64, 67, 68
*Calories Don't Count* (Taller), 65
Calvert, Stacey, 27–28
Campbell, Dr. Anne, 113
*Canadian Medical Association Journal,*
    251
cancer, 61, 224, 233, 343
    becoming pregnant after, 148, 156–57
    diet and, 15–17
    two-hit hypothesis, 256
    *see also specific forms of cancer*
Cancer Treatment Centers of America,
    267, 268
canola oil, 20, 69, 70, 247, 292, 295
Caplan, Dr. Arthur, 152
capsicum, 334
carbohydrates, 67, 68
    complex, 3, 16, 68, 285, 341
    low-fiber, diabetes and, 10–12, 15
    refined, 2, 223, 283, 292
    sugar, *see* sugar
cardiovascular fitness, 40
carpal tunnel syndrome, 349
Cascara sagrada, 336
Castelli, Dr. William, 21

Castlemen, Michael, 327, 328
Center for Complementary Medicine, 65
Center for Science in the Public
    Interest, 210
Centers for Disease Control and
    Prevention, 40, 56, 71, 144, 145,
    284, 337, 340
cereals, 2–3, 11, 15, 282, 296–97, 299
Chambliss, Catherine, 87
chaparral, 335
Chase, Bob, 143
cheese, 8, 283, 293
chemotherapy, 263–64, 268, 269, 270
    becoming pregnant after, 148
    parents choosing alternative medicine
        over, 324, 329
    vitamin C and, 343–44
childbirth, 147–48, 167–80
    birth assistants, 148, 169–71, 175–76
    comparison of nonhuman primate
        and human, 167–69
    elective Caesareans, 173–75
    natural, 147–48, 173
    pain relief, 148, 171–73
    sex after, 177–78
    *see also* pregnancy
children:
    with abusive stepfathers, 106, 114–16
    adopted, 151–52
    assisted fertility, telling them about,
        150–52
    with depressed parent, 91, 93–94
    exercise and, 43
    iron supplements and, 340
    missing, 103
    nutrition of, 3–4, 7, 199, 234
    rejection of mainstream medicine by
        parents, 324, 329
    teenagers, *see* teenage girls
    *see also* childbirth; pregnancy
chiropractors, 323, 325, 328
chlamydia, 145
cholesterol, blood, 54, 55, 68, 70, 293–94
    of French population, 281–83
    HDLs (high-density lipoproteins), 21,
        68, 218, 228, 280, 281, 288, 292,
        296, 298, 300, 340
    heart disease and, 284
    LDLs (low-density lipoproteins), 68,
        228, 282, 285–86, 297, 343
cholesterol, dietary, 67
Cholestin, 296
chondroitin, 349–51
chronic fatigue syndrome, 78, 89–91
Chu, Dr. Donald A., 47
cigarettes, *see* smoking

*Circulation,* 7, 286, 287, 291, 293
clinical trials:
    for bone marrow transplants, 265–70
    double-blind controlled, 327
Clinton, Bill, 144
Cloninger, Dr. C. Robert, 79
Cody, Dr. Hiram S., 3d, 250, 271–72
coffee, *see* caffeine
cognitive restructuring, 339
Col, Dr. Nananda, 225
Colb, Sherry, 122
Collins, Monique, 154
Colman, Dr. Eric, 71
colon (colorectal) cancer, 16, 17, 255,
    256, 343
    calcium and, 1, 4, 6
    fats and, 21
    fiber and, 12–14
    screening for, 12
comfrey, 331, 335
Commission E, Germany, 336, 337
Commonwealth Fund, 195, 196
compartmentalizing, 87
complementary medicine, *see* alterna-
    tive medicine
*Complete German Commission E
    Monographs,* 332
complex carbohydrates, 3, 16, 68, 285,
    341
conception, *see* pregnancy
congenital adrenal hyperplasia, 134–35
Connor, Dr. William, 21
contraception, 124
    birth control pill, 124, 127–29, 134,
        182
    morning-after, 124, 129–30
    teenagers' use of, 206, 208
Cooper, Dr. Susan, 151
Copel, Dr. Joshua, 178
Coppes, Dr. Max J., 329
Corfman, Dr. Philip, 129–30
Cornell University, 210
cosmetics, 304
cosmetic surgery, 301–302
    among teenage girls, 202–205
    breast implants, *see* breast implants
    demi-face lift, 320–21
    dentistry, cosmetic, 318–20
    liposuction, 302, 321–22
    on the neck, 320–21
    rhinoplasty (nose job), 302, 317–18
    selecting a surgeon, 302
    vision correction, *see* vision correction
Council on Responsible Nutrition, 329,
    332, 339
Cowan, Dr. Bryan, 184

cryomyolysis, 183
Cummings, Dr. Steven R., 236, 237, 238
Cunningham, Dr. Bruce, 308, 309
Cunningham, Michael, 306, 307
*Current Anthropology*, 215
Curry, Susie, 35
cycling, 29–30

**D**

dairy products, 219, 223
    calcium from, 7–8, 219, 232
    *see also specific products*
Daly, Dr. Martin, 115, 116
Darney, Dr. Philip D., 134
Darroch, Jacqueline E., 206
Darwin, Charles, 303
Das, Dr. Amal K., Jr., 350–51
DASH (Dietary Approaches to Stop
    Hyptertension) trial, 7
Daviglus, Dr. Martha, 295
Davis, Dr. Ann, 208
*Deal With It! A Whole New Approach to
    Your Body, Brain and Life as a Gurl*
    (Drill et al.), 189–90
de Becker, Gavin, 120
*Decade of the Brain, The* (Liebowitz), 230
DeCherney, Dr. Alan, 153, 155, 161
deep breathing, 327
Deland, Dr. Jonathan T., 30
de Lorgeril, Dr. Michel de, 293, 294
DeLuca, Dr. Hector F., 5
Denke, Dr. Margo, 68
dentistry, cosmetic, 318–20
depression, 78, 87, 91–99, 100, 102,
    117, 195, 200, 338, 357
    aging and, 228–30
    alternative medicine for, 325
    of loved one, coping with, 91–92
    post-partum, 180–82
    refractory or treatment resistant, 94–96
    St. John's wort for, 161–62, 328, 332,
        333–36
    winter, 97–99
dexfenfluramine, 71–72
DHEA (dihydroepiandrosterone),
    356–57
diabetes, 315, 316
    exercise and, 25
    fiber and, 1, 10–12, 15
    heart disease and, 280, 290
    high blood sugar and, 11
    micronutrients and, 11
    non-insulin dependent (Type II), 11,
        280
Diamond, Dr. Howard, 318
Diamond, Dr. Jared, 215

Dickinson, Dr. Annette, 329, 330, 332
diet, *see* nutrition
Dietary Supplement Health and
    Education Act of 1994, 329, 332,
    341, 356
dietary supplements, 323, 328–31
    herbal remedies, *see* herbal remedies
    regulation of, 324, 326, 329, 332–33,
        336–37, 352
    safety of, questioning, 326, 328–31
    vitamin and mineral supplements, *see*
        vitamin and mineral supplements
diet drugs, 47, 52, 54–56, 70–75
diets, weight loss, xiv, 196
    fads, 22–24, 64
    high-fat, high-protein, 64–67
    hip fractures and weight loss after 50,
        236–38
    sugar-free, fat-free foods, 62–64
    *see also* eating disorders
digitalis, 330
dinitrophenol, 74
DiPaola, Dr. Robert, 331
dipyrone, 330
diverticulosis, 14
docosahexaenoic acid (DHA), 293
*Doctors' Case Against the Pill, The*
    (Seaman), 129
*Doctor's Quick Weight-Loss Diet, The*
    (Stillman), 65
Domar, Dr. Alice, 339
domestic violence, 105–16
double-blind controlled clinical trials,
    327
doulas, 175–76
Dow Corning Corporation, 308
Dowling, Dr. James, 42
*Dr. Atkin's Diet Revolution* (Atkins), 64–65
Drill, Esther, 189–90
drugs:
    abuse of prescription drugs, 100
    addiction, 349
    bone loss and, 233
    breast-feeding and, 180
    diet, *see* diet drugs
    fertility, 148
    hormone replacement therapy, *see*
        hormone replacement therapy
    for impotence, *see* Viagra
    interactions, 326, 336
    for osteoporosis, 234–36, 238
    over-the-counter, 159–60
    during pregnancy, 159–60
    teenage experimentation with, 188, 196
    *see also specific drugs*
Duarte, Carol, 319

Duby, Deanna, 143
Dugatkin, Lee, 307
Duke University, Center for the Study
    of Religion, Spirituality and
    Health, 338
Dunlap-Kann, Carla, 35
Dunn, Dr. Andrea L., 40
Dutcher, Dr. Janice, 263
Dyson, Dr. Donald C., 163

**E**

eating disorders, 188, 195, 196, 199,
    200–201
    among ballerinas, 191–94
    peer counseling for, 188, 193–94
echinacea, 161–62, 328, 332, 334
Eckel, Dr. Robert H., 68, 69
egg donation, 148–52
eicosapentaenoic acid (EPA), 293
Eid, Dr. François, 136, 138
elderly:
    depression among, 228–30
    food pyramid for, 17–19
    strength training for, 43
Ellenbogen, Dr. Richard, 204
Elliot, Dr. Diane L., 212
Ely, Dr. Susan F., 321, 322
Emlen, Dr. Stephen T., 115–16
emotional health, 77–103
    of teenage girls, 199–200
    *see also specific emotional problems*
endometrial ablation, 183–84
endometrial cancer, 21, 261
Ensrud, Dr. Kristine, 237
*Enter the Zone* (Sears), 67
eosinophilia-myalgia-syndrome
    (E.M.S.), 76
ephedra, 52, 75–76, 328, 333, 335, 336
ephedrine, 75–76
*Epidemiologic Reviews*, 89
epilepsy, 233
Erickson, Dr. David, 162–63
Ernster, Dr. Virginia, 311, 312, 313
esophagus, cancer of the, 12, 16
*Essential Exercise for the Childbearing
    Year* (Noble), 27
estrogen, 81, 132, 133
    alcohol and, 249
    body fat and, 248
    bone density and, 218
    fibroids and, 182
    hormone replacement therapy, *see*
        hormone replacement therapy
    menopausal decline of, 218, 219
    post-partum depression, estrogen
        patch for, 180–82

*Estrogen: The Natural Way* (Shandler), 219
Etcoff, Dr. Nancy, 303–304, 305, 306–307
*Evolutionary Anthropology,* 169
Ewigman, Dr. Bernard G., 166
exercise, 25–50, 219, 292
  bone density and, 231, 234, 235
  breast cancer and, 247–48
  gadgets, 26, 41–42
  health benefits of, 25, 40–41
  heart disease and, 280, 284–85
  making time for, xiv, 41
  after menopause, 222
  percentage of population engaging in regular, 25, 39, 40
  personal trainers on the Internet, 48–50
  during and after pregnancy, 27–28
  technique and injury prevention, 28–30
  weight control and, 51–52, 55, 58, 62, 64
  *see also specific forms of exercise*
eyes, *see* vision correction

**F**

fad diets, 22–24, 64
Fahey, Dr. Thomas D., 43
*Family Planning Perspectives,* 208
Farley, Dr. Melissa, 112
farsightedness, laser surgery to correct, 313–17
fats, 15, 62–64, 67–70, 293
  benefits of, 70
  breakfast foods and, 3–4
  breast cancer and, 246–48
  heart disease and, 19–22
  high-fat, high-protein diets, 64–67
  low-fat diets, 67, 295, 341
  monounsaturated, 20, 21, 69, 70, 247, 293, 295
  polyunsaturated, 20, 21, 69, 70, 247, 283, 293, 295
  saturated, *see* saturated fats
  trans, *see* trans fatty acids
  triglycerides, *see* triglycerides
Fawcett, Dr. Jan, 95
fearfulness, 79–80
  of breast cancer, 243–45
Federal Trade Commission, 333
Federman, Dr. Daniel, 220
feet, caring for your, 29, 30–32
*Feisty Woman's Breast Cancer Book, The* (Ratner), 243–44

Feldman, Gayle, 278
fencing, 38–39
fenfluramine, 56, 71–72
fen-phen, 72, 74
Ferro, Mitch, 316
*Fertility and Sterility,* 161
fertility drugs, 148
fetal monitors, 163–64
feverfew, 334
fiber, 16, 18, 342
  blood sugar and, 1
  at breakfast, 3
  calcium absorption and, 8
  colorectal cancer and, 12–14
  diabetes and, 1, 10–12
  heart disease and, 14, 282
  insoluble, 14
  soluble, 14, 296
  weight control and, 15
fibroid embolization, 183, 184–85, 186
fibroid tumors, 148, 182–86
fibromyalgia, 78, 89–91, 349
Fibush, Judi, 278
fish, 232, 280, 293, 295, 296, 299
fish oils, 17, 70, 293
fitness competitions, 33–35
5-hydroxy-L-tryptophan (5-HTP), 76
flaxseed, 17, 70, 219, 296
Fleck, Dr. Steven, 43
Fletcher, Dr. Suzanne, 304
fluoride, 342
Flynn, Dr. Mary, 67, 68
Flynn, Dr. P. J., 258–59
foie gras, 283
folic acid (folate), 67, 280, 283, 296, 298–99, 340, 342, 343, 344, 346
food additives, xiv
Food and Drug Administration (FDA), 70–72, 73, 75, 76, 127, 129–30, 160, 173, 262, 263, 296, 299, 308, 313, 330, 356
  dietary supplements, regulation of, 324, 326, 328, 329, 332, 336–37, 340, 341, 352
  magnet therapy and, 353
Food and Nutrition Board, 342
  Committee on the Scientific Evaluation of Dietary Intakes, 342
food diary, 64
food pyramid, 11, 180
  for the elderly, 17–19
Forcade, Dr. Carlos, 185
Ford, Dr. Leslie, 258, 259, 262, 263
Fosamax (alendronate), 234, 235–36, 238
Fost, Dr. Norman, 149–50
Fox, Barry, 350

Framingham Heart Study, 286, 291
France, blood cholesterol levels in, 281–83
Francis, Bev, 34
Frank, Dr. Laurence, 171
Franz, Dr. Wanda, 83
Fraser, Laura, 65
Freiman, Dr. Jennie A., 175
Friedman, Debbie, 338
Friedman, Dr. Matthew J., 112
Frigoletto, Dr. Frederic D., Jr., 163
Frost, Dr. Marlene, 276
fruits, 1, 15, 16, 18, 219, 280, 285, 293, 341
Fuchs, Dr. Charles S., 12, 13
Fugger, Dr. Edward F., 153

**G**

Gaddy, Marcia, 175–76, 177
Gagnon, Dr. John, 125–26, 131–32
Gallagher-Thompson, Dolores, 100
gallbladder, cancer of the, 255
Galloway, Dr. Allison, 215
Galsworthy, Theresa, 231
gamma-butyrolactone, 330
Ganz, Dr. Patricia, 224, 245–46, 273
Gapstur, Dr. Susan M., 224
Garber, Dr. Alan, 270
Garcia, Dr. Jairo, 156–57
garcinia cambogia extract, 76
garlic, 297, 328, 334
Gaskin, Ina May, 172–73
gays, 142–43
Gebhart, Leslie Ingram, 244–45
Geer, Dr. James H., 125
Geller, Dr. Gail, 167
Genentech, 262, 264
Genetics & IVF Institute, 153, 155
germander, 335
Germany, research on herbal remedies in, 336, 351
Gharib, Dr. Soheyla D., 252
Gibala, Joan, 101
*Gift of Fear, The* (de Becker), 120
ginger, 334
ginkgo biloba, 161–62, 334, 336
ginseng, 332
Girls Inc., 208
*Girl Within, The* (Hancock), 195
Giuliano, Dr. Armando E., 272
Glantz, Dr. Stanton A., 287, 288
Glick, Dr. John, 268
glucosamine, 349–51
GnRH agonists, 184
Golant, Dr. Mitch, 91–92
Golant, Susan K., 91–92

Goldberg, Dr. Linn, 211, 212
Goldberg, Dr. Nieca, 289
goldenseal, 332
Goldman, Dr. Jan, 102–103
Goldrich, Sybil, 311, 312
golf, 29
Goodwin, Dr. Scott, 186
Gore, Al, 205
Gottman, Dr. John, 107–109, 110
grains, whole, 1, 14–15, 15, 16, 17, 219, 223, 280, 293, 296–97, 299
grandchildren, raising, 77, 87–89
Grandparents Information Center, 88
Grandparents Reaching Out, 88, 89
*Great Sex Weekend, The* (Schwartz), 135–36
Green, Dr. Joseph, 84–85
green tea, 17
Grey, Stella, 37
grief:
    after death of longtime partner, 99–102
    unresolved loss and, 102–104
Grifo, Dr. James A., 152
Grodstein, Dr. Francine, 225, 226
Groopman, Dr. Jerome, 270
Gruenwald, Dr. Joerg, 337
Guenther, Heidi, 191, 192
guided imagery, 327
Gulf War syndrome, 89, 90
Gurley, Dr. Bill J., 75–76
Guy, Dr. Roxanne, 309
Gynetics Inc., 129–30

**H**

Haas, Dr. Susan, 186
Haiken, Elizabeth, 304, 305
Hall, Dr. Doris M., 118, 120
Halmi, Dr. Katherine, 194
Halstead, Dr. Lauro, 354
Hamilton, Dr. Linda, 191–93
Hancock, Dr. Emily, 195
Hark, Dr. Lisa A., 295
Harper, Dr. Diane M., 251, 252
Harris, Dr. Tamara, 236–37
Harris, Herbert W., 230
Hartge, Dr. Patricia, 157
Hartmann, Dr. Lynn, 273, 274, 276, 277–78
Haseltine, Dr. Florence, 134
Haskell, Dr. William, 40
Haub, Carl, 205
Hauptman, Dr., 72, 73
Hawkes, Dr. Kristen, 215–16, 217
Hawkins, Alan, 86
Hawkins, Dr. Joy L., 172, 173
Hazlewood, Carlton F., 353

HCA (hydroxycitric acid) ("Citrimax"), 76
headaches, 327, 349
health and beauty, association between, 303–305
*Healthline,* 43
Health Professionals Follow-Up Study, 282
*Health Psychology,* 194
Heaney, Dr. Robert P., 8
heart attacks, 19, 20, 52, 70, 129, 131
    before age 50, 279, 288–90
    gender differences in survival of, 279
    smoking and, 280, 284
    statistics, xiv, 14
heart disease, 55, 61, 70, 211, 222, 227, 279–300, 343, 357
    alcohol and, 280, 281–82, 297–98, 300
    diet to prevent, 280, 292–95
    exercise and, 25, 280, 284–85
    fats and, 19–22, 280
    fiber and, 14, 282
    folic acid (folate) and, 280, 283, 296, 298–99
    lipoprotein (a), 285–86
    Mediterranean diet and, 292–95
    mortality statistics, xiii, xiv, 241, 244, 249
    risk after menopause of, 214, 218, 221, 224, 225, 241, 279
    secondhand smoke and, 280, 287–88
    triglyceride levels and, 290–92
    vitamin B-6, 280, 296, 297, 298, 299
    weight control and, 280
Heerdt, Dr. Alexandra, 246
height, 197, 199–200
    breast cancer risk and, 248
Heiman, Dr. Julia, 125–26
Helzlsouer, Dr. Kathy, 224, 242, 245
herbal remedies, 325, 331–37
    Asian, 324, 329–30
    to avoid, 335
    chart, 334–35
    combination of chemicals in, 333–36
    diet products, 75–76
    drug interactions, 326, 336
    labeling of, 332, 333, 337
    pregnancy risks of, 161–62
    quality standards, 331–32
    regulation of, 324, 328, 329, 331–33, 336–37
    safety of, questioning, 326, 336
    *see also specific herbs*
Herceptin, 262, 263–64
Herman-Giddens, Dr. Marcia E., 196
herpes, 145, 316

Hesse-Biber, Dr Sharlene, 196, 198, 199
Heymsfield, Dr. Steven B., 72, 73, 74, 75, 76
Heywood, Leslie, 35
"Hidden Epidemic, The," 145
high blood pressure, *see* hypertension
high-density lipoproteins (HDLs), 21, 68, 218, 228, 280, 281, 288, 292, 296, 298, 300, 340
Hill, Dr. Kim, 216–17
Hill, Dr. James O., 58–59
Hirsch, Dr. Jules, 71, 72–73, 74
Hirshaut, Dr. Yashar, 253
Hislop, Dr. T. Gregory, 252
Hobbins, Dr. John C., 166
Hobbs, Dr. Helen, 286
Hochman, Dr. Judith, 289–90
Hofer, Dr. Myron, 80
Hoffman, Dr. Eileen, 252
Hoffman, Dr. Robert S., 321
Hoffman-LaRoche, 54, 70, 71, 72
Hokanson, Dr. John E., 292
Hollidge, Margaret, 88
Holmes, Dr. King K., 144
Holmes, Dr. Lewis, 162
Holt, Dr. Peter R., 6
Holtzworth-Munroe, Amy, 107
homeopathic remedies, 323, 328
homocysteine, 296, 299, 300, 342
homosexuality, 142–43
*Hope in a Jar: The Making of America's Culture* (Peiss), 305
Horger, Dr. E. O., 3rd, 165
Horlick, Dr. Michael, 10
*Hormone of Desire, The* (Rako), 228
hormone replacement therapy, 214, 219, 220, 221–26
    bone density and, 231, 233, 234, 235, 238
    breast cancer and, 214, 221–24, 241, 245
    heart disease and, 214, 218, 221, 224, 225
    testosterone as part of, 133, 227–28
Horn, Mildred, 88
Hortobagyi, Dr. Gabriel, 266, 267, 268, 269
Houpt, Dr. Joseph B., 350
Hrdy, Dr. Sarah Blaffer, 171
Hu, Dr. Frank, 70
Huesmann, Dr. L. Rowell, 114
*Human Birth: An Evolutionary Perspective* (Trevathan), 168–69
human chorionic gonadotropin, 74
*Human Reproduction,* 153
Hummer, Robert, 338

Hunter, Bruce, 143
Hurtado, Dr. Magdalena, 216–17
Huston, Dr. James E., 218
Hyams, Capt. Kenneth C., 89, 90
Hyman, Dr. Steven, 96
Hynes, Dr. Noreen, 145
hypericin, 336
hyperopia, laser surgery to correct, 313–17
hypertension, 55, 298, 331, 338
  calcium and, 4, 7
  drugs to treat, 160
  exercise and, 25
  heart disease and, 284
  salt and, 7
hypnosis, 325, 327
  false memories and, 84–85
hysterectomy, 148, 182–83, 184
hysteroscopy, 185
*Hystories: Hysterical Epidemics and Modern Media* (Showalter), 90

**I**

Iams, Dr. Jay, 163–64
Imber-Black, Dr. Evan, 103
immune response, DHEA and, 357
impotence, 137–39
  Viagra for, *see* Viagra
Ingram, Carolyn, 244–45
insomnia, 325
Institute of Medicine, National Academy of Sciences, 310, 311, 312–13
insulin, 11, 283
  insensitivity, 67
insulin resistance, 11
insurance coverage:
  for alternative medicine, 325, 348
  for bone marrow transplants, 267–68
  for laser eye surgery, 316
  for Prometrium, 356
  for rhinoplasty, 318
*Internal Medicine News*, 87
Internet, personal trainers on the, 48–50
in vitro fertilization, 148
Iowa Women's Study, 282, 296
iron, 3, 9, 343, 347
  calcium's effect of absorption of, 340
  dangers of supplements to children, 340

**J**

Jacobson, Dr. Neil, 107–109, 110
Jarvis, Dr. William, 354
Jennings, Kevin, 142–43
Johnson, Dr. Lawrence A., 154
Johnson, Sheridan, 146

Johnston, Dr. Lloyd D., 211
Jones, Dr. Nicholas Blurton, 215
Jones, Justice Robert E., 310
Jordan, Dr. V. Craig, 259, 261
*Journal of Cardiovascular Risk*, 291–92
*Journal of Clinical Oncology, The*, 272
*Journal of Nutrition, The*, 19
*Journal of the American College of Cardiology*, 291
*Journal of the American Medical Association*, 6, 10, 14, 39, 71, 72, 130, 162, 224, 225, 248, 282, 286, 298
*Journal of the National Cancer Institute*, 252, 255
Jovanovic, Oliver, 122
Justice, Dr. Robert, 262, 263
"Just the Facts About Sexual Orientation & Youth," 142–43

**K**

Kaiser-Permanente, 325
Kalick, S. Michael, 304
Kaplowitz, Dr. Paul B., 197
Karlikaya, Dr. Guvene, 157
Kash, Dr. Kathryn, 251
Kassirer, Dr. Jerome P., 329
kava, 332, 334, 351–53
Kawachi, Dr. Ichiro, 287
Kearney-Cooke, Dr. Ann, 204
Kegel exercises, 27–28
Kennedy, Keith, 29
Kennell, Dr. John H., 177
Kerr, Dr. Michael, 116
Kessler, Dr. John F., 261
ketosis, 66
Keys, Dr. Ancel, 292
Khattak, Dr. Sohail, 162, 163
Kienlen, Dr. Kristine, 118, 119
Kindy, Joan and Hal, 99–101
King, Dr. Mary-Claire, 255
Kinsey, Dr. Alfred C., 125
Kirkland, Gelsey, 192
Kligman, Dr. Albert M., 305
Kling, Dr. Alan, 322
Klock, Dr. Susan, 151
knee pain, 350–51
Knight, Dr. Julia, 242–43
Knoll Pharmaceuticals, 72
Knopp, Dr. Robert H., 68
Knudson, Dr. Alfred, 256
Ko, Dr. Richard, 329–30
Koenig, Dr. Harold, 338, 339
Kolodny, Dr. Robert, 136, 137
kombucha tea, 335
Koren, Dr. Gideon, 162
Korsmeyer, Dr. Stanley, 220

Kraemer, Dr. William J., 29
Kramer, Dr. Peter, 91
Krauss, Dr. Ronald, 21
Kris-Etherton, Dr. Penny, 21
Krug, Larry, 46, 47
Kuney, Deb, 76
Kupfer, Dr. David, 95, 96
Kyffin, Dr. Robert, 174

**L**

lactose, 8, 232
*Lancet, The*, 129, 180, 263, 327, 338, 355
Landmark Healthcare Inc., 325
Landry, Dr. Susan H., 176, 177
Lanka, Dr. L. Darlene, 218
larynx, cancer of the, 12
laser eye surgery, 313–17
Lasik (laser in situ keratomileusis), 313–15
Laumann, Dr. Edward, 130–31
Law, Dr. Malcolm, 281
laxatives, 336
Leaf, Dr. Alexander, 294
Ledger, Dr. William, 175
Lee, Dr. Roberta, 352–53
Leffler, Dr. Christopher, 351
legumes, 293, 296, 299, 342
Lehnhardt, John, 170
Leiblum, Dr. Sandra R., 125
Levy-Koffer, Nathalie, 35–37
Lewy, Dr. Alfred, 97, 99
Lichtenstein, Dr. Alice H., 17, 68
Lichter, Dr. Allen S., 269
lidocaine, 322
Liebeskind, Dr. Doreen, 252–54
Liebman, Bonnie, 247
Liebowitz, Dr. Barry D., 229, 230
Liederbach, Marijeanne, 192
Lindsay, Dr. Robert, 233
Lindston, Kathie, 176
Lipkin, Dr. Martin, 6
lipoprotein (a), 285–86
liposuction, 302, 321–22
Lippiello, Dr. Louis, 351
liver cancer, 211
Lloyd-Hart, Margaret, 156, 157
lobelia, 335
Lockwood, Dr. Charles, 174, 175
Lomando, Russell M., 60
Longenbach, Lee Roy, 38, 39
longevity:
  spirituality and, 337–39
  vitamin and mineral supplements and, 340
*Losing It: False Hopes and Fat Profits in the Diet Industry* (Fraser), 65

Love, Dr. Lori A., 330
Love, Dr. Susan, 250, 275
LoVecchio, Dr. Frank, 330
low-density lipoproteins (LDLs), 68, 228, 282, 285–86, 297, 343
Lowe, Maria, 34
Lowe, Dr. Michael, 57
*Low-Fat Lies, High-Fat Frauds, and the Healthiest Diet in the World* (Vigilante and Flynn), 67, 68
Ludwig, Dr. David, 68–69
lumpectomy, 253, 272
lung cancer, 12, 16, 239, 244, 248, 343
  secondhand smoke and, 287
Lupron, 331
lupus, 357
Lynn, Dr. Steven Jay, 84
Lyon, Lisa, 33–34

**M**

McCaffrey, Maeve, 47
McCarron, Dr. David, 7
McCully, Dr. Kilmer S., 299
McDonald, Heather, 189–90
McGann, Nadine, 94–95
McGuire, Dr. William, 267
Mackenzie, Roderick, 129
McLaren-Hume, Mavis, 59
McLish, Rachel, 34
Magnaflex Inc., 354
magnesium, 342, 343, 347
  diabetes and, 11
magnet therapy, 353–55
Mahady, Gail, 355
ma huang, *see* ephedra
Maines, Dr. Rachel P., 139–41
malignant melanoma, 255
Malmstrom, Dr. Hans, 320
mammography, 252–54
  breast implants, interference of, 308
Mann, Dorothy, 145–46
Manson, Dr. JoAnn E., 60
Marchell, Dr. Tim, 210
margarine, 21, 246
Marin, Dr. Amy Dabul, 82–83
Markman, Dr. Maurie, 266
Marriott, Dr. Bernadette, 341, 342, 344
Martins, Peter, 192–93
massage therapy, 323, 325, 327
Mast, Coleen Kelly, 190
mastectomy, radical, xiii, 272, 277
Masters and Johnson, 137–38
*Maximizing the Arthritis Cure* (Theodosakis), 350
Mayer, Dr. Jean, 66
Mayo Clinic, 273–76

meats, red, 1, 15, 222–23, 280, 281, 297
media:
  coverage of health issues, xiii
  teenage girls, influence on, 187, 200–201, 208
medicalization, 130, 131
medicine ball, 46–47
meditation, 327, 337
Mediterranean diet, 69–70, 292–95
melatonin, 97–99
Melbye, Dr. Mads, 158
Meloy, Dr. J. Reid, 117, 118–19
Mendell, Patricia, 151
Meneses, Alex, 46
menopause and aging, 213–38
  of attractive women, 307–308
  blood pressure, and calcium, 7
  bone loss, 214, 218, 226, 231–38
  depression and, 228–30
  evolutionary theories of, 213–14, 215–17
  heart disease, risk of, *see* heart disease, risk after menopause of
  hormone replacement, *see* hormone replacement therapy
  life without, 219–21
  "natural" remedies for, 323, 336, 351
  perimenopause, 128, 218–19
  *see also* elderly
menstruation, 127, 197, 218
Meridia, 52, 72, 74–75
Messina, Dr. Mark, 223
Metabolife International, 75–76
methotrexate, 344
Meyerson, Rev. Beth, 144–45
Miacalcin (calcitonin), 234, 236
Michels, Karin, 158
Milbauer, Alan, 262
milk, 7, 8, 10, 17, 232
  breast, *see* breast-feeding
milk thistle, 335
Miller, Dr. Michael, 291
Miller, Jackie, 146
*Mind and Heart in Human Sexual Behavior, The* (Bell), 135
mind-body connection, 325
minerals:
  in breakfast foods, 4
  supplements, *see* vitamin and mineral supplements
  *see also specific minerals*
Mitchell, Dr. Allen, 162, 163
Molnar, Marika, 27–28
monounsaturated fats, 20, 21, 69, 70, 247, 293, 295
Moran, Jeffrey P., 190

Morley, Dr. Jeff, 318–20
Morrow, Dr. Monica, 224
Mortola, Dr. Joseph F., 81, 181, 182
Morton's neuroma, 31
Mount Sinai Medical Center, New York, 88
mouth, cancer of the, 12, 16
Ms. Olympia, 34, 35
Mullen, Dr. Paul E., 117
Munson, Tammy, 59–60
Murphy, Dr. Suzanne P., 343
muscular tension, 327
Muto, Dr. Michael G., 255
myolysis, 183
myomectomy, 182, 185–86
myopia, laser surgery to correct, 313–17

**N**

Nagin, Dr. Daniel, 113, 114
Naidu, Laveen, 193
Nanni, Dr. Christopher, 202–203, 318
National Academy of Sciences, calcium recommendations of, 6
National Alliance for the Mentally Ill, 230
National Association to Advance Fat Acceptance, 53, 54
National Breast Cancer Coalition, 269
National Cancer Institute, 14, 225, 241, 245, 261, 262, 263, 342
National Center for Health Statistics, 249
National Cholesterol Education Program, 291
National Coalition Against Domestic Violence, 111
National Council Against Health Fraud, 348
National Depressive and Manic Depressive Association, 230
National Domestic Violence Hotline, 110, 111
National Food Consumption Survey, 342–43
National Foundation for Depressive Illness, 230
National Health and Nutrition Examination Survey, 54
National Health Interview Survey, 337–38
National Heart, Lung and Blood Institute, 53
National Institute of Diabetes and Digestive and Kidney Disease, 53
National Institute of Drug Abuse, 210–11
National Institute of Mental Health, 96, 229, 230

National Institute on Aging, 236
National Institute on Drug Abuse, 212
National Institutes of Health, 8, 51, 53, 54, 332, 348
  calcium recommendations, 6
  Office of Alternative Medicine, 349, 354
  Office of Dietary Supplements, 336, 341
National Institutes of Mental Health, 81
National Organization for Victim Assistance, 121
National Osteoporosis Foundation, 232, 233, 234
National Resource Center on Domestic Violence, Battered Women's Justice Project, The, 111
National Victim Center, 121
National Violence Prevention Fund, 111
National Weight Control Registry, 58, 59, 76
"natural" remedies, cautions about, 323–24, 326, 328, 336
*Nature*, 216
Nature Conservancy, 352
*Nature Medicine*, 76
*Nature's Cures*, 327
Naylor, Stephen, 76
*Necessary Losses* (Viorst), 103
neck, cosmetic surgery on the, 320–21
Nelson, Dr. Anita L., 127
Nestle, Dr. Marion, 281, 283, 340
*Neurology*, 70
New, Dr. Maria I., 135
Newcomb, Dr. Polly A., 158
*New England Journal of Medicine*, 9, 12, 13, 20, 81, 137, 157, 163, 166, 225, 242, 246–47, 273, 288, 297, 321, 328
niacin (nicotinic acid), 346
nicotine, *see* smoking
Niebyl, Dr. Jennifer, 159
Nielsen, Rev. Barbara H., 339
Noble, Elizabeth, 27
Nolvadex, *see* tamoxifen
Northern California Cancer Center, 325
Norton, Dr. Larry, 224, 264, 265, 267, 268, 273, 343, 344
nose job (rhinoplasty), 302, 317–18
*Not-So-Scary Breast Cancer Book* (Ingram and Gebhart), 244–45
Nowak, Dr. Judith, 96
Nurses' Health Study, 10, 13, 14, 15, 60, 70, 226, 287–88, 295, 299, 300
nursing, 178–80, 181, 248
nutrition, 1–24, 199, 341, 344
  at breakfast, 3–4

food pyramid, *see* food pyramid
French diet and blood cholesterol levels, 281–83
weight control and, 55, 59, 62
*see also specific foods, nutrients, and diet-related diseases*
*Nutrition Action Health Letter*, 16, 40, 247, 357
*Nutrition Business Journal*, 351
nuts, 282–83, 293, 295

## O

Oberfield, Dr. Sharon E., 197
obesity, 51, 54, 67, 197, 238
O'Connell, Dr. James, 215
Odes, Rebecca, 189–90
Offit, Dr. Kenneth, 257
O'Hara, Dr. Michael W., 181
oils, *see specific types of oils*
Oktay, Dr. Kutluk, 156–57
Okuda, Dr. Wynn, 319
Olanow, Dr. C. Warren, 266
olive oil, 17, 20, 69, 70, 247, 280, 292, 293, 295
omega-3 fatty acids, 70, 292, 293
Ondrizek, Dr. Richard, 161
oral contraceptives, *see* birth control pills
orange juice, 296, 299
Orlistat, *see* Xenical
Ornish, Dr. Dean, 20–21, 67, 283, 293, 295
Orth-Gomer, Dr. Kristina, 286
O'Shaughnessy, Dr. Joyce, 270
osteoarthritis, 349, 350
osteoporosis, 1, 4, 7, 128, 220, 222, 232–34, 237, 342, 343
  drugs for, 234–36, 238
  exercise and, 25
  PMS as harbinger of, 5
  risk factors, 233, 234, 235
  vitamin D deficiency and, 9–10
ovarian cancer, 17, 128, 156–57, 273, 357
  bone marrow transplants for, 265–66
  inherited risk of cancer-causing mutations, 255, 256
ovarian tissue transplant, 148, 156–57
overweight, being, *see* obesity; weight and weight control
oxalic acid, 8
Oxford University, 297

## P

pancreatic cancer, 255
parathyroid hormone, 5
Parshall, Janet, 143

Pascali-Bonaro, Debra, 176
Paterson-Brown, Dr. Sara, 174
Patsky, Matthew, 341
Pauling, Dr. Linus, 343
Paulk, John, 143
PC-SPEC, 330, 331
Pearson, Cindy, 262
peas, *see* legumes
Pecora, Dr. Andrew, 268
*Pediatrics*, 68, 197, 199
Peiss, Kathy, 305
Pennington, Dr. Alfred, 65
*Penn State Sports Medicine Newsletter*, 28
Pennsylvania State University, 69
pennyroyal, 326, 328, 335
Perelman, Dr. Michael A., 136
perimenopause, 128, 218–19
*Perimenopause: Changes in a Woman's Health After 35* (Huston and Lanka), 218
*Perimenopause: Preparing for the Change* (Teaff and Wiley), 218
Perls, Dr. Thomas, 216
personal trainers on the Internet, 48–50
pesticides, xiv
Petrek, Dr. Jeanne, 277
Petro, Dr. Jane, 204
Pfizer, 126, 131
pharynx, cancer of the, 12
Phelan, Dr. Sharon, 178
phentermine, 71–72, 74
Philip Morris Companies, 287
Philippi, Dr. Alan, 351
phobias, 94
phosphorus, 342
*Physical and Rehabilitation Medicine*, 354
*Physicians' Desk Reference for Herbal Medicines*, 332, 337
Physicians' Health Study, 296
phytic acid, 8
phytoestrogens, 342
Pierce, Bill, 151–52
pilates, 44–45
Pilates, Joseph, 44
Pinkerton, Darlene and Thomas, 149
Pipher, Dr. Mary, 199
Pitman, Dr. Gerald H., 203, 317
placebos, 325, 338
plantain (herb), 330
plastic surgery:
  breast reconstruction, 277–78
  cosmetic, *see* cosmetic surgery
PMS, *see* premenstrual syndrome (PMS)
Pointer, Sam C., Jr., 310
poke root, 335
Poll, Heinz, 192

polycystic ovarian syndrome, 134
polyunsatured fats, 20, 21, 69, 70, 247, 283, 293, 295
Pope, Dr. Harrison G., Jr., 211–12
porcelain veneer, 319–20
*Postgraduate Medical Journal,* 177
*Postgraduate Medicine,* 295
post-traumatic stress syndrome, 106, 112, 117
prayer, 323, 337
pregnancy, 131, 147–48
    after cancer treatment, 148, 156–57
    childbirth, *see* childbirth
    choosing baby's sex, 153–55
    drugs during, 159–60, 259
    exercise and, 27–28
    fetal monitors, 163–64
    herbal remedies during, 161–62
    new technology aiding conception, 148
    solvents and birth defects, 162–63
    teenage, 196, 205–208
    ultrasound, 164–67
premenstrual syndrome (PMS), 78, 81–82
    calcium and, 1, 4, 5
presbyopia, 315, 317
President's Commission on Dietary Supplement Labels, 336
Pressman, Dr. Peter I., 253
Preven, 129–30
Pritchard, Dr. Kathleen I., 263
PRK (photorefractive keratectomy), 316
Progest, 355
progesterone, 81
    wild yams as source of natural, 355–56
progestin, *see* hormone replacement therapy
Prometrium, 355–56
Proscar, 333
prostate, enlarged, 333
prostate cancer, 21, 255, 343
    herbal remedies for, 331
prostitutes, 112
protein, 8, 16, 219, 232, 248
    high-fat, high-protein diets, 64–67
Prozac, 78, 82, 94, 95
*Psychiatric Research,* 99
*Psychology of Stalking: Clinical and Forensic Perspectives* (Meloy), 117, 118
*Psychosomatics,* 331
psyllium, 335

**Q**

Quade, Dr. Brad, 183
Quinn, Gail, 83

Quirk, Dr. Frances, 126

**R**

radiation therapy, 253
    parents choosing alternative medicine over, 324, 329
Rako, Dr. Susan, 228
raloxifene (Evista), 222, 234, 236, 261
Ramsay, Dr. David J., 348–49
Rao, Dr. Rama B., 321
rape, 122, 307
rape shield law, 122
Rasmussen, Helen, 17
Ratner, Elaine, 243–44
Rawlins, Dr., 155
Reardon, Dr. David, 83
Rebarber, Dr. Andrei, 173, 175
rectal cancer, *see* colon (colorectal) cancer
*Red Devil: To Hell With Cancer—and Back, The* (Rich), 271
Redmond, Dr. Geoffrey P., 133
Rees, Dr. Thomas D., 318
refined foods:
    flour, 2, 280
reflexology, 327
Regan, Claire, 21
relaxation response, 338
relaxation techniques, 327
religion and heath, 337–39
RenewTrient, 330–31
Response Oncology, 267, 269
*Reviving Ophelia: Saving the Selves of Adolescent Girls* (Pipher), 199
rheumatoid arthritis, 233
rhinoplasty, 302, 317–18
Rich, Kathy, 271
Rimm, Dr. Eric B., 281, 283, 297, 299, 300
Rittmaster, Dr. Roger S., 133, 134
Roberts, Miles, 170
Rogers, Dr. Alan, 217
Rolland, Dr. John, 103
Rosen, Dr. James C., 56
Rosen, Dr. Laura Epstein, 91, 92
Rosen, Dr. Raymond, 130–31
Rosenberg, Dr. Karen, 169
Rosenberg, Dr. Lynn, 225, 226
Rosenberg, Dr. Michael J., 227
Rosenblatt, Stanley, 287
Rosenthal, Dr. Larry, 319, 320
Roth, Dr. David M., 176
Ruddy, Dr. Shaun, 311
Rudorfer, Dr. Matthew, 96
running, 29
Russell, Dr. Robert M., 17, 18
Russo, Dr. Nancy Felipe, 82–83, 84

Ruzek, Dr. Sheryl Burt, 166

**S**

Sackheim, Dr. Harold, 95
Sahlins, Dr. Marshall, 201
St. John's wort, 161–62, 328, 332, 333–36, 336
salmon, canned, 8, 232
salt, 7, 8
Sampson, Dr. Wallace, 348
sardines, canned, 8, 232
sassafras, 331, 335
saturated fats, 2, 15, 19, 20, 21, 67, 68, 69, 70, 280, 292, 295
Sauer, Dr. Mark V., 149, 150
Saunders, Dr. Daniel, 108
Saunders, Rhonda, 117
saw palmetto, 161–62, 328, 333, 335, 336
Schairer, Dr. Catherine, 225
Schatzkin, Dr. Arthur, 13
schizophrenia, 102
Schmidt, Dr. Peter J., 81, 82
Schnall, Dr. Mitchell, 246
Schnur, Dr. Paul, 322
Schulman, Dr. Joseph, 153
Schultz, Dr. William B., 329
Schwartz, Dr. Arthur, 357
Schwartz, Dr. Pepper, 135–36
Scott, Dr. Susan Craig, 204
scullcap, 335
Seaman, Barbara, 129
Sears, Dr. Barry, 67, 68
seasonal affective disorder (SAD), 97–99
secondhand smoke, 280, 287–88
*Secret Life of Families, The* (Imber-Black), 103
Seedor, Dr. John, 313, 314–15
seeds, 293, 295
    as calcium source, 8
Seefeldt, Carol A., 86
Seidel, Dr. George, 155
selenium, 343, 344, 347
self-esteem of teenage girls, 195, 198–99, 208
Sellers, Dr. Thomas A., 223–24
Seltzer, Dr. Vicki L., 175
separation anxiety, 94, 200
SERMs (selective estrogen receptor modulators), 261
sexual abuse, 196
sexuality, 123–46
    contraception, *see* contraception
    female orgasm, 139, 140
    female sex drive, 124, 126, 130–32, 214, 219, 227–28

female sexual response, 125–26
homosexuality, 142–43
intercourse after childbirth, 177–78
sex education, 189–91
of teenage girls, 196, 205–208
testosterone and, *see* testosterone
transexuals, 141–42
Viagra's emotional impact, 135–36
vibrators, 139–41
sexually transmitted diseases, 124, 127, 144–46
teenagers and, 206, 207
Shandler, Nina, 219
Shepherd, Dr. Janet E., 255
Sherwin, Dr. Barbara, 228
Sherwin, Galen, 122
Shine, Dr. Kenneth, 312
*Should You Leave?* (Kramer), 91
Showalter, Dr. Elaine, 90
Shulman, Dr. Mark, 315, 317
sibutramine, *see* Meridia
Siscovick, Dr. David S., 295
skin care products, 304–305
Slamon, Dr. Dennis, 264
sleep, 87, 117
Sloan, Dr. Richard, 338–39
Smith, Ed, 351, 352
Smith, Michael, 42
SmithKline Beecham, 5, 332
Smith-Warner, Dr. Stephanie, 249
smoking, 159, 160, 222, 226, 233, 234, 235
breast cancer and, 249
heart attacks and, 280, 284
lung cancer and, 248
secondhand smoke, 280, 287–88
teenage, xiv, 188, 195, 196
*Social Organization of Sexuality, The* (Laumann et al.), 130–31
*Social Science Information*, 115
Society of Cardiovascular and Interventional Radiology, 185
sodium chloride, 7, 8
sodium fluoride, 236
solvents and birth defects, 162–63
Southwestern University Medical Center, 343
soybean oil, 20, 69, 70
soy foods, 8, 16–17, 219, 223, 261, 280, 296
Spain, Joan, 319
Spear, Dr. Scott, 309
sperm donation, 148, 151
Speroff, Dr. Leon, 129
Spiegel, Dr. David, 325
Spies, Dr. James B., 186

spinach, 8, 232, 299
spirituality, 323, 337–39
Spitzer, Dr. Robert, 81
sports, *see* exercise; *specific sports*
SSRIs (selective serotonin re-uptake inhibitors), 94, 160
stalking, 106, 117–21
Stampfer, Dr. Meir, 281, 282–83, 297, 298
Stanford University, 188, 193–94, 325
STAR (Study of Tamoxifen and Raloxifene), 261
Stein, Dr. Martin T., 200
stepfathers, abusive, 106, 114–16
steroids, 233
DHEA (dihydroepiandrosterone), 356–57
use by teenage girls, 210–12
Stillman, Dr. Irving, 65
Stoller, Dr. Melissa, 167–68
stomach cancer, 12, 16, 255
Stone, Robyn I., 100
strength training, 26, 29, 42–44, 212, 222, 231
stress, 327
of raising grandchildren, 87–89
of working mothers, 77, 85–87
stroke, 25, 52, 102, 129, 298, 349
Stuart, Richard B., 56
Studd, Dr. John W. W., 133, 181
Studin, Dr. Joel, 309
Stunkard, Dr. Albert, 56–57, 59, 74
sugar, 2, 223, 292
blood sugar, *see* blood sugar
-free foods, 62–64
Sultan, Dr. Mark, 202
sun exposure, vitamin D and, 9–10, 232
Surgical Eyes, 316
*Survival of the Prettiest: The Science of Beauty* (Etcoff), 303, 306
Survivors of Stalking, 121
Swain, Tony, 47
Sweda, Edward L., 287
swimming, 29
syphilis, 146

**T**

tai chi, 327
"Take Care of Your Feet for a Lifetime," 31–32
Talbot, Jan, 210
*Talking to Children About Their Conception: It's Easier Than You Think* (Wilkins), 152
Taller, Dr. Herman, 65
tamoxifen, 221, 222, 246–47, 253, 257–63

*Tamoxifen* (Kessler and Annussek), 261
Taylor, Dr. C. Barr, 194
Taylor, Judy, 35
Taylor, Dr. Maida, 128
tea, 280, 297
green, 17
*Teaching Sex: Shaping Adolescence in the 20th Century* (Moran), 190
Teaff, Dr. Nancy Lee, 218
teenage girls, 187–212
age at puberty, 196–97
cosmetic surgery among, 202–205
eating disorders among, *see* eating disorders
emotional problems and stunted growth, 199–200
media influence on, 187, 200–201, 208
parental guidance of, 188
pregnancies, 196, 205–208
self-esteem of, 195, 198–99, 208
sex and, 196, 205–208
sex education, 189–91, 208
sexually transmitted diseases among, 206, 207
smoking and drinking by, iv, 88, 195, 196, 209–10
steroid use by, 210–12
teeth:
calcium for, *see* calcium, for bones and teeth
cosmetic dentistry, 318–20
temperament, 79, 80
Temple Dr. Robert, 336
tennis, 28–29
tennis elbow, 349
Terman, Dr. Michael, 97, 99
testosterone, 43, 123, 131, 132–34, 219, 227–28
Theodosakis, Dr. Jason, 350
Thomas, Dr. Melissa K., 9–10
3M, 310–11
throat, cancer of the, 16
Thun, Dr. Michael, 12, 297, 298
thyroid deficiencies, 233
Thys-Jacobs, Dr. Susan, 5
Tilly, Dr. Jonathan L., 220, 221
tobacco, *see* smoking
Tobacco Institute, 287
Todd, Dr. Jan, 35
Tops (Take Off Pounds Sensibly), 76
Tracey, Margaret, 27–28
transexuals, 141–42
trans fatty acids, 19–20, 21, 70, 280, 295
Tremblay, Dr. Richard E., 114
Trepathy, Dr. Debu, 264
Trevathan, Dr. Wenda, 168–69

triglycerides, 21, 70, 283, 290–92
two-hit hypothesis, 256
Tyler, Dr. Varro E., 331–32, 333, 336

## U

ultrasound:
  of breast lumps, 253, 254
  scanning during pregnancy, 164–67
U.S. Department of Agriculture, 61, 343
United States Preventative Services
  Task Force, 250
University of Arizona Cancer Center, 344
University of North Carolina, 210
unresolved loss, 102–104
urushiol, 326
uterine cancer, 16, 128
  tamoxifen and, 247, 258, 259, 261,
    262, 263
Utiger, Dr. Robert D., 10, 137

## V

Vaccarino, Dr. Viola, 289, 290
valerian, 335
Vallbona, Dr. Carlos, 353–54
vegetables, 1, 15, 16, 18, 219, 223, 280,
  285, 293, 341
  as calcium source, 8
  dark green leafy, 70, 232, 296, 299, 342
Ventura, Stephanie, 205, 206
*Venus Envy: A History of Cosmetic
  Surgery* (Haiken), 304
Vermeil, Al, 47
Viagra, 123, 124, 125, 126, 131, 135–39
  emotional impact of, 135–36
  limitations and side effects of, 137–39
vibrators, 139–41
Vigilante, Dr. Kevin, 67, 68
violence, 105–22
Viorst, Judith, 103
Visco, Fran, 15, 269
vision correction:
  contact lenses, 305
  laser surgery, 313–17
  Lasik (laser in situ keratomileusis),
    313–15, 316
visualization, 327
vitamin A, 343, 344, 345
vitamin and mineral supplements, 19,
  323, 324, 339–47
  chart, 345–47
  dangers of, 340, 343–44
  dietary deficiencies and, 343
  efficacy of, 340
  government guidelines for, 341–42
  labeling of, 341
  regulation of, 324, 326, 329, 340

vitamin B-6 (pyridoxine), 280, 296, 297,
  298, 299, 343, 344, 346
vitamin B-12, 19, 346
vitamin C, 3, 66–67, 280, 343, 344, 345
  chemotherapy and, 343–44
vitamin D, 1, 3, 17, 67, 233, 234, 235,
  342, 344, 346
  calcium absorption and, 4, 5, 8, 9, 10,
    223, 232
  osteoporosis and deficiency of, 9–10
  sun exposure and, 9–10, 232
  supplements, 10, 232, 238
vitamin E, 222, 280, 343, 344, 346
vitamin K, 340
vitamins:
  in breakfast cereals, 4
  supplements, *see* vitamin and mineral
    supplements
  *see also specific vitamins*
Vondras, Father John, 83
Voog, Ana, 308, 309–10

## W

Wadden, Dr. Thomas, 58
Wadler, Dr. Gary I., 211
Wald, Dr. Nicholas, 281
walking, 29, 40, 222
Wallace, Alfred Russell, 303
Wallace, Dr. David, 315
Warner Lambert, 332
Warren, Dr. Michelle, 191, 193
Wasserheit, Dr. Judith N., 144, 145, 146
water, 17–18, 64
Weber, Dr. Barbara, 241, 242, 243,
  262–63, 273
Wechsler, Dr. Henry, 209, 210
weight and weight control, 51–77, 357
  behavior modification approach to,
    56–57
  body mass index (B.M.I.), 53–54
  danger of being moderately over-
    weight, 60–62
  diet drugs, *see* diet drugs
  diets to lose, *see* diets, weight loss
  eating disorders, *see* eating disorders
  exercise and, 51–52, 55, 58, 62, 64
  fiber and, 15
  guidelines, 61
  heart disease and, 280, 284, 285
  hip fractures and weight loss after 50,
    236–38
  maintaining weight loss, 58–60, 64, 76
  nutrition and, 55, 59, 62
  osteoporosis and, 233
  overweight in America, 39, 51–52,
    53–56, 60–62

triglyceride levels and, 292
  willpower and, 56–58
weight training, *see* strength training
Weisfuse, Dr. Isaac, 145
Weissman, Dr. Myrna M., 93–94
Wessely, Dr. Simon, 90, 91
West, Dr. William H., 266, 267, 269
Wetzel, Justice William A., 122
*What to Do When Love Turns Violent*
  (Betancourt), 110
*What to Do When Someone You Love Is
  Depressed* (Golant and Golant),
  91–92
*When Men Batter Women* (Jacobson and
  Gottman), 107, 110
Whiting, Dr. William C., 42
Wickerham, Dr. D. Lawrence, 261
widows, grief of, 99–102
Wild, Dr. Robert A., 132
wild yams, 332, 355–56
Wiley, Kim Wright, 218
Wilkins, Carole Lieber, 152
Willett, Dr. Walter C., 11, 15, 21
Williams, Dr. George C., 216
Williamson, Dr. David F., 56, 71, 73
willpower, 56–58
Wilson, Dr. Margo, 115
wine, *see* alcohol
Wing, Dr. Rena, 58–59
Winley, Diane Lacey, 337
Wolk, Dr. Alicja, 14
Wolkowitz, Dr. Owen M., 357
working mothers, 77, 85–87
World Cancer Research Fund, 16
World Health Organization, 53, 297
wormwood, 335
Wynne, Dr. Lyman, 102, 103

## X

Xenical, 52, 54–56, 70–75

## Y

Yang, Dr. Grace, 253
Yesalis, Dr. Charles E., 211, 212
yoga, 327
yogurt, 8, 232, 293
Youchah, Dr. Joan R., 181

## Z

Zeneca Pharmaceuticals, 262, 263
Zenilman, Dr. Jonathan, 146
zhong gan ling, 330
zinc, 340, 343, 347
Zirkin, Dr. Barry, 155
"Zone" diet, 67
Zuckerman, Dr. Diana, 309

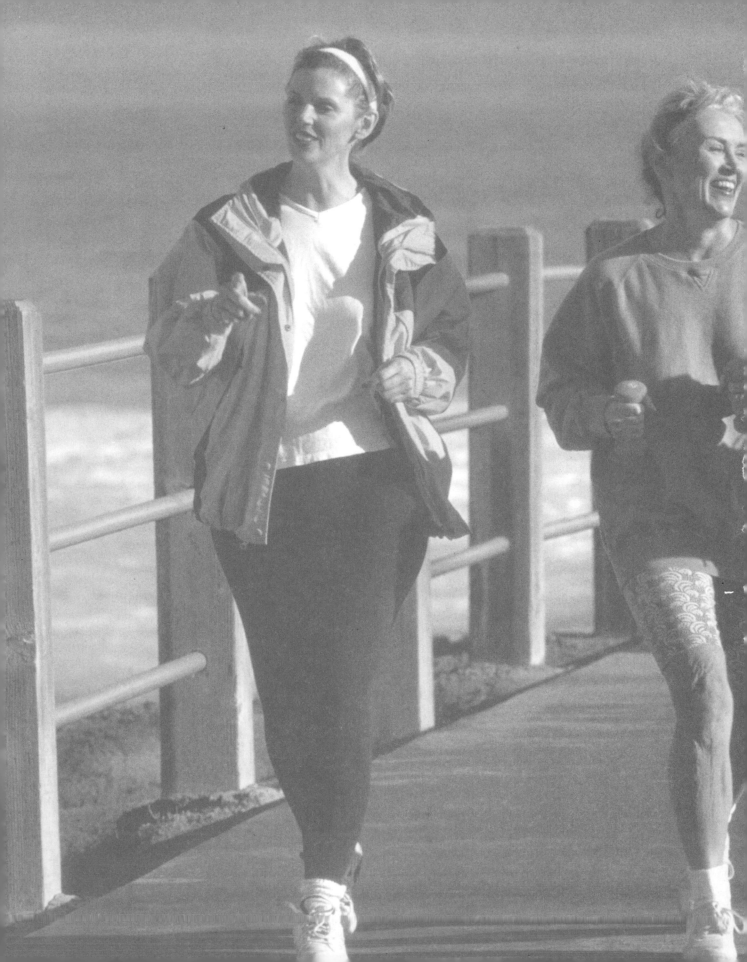